A. Carracedo   B. Brinkmann   W. Bär   (Eds.)

Advances in Forensic Haemogenetics 6

Springer

Berlin
Heidelberg
New York
Barcelona
Budapest
Hong Kong
London
Milan
Paris
Santa Clara
Singapore
Tokyo

Advances in Forensic Haemogenetics 6

16th Congress of the
International Society for Forensic Haemogenetics
(Internationale Gesellschaft für forensische Hämogenetik e.V.)
Santiago de Compostela, 12–16 September 1995

Edited by
A. Carracedo, B. Brinkmann and W. Bär

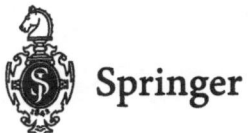 Springer

Professor Dr. med. ANGEL CARRACEDO
University of Santiago de Compostela
Institute of Legal Medicine
c/San Francisco s/n
E-15705 Santiago de Compostela

Professor Dr. med. BERND BRINKMANN
Universität Münster
Institut für Rechtsmedizin
Von-Esmarch-Straße 86
D-48149 Münster

Professor Dr. med. WALTER BÄR
University of Zurich
Institute for Legal Medicine
Winterthurerstraße 190
CH-8057 Zurich

ISBN-13: 978-3-540-60492-1   e-ISBN-13: 978-3-642-80029-0
DOI: 10.1007/978-3-642-80029-0

Die Deutsche Bibliothek – CIP-Einheitsaufnahme
International Society for Forensic Haemogenetics: ...Congress of the International Society for Forensic Haemogenetics (Internationale Gesellschaft für Forensische Hämogenetik e.V.) – Berlin; Heidelberg; New York; London; Paris; Tokyo; Hong Kong, Barcelona; Budapest: Springer.
Bis 12 (1988) u.d.T.: Society for Forensic Haemogenetics: ... Congress of the Society for Forensic Haemogenetics
16. Santiago de Compostela. – 1996
(Advances in forensic haemogenetics; 6)

NE: GT

Typesetting: Camera ready by authors
SPIN: 10510780   19/3133-5 4 3 2 1 – Printed on acid-free paper

Preface

The 6th volume of "Advances in Forensic Haemogenetics" comprises the scientific contributions to the 16th Congress of the International Society for Forensic Haemogenetics ISFH held on Sept., 12–16, 1995 at Santiago de Compostela, Spain. The numerous papers mainly deal with the applicability of DNA technology to forensic questions. The invited speakers approached important topics such as variation of mitochondrial DNA in ancient and modern humans, the "STR approach" to solve forensic questions, the statistical analysis of STR data, automation of DNA analysis, long PCR and its applications, national DNA databases and ethical and legal aspects of DNA analysis.

It has become obvious that PCR based polymorphic systems clearly dominate the scene of forensic DNA analysis worldwide. It will however be necessary to make efforts to standardize the still increasing number of systems with regard to nomenclature to achieve a universal comparability of results.

Legal systems differ from country to country which has to be taken into account when reporting DNA results. There is still controversy about the way DNA results are to be presented in court-rooms. We should make efforts to assess the value of DNA evidence by a common scientifc statistical approach that is comprehensive enough to treat all possible hypotheses such as involved relatives, different ethnics and/or the not so rare situations with mixed stains.

On behalf of the Executive Committee of our society I would like to thank all the authors of the articles of this volume and Springer-Verlag for having made such a quick publication possible. A special thank you goes to the organizing committee of this congress and his president Prof. Luis Concheiro and to the Congress president Prof. Angel Carracedo and the rector of the University of Santiago de Compostela for their enormous hospitality.

WALTER BÄR
President ISFH

Contents

1 Mitochondrial DNA

Mitochondrial DNA Variation in Ancient and Modern Humans 3
E. Hagelberg

A Two Stage Strategy for the Automated Analysis of Mitochondrial DNA 11
K.M. Sullivan, G. Tully, R. Alliston-Greiner, A. Hopwood, J.E. Bark, and P. Gill

Mixing and Thermic Treatment of Mitochondrial PCR Fragments Reveal Sequence
Differences by Heteroduplex Formation – A Rapid Method
for Forensic Identity Testing 14
R. Szibor, I. Plate, E. Kirches, and D. Krause

Genetic Analysis of Single Hair Shafts by Automated Sequence Analysis
of the Mitochondrial D-Loop Region 17
R. Decorte, E. Jehaes, F.-X. Xiao, and J.-J. Cassiman

Mitochondrial HVR1 Polymorphism in Italy 20
E. d'Aloja, I. Boschi, A. Moscetti, M. Dobosz, V.L. Pascali, and A. Fiori

mtDNA Sequences in Norwegian Saami and Main Populations 23
B.M. Dupuy and B. Olaisen

Mitochondrial DNA Quantification in Animal Blood and Hair by Slot Blotting 26
F. Fridez and R. Coquoz

Detection of Sequence Variants in Hypervariable Segments of Mitochondrial DNA
in the Asian Population 29
K. Honda, M. Nakatome, S. Hanhara, Zaw Tun, M.N. Islam, H. Bai, Y. Ogura,
H. Kuroki, M. Yamazaki, M. Terada, S. Misawa, and C. Wakasugi

Routine Mitochondrial DNA Identification 32
C. Tesson, A. Penaud, M.G. Le Roux, A. Millaseau, V. Guibert, J.P. Moisan,
and O. Pascal

Automated Fluorescent Sequencing of Mitochondrial DNA
for Italian Population Frequency Data 35
P. Montagna, R. Biondo, S. Tavano, S. Giuliacci, A. Pezza, and A. Spinella

2 DNA Sequencing Data

The STR Approach 41
B. Brinkmann

Analysis of Sequence Variations in the Alleles From Three STR Loci 52
L. Perlee, J. Neuweiler, and I. Balazs

AMPFLP Typing for the HUMCD4 STR Polymorphism in an Austrian Caucasoid
Population Sample: Sequence Data and Allele Distribution 55
B. Glock, D.W.M. Schwartz, E M. Dauber, E.M. Schwartz-Jungl, and W.R. Mayr

Typing of the HUMVWA Microsatellite Polymorphism: Allele Frequencies and
Sequencing Data 58
D.W.M. Schwartz, E.M. Dauber, B. Glock, and W.R. Mayr

Sequencing and Size Determination of the D1S80 Interallele 60
H. Fukushima, N. Harashima, Y. Katsuyama, M. Ota, C.Y. Liu, and Y. Hama

Analysis of the Short Tandem Repeat Polymorphism D18S51: Allele Frequencies
and Sequence Studies 63
P. Berschick and J. Reinhold

Investigation of the STR HUMLIPOL in Austrian Caucasoid Individuals: Sequence Data
and Allele Frequencies 66
B. Glock, D.W.M. Schwartz, E.M. Dauber, E.M. Schwartz-Jungl, and W.R. Mayr

D12S391: A Highly Useful STR for Forensic Purposes 69
*M.V. Lareu, F. Barros, A. Salas, C. Pestoni, I. Muñoz, M.S. Rodríguez-Calvo,
and A. Carracedo*

DNA Sequence Analysis of PCR Products of MCT118 Locus
in Japanese DNA Samples 72
K. Sekiguchi, I. Sakai, N. Mizuno, K. Yoshida, K. Kasai, H. Sato, and S. Seta

3 Statistics

Statistical Analysis of STR Data 79
I.W. Evett and J S. Buckleton

The Use of Likelihood Ratios in Reporting Difficult Forensic Cases 87
D.L. Monahan, S J. Cordiner, and J S. Buckleton

Identification of Biological Stains: Probability of Identity or of Kinship 90
K. Hummel, W. Bär, and N. Fukshansky

Decision-Making in Paternity Diagnostics Using SLPs. 93
B. Olaisen and M. Stenersen

Hardy-Weinberg Equilibrium in RFLP Databases 96
C.H. Breener

Sedna: A Computer Program for Semiparametric Estimation of Densities
and Match Probabilities in DNA Forensic Identification and Paternity Cases 99
D. Alonso, R. Cao, A. Carracedo, and E. Valverde

DNA PCR Polymorphisms in Paternity Test Protocols: A Biostatistical Approach . . 102
R. Domenici, S. Fornaciari, M. Nardone, A. Rocchi, I. Spinetti, M. Venturi,
and M. Bargagna

4 DNA Polymorphisms

Methods for Typing the STR Triplex CSF1PO, TPOX, and HUMTH01 That Enable
Compatibility Among DNA Typing Laboratories 107
B. Budowle, B.W. Koons, K.M. Keyes, and J.B. Smerick)

Selection of STR Loci for Forensic Identification Systems 115
A.J. Urquhart, N.J. Oldroyd, T. Downes, M. Barber, R. Allison-Greiner,
C.P. Kimpton, and P.D. Gill

PCR Typing of Alu Elements: Molecular Genetics and Forensic Application 118
P.M. Schneider, L. Zhang, C. Esdar, G. Rittner, M.A. Batzer, and C. Rittner

An Investigation of Variation in the Sizing of Short Tandem Repeat Loci 121
D. Syndercombe Court, C. Phillips, J. Thomson, and P. Lincoln

Male Identification Using Y Chromosomal STR Polymophisms 124
L. Roewer, M. Kayser, M. Nagy, and P. de Knijff

Corresponding Repeats in STRs and Internal Standard in Fragment Analysis 127
B.M. Dupuy and B. Olaisen

Construction and Calibration of Allelic Ladders for the PCR-Based Systems D8S320
and AR 130
P. Huber, W. Schmidt, and J. Holtz

Establishment of a Highly Discriminating Pentaplex PCR System for Detection
of PCR Fragments in Silver-Stained Polyacrylamide Gels 133
H. Haas and G. Weiler

Multiplex Amplifications and Automated Fluorescent Typing
of Short Tandem Repeat (STR) Loci: The French Experience 139
F. Rousselet, H. Pfitzinger, and P. Mangin

A Tetraplex PCR System for the Analysis of Paternity Cases 142
C. Seidl, O. Jäger, and E. Seifried

Development and Applications of High Throughput Multiplex STR Systems 145
J. Schumm, C. Sprecher, A. Lins, and K. Micka

Properties of an STR Muliplex Marker System Suitable for Paternity
and Forensic Determinations 148
J. Neuweiler, L. Perlee, J. Venturini, and I. Balazs

Analysis of D1S80 VNTR Allele Polymorphisms and Association
with a Nearby Flanking Sequence Polymorphism in Two Spanish Populations . . . 151
C. Albarrán, O. García, R. Deka, A. Alonso, P. Martín, M. Sancho, D.N. Stievers,
and R. Chakraborty

Somatic Instability in Cancer at Seven Tetrameric STR Loci Used
in Forensic Genetics 154
A. Alonso, P, Martín, C. Albarrán, A. Guzmán, B. Aguilera, H. Oliva, and M. Sancho

Null Alleles Detection in Loci D1S7, D7S21, and D12S11 by PCR 157
S. Alonso, A. Castro, I. Fernández-Fernández, A. García-Orad, G. Tamayo,
and M.Martínez de Pancorbo

Mutation Rate Variation in the Hypervariable VNTR g3 (D7S22) is Associated with a
Flanking DNA Sequence Polymorphism near the Repeat Array 160
R. Andreassen and B. Olaisen

The Approach of Using Random Priming for Small Forensic DNA Samples 163
A. Baasner, M. Prinz, and C. Schmitt

Use of PCR Triplex System for DNA Typing of Forensic Samples 167
M.L. Baird, L. Perlee, J. Neuweiler, L. Galbreath, and I. Balazs

Evaluation of New STR Loci for Forensic DNA Typing 171
R. Coquoz

Automated Profiling of Multiplexed DNA Markers: An Italian Database of Four
Co-Amplified STR Loci 174
F. De Stefano, L. Casarino, M.G. Costa, A. Mannucci, and G. Bruni

Microbial DNA Challenge Studies of PCR-Based Systems Used
in Forensic Genetics 177
A. Fernández-Rodríguez, A. Alonso, C. Albarrán, P. Martín, M.J. Iturralde,
M. Montesino, and M. Sancho

Some Critical Comments and Experimental Calculations Used
as Validation Standards in the Implementation of RFLP Analysis 180
I.C. Flores, G. Repetto, and P. Sanz

Analysis of Somatic Mutations at Short Tandem Repeat Loci
in Colorectal Carcinomas 183
P. Hoff-Olsen, G.I. Meling, and B. Olaisen

Simple and Rapid Duplex PCR for Forensic and Paternity Testing 186
K. Lalu and M. Lukka

Genetic Studies of a STR at the UGB Locus 189
P. Leyenda and B. Caeiro

Tumor Inoculation between Two Unrelated Human Individuals: STR Analysis
of Paraffin-Embedded Tissue Section 192
C. Luckenbach, V.H. Gärtner, C. Seidl, and H. Ritter

Molecular Phenotyping of Two Trinucleotide Repeats (XT00444 and D5S373):
Experimental Conditions 195
J.R. Luis and B. Caeiro

Development and Optimisation of a Highly Discriminating Multiplex PCR System
Suitable for Forensic Identification 198
N.J. Oldroyd, A.J. Urquhart, C.P. Kimpton,E.S. Millican, S.K. Watson, R.E. Frazier,
and P.D. Gill

Manual DNA Typing via the Short Tandem Repeats (STRs): KW 426, TH and hTPO   201
R. Pöltl, C. Luckenbach, and H. Ritter

A Multiplex Amplification Approach for Simultaneous Typing of Five Loci in DNA
of Ancient Basque Populations 204
*L. Prieto, E. Arroyo, A. Pérez-Pérez, C. Asperilla, I. Arenal, J.M. Ruíz de la Cuesta,
and D. Turbón*

Triplex PCR of Three STR Loci with Nonoverlapping Allele Sizes 207
I. Rostedt and M. Lukka

Visualization of Epigenetic Toxicological DNA Changes 210
T. Sawaguchi, S. Nakamura, X. Wang, and A. Sawaguchi

The 3 Hypervariable VNTR Locus APO B:
Three Different Analysing Methods Revealing Different Alleles
and Large Family Studies 213
S. Sedlmayr, R. Pöltl, C. Luckenbach, and H. Ritter

Automated Fluorescent PCR Based Analysis of the STR Polymorphism
at Locus D8S639 and at the CYP19 Gene 216
C. Seidl, O. Jäger, M. Kilp, and E. Seifried

Mutations of D2S44 and D4S139 Alleles and Presence of Two-Fragment Alleles for
D4S139 219
A. Vandenberghe, N. Mommers, I. Peeters, M. Vandenbroeck, and L. Muylle

Nonautomatic Multiplex Analysis and Detection of Six STR-Loci:
HPRT, FABP2, CD4, F13A1, CYP19 and LPL 223
R. Weispfennig, C. Luckenbach, and H. Ritter

DNA Analysis of Polymorphism in Drug or Xenobiotic Metabolism 226
M. Yamada, M. Sato, I. Ushiyama, Y. Yamada, A. Nishimura, and K. Nishi

Forensic Efficiency and German Population Data
for the Tetrameric STR Polymophism DHFRP2 (HUMFOLP23) 229
M. Benecke, C. Schmitt, and M. Prinz

5 Forensic Applications

Criminal Intelligence Databases and Interpretation of STRs 235
*P. Gill, A.Urquhart, E. Millican , N. Oldroyd, S. Watson, R. Sparkes,
and C.P.Kimpton*

Identification Through Genetic Typing of the Victims of the Sect of the Solar Temple
(Cheiry/Salvan, Switzerland) 243
C. Brandt-Casadevall, N. Dimo-Simonin, and T. Krompecher

Design of Novel Oligonucleotide Probes for Sex Determination and Its Forensic
Application 246
R. Kobayashi, N. Iizuka, and Y. Itoh

Casework Experiences with a Multiplex STR System 249
M. J. Greenhalgh

Multiplexed DNA Markers from Cigarette Butts in Forensic Casework 252
F. De Stefano, G. Bruni, L. Casarino, M.G. Costa, and A. Mannucci

DNA Polymorphisms in Dental Pulp: Effect of Environmental Factors 255
A. Alvarez García, I. Muñoz, C. Pestoni, M. V. Lareu, M. S. Rodríguez-Calvo,
F. Barros, and A. Carracedo

Identification of Human Remains Using DNA Amplification (PCR) 258
J. Andradas, E. García, T. Cámara, L. Prieto, and J. López

The So-Called Alcohol-Blood Sample Identity Expertise 261
W. Huckenbeck and W. Bonte

Application of the STR Androgen Receptor (HUMARA) Polymorphism
to Paternity Cases 264
L. Caenazzo, E. Ponzano, C. Crestani, G. Bonan, and P. Cortivo

Multiplex Genetic Typing of CSF1PO, TPOX, and HUMTH01 in Forensic Samples . 266
A. Castro, I. Fernández-Fernández, S. Alonso, A. García-Orad, G. Tamayo,
and M.M. de Pancorbo

A Five Minute Procedure for Extraction of Genomic DNA from Whole Blood,
Semen and Forensic Stains for PCR 269
J. Dissing, L. Rudbeck, and H. Marcher

False Results in the HLA-DQα Typing: Two Cases Reported 272
P. Fattorini, N. Malusa, A. Junge, F. Cossutta, F. Florian, B.M. Altamura, G. Furlan,
and G. Graziosi

Forensic Use of PCR DNA Analysis in Hairs, Envelopes, and Cigarette Ends 275
R. Fernández, E. Ramírez, M. Crespillo, J.A. Luque, P. García, and J.L. Valverde

PCR-DNA Typing from Beard Samples 278
L. Garofano, G. Lago, C. Zanon, M. Bruno, P. Carresi, G. Zignale, S. Gino,
and C. Torre

PCR-Based Analyses of Epidermal Cells Found on Adhesive Tape 281
L. Garofano, G.Lago, C. Zanon, A. Virgili, G. D'Errico, G. Vespi, S. Gino,
and C. Torre

Determination of Sex in Dental Pulp Using PCR 284
A. Gremo, M.A. Martínez, J. Sánchez, and C. Landete

Use of PCR in Forensic Casework in the Area of Berlin-Brandenburg:
Allele Frequency Distribution of Six Microsatellites 287
G. Bläß, B. Jauert, W. Oesterreich, E. Ackermann, A. Pieper, and S. Herrmann

The Never Ending Story: A New Tsarevitch? 290
W. Huckenbeck, W. Bonte, V. Hees, S. West, and K.W. Alt

Influence of Mediaeval Clothes Colour Pigments on DNA Extraction
and Amplification 292
C. Keyser, D. Montagnon, B. Ludes, E. Crubezy, D. Cardon, P. Walton Rogers,
J. Wouters, and P. Mangin

Forensic Investigations After Sexual Abuse of Several Infants:
A Criminal Case Report 295
J. Kreike, A. Lehner, E. Friedrich, and O. Tauscher

Sex Determination on Ancient Bones 298
K. Kuntze, W. Huckenbeck, W. Bonte, and K.W. Alt

Identification of the Skeletal Remains of Two 12-Year Old Bodies by Nuclear DNA
Polymorphisms Analysis 301
P. Martín, A. Alonso, C. Albarrán, and M. Sancho

Identification of Vestiges from Diverse Biological Sources
Using Duplex Amplification of Short Tandem Repeat Loci 304
M A. Martínez, S. San José, A. Rojas, and A. Gremo

A Rare Paternity Case with PP 99.99% and Exclusion at Three Loci 307
E. Seifried, C. Seidl, R. Grigorean, E. Brude, O. Jäger, U. Langenbeck,
and K. D. Zang

Three Intriguing Identification Cases 310
B. Mevåg, S. Jacobsen, and B. Olaisen

Forensic DNA Typing in the Spanish Police Using VNTR Single Locus Probes . . . 313
E. Rivas, T. Vicente, C. Gamella, J. González, J. Andradas

PCR Typing of DNA Extracted from Epidermal Particles Won by Scratching 316
M. Sánchez-Hanke, K. Püschel, C. Augustin, P. Wiegand, and B. Brinkmann

PCR Genotyping in Dental Pulp from Old Human Skeletal Remains
and Fire Victims 319
P. Sanz, V. Prieto, and M.I. Andres

ABO Genotyping of the Suspects Using Their Sperm DNA 322
M. Sasaki, K. Shimizu, T. Fukushima, and H. Shiono

Forensic Identification Using DNA Recovered from Saliva on Human Skin 325
D.J. Sweet, J. A. Lorente, M. Lorente, A. Valenzuela, and E. Villanueva

Analysis of STR Loci in Old Blood Stains Using Automated and Manual Genotyping
Systems 328
J. Thomson, C. Phillips, D. Beckett, O. Summerfield, and P. Lincoln

Microsatellite DNA Polymorphism Analysis in a Case of Illegal Cattle Purchase . . . 331
D. Beamonte, E. Valverde, A. Guerra, B. Ruíz, and J. Alemany

Disaster Victim Identification by Using the DNA Technology on Dental Pulp:
Preliminary Results 334
A. Marcotte, B. Hoste, M. Fays, E. De Valck, and A. Leriche

Combined STR VNTR and MVR Typing and mtDNA Sequencing Led to the
Identification of Human Remains Emergent from the AMIA Explosion
in Buenos Aires 337
D. Corach, A. Sala, G. Penacino, and A. Sotelo

6 Methodology

Rapid Sex Typing by Fluorescent Based PCR
of the X-Y Homologous Amelogenin Gene and Analysis by CGE 343
A.D. Kloosterman, M.J. van der Schans, H.J.T. Janssen, and F.M. Everaerts

Heteroduplex Analysis Is a Rapid Method for Detection of Suballeles Caused
by Mixed Length and Sequence Variability in STR Systems 346
R. Szibor, I. Plate, and D. Krause

Use of CDP-STAR in a Fast and Highly Sensitive Chemiluminescent
Detection Procedure of VNTR Loci with Neutral or Charged Membranes 349
S.L. Leary, J. Victor, and I. Balazs

Evaluation of Primer Extension Preamplification (PEP) in Forensic Studies 353
Y. Itoh and R. Kobayashi

Sequential Multiplex Amplification (SMA) in Cases with Minimal Amounts
of DNA 356
M. Lorente, J.A. Lorente, J.C. Alvarez, B. Budowle, and E. Villanueva

Detection of Single Base Changes in PCR Amplified DNA Using Double and Single
Strand Conformational Polymophisms (SSCP and DSCP) 359
F. Barros, M.S. Rodríguez-Calvo, I. Muñoz, C. Pestoni, M.V. Lareu,
and A. Carracedo

Evaluation of Hybridisation Equipment for Use
with Nonisotopically Labelled Probes 362
W.P. Childs and G. Rysiecki

CDP-Star^TH as a Chemiluminescent Substrate for Use
with Alkaline Phosphatase Labelled Probes 365
W.P. Childs, G. Rysiecki, and P. Elsmore

Simple and Rapid Typing of STRs on an Automated DNA Sequencer 368
R. Decorte and J.-J. Cassiman

A Modification to the "Chelex" DNA Extraction Method for Casework Samples . . . 371
M.J. Greenhalgh

Application of HLA-DR Typing by PCR-SSP to Forensic Samples 374
M. Ota, Y. Katsuyama, Y. Hama, N. Harashima, C.Y. Liu, and H. Fukushima

The MVR-PCR Approach for the Typing of the MS32 Locus: Usefulness
and Technical Problems 377
M S. Rodríguez-Calvo, S. Bellas, M.V. Lareu, I. Muñoz, C. Pestoni, F. Barros,
and A. Carracedo

Introduction of Two New Electrophoresis Gel Systems for Screening and High
Resolution Identification of STRs Under Native Conditions 380
H.P. Schickle and R. Westermeier

Oligo-AP Probes and Chemiluminescence: Sensitivity for Stains Analysis 383
A. Teyssier

Automation of In Situ DNA Sample Preparation for PCR Using the FTA^TM DNA
Collection System, Oral Swabs, and the Rosys Laboratory Workstation 386
P. Williams, S. Seim, L. Wiessner, P. Stover, H. Polesky, E. Heath, and L. Hammer

STR Typing without DNA Extraction Using an Infrared-Based Nonradioactive
Automated DNA Sequencer 390
R. Roy, D.L. Steffens, B.O. Gartside, G.Y. Jang, and J.A. Brumbaugh

Evaluation of Hereditary Distance
by Restriction Landmark Genomic Scanning (RLGS) 393
T. Sawaguchi, X. Wang, Y. Okazaki, S. Nakamura, O. Ohue, Y. Hayashizaki,
S. Sawaguchi

7 Conventional Markers

The PI System: Genetic Variation, Forensic Application and Clinical Aspects 399
S. Weidinger

A Parentage Testing Study Revealing a Possible Deletion at the PLG Locus 405
H. Polesky, M. Mount, S. Seim, and L. Wiessner

Detection of the ABO, GC, ACP, and HLA-DQA1 Polymorphisms
at the DNA Level Using PCR and SSCP 407
J. Dissing and D. Christiansen

Novel Polymorphisms in the Coding Sequence
of the Coagulation Factor XIII A-Subunit and Their Halotype Diversity 410
K. Suzuki, M. Iwata, T. Fukunaga, G. Ishimoto, J. Henke, L. Henke, M. Szekelyi,
S. Ito, H. Tsuji, and A. Tamura)

Nucleotide Changes in Various Variants of the Coagulation Factor XIII A-Subunit . 413
K. Suzuki, J. Henke, M. Iwata, L. Henke, M. Szekelyi, S. Ito, and A. Uchida

ABO Genotyping with PCR 416
U. Schacker, P. M. Schneider, and M. Zapata

Indication for a Silent Allele of Properdin Factor B Polymorphism (BF*Q0)
in a Paternity Case 418
R. Domenici, S. Fornaciari, M. Nardone, A. Rocchi, I. Spinetti, M. Venturi,
and M. Bargagna

Preliminary Studies on the Population Substructure for C1R Protein in Chinese
Populations 421
Q. Gou, Z. Jin, Y. Hou, J. Wu, Y. Xu, and M. Wu

A Study of Polymorphism of Antithrombin III at the Level of Both Protein
and DNA in a Chinese Population 424
Q. Gou, Y. Hou, Y. Zhang, and M. Wu

Genetic Polymorphisms of Alpha-1-Antitrypsin and Group-Specfic Component in
Spanish Gypsy Population 427
A. Guisán, I. López-Abadía, J.M. Ruíz de la Cuesta, and F. Bandrés

Studies on Blood Genetic Markers in Some Mongoloid Populations
of Eastern Siberia 429
G. Ishimoto, K. Suzuki, H. Matsumoto, V.P. Wiebe, and V. Valentina

PI Subtyping in Dental Pulps 432
A. Kido and M. Oya

GC Subtyping in Serum and Semen after Neuraminidase Treatment 435
A. Kido, M. Oya, and M. Hara

Simultaneous Focusing of PGM1 and ACP Phenotypes Using Miniaturized Gels
and Three Electrode Technique 438
W. Kuchheuser and D. Krause

Platelet and Granulozyte Alloantigen Typing Using Sequence-Specific Primer
(SSP) PCR Amplification 441
C. Phillips, P.J. Lincoln, T. Annan, A. Waters, J. Chapman, and M. Murphy

Plasma Protein Markers in S. Tomé e Principe 444
M.F. Santos, A. Amorim, L. Manco, and M.J. Trovoada

Detection of a Silent GC Allele in a Danish Mother and Child 446
M. Thymann, H.E. Hansen, and J. Dissing

ABH-Related Antigens Participate in the Spermatogenesis of Cats and Rats 449
I. Ushiyama, M. Yamada, A. Tanegashima, A. Nishimura, M. Kane, Y. Yamamoto, and K. Nishi

Species Identification by Analysis of the Genes for ABO Blood Group 452
M. Yamada, I. Ushiyama, M. Sato, H. Ueyama. I. Ohkubo, A. Nishimura, and K. Nishi

8 Population Genetics

Statistical Issues in DNA Profiling 457
B.S. Weir and J.S. Buckleton

Population Genetics of D1S80, HUMVWA31 A, and HUMF13A1
from Portugal and Goa (India) 465
H. Geada, R. Espinheira, T. Ribeiro, and L. Reys

Genetic Substructure at the STR Loci HUMTH01
and HUMVWA in Han Populations, China 468
Y. Hou and H. Walter

Collaborative Study on the Polymorphism of the D1S80 Locus
in the Italian Population 471
G. Graziosi

DNA Fingerprinting in Balearic Populations 475
I. Albalá, A. Picornell, J.A. Castro, and M.M. Ramon

HLA-DQA1 and D1S80 in the Population of Valencia (Spain) 478
M. Aler, M.V. Lareu, F. Verdú, C. Pestoni, and M.S. Gisbert

Gene Frequencies of Human Populations along Pyrenean Chain 480
M.P. Aluja,. R.M. Nogués, A. Sevin, and G. Larrouy

Multiplex PCR and Automated Flourescence Detection of Four Tetrameric STRs
in an West-Austrian Population 483
E. Ambach, W. Parson, H. Niederstätter, and B. Budowle

Population and Formal Genetics of the STRs TPO, TH01 and VWFA31/A in North
Portugal 486
A. Amorim, L. Gusmão, and M.J. Prata

Population Genetics of Three STRs: TH01, CSF1PO , and TPOX in Southern Spain . 489
M.I. Andres, V. Prieto, I.C. Flores, and P. Sanz

Frequency Multivariate Analysis of LDLR, GYPA, HBGG, D7S8, and GC
in 12 Different Populations 492
E. Arroyo, C. Asperilla, L. Prieto, M. Herrera, and J.M. Ruíz de la Cuesta

Worldwide Distribution of D1S80 Polymorphism: Comparison
of Genetic Distances and Cluster Analysis 495
C. Asperilla, E. Arroyo, L. Prieto, and J.M. Ruíz de la Cuesta

Allele Frequency Distributions of 3 STR-Loci in a Population Sample from Northern
Germany 498
C. Augustin, M. Sánchez-Hanke, and K. Püschel

Allele Frequency Distribution of Three STRs Loci: HUMARA, HUMPLA2,
and VS17T in the Spanish Population 501
C. Cabrero, A. Díez, E. Valverde, and J. Alemany

Determination of the Allele and Genotype Frequencies of Loci HLA-DQA1, LDLR,
GYPA, HBGG, D7S8, and GC in Bogota (Colombia) 503
M. Castillo, M. Paredes, C. Peñuela, I. Bustos, M. Jiménez, and A. Galindo

Allele Distribution of the Amplitype PM Coamplification System in a Population of
Northern Italy 506
N. Cerri, R. Mignola, and F. De Ferrari

Characterization of YNZ22 Locus for Forensic Purposes, Allele and Genotype
Frequencies in a Northern Italian Population 510
N. Cerri, S. Pivetti, and F. De Ferrari

D1S80 Population Data in the North East of Spain 514
M. Crespillo, J.A. Luque, R.M. Fernández, P. García, E. Ramírez, and J.L. Valverde

Population Study for the HLA-DQA1, LDLR, GYPA, HBGG, D7S8, and GC Loci in North
East of Spain 517
M. Crespillo, J.A. Luque, P. García, E. Ramírez, R.M. Fernández, and J.L. Valverde

Allele Frequencies of Four STRs (HUMTH01, HUMVWFA31, HUMF13A01,
HUMFESFPS) in the North East of Spain 520
M. Crespillo, J. A. Luque, E. Ramírez, P. García, R.M. Fernández, and J.L. Valverde

German Data on the Loci of Low-Density Lipoprotein Receptor, Glycophorin A,
Hemoglobin γ, D7S8, Group-Specific Component and HLA-DQα 523
W. Huckenbeck, H.G. Scheil, U. Cremer, D. Makuch, T.H. Eiermann, K. Kuntze,
and W. Bonte

Allele Frequencies of VWA, FESFPS, FXIIIA1, and D21S11 in an Italian Population
Sample 526
M. Dobosz, M. Pescarmona, A. Moscetti, A. Caglià, E. d'Aloja,. L. Grimaldi,
and V.L. Pascali

STR Analysis : HUMTHO1 and HUMFESFPS for Forensic Application 528
R. Espinheira, H. Geada, T. Ribeiro, and L. Reys

Profiling the North East Italian Population
by Four Highly Polymorphic DNA Probes 529
P. Fattorini, F. Florian, S. Tafuro, F. Cossutta, B.M. Altamura, and G. Graziosi

Allele Frequencies of HLA-DQ, LDLR, GYPA, HBGG, D7S8, and GC in the Resident and
Autochthonous Populations of the Basque Country 532
O. García, P. Martín, B. Budowle, C. Albarrán, and A. Alonso

Study of HUMACTBP2 STR Polymorphism, Performed by PCR and Automated Laser
Flourescence (ALF) Sequencer in a Population Sample of Catalonia 535
M. Gené, E. Huguet, M. Luna, P. Moreno, M.V. Lareu, and A. Carracedo

Aymara and Quechua Amerindian Populations Characterized by HUMTH01
and HUMVWA STR Polymorphisms 537
M. Gené, E. Huguet, P. Moreno, M. Fuentes, J. Corbella, and J. Mezquita

Suitability of the HUMTH01, HUMCD4, and HUMVWA STR Polymorphisms
for Legal Medicine Investigations in the Population of Catalonia (North East Spain) 540
M. Gené, E. Huguet, P. Moreno, C. Sánchez, J. Corbella, and J. Mezquita

Population and Formal Genetics of the STR System MBP-Locus B in North Portugal 542
L. Gusmão, M. J. Prata, and A. Amorim

Allele Frequency Distributions of Five Loci (LDLR, GYPA, HBGG, D7S8 and GC)
in a Japanese Population 544
M. Hara, A. Kido, K. Saito, A. Takada, K. Yabe, T. Murai, and H. Watanabe

Frequency Data on the Loci LDLR, GYPA, HBGG, D7S8, and GC
in a Population Resident in Madrid (Spain) 547
*M. Herrera, C. Asperilla, M.A. Aumente, L. Prieto, E. Arroyo,
and J.M. Ruíz de la Cuesta*

German Data on the PCR-Based Loci HUMVWA 31, HUMTH01, HUMES/FPS,
HUMF 13B, and D1S80 549
*W. Huckenbeck, H.-G. Scheil, S. West, K. Demir, J. Kanja, A. Kaiser, V. Hees,
W. Meyer, K.W. Alt, D. Scholten, V. Stancu, M. Bronczek, and W. Bonte*

D1S80 Alleles in Wielkopolska Population (Poland) 552
*J. Jaroszewski, U. Schütte, M. Schurenkamp,P. Krajewski, J. Kempa, Z. Przybylski,
and S. Rand*

A Study on the Short Tandem Repeat System ACTBP2 (SE33)
in an Austrian Population Sample Using Nondenaturing Electrophoresis
and a Sequenced Allelic Ladder 555
M. Klintschar and R. Crevenna

HLADQA1 Allele Frequencies in the World Using a Biplot to Visualize Alleles
and Populations Simultaneously 557
A.D. Kloosterman, M. Sjerps, D. Eerhart, and N. Dimo

Efficiency of 6 STR Systems, HLADQα and the Polymarker Systems (PM) in Paternity
Testing 560
A. Kratzer and W. Bär

Swiss Population Data for the STR Systems HUMVWA, HUMF13A1,
and HUMFES 563
A. Kratzer and W. Bär

Studies on the HUMTH01 and HUMVWA Polymorphisms
in a South West German Population 566
K. Leim, S. Degenhartt, W. Reichert, and R. Mattern

Spanish Population Data on Seven Loci (D1S80, D17S5, HUMTH01, HUMVWA,
ACTBP2, D21S11, and DQA1): Equilibrium and Independence 569
M. Lorente, J.A. Lorente, J.C. Alvarez, B. Budowle, and E. Villanueva

Two Highly Polymorphic VNTR Loci D5S110 (LH1) and D4S139 (PH30): Analysis, Formal and Population Genetic Data 572
C. Luckenbach, A. Luckenbach, V. Almeida, M. Mainka, J. Jung, and H. Rittner

Allele Frequency Distribution of Five VNTR Loci and Paternity Testing in the North East of Spain 575
J.A. Luque, P. García, R.M. Fernández, M. Crespillo, E. Ramírez, and J.L. Valverde

Spanish Population Data on 13 PCR-Based Systems 578
P. Martín, A. Alonso, B. Budowle, C. Albarrán, O. García, and M. Sancho

Allele Frequencies of D1S80, LDLR, GYPA, D7S8, GC, HBGG, and SE 33 in Polish Population Sample 581
D. Miscicka-Sliwka, K. Sliwka, A. Syroczynska, T. Grzybowski, B. Baranowska, and J.A. Berent

Haplotype Frequencies of Two STRs of the Chromosome 8q (D8S344 and D8S323) 584
S. Mourelo, S. Dios, and B. Caeiro

Japanese Population Data on Six STR Loci 587
A. Nagai, S. Yamada, Y. Watanabe, Y. Bunai, and I. Ohya

Forensic Application of STR Polymorphic Markers 589
S. Nakamura, T. Sawaguchi, and A. Sawaguchi

Population Studies of Two AMPFLPS and Two STRs Systems in a North Polish Population 592
R. Pawlowski, A. Welz, A. Maciejewska, and R. Paszkowska

Allele Frequency Distribution of 15 PCR-Based DNA Polymorphisms in the Population of Galicia (NW Spain) 595
C. Pestoni, A. García Rivero, S. Bellas, M.V. Lareu, M.S. Rodríguez-Calvo, F. Barros, I. Muñoz, and A. Carracedo

The Allelic Distribution of Five STRs Systems in a North Italian Population 598
A. Piccinini, S. Rand, and B. Brinkmann

Population Study of Three STR Loci in the North of Portugal 601
M.F. Pinheiro, M.L. Pontes, M. Gené, E. Huguet, and J. Pinto da Costa

Population Genetics of the STRs TPO, TH01, and VWFA31/A in S. Tomé e Príncipe 604
M.J. Prata, A. Amorim, L. Gusmão, and M.J. Trovoada

Automated Analyisis of Five STR Loci: Allele Frequencies and Family Studies in the German Population 607
J. Reinhold and J. Arnold

Southern Spain Population Frequencies of the Loci LDLR, GYPA, HBGG, D7S8, and Gc:A Comparison between Andalusian and Canary Islands Frequencies 610
V. Prieto, M.I. Andres, I.C. Flores, and P. Sanz

Allele Frequency Distribution of D2S44, D12S11, D7S21, D7S22, and D5S43 Loci in Southern Spain 613
G. Repetto, I.C. Flores, and P. Sanz

HLA-DQA1 Polymorphism in Two Portuguese Population Samples from Lisbon
and the South of Portugal 616
S.M. Santos, F. Simões, A. Armada, A. Clemente, and M.C. Correia

D1S80 Locus Polymorphism in a Population Sample from Lisbon 617
S.M. Santos, F. Simões, A. Armada, A. Clemente, and M.C. Correia

AMPFLP Typing of the D21S11 Microsatellite Polymorphism: Allele Frequencies
and Sequencing Data in the Austrian Population 622
D.W.M. Schwartz, E.M. Dauber, B. Glock, and W.R. Mayr

Typing for the HUMFES/FPS Short Tandem Repeat Polymorphism in an Austrian
Caucasoid Population Sample 626
D.W.M. Schwartz, B. Glock, E.M. Dauber, E.M. Schwartz-Jungl, and W.R. Mayr

Analysis of the SR Polymorphism VWA and FES: Allele Frequency
and Family Studies in an Italian Population Sample 628
E. Ponzano, L. Caenazzo, C. Crestani, G. Bonan, and P. Cortivo

Analysis of the Short Tandem Repeat Polymorphism D2S11 in German Caucasians   630
C. Seidl, O. Jäger, and E. Seifried

Population Data of the VNTR Loci D10S28,D4S139, D16S309, and D5S110
in German Caucasians 632
C. Seidl, U. Rabold, B. Brüggemann, M. Kilp, D. Teixidor, and E. Seifried

A Population Study of 5 PCR Genetic Markers: LDLR, GYPA, HBGG, D7S8,
and GC in Italy 635
A. Tagliabracci, L. Buscemi, N. Cucurachi, R. Mencarelli, R. Giorgetti,
and S.D. Ferrara

Allele Frequencies of the HUMFES/FPS System in Northern and Central Italy 637
A. Tagliabracci, M. Paoli, D. Rodríguez, N. Cucurachi, L. Buscemi, S.D. Ferrara,
C. Previderè, G. Peloso, A. Riva, G. Pierucci, R. Domenici, S. Fornaciari, I. Spinetti,
M. Nardone, and M. Bargagna

The Y-Linked Locus Y27H39 (DYS19), Frequency Distribution in South Bavarian
and Application to Paternity Testing 641
G.M. Weichold, W. Keil, and B. Bayer

Studies on the HUMACTBP2 (SE33) 644
G.M. Weichhold, W. Keil, and B. Bayer

Hungarian Population Data for 11 PCR-Based Polymorphisms 647
Woller, S. Füredi, and Z. Pádár

Allele Frequency Distribution of the STR System ACBP2 (SE33) in a Population
of Portugal (Central Area) 650
L. Souto and M.C. Vide

Allele Frequencies in Four STRs for a Population of Portugal (Central Area) 652
L. Souto, D.N. Vieira, F. Corte-Real, and M.C. Vide

DNA Profiling: A Genetic Study of Two VNTR Loci in the East Midlands 655
V.J. Stinton and S.S. Mastana

Comparison of Turkish Subpopulations Using Two STRs 658
S. Atasoy, E. Abaci-Kalfoğlu, P. Wiegand, and B. Brinkmann

The Genetic Structure of Four Argentine Ethnic Groups Reflected by the Analyses
of Ten STRs 662
A. Sala, G. Penacino, A. Goycoechea, F. Carnese, A. Tomeo, and D. Corach

D1S80 AMP-FLP Attributes in Two Different Ethnic Groups
of Argentine Populations 665
G. Penancino, A. Sala, J. Smerick, J. Pérez Calvo, S. Baechtel, B. Budowle,
and D. Corach

9 Standardization , Ethics

Ethical and Legal Aspects 671
S. Grisolía

The Development of Quality Assurance Measures in Forensic DNA Typing 675
L.A. Presley and J. Mudd

The American Association of Blood Banks Inspection and Accreditation Program
for Parentage Testing Laboratories 678
R.H. Walker

Parentage Testing Survey Program of the College of American Pathologists:
Red Cell Antigens, Serum Proteins an Red Cell Enzymes Testing Results 681
H. Polesky, D. Endean, C. Harrison, J. Morris, R. Roby, and R. Walker

A Review of the 1991-1994 Paternity Testing Workshop
of the English-Speaking Working Group 683
D. Syndercombe Court and P. Lincoln

DNA Legislation in the Netherlands 686
H.J.T. Janssen and A D. Kloosterman

Science and Conscience: Regulation or Guidelines for Forensic Haemogenetics? . . 689
M. Lorente, J.A. Lorente,B. Budowle, and E. Villanueva

HUMTHO1 Allele Frequencies in Italy - Report of the GEFI Collaborative Study . . 692
E. d'Aloja and R. Domenici

A Review of the Collaborative Exercises of the Spanish
and Portuguese ISFH Working Group 695
J. Gómez and A. Carracedo

Comparability of RFLP Results between Laboratories: AABB/CAP Survey Data . . . 699
C. Harrison, R. Allen, D. Endean, J. Morris, H. Polesky, R. Roby, and R. Walker

Proficiency Testing in Forensic DNA Analysis 702
A. S. Riordan, M. Parker, and G. Rysiecki

1 Mitochondrial DNA

Mitochondrial DNA Variation in Ancient and Modern Humans

Erika Hagelberg

Department of Biological Anthropology, University of Cambridge, Downing Street, Cambridge CB2 3DZ, U.K.

INTRODUCTION

Mitochondrial DNA (mtDNA) has been used extensively in recent years as a tool for the study of human evolutionary history. The human mtDNA genome is a closed circular molecule of approximately 16,569 base pairs in length (Anderson *et al*. 1981) located in the cellular cytoplasm. It is relatively simple, containing only 37 genes with no introns, and little other non-coding DNA besides the 1 Kb (Kilobase) control region. The simplicity and rapid rate of evolution of mtDNA make it suitable for phylogenetic studies over recent time scales, while the presence of thousands of copies of mtDNA in each cell favours their survival in compromised biological samples. The mtDNA genome is inherited in a strictly maternal fashion and evolution occurs by the accumulation of mutational changes through generations. The very high rate of accumulation of mutations (mtDNA evolves on average about 10 times faster than nuclear DNA) means that deleterious mtDNA mutations are important in human disease and ageing (Wallace 1995). It also means that there are numerous harmless mutations, either silent or in non-coding regions, which can provide convenient genetic markers for the reconstruction of human evolutionary history.

The study of the patterns of genetic diversity in modern human populations can help reconstruct past events, such as ancient migrations, population expansions, and bottlenecks. All humans have ancestors, so each person carries in his or her genes a record of their past history. However, the patterns of genetic diversity in present-day populations may occasionally obscure past events, for instance in the case of multiple migrations, recent invasions, or demic collapse resulting from infectious diseases or genocide. In order to achieve an accurate understanding of what happened in the past it becomes necessary to rely on additional information provided by historical reports or the archaeological record. Nevertheless, with the development of powerful techniques for DNA analysis, notably the polymerase chain reaction, the possibility of recovering genetic information directly from the bones or mummified remains of ancient peoples promises to provide exciting new insights into past historical events. The application of novel molecular biology methods to the analysis of compromised biological samples has been particularly relevant for forensic identification and has also helped to increase the rate of acquisition of valuable population genetic data.

MITOCHONDRIAL DNA AND HUMAN EVOLUTION

A notable example of the use of genetic markers, and specifically mtDNA, for the reconstruction of human evolutionary history was the 1987 study by the late Allan Wilson and colleagues at the University of California in Berkeley (Cann *et al*. 1987). These workers used high resolution restriction mapping of mtDNA from humans of different geographical origins to generate data to test the two contrasting models for the evolution of anatomically modern humans. In the first of these models, known as the regional continuity model, modern humans are thought to have evolved in parallel from archaic *Homo erectus* in different parts of the world, with enough gene flow between populations of different continents to ensure that modern *Homo sapiens* evolved into a single biological species. The opposing hypothesis, known as the Out of Africa model, agrees with the view that archaic humans spread throughout the Old Word, but proposes that anatomically modern humans originated solely in Africa and eventually replaced the different species of archaic humans in the course of a second, more recent, expansion from Africa. Before this study was published, most palaeontologists tended to support a middle view between the two extremes and containing elements of both theories, but the mtDNA data, frequently misunderstood or overinterpreted, caused a deep polarization of views (Wolpoff 1989).

Wilson and colleagues observed markedly little variation in modern human mtDNA types, suggesting a recent common origin, as well as more variation in African mtDNA types than anywhere else, consistent with the view that African lineages are the oldest and had more time to accumulate mutations. Phylogenetic analysis by maximum parsimony suggested that all modern mtDNAs could be traced to a single individual, known as the African Eve, who lived in Africa about 200,000 years ago. The term African Eve, suggesting a single female ancestor for modern humans, undoubtedly contributed to some the controversy that greeted the results (Lewin 1987; Wainscoat 1987). Further studies by the Wilson group, based on sequencing of the hypervariable control region of mtDNA, confirmed that the coalescence time (origin of the single common ancestor) of the maximum parsimony tree was about 200,000 years ago, and that the deepest branches of the tree were in Africa, giving further support to the Out of Africa model (Vigilant *et al.* 1991). This model also agreed with the conclusion reached by the studies by Wainscoat *et al.* (1986) of β-globin gene variation in different human populations.

Although later studies have questioned the statistical validity of the mitochondrial DNA tree (Templeton 1992), genetic studies on modern human populations have generally revealed more variation in Africa than elsewhere. A recent restriction enzyme analysis of mtDNA variation revealed the most ancient of all the continent-specific lineages in African populations (Chen *et al.* 1995). On balance, although there are still many problems in the interpretation of phylogenetic data, the DNA evidence seems to point to Africa as the place of origin of modern humans.

MITOCHONDRIAL DNA POLYMORPHISMS AS ANTHROPOLOGICAL MARKERS

While these studies have helped clarify the general patterns of recent human evolution, more detailed studies of human populations of different geographic locations are required to address specific anthropological questions. In recent years much work has been done on the analysis of human mtDNA variation by restriction mapping and DNA sequencing to help shed light on the patterns of migrations of humans in different geographical regions, such as Africa, Europe, the Pacific and the Americas.

The Pacific area was one of the first regions of the world to be studied in detail by molecular anthropologists as it was settled relatively recently and provides an excellent scenario for testing models of human colonization. Although Australia and Papua New Guinea (PNG) were probably occupied as early as 50,000 years ago, the remote archipelagos of eastern Polynesia were only settled for the first time by humans in the last 1,000 years (Bellwood 1989). By measuring the degree of genetic diversity in present day populations of PNG and assuming that this diversity had accumulated since the first human settlement, the Wilson group had a convenient method to calibrate the mitochondrial DNA clock. Unfortunately, this calibration assumed that all the variation in PNG had arisen since the first settlement and disregarded the effects of multiple migrations, problems inherent in most attempts to determine the rate of evolution of mtDNA. Estimates of the rate of mutation of mtDNA in humans have a very wide margin of error . This causes significant problems for the interpretation of relatively recent events in human prehistory, such as the settlement of the Pacific and the New World (Stoneking 1993).

One of the first anthropologically useful mtDNA markers to be identified was a deletion of 9 base pairs (9-bp) in a small non-coding region between the genes for cytochrome oxidase II and lysil transfer RNA (Wrischnik *et al.* 1987). The 9-bp deletion was observed at relatively high frequencies (5-40%) in individuals of Asian origin and was later found to be present in Polynesians at frequencies reaching fixation (100%). The occurrence of the 9-bp deletion throughout Asia and the Pacific, and its fixation in Polynesians, has been presented as evidence of the ultimately Southeast Asian ancestry of the Polynesians. This interpretation of the data is supported by the fact that the deletion is absent or virtually absent in Australia and in the highlands of PNG, areas which are presumably inhabited by the descendants of the first Australoid and Papuan settlers of the Pacific (Hertzberg *et al.* 1989; Stoneking & Wilson 1989).

Although the 9-bp deletion was originally thought to occur only in populations of Asian origin, including native Americans, it has subsequently been observed in African populations. It is now known that the deletion has occurred independently in different parts of the world, and that this region of the mtDNA genome is particularly sensitive to mutation. We have detected both the deletion of one of the 9-bp motifs as well as a 9-bp triplication in several European individuals.

In recent studies, we have observed the 9-bp deletion in the following Pacific populations, *inter alia*:

Eastern Polynesia:	Tahiti	96%
Central Pacific:	Samoa	100%
	Tonga	88%
	Fiji	66%
PNG Coast		42%
PNG Highlands		4%
Island SE Asia	Taiwan	35%
	Borneo	33%

Sequence data from the hypervariable region of mtDNA of Circum-Pacific populations have revealed further mtDNA polymorphisms that seem to be present exclusively in Polynesians (Hagelberg & Clegg 1993; Lum *et al.* 1994; Melton *et al.* 1995). This Polynesian mtDNA type is characterized by the 9-bp deletion and by base substitutions at positions 16,189, 16,217, 16,247 and 16,261 of the control region of the mtDNA genome. The Polynesian mtDNA type seems to derive from an ancestral type present in Asia and characterized by the 16,189 substitution and the 9-bp deletion. A second mutation occurred on this background, characterized by the additional substitution at 16,217. This mtDNA type is present in Taiwan and Borneo and also in the Americas (Schurr *et al.* 1990; Ballinger *et al.* 1992; Horai *et al.* 1991; our unpublished observations), reflecting the Asian origin of the populations of the New World. The additional two substitutions 16,247 and 16,261 appear eastwards in the Pacific, with the Polynesian type accounting for about 80% of individuals sampled. The Polynesian mtDNA motif is also present at high frequency in Malagasy, showing that migrations from Southeast Asia did not only lead to the colonization of Oceania in the east, but also to Madagascar in the west (Soodyall *et al.* 1995).

MtDNA control region polymorphisms associated with the 9-bp deletion. The Polynesian mtDNA type (type i) derives from an ancestral type that can be traced back to Asia:

i)	16 189	16 217	16 247	16 261
ii)	16 189	16 217		16 261
iii)	16 189	16 217		
iv)	16 189			

Interestingly, we have observed the Polynesian mtDNA type in bone samples from prehistoric sites in Polynesia, although we failed to detect the polymorphisms in several bones from archaeological sites in Melanesia and the central Pacific that were occupied by supposedly proto-Polynesian Lapita settlers (Hagelberg & Clegg 1993). This would tend to argue against the simple scenario of a recent expansion of people from island Southeast Asia into Polynesia and would support the contention that the earlier settlers of island Melanesia may have expanded gradually into the central Pacific before the arrival of the Polynesians (Terrell 1986). Further research on ancient bone samples is needed before this question can be settled. This and other problems relating to the migration patterns of ancient peoples can only really be addressed using direct genetic evidence based on ancient DNA.

We recently carried out analyses on prehistoric skeletal remains from two archaeological sites in Easter Island to help resolve the long-standing question of the origin of the prehistoric Easter Islanders (Bahn & Flenley 1992). Twelve ancient individuals were analysed and in every case we detected the 9-bp deletion and the Polynesian-specific base substitutions, confirming the Polynesian ancestry of the original inhabitants (Hagelberg *et al.* 1994). Despite these results, evidence from archaeology and botany seems to suggest a certain amount of contact between Polynesia and South America. We are now embarked on a new ancient DNA project to investigate the genetic origins of the prehistoric inhabitants of the Pacific coast of South America.

ANCIENT DNA STUDIES

The field of ancient DNA was born in 1984 with the report by Wilson's group of the cloning of DNA from the skin of an extinct quagga (Higuchi *et al.* 1984). Initially, developments were slow due to the technical problems associated with the analysis of ancient DNA sequences, but the subject has enjoyed rapid growth in the last few years (three international conferences on ancient DNA studies have taken place, and the first issue of a journal dedicated to ancient DNA research will be published in Spring 1996), as well as an unprecedented amount of attention from the news media.

From early on, the polymerase chain reaction (Saiki *et al.* 1985) became the technique of choice in ancient DNA studies, as it permits the amplification of a specific DNA fragment from degraded organic samples, even in the presence of vast amounts of microbial DNA and other contaminants, and avoids some of the sequence artefacts associated with DNA cloning (Pääbo & Wilson 1988; Pääbo *et al.* 1989). Ancient DNA studies have been burdened from the start by technical problems, including the difficulty of extracting usable DNA from some types of tissues, contamination by modern DNA, and PCR inhibition by unknown compounds in the tissue extracts. Despite this, DNA has been extracted from plant and insect tissues of considerable antiquity (DeSalle & Grimaldi 1994) and there is even a debated claim of DNA isolated from dinosaur bones (Woodward *et al.* 1994).

Because of the interest generated by ancient DNA research, scientists are pressed to produce exciting results on very old and exotic materials, and much of the research has been of a headline-catching type, rather than of real scientific interest. Some research groups have shied away from work on human remains because of the contamination problems. Samples can become contaminated by people handling the bones or by small amounts of human DNA in common dust, as well as by the sequences generated in previous PCR reactions. Whereas in animal studies one can rely on phylogenetic inference for checking the validity of the results, in the case of human studies it may be difficult to distinguish between a genuine DNA sequence and one resulting from contamination (Hagelberg & Clegg 1991; Hagelberg 1994).

The forensic identification of human remains became an early target of ancient DNA techniques, as well as providing a way to test the validity of the analyses by comparing DNA extracted from the remains with DNA from close relatives of a presumed victim. Bone DNA typing by analysis of polymorphic nuclear microsatellite DNA has been used successfully in a number of forensic cases (Hagelberg *et al.* 1991; Jeffreys *et al.* 1992; Gill *et al.* 1994). In addition, despite the difficulty in calculating likelihood ratios based on mtDNA data, the analysis of mtDNA can be applied usefully to the identification of samples like single hairs, or skeletal remains that are too old or decayed to permit the amplification of single-copy nuclear sequences (Higuchi et al. 1988; Stoneking *et al.* 1991; Ginther *et al.* 1993; Holland *et al.* 1993).

To conclude, mtDNA provides a unique tool for the study of the genetic relationships of ancient and modern human populations, as well as for forensic identification. Although the strictly maternal inheritance of mtDNA means that it is highly susceptible to genetic drift and any results must be interpreted with caution, the relative simplicity of mtDNA and its usefulness in ancient DNA research will undoubtedly help maintain its important role in anthropology and forensic science.

REFERENCES

Anderson S, Bankier A T, Barrell B G, de Bruijn M H L, Coulson A R, Drouin J, Eperon I C, Nierlich D P, Roe B A, Sanger F, Schreier P H, Smith A J H, Staden R, Young I G (1981) Sequence organisation of the human mitochondrial genome. Nature 290 :457-465

Bahn P, Flenley J (1992) Easter Island, Earth Island. Thames and Hudson, London

Ballinger S W, Schurr T G, Torroni A, Gan Y-Y, Hodge J A, Hassan K, Chen K-H, Wallace D C (!992) Southeast Asian Mitochondrial DNA analysis reveals genetic continuity of ancient mongoloid migrations. Genetics 130:139-152

Bellwood P S (1989) The colonization of the Pacific: Some current hypotheses. In: Hill A V S and Serjeantson S W (eds) The colonization of the Pacific: A genetic trail. Oxford University Press, Oxford, p 1

Cann R L, Stoneking M, Wilson A C (1987) Mitochondrial DNA and human evolution. Nature 325:31-36

Chen Y-S, Torroni A, Excoffier L, Santachiara-Benerecetti A S, Wallace A C (1995) analysis of mtDNA variation in African populations reveals the most ancient of all human continent-specific haplogroups. Am J Hum Genet 57:133-149

DeSalle R, Grimaldi D (1994) Very old DNA. Current Opinion in Genetics and Development 4:810-815

Gill P, Ivanov P L, Kimpton K, Piercy L, Benson L, Tully G, Evett I, Hagelberg E, Sullivan K (1994) Identification of the remains of the Romanov family by DNA analysis. Nature Genetics 6:130-135

Ginther C, Issel-Tarver L, King M C (1992) Identifying individuals by sequencing mitochondrial DNA from teeth. Nature Genetics 2:135-138

Hagelberg E (1994) Mitochondrial DNA from ancient bones. In: Herrmann B, Hummel S (eds) Ancient DNA. Springer-Verlag, New York, p 195

Hagelberg E, Clegg J B (1991) Isolation and characterisation of DNA from archaeological bone. Proc R Soc Lond B 244:45-50

Hagelberg E, Clegg J B (1993) Genetic polymorphisms in prehistoric Pacific islanders determined by analysis of ancient bone DNA. Proc R Soc Lond B 252:163-170

Hagelberg E, Gray I C, Jeffreys A J (1991) Identification of the skeletal remains of a murder victim by DNA analysis. Nature 352:427-429

Hagelberg E, Quevedo S, Turbon D, Clegg J B (1994) Genetic affinities of prehistoric Easter Islanders. Nature 369:25-26

Hertzberg M, Mickleson K P N, Serjeantson S W, Prior J F and Trent R J (1989) An Asian-specific 9-bp deletion of mitochondrial DNA is frequently found in Polynesians. Am J Hum Genet 44: 504-510

Higuchi R, Bowman B, Freiberger M, Ryder O A, Wilson A C (1984) DNA sequences from the quagga, an extinct member of the horse family. Nature 312:282-284

Higuchi R, von Beroldingen C H, Sensabaugh G F, Erlich H A (1988) DNA typing from single hairs. Nature 332:543-546

Holland M M, Fisher D L, Mitchell L G, Rodriguez W C, Canik J J, Merril C R, Weedn V W (1993) Mitochondrial DNA sequence analysis of human skeletal remains from the Vietnam War. J For Sci 38:542-553

Horai S, Kondo R, Murayama K, Hayashi S, Koike H, Nakai, N (1991) Phylogenetic affiliation of ancient and contemporary humans inferred by mitochondrial DNA. Phil. Trans. R. Soc. Lond. B 333:409-417

Jeffreys A J, Allen M, Hagelberg E and Sonnberg A (1992) Identification of the skeletal remains of Josef Mengele by DNA analysis. Forensic Science International 56:65-76

Lewin R (1987) The unmasking of Mitochondrial Eve. Science 238:24-26

Lum J K, Rickards O, Ching C, Cann R L (1994) Polynesian mitochondrial DNAs reveal three deep maternal lineage clusters. Hum Biol 66:567-590

Melton T, Peterson R, Redd A J, Saha N, Sofro A S M, Martinson J, Stoneking M (1995) Polynesian genetic affinities with Southeast Asian populations as identified by mtDNA analysis. Am J Hum Genet 57:403-414

Pääbo S, Higuchi R G, Wilson A C (1989) Ancient DNA and the polymerase chain reaction. J biol Chem 264:9709-9712

Pääbo S, Wilson A C (1988) Polymerase chain reaction reveals cloning artefacts. Nature 334:387-388

Saiki R K, Scharf S, Faloona F, Mullis K B, Horn G T, Erlich H A, Arnheim N (1985) Enzymatic amplification of ß-globin genomic sequences and restriction site analysis for diagnosis of sickle cell anemia. Science 230:1350-1354

Schurr T G, Ballinger S W, Gan Y-Y, Hodge J A, Merriweather D A, Lawrence D N, Knowler W C, Weiss K M, Wallace D C (1990) amerindian mitochondrial DNAs have rare Asian mutations at high frequencies, suggesting they derived from four primary maternal lineages. Am J Hum Genet 46:613-623

Stoneking M (1993) DNA and recent human evolution. Evol Anthropol 2:60-73

Stoneking M, Hedgecock D, Higuchi R G, Vigilant L, Erlich H A (1991) Population variation of human mtDNA control region sequences detected by enzymatic amplification and sequence-specific oligonucleotide probes. Am J Hum Genet 48:370-382

Stoneking M, Wilson A C (1989) Mitochondrial DNA. In: Hill A V S and Serjeantson S W (eds) The colonization of the Pacific: A genetic trail. Oxford University Press, Oxford, p 215

Soodyall H, Jenkins T, Stoneking M (1995) 'Polynesian' mtDNA in the Malagasy. Nature Genetics 10:377-378

Templeton A R (1992) Human origins and analysis of mitochondrial DNA sequences. Science 255:737

Terell J (1986) Prehistory in the Pacific Islands. Cambridge University Press, Cambridge

Vigilant L, Stoneking M, Harpending H, Hawkes K, Wilson A C (1991) African populations and the evolution of human mitochondrial DNA. Science 253:1503-1507

Wainscoat J (1986) Out of the garden of Eden. Nature 325:13

Wainscoat J S, Hill A V S, Boyce A J, Flint J, Hernandez M, Thein S L, Old J M, Falusi A G, Weatherall D J, Clegg J B (1986) Evolutionary relationships of human populations from an analysis of nuclear DNA polymorphisms. Nature 319:491-493

Wallace D C (1995) Mitochondrial DNA variation in human evolution, degenerative disease, and aging. Am J Hum Genet 57:201-223

Wolpoff M H (1989) Multiregional evolution: The fossil alternative to Eden. In Mellars P, Stringer C (eds) The human revolution. Edinburgh University Press, Edinburgh, p 62

Woodward S R, Weyand N J, Bunnell M (1994) DNA sequence from Cretaceous period bone fragments. Science 265:1229-1232

Wrischnik L A, Higuchi R G, Stoneking M, Erlich H A, Arnheim N, Wilson A C (1987) Length mutations in human mitochondrial DNA: direct sequencing of enzymatically amplified DNA. Nucl Acids Res 15:529-542

A Two Stage Strategy for the Automated Analysis of Mitochondrial DNA

K.M. Sullivan, G. Tully, R. Alliston-Greiner, A. Hopwood, J.E. Bark, P. Gill.

The Forensic Science Service, Priory House, Gooch Street North, Birmingham, U.K. B5 6QQ

INTRODUCTION

DNA amplification and sequencing of the mitochondrial (mt) non-coding region provides a highly sensitive and discriminating test for individual identification which is ideal for the analysis of severely degraded human remains (Sullivan et al. 1994, Gill et al. 1994). A major drawback with DNA sequencing as a forensic tool is the labour-intensive nature and therefore high cost of the technique, which presently limits its application to the investigation of serious crime. Alternative strategies to DNA sequencing have been developed to characterise sequence polymorphisms in mtDNA products including hybridisation with allele-specific probes (Stoneking et al. 1991), detection of length polymorphisms (Bodenteich et al. 1992) and oligonucleotide ligation assay (Sullivan et al 1993). More recently, the novel technique of multiplex solid phase fluorescent minisequencing has been developed (Tully et al. 1995) which detects both sequence and length polymorphisms. The latter is being developed by our laboratory as a primary screen in a two stage strategy for the automated analysis of mtDNA. The minisequencing technique enables the majority of non-related individuals to be eliminated in a rapid and straightforward test so that the remaining samples can then be distinguished further by the application of full DNA sequencing, which is more discriminating than minisequencing but also much more labour-intensive to perform.

MULTIPLEX FLUORESCENT SOLID PHASE MINISEQUENCING

Sections of the non-coding region are amplified using biotinylated primers, and the PCR product is immobilised on magnetisable streptavidin-coated beads and used as the template for minisequencing. The concept of fluorescent minisequencing is to characterise a particular polymorphic site within the PCR product by annealing to it a primer whose 3' end is 1 base upstream from the site in question. A single base extension reaction is then performed utilising dideoxynucleotides labelled with 4 distinguishable dyes (Perkin Elmer). The resultant dye-labelled extension product can then be characterised by eluting the primer from the DNA followed by electrophoresis and analysis on an ABD 377 automated DNA sequencer. It is possible to characterise simultaneously several informative sites by designing a detection primer for each site with appropriate mobility-modifying homopolymer tails such that all products can be resolved by electrophoresis through a 12cm long 19% acrylamide gel.
From previously constructed British Caucasian and Afro-Caribbean mitochondrial sequence databases, minisequencing primers were designed for the characterisation of 10 highly polymorphic point mutation sites (L73, 146,

152, 195, 247, 16069, 16129, 16189, 16224, and 16311), plus one site of oligo(G) length variation (L302), and a dinucleotide repeat within the mtDNA. The latter is characterised with two oligonucleotides for sites L523 and 525, making it possible to determine whether 4,5 or >5 dinucleotide repeats are present within the polymorphic region. Preliminary results from 120 unrelated British Caucasians have been determined for which 53 different mitotypes i.e. variants at the 12 loci were detected with the commonest type present in 16.8% of the population, 34% of mitotypes are unique and the overall probability of random match (pM) is approximately 0.05.

DNA SEQUENCING OF SEVERELY DEGRADED SAMPLES

For the more detailed comparison of samples which cannot be distinguished by minisequencing, a full sequencing strategy can be used that generates sequence of excellent quality from forensic samples in a highly automated procedure. Routine analysis comprises amplification of the entire non-coding region followed by a second nested PCR reaction in which either the HV1 (403bp) or HV2 (383bp) segments of the mt non-coding region are amplified (Sullivan et al 1994). However, for highly degraded samples a single round of amplification is employed using closely spaced primers. In total 8 different pairs of primers each of which amplifies only part of 1 hypervariable section are utilised in 35 cycle reactions: (-21M13)L15997 with (Biotin)H16239; (-21M13)H16239 with (Biotin)L15997; (-21M13)H16401 with (Biotin)L16159; (-21M13)L16159 with (Biotin)H16401; (-21M13)H255 with (Biotin)L29; (-21M13)L29 with (Biotin)H255; (-21M13)L164 with (Biotin)H408; (-21M13)H408 with (Biotin)L164. This enables both strands of both hypervariable regions to be determined in solid phase sequencing reactions using universal M13 sequencing primers in conjunction with an ABD 377 sequencer. Up to 243bp of data is generated from each PCR product with sequence comparisons between complementary or overlapping strands performed using the SeqEd™ computer program to confirm the data. Comparison of different sequencing strategies indicates that use of modified T7 polymerase plus dye-labelled primers for the sequencing reaction yields data with the lowest background noise and minimal sequence context-specific variation, enabling subtle sequence characteristics such as heteroplasmy to be detected reliably.

CASEWORK APPLICATIONS

Full automated DNA sequencing is now being used on a routine basis in forensic casework within our laboratory. Applications are restricted to discrete evidential samples such as severely degraded bones, faeces and hair shafts which are refractory to chromosomal DNA analysis. Analysis of DNA from faeces has been facilitated by the magnetic capture and washing of the template in solid phase, using the Dynal DNA Direct™ kit, prior to amplification. Results are obtained from as little as 10mg wet weight of starting material (Fig. 1) Analysis of DNA from hair shafts typically requires a one round amplification of short PCR products in order to generate sufficient template for successful sequencing. In general, 2 to 4cms of head hair shaft is used per DNA extraction and where possible all casework samples are subjected to duplicate extractions, amplifications and sequence analyses to confirm the sequence for casework reporting purposes. It is envisaged that the minisequencing technique, when introduced into casework, will provide a rapid and cheap screen making the analysis of large numbers of samples recovered from a scene of crime a more economically feasible proposition.

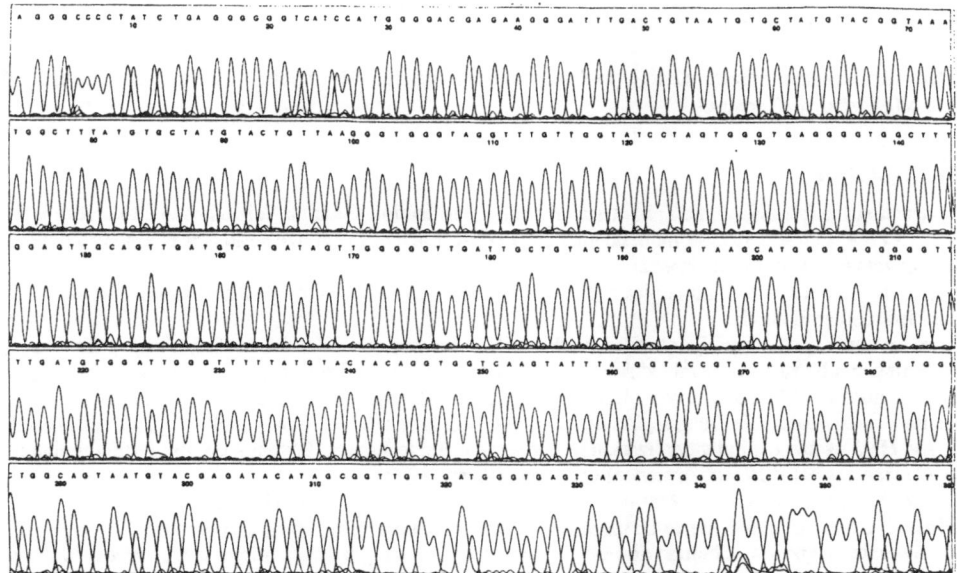

Fig 1. Mitochondrial DNA sequence from human faeces. DNA extracted from 20mg (wet weight) of material was amplified with HV1-specific primers then bound to Dynal beads and sequenced with Sequenase.

REFERENCES

Bodenteich A, Mitchell LG, Polymeropoulos MH and Merril CR.   (1992).
  Dinucleotide repeat in the human mitochondrial D-loop. Hum. Mol. Genet.
  1(2): 140.
Gill P, Ivanov P, Kimpton C, Piercy R, Benson N, Tully G, Evett I, Hagelberg E.
  and Sullivan K. (1994) Identification of the remains of the Romanov family by
  DNA analysis. Nature Genet. 6(2): 130-135.
Stoneking M, Hedgecock D, Higuchi RG, Vigilant L and Erlich HA (1991).
  Population variation of human mtDNA control region sequences detected by
  enzymatic amplification and sequence-specific oligonucleotide probes.
  Am.J.Hum.Genet. 48: 370-382.
Sullivan KM, Piercy R, Benson N, Faulkner K and Gill P. (1993)
  Mitochondrial DNA analysis as a tool for forensic investigations.
  Proceedings of the 2nd International Symposium on the Forensic Aspects of
  DNA Analysis. In press.
Sullivan KM, Piercy R, Benson N, Ivanov P, Mannucci A and Gill P.
  (1994) Solid phase sequencing of mitochondrial DNA: towards a fully
  automated forensic DNA test. p135-148 In M Uhlen, E Hornes and O Olsvic
  (Eds.) Advances in Biomagnetic Separation. Eaton Publg., Natick MA,USA.
Tully G, Sullivan KM, Nixon P, Stones R and Gill P. (1995) Detection of
  mitochondrial sequence polymorphisms using multiplex solid-phase
  fluorescent minisequencing. Manuscript in preparation.

MIXING AND THERMIC TREATMENT OF MITOCHONDRIAL PCR FRAGMENTS REVEAL SEQUENCE DIFFERENCES BY HETERODUPLEX FORMATION –A RAPID METHOD FOR FORENSIC IDENTITY TESTING

R. Szibor, I. Plate, E. Kirches and D. Krause

Institut für Rechtsmedizin, Otto-von-Guericke-Universität Magdeburg, Leipziger Strasse 44 39120 Magdeburg, Germany

INTRODUCTION

For extracting the full information about stains or an identification situation, it is advisable to investigate karyotic STR systems as well as mitochondria (mt) DNA. Each of the above strategies is associated with special advantages and disadvantages:
1. Due to the high number of mt copies per cell, it is a much higher sensitivity what distinguishes mt testing from other methods.
2. Since mt concerns maternally inherited markers, it avoids wrong results due to illegitamate paternities.
3. mt testing can be superior if mixed stains have to be investigated. Stain sorting by cloning is possible.
Within the human mt D-Loop, a considerable potential for information concerning individualization is condensed on an assessable DNA region of about 800 bp. There are two hypervariable regions designated HV1 and HV2 usable for individualization by the sequencing technique. Within a group of 100 unrelated white Caucasians, 91 different sequences were seen (Piercy 1993).
We suggest that the application of mt testing needs a simple screening method for detecting identities and nonidities if a mass of stains has to be investigated or if stain sorting has to be carried out.
In the genomic diagnostic of human diseases, sequence heterogenity between alleles can be recognized by using techniques such as heteroduplex (HD) analysis (HDA), single strand confirmation polymorhism (SSCP) investigation and chemical cleavage.
The PCR product of a karyotic gene fragment produces a HD if the genotyp is heterozygous with regard to the sequences and / or to the repeat numbers in STRs. Leaving aside the fact that there are some infrequent mt heteroplasmatic disturbances, e.g. deletions, mt population of a human induviual is usually uniform. Therefore, D-loop amplification of polymorphic regions of a certain proband or a pure stain normally cannot produce any HDs. Likewise, if D-loop products stemming from the same source are submitted to mixing and thermic treatment, they should provide only homoduplexes. Thus, if D-Loop products from a stain and the stain causer or from a proband and his maternal relatives are treated in the mentioned manner, it is expected that no HD formation takes place. On the other hand, if nonidentical sequences were mixed and thermically treated, reciprocal rearrangements - beside homological reassociation - take place resulting in HD formation. HDs migrate markedly slower than homoduplexes if native PAGE is used for separation. Therefore, HDA can reveal sequence differences in D-Loop fragments.

MATERIAL and METHODS:

For amplifying the fragments of interest we use the following primers:
HV 1*   L 15996 / H 16498   (544 bp)   HV 2* L 29 / H 408   (431 bp)
Whole D-loop* :L 15926 / H   580   (1280 bp)[*PCR was carried out according to Sullivan (1991)

mt-HDA PROTOCOL:

1. Amplify the D-loop fragments from the different sources and check the PCR success by PAGE.
2. Mix the samples of question (e. g. stain vs. possible causer   or   corpse vs. maternal related relatives).
3. Carry out 5 PCR cycles omitting the enzyme and chill immediately on ice.
4. Separate the mixtures as well as the pure mixture components using vative PAGE and silver staining.

For introducing mt HDA, mixing experiments were performed using amplified HV1 as well as HV2 fragments. Mother/child and sibling/sibling combinations were regarded as mixtures of identical sequences. Father/child and wife/housband pairs were seen as mixtures of non identical fragments.

Sequences were read using the A373 sequencer and the Taq dye terminator cycle sequencing kit (ABI).

RESULTS and DISCUSSION

If HV1 fragments stemming from 50 mother/child pairs were mixed and thermically treated, HDs could never be seen. In opposite, if the procedure was carried out in 50 father / child pairs, HDs were seen in 48 cases. As it is demonstratad by mixing HV1 fragments of siblings with those from their father, each mixture provides the same HD shape. (Fig.1)

In parallel, when we mixed HV2 products within 100 mother/child pairs we did not see HDs, but we did in 85% of father/child pairs. HDA in families using HV2 is depicted in Fig. 2.

If the HV2 fragments of any proband are mixed with those of unrelated persons, about 85 % of mixtures produce HDs again (Fig. 3). Furthermore, there is a high variability in the HD patterns.

The following conclusions can be drawn from Fig. 4 and 5:

1. HV fragments of different source but with equal sequences (e.g. siblings) produce identical HD patterns if they are mixed with their counterpart fragments stemming from the same probands.

2. A prominent HD is caused by a high number of missmatches, no or a discrete HD indicates that there are no or only sporadic missmatches. Additionally, we suppose that the missmatch positions may play a significant role, too (This assumption has not been systematically investigated until now).

3. HDA in the HV 1 and the HV2 region have an independent chance to indicate nonidentities of mt of persons or stains.

In addition to HDA, for the same purpose, we tried the SSCP technique. Here is again a good chance that heterogenity in mixed fragments becomes visibel by doubleband formation. However, in our hands, the SSCP technique seems to be much less effective than HDA.

Ending Statement: HDA is a suitable technique to detect the majority of the nonidentities of sequences if mtDNA stemming from different sources is mixed. Thus, if a mass of stains has to be investigated or if stain sorting has to be done by HV1 and HV2 cloning, this method may help to focus the more expensive sequencing techniques onto highly interesting samples or stains.

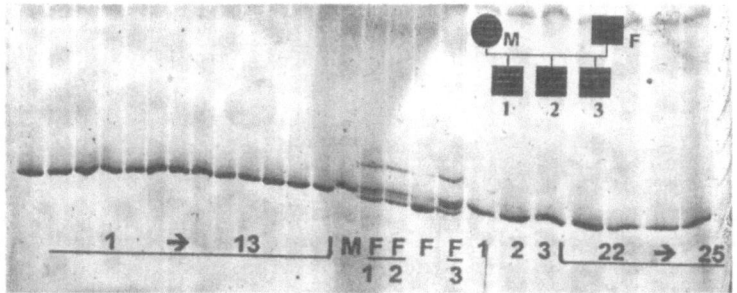

Fig 1: HDA experiment using VH1 fragments of mother/child pairs and of a famliy depicted in the pedigree. lanes 1–13 and 22–25 contain mixed HV 1 fragments of 17 mother/child pairs. In the middle of the gel, there are pure and mixed HV1 fragments stemming from the pedigree. Clear HDs were formed in father/child pairs. Due to the identity of the father/child combinations, all HDs show the same shape.

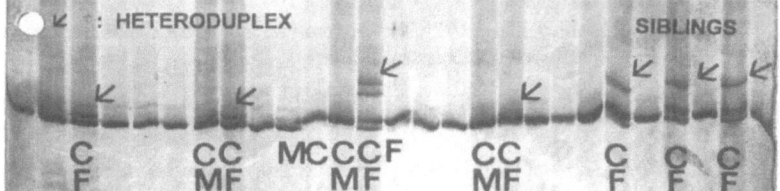

Fig 2: HDA of the D-loop HV2 region in five families. Full lettering is given only for the family in the middle of the gel: M (unmixed fragment of the mother), F (unmixed fragment of the father), C (unmixed fragment of the child), letter combination (mixed fragments).

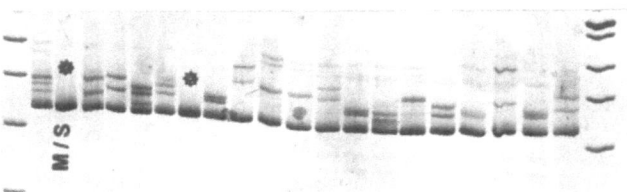

Fig 3: HDA in HV2: All lanes contain the same HV2 product of a woman mixed with the counterparts stemming from her son (M/S) and 19 unrelated donors. *= none HD formation.

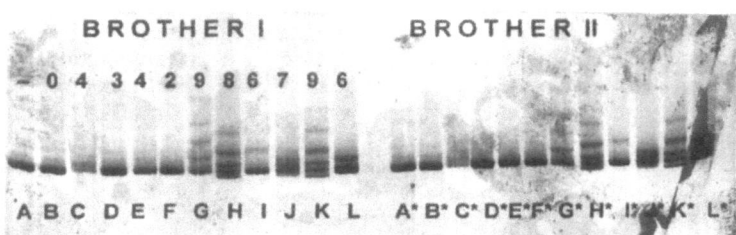

Fig 4: HDA in HV2: PCR fragments stemming from two brothers were mixed with those from 100 unrelated probands giving two identical series of HV2 mixtures. Out of both series four mixtures were chosen producing no or weak HDs (C–F and C*–F*) and six pairs creating powerful HDs (L–G and L*–G*). Sequencing revealed the number of missmatches between the mixture components (figures). Lanes A and B contain the pure and mixed HV2 fragments of the brothers, respectively.

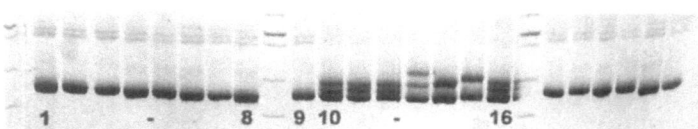

Fig 5: HDA in HV1: Fragments were mixed using products from probands wich were chosen bacause of lacking HDs in mixtures of HV2. (Compare with Fig 4 !) Lanes 1 to 8 contain pure HV1 products, lanes 10 to 16 show pairs which were tested with regard to HD production in HV2 (equal tolanes C–I in fig. 4).

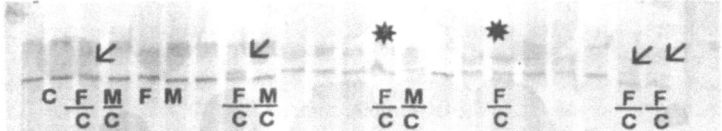

Fig 6: SSCP study in five families using HV2: . Heterogenity in mixed fragments becomes visibel by doubleband formation in three of five nonidentical mixtures.
↙= sequence heterogenity detected, *= sequence heterogenity not detected.

References :
Piercy R, Sullivan KM, Benson N, Gill P (1993) The application of mitochondrial DNA typing to the study of white Caucasian geneticc identification. Int J Med 106: 85-90
Sullivan KM, Hopgood R, Gill P (1991) Automated amplification and sequencing of human mitochondrial DNA. Electrophoresis 12: 17-21

GENETIC ANALYSIS OF SINGLE HAIR SHAFTS BY AUTOMATED SEQUENCE ANALYSIS OF THE MITOCHONDRIAL D-LOOP REGION

R. Decorte, E. Jehaes, F.-X. Xiao and J.-J. Cassiman

Center for Human Genetics, K.U.Leuven, Herestraat 49, B-3000 Leuven, Belgium

INTRODUCTION

Hair samples found at a crime scene can be important as evidence material in the identification of the offender. Sometimes, it represents the only biological evidence sample which connects a suspect to a crime. However, most hairs submitted for DNA analysis are shed hair which do not contain a hair root. Analysis with VNTR or STR markers is therefore problematic and in most cases no DNA profile is obtained. In contrast to nuclear DNA, sufficient amounts of mito-chondrial DNA can be extracted from hair shafts to allow the analysis of the highly polymorphic mt d-loop region.

Here, we present a strategy for the analysis of the two hypervariable regions in the mt d-loop by PCR and automated sequence analysis on the A.L.F. DNA sequencer. A population database was constructed with 51 unrelated Caucasians of Belgian descent.

MATERIALS AND METHOD

DNA was extracted from hair shafts according to the procedure described by Gill (1985) except for concentration of the DNA extract. which was done by filtration on Microcon 30 or 100 devices (Amicon).

Five microliter of the DNA extract was added to a PCR reaction containing 2.5 units of Taq DNA-polymerase (Perkin-Elmer), 2.5 mM $MgCl_2$, 0.2 µM of oligodeoxyribonucleotides (dTTP, dATP and dCTP), 200 µM of dITP, 40µM dGTP, 0.2 mM of each primer (Fig. 1) and PCR buffer 50 mM KCl, 10 mM Tris-HCl (pH 8.4), 200 mg/ml gelatin and 170 µg/ml of BSA in a volume of 100 µl. The reactions were processed for 35 cycles to denaturation at 94°C for 45 sec., annealing at 60°C for 30 sec. and extension at 72°C for 30 sec in a GeneAmp 2400 or 9600 Cycler (Perkin-Elmer).

Semi-nested PCR was performed as follows: a first PCR was done with primer pair L15996 and H16401-B or primer pair L20 and H408-B under the conditions described above except for the number of cycles which was reduced to 30. In a second PCR reaction 5 µl of the first PCR was used as a template with one of the two primers replaced by an internal primer. Quality control of the PCR products was done on 6% polyacrylamide gels in Tris-borate-EDTA buffer at 200 volt.

Single stranded templates were generated by binding of 70 µl of the biotinylated PCR products to streptavidin-coated beads (Dynabeads™, Dynal), as described by the manufacturer, followed by denaturation with 1N NaOH. Enzymatic sequencing with T7 DNA polymerase was done with the AutoRead Sequencing kit (Pharmacia-Biotech). In all the sequencing reactions, a single fluorescein-labelled primer (U.P.) was used which was complementary to the 3'end of the 3'PCR primer (Fig. 1).

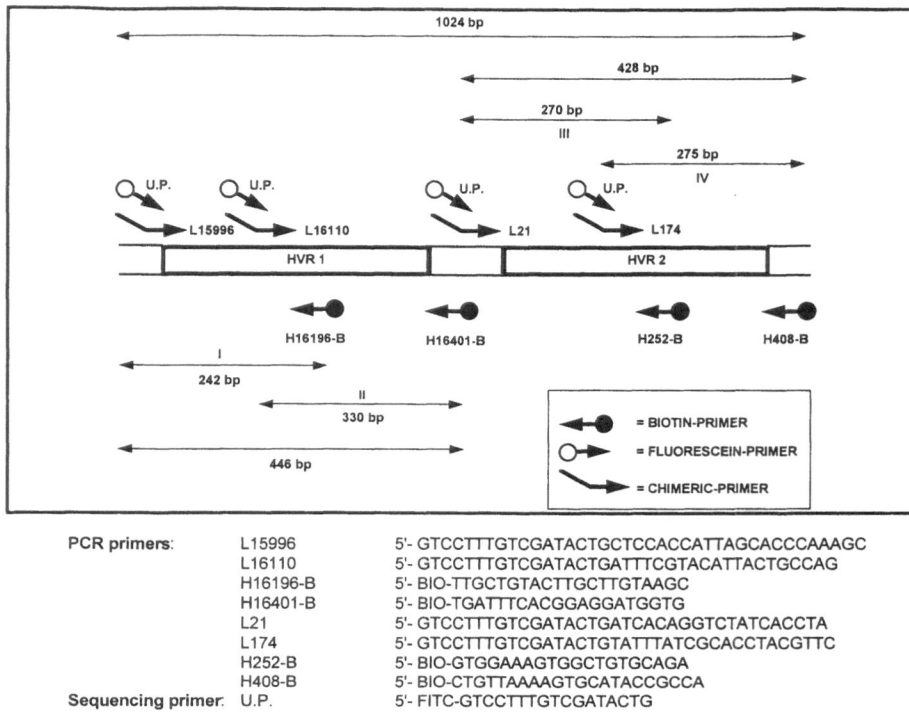

PCR primers:	L15996	5'- GTCCTTTGTCGATACTGCTCCACCATTAGCACCCAAAGC
	L16110	5'- GTCCTTTGTCGATACTGATTTCGTACATTACTGCCAG
	H16196-B	5'- BIO-TTGCTGTACTTGCTTGTAAGC
	H16401-B	5'- BIO-TGATTTCACGGAGGATGGTG
	L21	5'- GTCCTTTGTCGATACTGATCACAGGTCTATCACCTA
	L174	5'- GTCCTTTGTCGATACTGTATTTATCGCACCTACGTTC
	H252-B	5'- BIO-GTGGAAAGTGGCTGTGCAGA
	H408-B	5'- BIO-CTGTTAAAAGTGCATACCGCCA
Sequencing primer:	U.P.	5'- FITC-GTCCTTTGTCGATACTG

Figure 1: Strategy of the amplification and sequencing procedure for the analysis of mtDNA variation in the d-loop region.
Primers are identified by a letter designating the strand of mtDNA (L is the non-coding and H is the coding strand) and a number corresponding to the reference sequence (Anderson 1981) of the base at the 3' end of the primer. U.P. is a universal primer not complementary to mtDNA.

Seven microliter of the sequencing reactions were loaded on a 7% Urea-Hydrolink Long Ranger gel (J.T. Baker) after denaturation for 3 min. at 85°C. Electrophoresis was done on the automated A.L.F. DNA sequencer (Pharmacia-Biotech).

RESULTS AND DISCUSSION

The developed strategy for the analysis of the d-loop region is outlined in Fig. 1. Depending on the source and the constitution of the biological sample either the two hypervariable regions (HVR1 or HVR2) or four overlapping segments (I to IV) are amplified. This approach allows also for a semi-nested PCR where one of the two hypervariable regions (HVR1 or HVR2) is amplified in a first PCR followed by a second amplification reaction of the two overlapping segments. The primers complementary to the H-strand are biotinylated which after capture with Dynabeads and alkali denaturation results in single stranded templates for enzymatic sequence analysis (solid-phase-approach). The non-biotinylated strand can be collected for further sequencing which will confirm the obtained sequence data from the biotinylated DNA strand. The unlabelled PCR primers are chimeric with a universal sequence (5') and a specific sequence complementary to the L-strand (3') (Fig. 1). This approach has the advantage that the sequence can be read

Table 1: Distribution of the mtDNA types observed in this study

| Frequency (%) | Number of mtDNA types | | |
	HVR1	HVR2	d-loop
19.6	1	-	-
9.80	-	1	-
7.84	-	1	-
5.88	3	-	-
3.92	2	4	2
1.96	28	34	47

starting from the beginning of the amplified fragment. Sequence analysis of the PCR products revealed a number of 'stops' in the obtained sequence which was probably due to 'pausing' of the enzyme at regions with secondary structure. These 'stops' were resolved mainly by the inclusion of dITP, a nucleotide analogue for dGTP, in the PCR reaction (Dierick 1993).

Amplification of mtDNA from fresh hair shafts showed that it was possible to amplify a fragment of 1024 bp containing the complete d-loop with 40 cycles (data not shown). Evaluation on forensic hair samples resulted, however, in a low success rate of amplification even for the two hypervariable regions of 430 bp when a single amplification step was used. By using the semi-nested approach a success rate of 95-100% was obtained. This was a two to three fold increase of the success rate compared to the analysis with VNTR or STR markers.

In order to provide a statistical value in case of a match, we started with a survey for mtDNA variation in a small population of 51 unrelated Caucasians of Belgian descent. On average between 700 and 800 nucleotides were obtained for each individual. Differences with the reference sequence (Anderson 1981) were observed at 50 positions in the first hypervariable region (HVR1) and at 28 positions in the second (HVR2). In total, 49 different mtDNA types were identified: 47 sequences were observed only once in the population of 51 individuals while 2 mtDNA types were observed each 2 times (Table 1).

The mean pairwise sequence difference within the database was 3.52 for HVR1, 3.86 for HVR2 and 7.38 for the complete d-loop region. Therefore, a possible strategy for routine use in forensic analysis could be based on the analysis of HVR2 which is the most variable region (Table 1). In case of a match between the evidence sample and the reference sample from suspect or victim, further analysis of HVR1 will confirm or exclude a match. This approach has until now been used with success in several forensic cases. However, in those cases where close maternal relatives (brothers) may be suspected of a crime it is not possible to identify the offender between the relatives with mtDNA analysis alone. Only exclusion analysis with mtDNA is possible with 100% reliability.

REFERENCES

Anderson S, Bankier AT, Barrell BG, De Bruijn MHL, Coulson AR, Drouin J, Eperon IC, Nierlich DP, Roe BA, Sanger F, Schreir PH, Smith AJH, Staden R, Young IG (1981) Sequence and organization of the human mitochondrial genome. Nature 290:457-465

Dierick H, Stul M, De Kelver W, Marynen P, Cassiman JJ (1993) Incorporation of dITP or 7-deaza dGTP during PCR improves sequencing of the product. Nucleic Acids Research 21:4427-4428

Gill P, Jeffreys AJ, Werrett DJ (1985) Forensic applications of DNA 'fingerprints'. Nature 318:577-579.

MITHOCONDRIAL HVR1 POLYMORPHISM IN ITALY

E.d'Aloja, I.Boschi, A. Moscetti, M.Dobosz, V.L.Pascali * and A. Fiori

Immunohematology laboratory, Istituto Medicina Legale, Università Cattolica, Largo F.Vito 1, 00168 Roma, Italy; (*) Istituto Medicina Legale, Università di Verona

INTRODUCTION

Polymorphism within the mainframe of mitochondrial DNA sequence (mtDNA) is an interesting source of human molecular diversity. Most of the mtDNA sequence variation occurs at two regions (namely, HVRI and HVRII) encompassing a relatively short area (800 base pairs) of the entire mtDNA genome. Both have been used in studies addressing the structure and relationships of human populations (Vigilant 1989).
Recently, evidence has been given that there is considerable advantage in using mtDNA for forensics (Holland 1993, Piercy 1993), two hyperpolymorphic domains have been used to solve special problems of identification which would have not been possible to deal with nuclear loci. To properly exploit the potential informativeness of mtDNA, an adequate database of the appropriate population should be available as reference for statistical analysis. We recently undertook a study aimed at determining the sequence polymorphism shown by our reference population (Central and Southern Italy) at HVRI domain of d-loop region. In this report, we give information on 74 individual sequences.

MATERIALS AND METHODS

MtDNA was extracted from whole blood samples from 74 unrelated individuals. To amplify HVRI fragment, two separate sets of primers were used (L15990 and H16239 for set 1 and L16159 and H16410 for set 2; primers sequence is summarized in table n.1), each generating a 280 base pair length fragment. The two segments overlapped on a 50 base pair long region in the middle. All fluorescent primers were synthesized on a 391 PCR-mate (ABI) using a slightly modified cycle to label the 5'-end of one primer of any given pair by a fluorescein-amidite (FluorPrime TM, Pharmacia).
The PCR products were controlled on agarose, then they were purified and concentrated by a Microcon 30 spin-dialysis column to remove unincorporated primers. An aliquot of 50 nanograms template was administered to the TAQ cycle sequencing reaction and forward\reverse sequences were produced (sequencing primers as follow: L15997, H16236, L16163 and H16395; primers sequence is summarized in table n.1). Sequencing cycles (15 on average for good quality DNA) were specifically designed for each fluorescent-primers (1 µM each). The reaction products were denatured for 10 minutes at 95°C, then loaded onto the ALF DNA sequencer (Pharmacia); electrophoresis was performed on a denaturing polyacrilamide gel (7M urea, 6%T) for 4-5 hours depending on the fragment length to sequence. The sequencing data were analyzed by internal ALF software facilities and sequences were alligned on the original Cambridge consensus sequence (Anderson 1981).

RESULTS AND DISCUSSION

All collected data and a shortenend version of the resulting database are shown in Fig. 1 and Table 2. As internal controls, mother-child samples were processed whenever possible. No mutation was observed in these cases.

A total of 55 different haplotypes were identified, containing 55 overall mutation sites. The majority of sequences were represented only once in the database. The most common genotype (identical to the Cambridge consensus sequence) was observed with a frequency of 12%. Except for eleven transversion, all polymorphisms were transitional events (with pyrimidine mostly involved). No insertion/deletion was documented. Most mutations (76 %) were C➔T or T➔C.

A comparison with previously published Caucasian data is in progress and will be detailed elsewhere.

REFERENCES

Anderson S, Bankier AT, Barrell BG, de Bruijn MHL, Coulson AR, Drouin J, Eperon IC, Nierlich DP, Roe BA, Sanger F, Schreier PH, Smith AJH, Staden R, Young IG 1981 Sequence and organization of the human mitochondrial genome. Nature 290: 457-465.

Holland MM, Fisher DL, Mitchell LG, Rodriguez WC, Canick JJ, Merril CR, Weedn VW (1993) Mitochondrial DNA sequence analysis of human skeletal remains: identification of remains from the Vietnam War. J. For. Sci. 38: 542-553.

Piercy R, Sullivan KM, Benson N, Gill P (1993) The application of mitochorndrial DNA typing to the study of white Caucasian genetic identification. Int. J. Leg. Med. 106: 85-90.

Vigilant L, Pennington R, Harpending H, Kocher TD, Wilson AC (1989) Mitochondrial DNA sequences in single hairs from a Southern African Population. Proc. Natl. Acad. Sci. USA 86:9350-9354

Fig.1. Position of mutant nucleotides

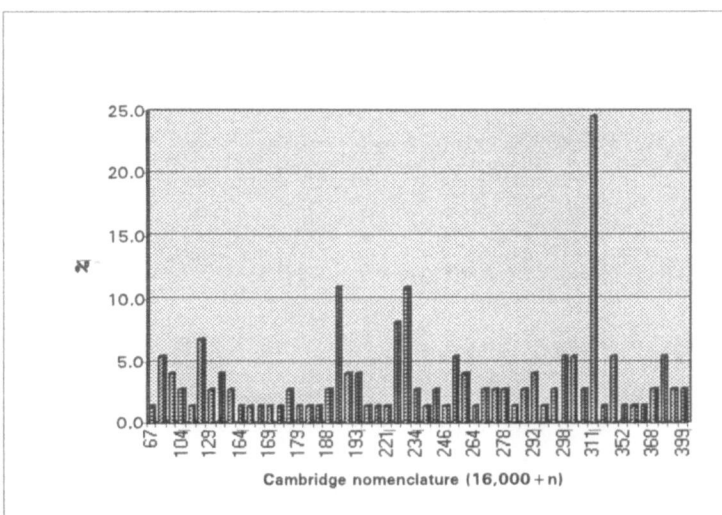

Table 1. PCR primers for the amplification and the sequencing reaction

Primers set		Forward primer L strand	Reverse primer H strand
I round	I set	L15990: TTAACTCCACCATTAGCACC	H16239: TGCCTTTGGAGTTGCAGTTG
I round	II set	L16159: TACTTGACCACCTGTAGTAC	H16401: TGATTTCACGGAGGATGGTG
Sequencing I set		L15997: CACCATTAGCACCCAAAGCT	H16236: CTTTGGAGTTGCAGTTGATG
Sequencing II set		L16163: TGACCACCTGTAGTACATAA	H16395: CACGGAGGATGGTGGTCAAG

Table 2. Most common haplotypes in 74 Italians

position	obs	%	16001	16224	16260	16304	16311	16410
Cambridge			A	T	C	T	T	A
hapl. 1	9	12.2	-	-	-	-	-	-
hapl. 2	6	8.1	-	C	-	-	C	-
hapl. 3	5	6.7	-	-	-	-	C	-
hapl. 4	2	2.7	-	-	T	-	-	-
halpl. 5	2	2.7	-	-	-	C	-	-
others	1 x 50	1.35 X 50						

mtDNA sequences in the Norwegian Saami and main populations

B. M. Dupuy and B. Olaisen

Institute of Forensic Medicine, University of Oslo, Noway

INTRODUCTION

The mitochondrial DNA has several properties useful for the reconstruction of human population history. The origin of the Saami people is still not known, even if much have been done to unravel the secrets of the past. One hypothesis is that Saami are the ancient Nordic people, another that they have a strong Mongolian component among their ancestors, and a third that they are mainly of European descent (for a comprehensive review, see Eriksson 1988). In a recent report, Sajantila et al. (in press 1995) show that Saami are distinct from other Europeans by characteristic patterns in mtDNA D-loop sequence, and they conclude that the Saami seem to have a long history distinct from other European populations.

A considerable proportion of Saami live in Norway, with Karasjok and Kautokeino as two main, geographically separated communities (Fig. 1). We have a rather large, 25 years old material of serum samples from Karasjok and Kautokeino.

The aim of the present study was to find out if these samples could be used as a source for mtDNA sequencing. Having shown that this is indeed the case, we have embarked on a study of D-loop variation in Norwegian Saami and main populations. This is a preliminary report of this study.

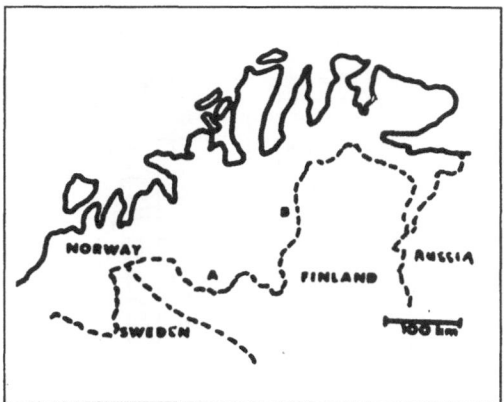

Figure 1 Map showing the northern parts of Norway. The letters indicate the administrative centers of Kautokeino (A) and Karasjok (B).

MATERIALS

The Saami material consists of serum from 201 Saami from the Karasjok and Kautokeino communities. 159 samples (92 from Karasjok, 67 from Kautokeino) were collected in 1970. The criteria as to the Saami origin and unrelatedness are described by the collector (Teisberg 1971). In 1989 another 42 samples from Karasjok were collected. 20 of these are from individuals which may be related to/identical with persons in the old material.

The material from the main Norwegian population consists of blood samples from 30 unrelated individuals from all over Norway. They all have four Norwegian grandparents.

METHODS

DNA extraction: Serum samples were spun in an Eppendorf centrifuge 12000 rpm, 30 min. The pellets were digested overnight by proteinase K, and DNA extracted by phenol/chloroform, pelleted by 100% ethanol and resuspended in 50 microliter TE buffer. Blood samples (EDTA) were extracted by the salting out method (Miller et al. 1988).

Primers and PCR: Amplification conditions for the 9 bp deletion: Hertzberg et al. 1989.
Electrophoretic procedures: 6% PAGE, ABI 373A Sequencer, Software: 673 Genescan, 373 Sequencer, and Sequence Navigator. **Sequencing reactions:** PRISM™ Solid Phase Sequenase Dye Terminator DNA Sequencing Kit (Perkin Elmer).

RESULTS AND DISCUSSION

Table 1: Distribution of mtDNA sequences in 30 main population Norwegians.

HAPLOTYPES	16113	16129	16145	16162	16171	16185	16189	16192	16213	16215	16221	16223	16224	16256	16260	16263	16270	16271	16275	16278	16291	16292	16293	16298	16304	16311	16362	16391
Anderson-81	G	G	G	A	A	C	T	C	G	A	C	C	T	C	C	T	C	T	G	C	C	C	A	T	T	T	T	G
Norwegians:																												
No. of obs																												
6																												
2																									C			
1										A															C			
2													C													C		
1											G		C													C		
1						C							C										G			C		
1		A		G								T														C	A	
2																							G			C		
1						C											T											
1						C											T											
1												T									T							
1		A			T							T	C	T											C			
1												T										T						
1	T																											
1									A																C			
1								T						T			T				T							
1				G																								
1			A																									
1																C												
1						C										C												
1																									C			
1												T							A									
TOTAL:30																												

Table 2: Distribution of mtDNA sequences in Norwegian Saami populations.

		HAPLOTYPES	16013	16126	16136	16144	16148	16149	16154	16162	16189	16223*	16256	16261	16270	16294	16298	16335	16358	16360	16362*	16400
		Anderson-81	A	T	T	G	A	C	G	A	T	C	C	C	C	C	T	A	A	C	T	C
SAAMI	**SAAMI**	Obs. in																				
KARASJOK	**KAUTOKEINO**	**NORWEGIANS**																				
No. of obs	No. of obs	No. of obs																				
50	13	1															C					
41	29	0					C			C					T							
7	2	0					C	T		C					T							
19	17	0					C			C					T			G				
1	0	0					C	T		C	T											
5	0	0				C	C			C	T										T	C
5	0	0									G											
1	0	0									G	C										
3	0	0													T							
0	1	0				C			A									T				
0	2	0												T		T						
1	0	6																				
TOTAL:133	**TOTAL:64**	**TOTAL:7**																				

PCR products were obtained from all samples. All 201 Saami lacked the 9 bp deletion commonly seen in Asians (Hertzberg et al. 1989).

mtDNA sequences (15997-16401, primers included) for 197 individuals (four are still not typed) are depicted in Tables 1 and 2 for the main population and the Saami, respectively. Ordinarily, about 350 bp could be read. In the 30 individuals from the main population, the Cambridge sequence (Anderson 1981) was experienced in 20 % (6 individuals), otherwise no particular sequence was seen more than twice (7%), a total of 22 different sequences being observed. In the 197 Saami, only twelve different sequences were observed. 57% of the Saami shared a main theme with C in positions 16144 and 16189, and T in 16270 (Motif A, not seen in the main population), while another 31% shared a sequence differing from the Cambridge sequence only by a C in position 16298 (Motif B, seen once in the main population). These findings are in good accordance with those of Sajantila et al. (in press 1995). In the present material, motif A is divided in two groups by a A->T transversion in 16148, and a further subdivision by a A->G transition in 16335 was also observed. While Motif A thus includes several variants, Motiv B does not. These findings might indicate that Motif B represents an admixture of a population with a mtDNA sequence closely related to the most common European sequence into a population already exhibiting multiple variants of Motif A.

There are significant differences in sequence distribution between the Kautokeino and Karasjok Saami subpopulations (p=0.005). In particular, Kautokeino Saami have a higher proportion of Motif A and a lower proportion of Motif B than Saami from Karasjok. Moreover, the number of different mtDNA lineages may seem to be even less in Kautokeino than in Karasjok.

Comparing the Saami mtDNA sequences with those of other populations (see e.g. Stoneking et al. 1991), no obvious close relationships are found. The C in 16298 as well as the C in 16189 are each found in one of four sequences characteristic for Amerind populations, but with several site differences elsewhere (Ginther et al. 1993).

The remarkable differences in sequence distributions between Saami and neighbouring populations have already proved that mtDNA is a particularly efficient tool for population studies in arctic north-western Europe. We have started studies of ancient bones which hopefully will add valuable contributions to the knowledge of the history of people living in these areas.

REFERENCES:

Anderson S, Baker AT, Barrell BG, de Bruijn MHL, Coulson AR, Drouin J, Eperin IC, Nierlich DP, Roe BA, Sanger F, Schreier PH, Smith AJH, Staden R, Young IG (1981) Sequence and organization of the human mitochondrial genome. Nature 290: 457-465

Eriksson AW (1988) Anthropology and health in Lapps. Coll. Antropol. 12 (2): 197-235

Ginther C, Corach D, Penacino GA, Rey JA, Carnese FR, Hutz MH, Anderson A, Just J, Salzano FM, King M-C (1993) Genetic variation among the Mapuche Indians from the Patagonian region of Argentina: Mitochondrial DNA sequence variation and allele frequencies of several nuclear genes. In: DNA fingerprinting: State of the science, ed: Pena SDJ, Chakraborty R, Epplen JT, Jeffreys AJ (Bonhäuser Verlag, Basel)

Hertzberg M, Mickleson KNP, Serjeantson SW, Prior JF, Trent RJ (1989) An Asian-specific 9-bp deletion of mitochondrial DNA is frequently found in Polynesians. Am J Hum Genet 44: 504-510

Miller SA (1988) A simple salting out procedure for extracting DNA from human nucleated cells. Nucleic Acid Res 16(3): 1215-1217

Sajantila A, Lahermo P, Anttinen T, Lukka M, Sistonen P, Savontaus M-L, Aula P, Beckman L, Tranebjaerg L, Gedde-Dahl T, Issel-Tarver L, DiRenzo A, Pääbo S (1995) Genes and languages in Europe: An analysis of mitochondrial lineages. Genome Research, in press.

Stoneking M, Hedgecock D, Higuchi RG, Vigilant L, Erlich HA (1991) Population variation of human mtDNA control region sequences detected by enzymatic amplification and sequence-specific oligonucleotide probes. Am J Hum Genet 48: 370-382

Sullivan KM, Hopgood R, Gill P (1992) Identification of human remains by amplification and automated sequencing of mitochondrial DNA. Int J Leg Med 105: 83-86

Teisberg P (1971) C3 types of Norwegian Lapps. Human Heredity 21: 162-167

Mitochondrial DNA Quantification in Animal Blood and Hair by Slot-Blotting

F. Fridez, R. Coquoz

Institut de Police Scientifique et de Criminologie, University of Lausanne, Bâtiment de Chimie, 1015 Lausanne-Dorigny, Switzerland

INTRODUCTION

The hairs of cats and dogs easily cling to various objects whose surfaces are not entirely smooth; the result is that hairs are constantly found on clothes, furnitures, carpets, etc. which are in contact with the everyday life of these animals. This type of evidence could become an extremely important evidential value in the investigations of certain crimes and offences. By their interesting unusual presence in certain places, they may give interesting informations on the circumstances of the crime. Hairs are potential sources of DNA. However, the samples which are analysed often have roots of bad quality or even no roots at all, this means that there is a great risk of not having enough genomic DNA to carry out an analysis, even by PCR. It is therefore interesting to analyse the mitochondrial DNA (mtDNA) of the shaft of the hair. As for the analysis of genomic DNA, to know the amount of DNA available would be a precious information.
A quantification of mitochondrial DNA by slot-blotting has therefore been attempted by using oligonucleotide probes coupled to alkaline phosphatase.

MATERIALS AND METHODS

Blood: total DNA was extracted from cat, dog and human blood by using the phenol/chloroform method: extraction overnight at 37°C in a solution of 10mM Tris-HCl pH7.5, 10mM EDTA pH7.5, 100mM NaCl, 2% SDS, containing 6mM DTT and 1.5mg/ml proteinase K. DNA was then precipitated with alcohol in presence of 0.022mg/ml glycogen and 2M NH_4Ac and dissolved in water (Piercy et al., 1993).

Hair: 50 cat hairs per sample were used for the extraction of the total DNA, roots and shafts being separated. The same procedure was carried out for dog hair. A purification process using Microcon™ 30 microconcentrators (Amicon, Beverly, MA, USA) has been attempted on a few samples.
The most coarse hair, having roots of average to good quality, were taken by stroking the animal.
Before extraction, shafts were washed in sterile water. Both roots and shafts were extracted overnight at 56°C in a solution of 50mM Tris-HCl pH8, 10mM EDTA pH8, 0.1M NaCl, 2% SDS, 0.2M DTT and proteinase K 3.2mg/ml (for the roots) and 0.27mg/ml (for the shafts). DNA was then precipitated in the same way as abovementioned.

Preparation of pure mtDNA: mtDNA was isolated after extraction of a cats liver, respectively of a dogs liver by following the procedure described by White and al. (1992) uses differential centrifugation of the mitochondria and DNA purification by salt-precipitation of the proteins followed by an organic extraction (White *et al.*, 1992).

DNA quantification: The mitochondrial DNA quantification was attempted by slot-blot hybridization using a nylon membrane in a non-radioactive format. The procedure was similar to the "Human Quantification System" (Gibco-BRL, Gaitherburg, MD, USA). The detection buffer was substituted by a solution of 0.1M diethanolamine, 1mM magnesium chloride pH9.5 and the chemiluminescent substrate used was CDP-Star™ (Tropix, Bedford, USA). The totality of each extract containing the 50 shafts, respectively the 50 roots were deposited on the membrane.

Probes: 4 cat probes and 3 dog probes were tested at different temperatures:

Probe name	Sequence	Hybridization temperatures tested
(Cat) B17	5'- AAT CAC ACC CCC TTA TCA -3'	52; 50; 44°C
(Cat) F207	5'- CTG TCG CGA CGT TAA TT -3'	50; 44°C
(Cat) F385	5'- ATG GGA TAC GTC CT -3'	50; 44; 33°C
(Cat) F241	5'- TAT TTA CAC GCC AAC GGA GC -3'	52; 50; 46°C
(Dog) C230	5'- GAA TTA TCC GCT ATA T -3'	50; 46; 40°C
(Dog) C243	5'- TAT GCA CGC AAA TGG CGC -3'	54; 50; 45°C
(Dog) B291	5'- TGT AGG ACG AGG CCT ATA-3'	50; 48; 45°C

The sequences belong to the cytochrom b of the mtDNA of these animals. They were chosen after consultation in the Genbank (The National Center for Biotechnology Information, Bethesda, Maryland). They were conjugated to an alkaline phosphatase enzyme according to an E-Link™ Oligonucleotide Labelling kit (Cambridge Research Biomedicals Ltd, Cheshire, UK) except for two probes (C230; C243) which were synthetized and conjugated by Genset SA (Paris, France).

Southern blotting: cat and dog DNA extracts were analysed on 0.6% agarose gel followed by staining with ethidium bromide and transferred on a nylon membrane. They were then hybridized with the probes in order to verify the specificity for mtDNA.

RESULTS AND DISCUSSION

The most sensitive and specific probe for cat DNA was found to be the F241 probe at an hybridization temperature of 50°C. Southern blotting demonstrated the specificity of the probe and the absence of cross-hybridization with genomic DNA (fig. 1).
The concentration of the mtDNA isolated from liver was estimated by comparison with DNA marker on a minigel stained with ethidium bromide. This mtDNA extract could then be used as a standard for slot-blotting quantification. It was then possible to estimate the amount of mtDNA in blood and hair (fig. 2) :

Cat samples	Estimation of the mitochondrial molecules number [1]
1 μl blood	about 2'000 000
1 hair root	about 200'000
1 hair shaft	about 200'000

[1]As an element of comparison, it is interesting to note that the 200'000 copies of the mitochondrial genome detected in a hair shaft would correspond to 1.2 μg of DNA if this was nuclear DNA instead of mtDNA.

The estimation of the mtDNA amount in hair shafts was difficult because of interference in the detection of the signal. This phenomenon mainly occured while using dark-coloured hair, meaning that melanin might well be the interfering molecule. A purification process (filtration over Microcon™ 30 microconcentrators) was attempted in order to remove this inhibition but no better results were obtained and some DNA was even detected in the filtrate (fig. 2).

The most sensitive and specific probe for dog DNA was found to be the B291 probe at an hybridization temperature of 48°C. The chosen sequence is complementary to a mitochondrial sequence and not genomic but this was not totally confirmed. This probe is less sensitive compared to the cat probe and the same inhibition phenomenon was observed.
The amounts of mtDNA which were detected in blood, in a root and in a shaft of a dogs hair are similar to those determined for the cat.

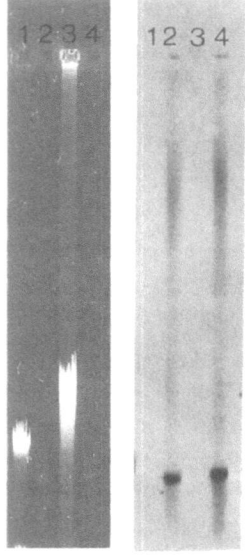

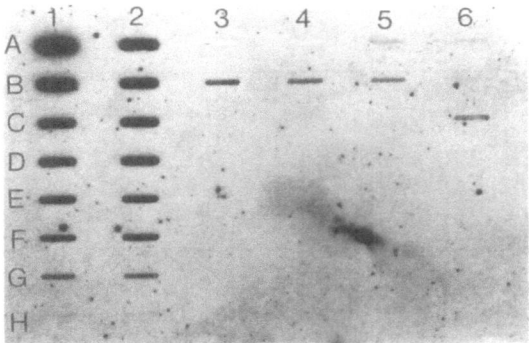

Figure 2. An example of the quantification of mitochondrial DNA present in blood, hair roots and hair shafts of cats.
Column 1: standards (liver extract) containing 1A = 6 ng, 1B = 3 ng,1C = 1 ng, 1D = 0.8 ng, 1E = 0.4 ng, 1F = 0.2 ng, 1G = 0.1 ng, 1H = 0 ng of mitochondrial DNA.
Column 2: Total DNA extracted from 60 µl (2A), 42 µl (2B), 30 µl (2C), 18 µl (2D), 12 µl (2E), 6 µl (2F), 3 µl (2G) of blood.
Samples 3A, 4A, 5A : amount of mtDNA present in 50 hair shafts of three different cats after purification with Microcon™30 microconcentrators.
Samples 3B, 4B, 5B: amount of mtDNA present in each 50 corresponding roots without purification.
Sample 6A: filtrate of sample 3A, 6B: filtrate of sample 4A, 6C: filtrate of sample 5A.

Figure 1. *Left::* agarose gel stained with ethidium bromide. *Right::* DNA transferred on a membrane and hybridized with the cat probe F241
1. Hind III Digest of Lambda DNA marker (band 1: 23'130 base pairs)
2. Cat mitochondrial DNA
3.Total DNA extracted from 12 µl of cat blood
4.Cat mitochondrial DNA

Blood is a relatively rich source of mitochondrial DNA and not surprisingly, the roots contain more mitochondrial DNA molecules than the shafts. According to the estimations, the cats hair, respectively the dogs hair, contain enough mitochondrial DNA to carry out an analysis in the aim of an individual identification by identical methods to those used in human identification.

We were hoping to be able to estimate the amount of mtDNA in hair and to devise a quantification method which might help in routine mtDNA analysis. Regarding to the results, this second goal could not be reached because of insufficient sensitivity. Therefore, in order to quantify mtDNA in single hair, it would then be necessary to look for other methods than slot-blotting.

REFERENCES

Piercy R, Sullivan KM, Benson N, Gill P (1993) The application of mitochondrial DNA typing to the study of white Caucasian genetic identification. Int J Leg Med 106: 85-90
White PS, Densmore LD (1992) Mitochondrial DNA isolation. In: Hoelzel AR (ed) Molecular Genetic analysis of populations: a practical approach. IRL Press, p 29-58.

Detection of Sequence Variants in Hypervariable Segments of Mitochondrial DNA in the Asian Population

K. Honda*, M. Nakatome*, S.Harihara**, Zaw Tun*, M.N. Islam*, H. Bai*, Y. Ogura*
H. Kuroki*, M. Yamazaki*, M. Terada*, S. Misawa*** and C. Wakasugi*

*Dept of Legal Med, Osaka Univ Med School, 2-2 Yamadaoka, Suita, Osaka 565, Japan
**Dept of Biological Sciences, Graduate School of Science, The Univ of Tokyo, Tokyo 113, Japan
***Dept of Legal Med, Univ of Tsukuba, 1-1-1 Tennodai, Tsukuba 305, Japan

Introduction

The analysis of highly polymorphic regions of mitochondrial DNA is one of the most commonly used methods for personal identification. The recent advances of fluorescent detection in automated DNA sequencing (Smith et al. 1986) has made it possible a rapid analysis of sequence variants without using isotopic labeling.

We chose to analyze the control region in mitochondrial DNA because it displays many polymorphisms (Aquadro et al. 1983, Sullivan et al. 1992)

Materials and method

We collected saliva as samples from total 171 individuals of Asian population (Japan, China, Mongolia, Myanmar, Bangladesh, and Europe).

DNA extraction - one drop of saliva (3μl)was collected in 500μl microtube by the straw from the oral cavity. Next, 250 μl of 5 % chelex was added into the tube, incubated at 56℃ for 30 minutes and at 94℃ for 10 minutes after vortex mixing. DNA were extracted in 45 minutes by chelex based method.

After microcentrifugation for 5 minute at 5000g, 5μl of supernatant was added to PCR mixture.

The following primers and thermocycle were used for Segment I and II amplifications (Stoneking et al. 1991)

Seg I	L15996: 5'-CCACCATTAGCACCCAAAGC	20mer
	H16401: 5'-TGATTTCACGGAGGATGGTG	20mer
Seg II	L29: 5'-TCTATCACCCTATTAACCAC	20mer
	H408: 5'-GTTAAAAGTGCATACCGCCA	20mer
Thermocycle	94℃-45s/ 56℃-1m/ 74℃-1m (27+20 cycles)	

The two hypervariable segments of mitochondrial control region were amplified separately by the method of semi-nested PCR (Honda et al. 1994; 1995). In the first PCR, the 982 bp segment was amplified with the primers L15996 and H408. In the second PCR, 406bp segment was amplified with primers of L15996 and H16401 (Segment I), and 380bp segment was amplified with primers of L29 and H408 (Segment II). The sequence variants of the two hypervariable segments were examined by the one-lane-direct-sequencing labeled by dye-deoxy-terminator using DNA- sequencer (ABI; model 373A).

Results

The seminested PCR is extremely sensitive and specific so that as low as 0.01pg. concentration of the template DNA can be amplified without unspecific band (Fig.1).

In our result, more than 12% of sequence variants were detected in each segment (Fig.2). Some of them were suspected to be Asian specific (e.g.16085: C to G change, 150: C to T change) because they were rarely found in Caucasians. About 4 to 18 of each sequence variants per individual were found in comparison with full sequence data by Anderson et al. (1981). In both segments, Cytosine to Guanine replacement was most frequently found, and the next was Cytosine to Thymine.

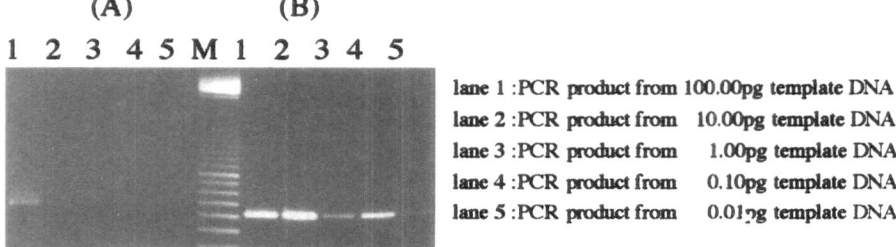

(A)   **(B)**

1 2 3 4 5 M 1 2 3 4 5

lane 1 :PCR product from 100.00pg template DNA
lane 2 :PCR product from 10.00pg template DNA
lane 3 :PCR product from   1.00pg template DNA
lane 4 :PCR product from   0.10pg template DNA
lane 5 :PCR product from   0.01pg template DNA

Fig 1 - Comparison of sensitivity between Simple PCR and Nested PCR
  (A) Agarose gel electrophoresis of Mitochondrial Control Region Seg.I amplification products after 30 cycles
      of standard PCR with decreasing concentration of template DNA. M : 100 bp ladder
  (B) Agarose gel electrophoresis of Nested PCR (using 1μl aliquot from first amplification mixture and 20
      cycles further amplification). Concentrations of template DNA correspond to that of (A).

Position No.	16085 (C)	16091(A)	73(A)	150(C)	152(T)
Japanese	G: 50%	T: 28%	G:95%	T:27%	C:27%
Chinese	G:95%	T: 5%	G:75%	T:13%	C:25%
Mongolian	G:95%	T: 90%	G:80%	rare	C:60%
Myanmar	G:70%	T: 40%	G:67%	T:17%	C:35%
Bangladeshi	G:97%	rare	G:95%	T:18%	C:33%
European	rare	rare	G:45%	rare	C:20%

Table 1 - Percentage of nucleotide replacements observed in various population

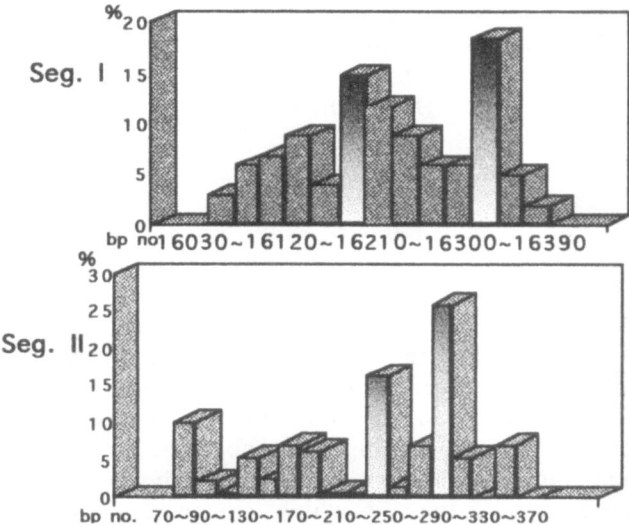

Fig.2 Distribution of sequence variants in segment I and II

References

Aquadro CF, Greenberg BD (1983) Human mitochondrial DNA variation and evolution: analysis of nucleotide sequences from seven individuals. Genetics 103: 287-312

Anderson S, Bankier AT, Barrell BG, de Bruijn MHL, Coulson AR, Drouin J, Eperon IC, Nierlich DP, Sanger F, Schreier PH, Smith AJH, Staden R, Young IG (1981) Sequence and organization of the human mitochondrial genome. Nature 290: 457-465

Honda K, Sugiyama E, Tsutikane A, Katsuyama Y, Harashima N, Ota M, and Fukushima H (1994) Nested amplification of COL2A1 3' variable region in skeletal remains. Jpn J Legal Med 48: 156-160

Honda K, Bai H, Terada M, Nakatome M, Islam MN, Ogura Y, Kuroki H, Yamazaki M, Misawa S, Wakasugi C (1995) Detection of semi-nested D1S80 (pMCT118) locus polymorphism using polymerase chain reaction in skeletal remains. J Forensic Sci 40 (4): 637-640

Smith LM, Sanders JZ, Kaiser RJ, Hughes P, Dodd C, Connell CR, Heiner C, Kent SBH, Hood LE (1986) Fluorescence detectrion in automated DNA sequence analysis. Nature 321: 674-679

Stoneking M, Hedgecock D, Higuchi R, Vigilant L, Erlich HA (1991) Population variation of human mtDNA control region sequences detected by enzymatic amplification and sequence-specific oligonucleotide probes. Am J Hum Genet 48, 370-382

Sullivan KM, Hopgood R, Gill P (1992) Identification of human remains by amplification and automated sequencing of mitochondrial DNA. Int J Legal Med 105 (2): 83-6

ROUTINE MITOCHONDRIAL DNA IDENTIFICATION

Tesson C., Penaud A., LE ROUX M.G., Millasseau A., Guibert V., Moisan J.P., Pascal O.
Laboratoire de Génétique Moléculaire . Hotel Dieu BP 1005 44035 Nantes Cedex France

DNA typing is a common technique in Forensic sciences used for the characterisation of body fluids. The analysis of genomic DNA may be limited if DNA is highly degraded or in low abundance (rootless hair and bones for example). On the other hand some biological tools (such as anti sera) could be used to exclude human origin but few could easily establish the animal origin. Mitochondrial DNA could be used to overcome these problems. Indeed mitochondrial DNA is composed of different areas, two of which are particulary interesting : the first one encodes the cytochrome b gene and show interspecies mutations. Amplification and sequencing of this region allows us to determine the animal origin (this technique is licenced from BioID compagny - St John's Canada). The second one encodes hypervariable regions with point mutations differing from one individual to another. We make routine use of these two techniques to resolve Forensic caseworks.

Materials and Methods

A/ DNA extraction

DNA extraction is performed routinely for caseworks applying techniques as previously described (Pascal 1991) except for hairs and bones. Hairs are dissolved by incubation in the presence of proteinase K and DTT followed by phenol chloroform purification, and bones using Guanidium thyiocyanate (Hoss 1993).

B/ Amplification:

*Animal identification : the primers used are those described by Bartlett (1992). In case of highly degraded DNA, shorter sequences are amplified.

*Mitochondrial Hypervariable regions :
the primers used are :

From 15 to 270 :	CAC CCT ATT AAC CAC TCA CG
	TGT GTG GAA AGT GGC TGT GC
from 145 to 389	CTC ATC CTA TTA TTT ATC GC
	CTG GTT AGG CTG GTG TTA GG
From 1591 to 16258	TTA ACT CCA CCA TTA GCA CC
	TGG CTT TGG AGT TGC AGT TG
From 16140 to 16420	TAC TTG ACC ACC TGT AGT AC
	TGA TTT CAC GGA GGA TGG TG

38 cycles are performed.

Sequencing is performed with Sequenase[R] (Amersham). Fragments are analysed either manually or in an IBI automatic sequencer.

C/ Interpretation :

Animal identification : the sequences are analysed by a specific comparison program by BioID in St John (Canada).

Human hypervariable regions : the sequences obtained are compared to the reference sequence (Anderson 1981) and the mutation frequencies used are those published by Piercy et al (1993).

RESULTS

Animal identification

Animal identification is a powerful tool used to ascertain the origin of biological samples, and may also be used to confirm or to disregard witness statements. We used, for example, this technique for a murder where four people of the same family were killed. An animal food bag, a bowl and a knife all containing blood stains, were found in the house of the suspect . The grandmother said that she had killed a mouse in the bag. Analysis of the DNA showed that the bloodstains found on the bag were from "mus domesticus" (mouse), the bloodstains from bowl were from "Gallus gallus" (chicken) and the bloodstains from the knife were from "Sus scrofa" (pig).

Human identification

In the past DNA, extracted from bones or from rootless hair have been very difficult to type. We currently use mitochondrial DNA for exclusion or identification.

Two main problems have to be considered :

-Contaminations

DNA is present in every nook of a molecular biology laboratory and we have to avoid the contamination of the sample by exogenous DNA and amplification products. Extractions from bones and hairs were performed in a separate room, using specific material set aside for these techniques (centrifuge, automatic pipettes, and so on). Preparation of the samples for PCR amplification is performed in a second room and sequencing in a third one. The cycle number is limited to 38. Negative extraction samples and negative amplification samples are included in each experiment. If contamination is seen in the negative samples, then we also sequence these PCR products. A single technician is appointed to Mitochondrial DNA typing and does not use other techniques.

INTERPRETATION:
Two major questions are in discussion:
a/ The fidelity of amplification : we use Sequenase[R] sequencing kit, which is supposed to be the most faithful enzyme.
b/ The neomutation rate : which seems to be very low from one generation to the other. However no extensive work has been carried out which could permit us to confirm this assumption.
Therefore in order to compare (exclude or include) two samples from different origins we require at least three point mutations. In the case of identity, error risks are calculated using the mutation rate published by Piercy et al. Absence of point mutations are included in these calculations.

CONCLUSION
Mitochondrial DNA analysis is a very powerful technique which permit the tools of molecular biology to be used for legal purposes. Recently these techniques has been used successfully to identify Romanov family remains (Gill 1994 - Stoneking 1995). However these techniques are very long and a high degree of safety must be exercised in order to exclude contaminations. Personnel and materials must be perfectly adapted. Finally, the interpretation of results must be carried out carefully with regards to the fidelity of amplification and the neomutation rate.

Anderson S., Bankier A., Barrell B., De Bruijn M, Coulson A., Drouin J., Eperon I., Nierlich D., Roe B., Sanger F., Schreier P., Smith A., Staden R., Young I. (1989) Sequence and organisation of the human mitochondrial genome. Sciences 290 : 457-465
Bartlett S., Davidson W. (1992) FINS (Forensic Informative Nucleotide Sequencing) : a procedure for identifying the animal origin of biological specimens. Biotechniques 12 : 408-411
Gill P., Ivano P., Kimpton C., PiercyR., Benson N., Tully G., Evett I., Hagelberg E., Sullivan K. (1994) Identification of the remains of the Romanov family by DNA analysis. Nature Genetics 6 : 130-135
Hoss M., Paabo S. (1991) DNA extraction from pleistocene bones by a silica-based purification method. Nucleic Acids Res. 21 : 3913-3914
Pascal O., Aubert D., Gilbert E., Moisan J.P. (1991) Sexing of forensic samples using PCR. Int. J. Leg. Med. 104 : 205-207
Piercy R.,Sullivan K., Benson N., Gill P. (1993) the application of mitochondrial DNA typing to the study of white caucasian genetic identification. Int. J. Leg. Med. 106 : 85-90
Stoneking M., Melton T., Nott J., Barritt S., Roby R.,Holland M., Weedn V., Gill P., Kimpton C., Aliston-Greiner R., Sullivan K. (1995) Establishing the identity of Anna Anderson Manahan. Nature Genetics 9 : 9-10

AUTOMATED FLUORESCENT SEQUENCING OF MITOCHONDRIAL DNA FOR ITALIAN POPULATION FREQUENCY DATA.

P. Montagna, R. Biondo, S. Tavano, S. Giuliacci, A. Pezza and A. Spinella.
Direzione Centrale Polizia Criminale, Servizio Polizia Scientifica, Divisione III,
Viale dell'Aeronautica, 7 - 00144 Roma, Italy

Introduction

The analysis of mitochondrial DNA (mt DNA) sequence is a method to establish mtDNA type. In the context of forensic science a determination of the frequency of the different mtDNA types in the population must be done.

In this study we present population databases from 100 unrelated individuals representative of all italian regions. The mtDNA regions subjected to analysis was HVI (16.024-16365) and HVII (73-340). In both HVI and HVII, two sets of primers was used to amplify the regions of the mtDNA control region.

Mitochondrial DNA sequencing was performed with fluorescence-basd automated sequencer (373 A, ABD of P.E.,CA) from PCR products purified by filtration in a Microcon-100. Two different types of chemistries was employed.

A calculation of the frequency of a mtDNA type is the number of times the specific sequence has been observed, divided by the number of samples in the databases. This counting method was adopted only with DNA sequence information that was free from ambiguities within the region of comparison.

Material and Methods

DNA Preparation
Whole Blood
Genomic DNA, extracted from 500 μl of whole blood with phenol/clorophorm procedure, was quantified by spectrophotometry.

DNA Amplification
Mitochondrial DNA

Oligonucleotides primer specific for HV1 (16,024-16,365) and HV2 (73-340) regions were prepared.Two chimeric primers combining the M13-21 primer sequence with the mt-specific sequences and a primer with biotin at the 5' end were also synthesized.
All PCRs were performed in two-stage amplification. In the first-stage primers A and B were used to amplify a 1333-bp segment of human mtDNA of the hypervariable region 1 (HV1). Primers C and B were used to amplify a 1200-bp segment of the hypervariable region 2 (HV2). The PCR conditions were: in a total volume of 25 μl were mixed 50 ng whole blood DNA or 5 μl of nonquantitated bone DNA as template, primers at 1μM concentration. Amplification products were analyzed on 5% horizontal polyacrylamide gel stained with silver. In the second stage primers C and F were used to amplify a 400-bp segment of the hypervariable region 1 (HV1). Primers P1 and P2 were used to amplify a 395-bp segment of the hypervariable region 2 (HV2) at 0.5 μM final concentration. The primers F and P2 were chimeric.

REGION HV1 (16024-16365)		REGION HV2 (20-340)	
PRIMERS	POSITION	PRIMERS	POSITION
A	L15926	B	H00580
B	H00580	C	L15997
C	L15997	P1	L20
F	H16401	P2	H00395

DNA Sequencing

6µl of bone and 4 µl whole blood of the PCR solution with and without purification in Centricon 100 (Amicon Corp.) were used . for sequencing reactions. The sequencing was carried out according to the DyeDeoxy™ -Terminator and Dye-Primer Cycle Sequencing Kit (ABD,PE). The reactions were denatured for 4 min at 95° C and loaded onto a 6% acrylamide gel. Electrophoresis and sequencing analysis were performed with an Applied Biosystems Mod. 373A DNA sequencer. Sequence comparisons were made using ABD SeqEd (sequence editing) software.(FIG. 1)

```
                         10         20         30         40         50
                          |          |          |          |          |
1   1... 50 HV2   CTATTAACCA CTCACGGGAG CTCTCCATGC ATTTGGTATT TTCGTCTGGG
7E  1... 50 I.    CTATTAACCA CTCACGGGAG CTCCCCATGC ATTTGGTATT TTCGTCTGGG
8   1... 50       ---------- ---------- ---*------ ---------- ----------

                         60         70         80         90        100
                          |          |          |          |          |
1   51..100 HV2   GGGTATGCAC GCGATAGCAT TGCGAGACGC TGGAGCCGGA GCACCCTATG
7E  51..100 I.    GGGTATGCAC GCGATAGCAT TGCGAGACGC TGGAGCCGGA GCACCCTATG
8   51...100      ---------- ---------- ---------- ---------- ----------

                        110        120        130        140        150
                          |          |          |          |          |
1  101..150 HV2   TCGCAGTATC TGTCTTTGAT TCCTGCCTCA TCCTATTATT TATCGCACCT
7E 101..150 I.    TCGCAGTATC TGTCTTTGAT TCCTGCCTCA TCCTATTATT TATCGCACCT
8  101...150      ---------- ---------- ---------- ---------- ----------

                        160        170        180        190        200
                          |          |          |          |          |
1  151..200 HV2   ACGTTCAATA TTACAGGCGA ACTTACTTAC TAAAGTGTGT TAATTAATTA
7E 151..200 I.    ACGTTCAATA TTATAGGCGA AGATACTTAC CCAAGTGTGT GATCTATCTA
8  151...200      ---------- ---*------ --**------ --**------ *-**--**--

                        210        220        230        240        250
                          |          |          |          |          |
1  201..250 HV2   ATGCTTGTAG GACATAATAA TAACAATTGA ATGTCTGCAC AGCCACTTTC
7E 201..250 I.    ATGTCTGTAG GACATTATTA TTACAATTGA ATGTCTGCAC AGCCGCTTTC
8  201...250      ---**----- ----*--*-- -*-------- ---------- ----*-----

                        260        270        280        290        300
                          |          |          |          |          |
1  251..300 HV2   CACACAGACA TCATAACAAA AAATTTCCAC CAAA-CCCCC CCTCCCCC-G
7E 251..300 I.    CACACAGACA TCATTACAAA AAATTTCCAC CAAACCCCCC CCTCCCCCCG
8  251...300      ---------- ----*----- ---------- ----*----- -------*-

                        310        320        330        340        350
                          |          |          |          |          |
1  301..308 HV2   CTTCTGGC
7E 301..308 I.    CTTCTGGC
8  301...308      --------
```

Figure 1 . Sequence information generated by directly comparison with reference sequence (ANDERSON) using Seq ED Software.

Results

Several strategies are currently available for the analysis of a DNA profile. Last tecnique used in forensic caseworks involves the direct sequencing of amplification product of the control region of mitochondrial DNA (HVR1 - HVR2). This region is highly polymorphic and presents different types of single nucleotide substitutions. In this case a single base substitution represents a different mtDNA type. In order to defined the different mtDNA type in Italian population, the hypervariable Region 1 and hypervariable Region 2 have been sequenced.

The region HV1 is between 16,000 to 16,400, and HV2 is located on the other side, approximately 10 to 320.

Therefore, a list of the mtDNA types of the individuals in Italian population has been done with respect to Anderson sequence. A calculation of the frequency of a mtDNA type is the number of times the specific sequence has been observed, divided by the number of samples in the databases. This counting method was adopted only with DNA sequence information that was free from ambiguities within the region of comparison.

This database include a sample of about 100 individuals collected from different regions of Italy. An example of some data from our database is show in figure 2.

We have found no deviation from Anderson sequence in only one sample. A statistical estimate of the results showed that 100 individuals defined 100 different mtDNA type. Therefore the frequency of a mtDNA type is about 0.01. This frequency might be multipled by allele frequencies of polymorphic nuclear loci to increase the power discrimination of the DNA test.

Reference

Sanger,F., Nicklen, S. and Coulson, A.R. " DNA sequencing with chain- trminator inhibitors ".1977 Proceeding of the National Academy of Science of the U.S.A 74 : 5463-5468

Monnat, R. J. and Loeb, L. A. "Nucleotide sequence preservation of human mitochondrial DNA ". 1985. Proceeding of the National Academy of Science of the U.S.A 82: 2895-2899

Anderson S., Bankier A.T., Barrell G.B. et al. "Sequence and organization of the human mitochondrial genome"1981.Nature 290:457-465

Sullivan K.M., Hopgood R., Lang B. Gill P. "Automated amplification and sequencing of human mitochondrial DNA."1991.Electrophoresis 12:17-21

Hopgood R., Sullivan K.M., Gill P. "Strategies for Automated Sequencing of Human Mitochondrial DNA directly from PCR Products."1992 BioTechniques 13:82-92

Gill P. et al. "Identification of the remain of Romanov family by DNA analysis" 1994. Nature genetics 6: 130-135.

Figure 2

Region HV1

Sequences	16094	16108	16142	16145	16152	16158	16162	16176	16177	16179	16189	16198	16205	16209	16214	16216	16218	16223	16225	16245	16256	16280	16282	16298	16325	16332	16348	16382	16390	16401
Anderson	T	C	A	G	T	A	A	C	A	A	C	T	T	C	T	C	A	C	C	C	C	C	C	C	T	T	C	C	G	C
Sample 1		C									C																			
Sample 2						T		T	G	G																		T		
Sample 3																				G					G	G				
Sample 4																	G								G	G				
Sample 5			G																											
Sample 6																	G		G	G		C				G				G
Sample 7										T		T				G								C						
Sample 8										T	C	T	G		G							C								
Sample 9											C		G							G		C		C						
Sample 10											C		G	G	G						G		G							G

Region HV2

Sequences	10	14	21	25	30	32	42	48	49	55	57	60	73	75	77	79	85	90	97	110	122	127	131	146	152	164	172	173	181	182	188	191	192	195	200	201	210	211	215	222	223	233	234	237	241	256	263	271	285	286	291	306.1	315.1
Anderson	T	T	A	A	T	A	T	C	A	A	T	T	T	G	A	G	G	G	A	G	C	C	T	T	T	T	C	T	T	C	A	A	T	T	C	C	T	A	A	A	C	C	A	A	A	A	C	C	C	A	A	--	--
Sample 1					C																								T	T			G		C	C						C		T			G	G		T		+C	+C
Sample 2																																					C															+	+
Sample 3			C				C			C		C	G									C	C		C	G	G																			G	G	G				+C	+C
Sample 4		C																					C								G		G													G	G					+	+
Sample 5												G	G										C									G	G													G	G						
Sample 6		G										C	G			C					G		C				G					G															G		T				
Sample 7				C		C	C		C											G	G																										G					+C	+C
Sample 8																													A																		G		G				
Sample 9													G							C														A													G		G		T	+C	+C
Sample 10											G	C	G					C	C					C					T																		G		G		C	+C	+C

Example of same multiple sequences from HV1-HV2 Regions that are aligned and presented together. The Anderson sequence is show on the first box. All deviation from the standard are show as the corresponding letter of the nucleotide which differs from the Anderson.

2 DNA Sequencing Data

The STR approach
B. Brinkmann, Institute of Legal Medicine, Münster, Germany

Introduction

Since the beginning of forensic hemogenetics, forensic scientists have been dreaming of a technology which should ideally fulfill a few basic requirements.
A high statistical efficiency is needed as well as a high suitability to the quality of the stain with its properties: degradation, contamination, inhibition etc. Also, an extreme sensitivity is desired especially if only microstains are present. Furthermore, the whole process involved needs a good success rate.
The invention/introduction of VNTR polymorphisms by Jeffreys has opened a wide door to these dream castles but we were still miles away from the ideal. There existed problems with the reproducibility especially of MLPs and there existed and still exist problems relative to the accuracy and precision of the SLPs. Although these technologies are statistcally unbelievably efficient, there are further problems concerning the sensitivity and degradation.
Microsatellite polymorphisms have been introduced by Edwards et al. (1991), Polymeropoulos et al. (1992), Tautz (1991) and others in the early nineties. At least theoretically, this DNA generation seems to easily resolve many of the disadvantages of earlier technologies. This will be investigated further.
By definition microsatellites or STRs (short tandem repeats) vary by repeat size between 2 and 7 bp (Edwards at al. 1991) with fragment sizes < 350 bp. Out of these dinucleotide polymorphisms suffer from the disadvantage of quite intensive slippage bands leading to patterns which are difficult to interpret in stain work. Tetranucleotide polymorphisms – thousands have been predicted to be present in the human genome (Weber and May 1992, Tautz and Rentz 1991) – have the advantages of no or negligable slippages and consecutive alleles can be more easily resolved. Therefore among those which have been elaborated for forensic application, tetra- and pentanucleotide polymorphisms

appear to be most promising.

Categories of microvariation

We subdivide into three categories of STR systems : (1) STRs with low microvariation mainly consisting of repeat related length variants. (2) STRs with intermediate microvariation where in addition to category (1) structure and length variations exist. (3) STRS with high microvariation showing extensive structure and length variations.

(1) Low microvariation: CD4 is a system of the first category with pentameric repeat units as basic motif (Fig. 1a). From allele 9 onwards the 4th repeat unit shows a T to C transition which is the only minor variation in this system. 11 consecutive alleles have been observed. - Black Africans show this multiplicity of 11 alleles, only 2 of them reaching the 20%-level (Fig. 2). Three rather different Caucasian populations (Germans, Turks, Moroccans) show quite similar profiles but are nearly reduced to a 3-allele model. Especially the German population nearly lacks all other alleles while the 2 other populations show some admixture of African alleles. Again the 3 Asian populations are very similar but are nearly reduced to a 2-allele model. From these differences one could conclude that these uneven distributions reflect different allele pools in the respective founder groups (Brinkmann et al. 1995).

Fig. 1a) Schematic presentation of HumCD4 alleles 5 - 15. Nomenclature according to the number of repeats.
FR = flanking region.

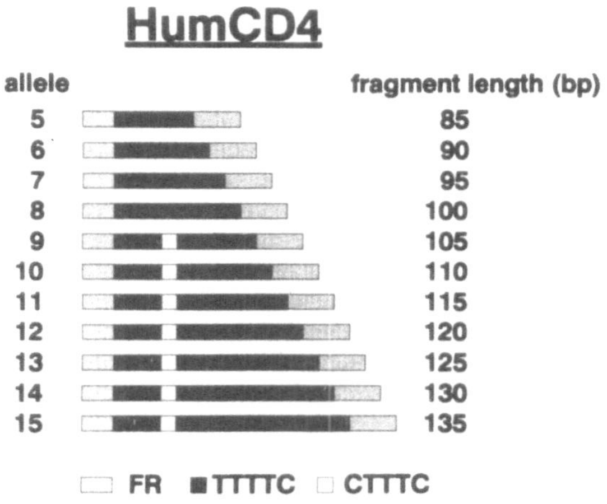

HumCD4

allele		fragment length (bp)
5		85
6		90
7		95
8		100
9		105
10		110
11		115
12		120
13		125
14		130
15		135

☐ FR ■ TTTTC ☐ CTTTC

43

Fig. 1b) Allele distribution of CD4 alleles in 9 populations differentiated into 3 major ethnic groups. The figure preceding each population = number of individuals.

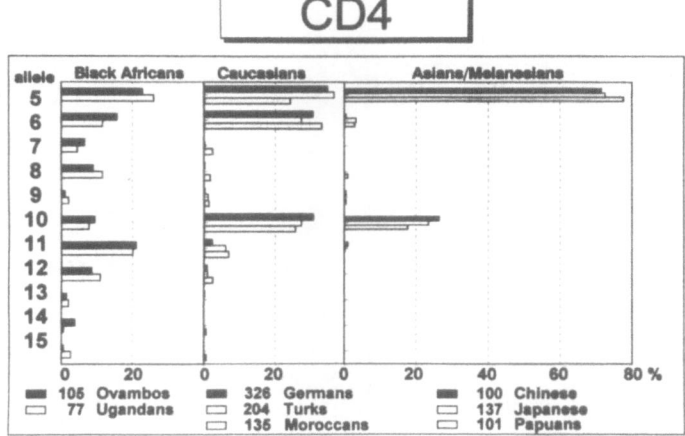

HumF13B is an example of a tetranucleotide STR with low microvariation (Fig. 1b). There exist 6 regular alleles differing by one repeat unit and 2 rare A to C transversions in the 3' flanking region of 2 alleles and a further T to A transversion in allele 12 (Alper et al. 1995).

These variant alleles - all point mutations - can be easily resolved in native gels, not of course under denaturing conditions.

Fig. 2a) Schematic presentation of HumF13B alleles 6 - 12A detectable usinga non-denaturing gel system.
FR = flanking region;
C = cathodal;
A = anodal.

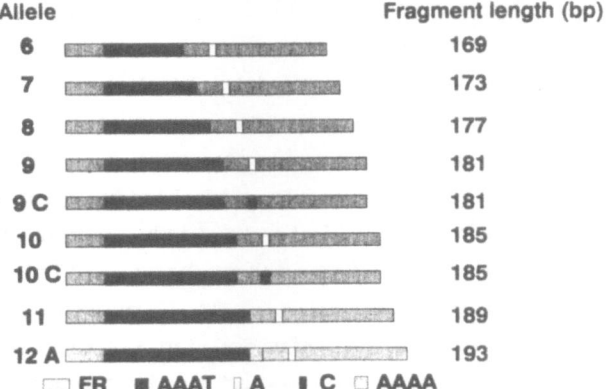

Fig. 2b) Allele di-
stribution of
HumF13B alleles.
Mode of representa-
tion as in Fig. 1b.

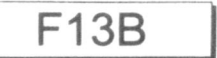

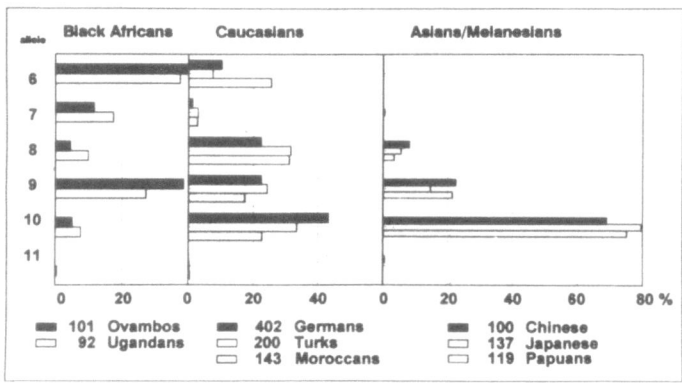

Africans have 5 alleles with appreciable frequencies. Caucasian
are reduced to 4 frequent alleles and a rare allele 7 with 2 %
only in Germans. The 3 Asian populations are reduced to a 3-
allele model. At least this looks like another founder effect.
HumFES is an example of low microvariation with similarities to
HumF13B. In addition to 6 regular repeat related variants there
exist variants 10A and 11A with A to C transversion in the 5'
flanking region (Möller et al. 1994). (A stands for anode and C
for cathode because these alleles migrate either slower or
faster relative to the consensus alleles of same length).
(2) Intermediate microvariation: VWA belongs to the intermediate
microvariation group. There exist 2 alleles that differ basically. The consensus allele has a composite repetitive structure
starting with 1 TCTA, continuing with 3 to 5 TCTGs and ending
with the proper variable TCTA part. Allele 14 is unique and
differs from the consensus at these 3 sites (Fig. 3a).
It seems to show until now only very few stepwise mutated daugh
ter alleles in either population (Barber et al. 1995). There
exists also no allele 14 with a consensus structure in either
population. On the other hand, alleles 15 upwards show some
length variation of the TCTG proportions (Fig. 3b). Therefore
VWA alleles can be divided into 2 groups: 11 to 14 with considerable conservativeness of their structure and length with no or
at most extremely low new mutations. Alleles 15 to 22 where we

have already observed 2 new mutations with either insertions or deletions of single repeats (Brinkmann et al. 1995) and a third one more recently.

Fig. 3a) Comparison be-
tween HumVWA consensus
alleles and variant
allele 14

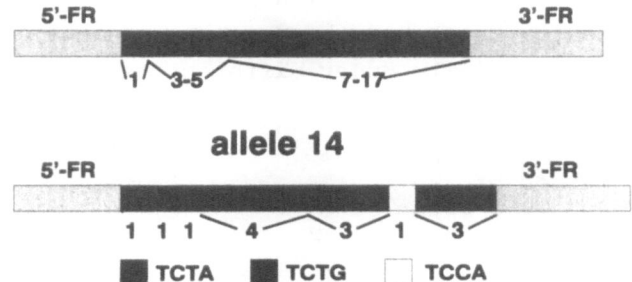

Fig. 3b) schematic presentation of known VWA alleles.
Further explanation see text.

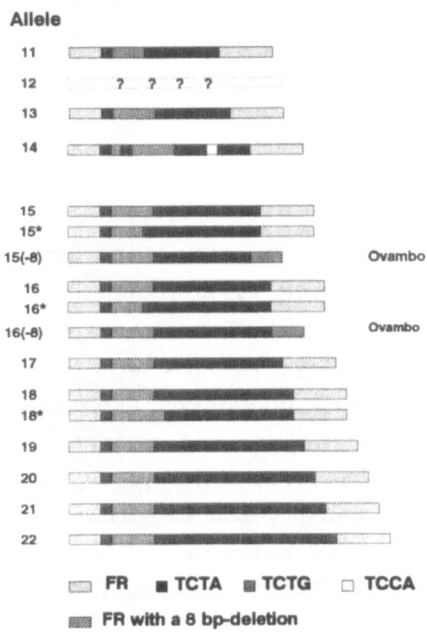

(3) High microvariation: ACTBP2 or SE33 belongs to group 3 and
is one of the most complex systems. There are at least 3 series
of alleles: Series 1 ranging between 12 and 21 with a more or
less regular repeat structure (Fig. 4). Series 2 with the appearance of a hexamer within the repeat structure, but at different
sites. These alleles range between 22 and 32. Series 3 with the
insertion of 2 hexamer units, again at different sites within
the repeat structure. Range 32 to 33. Because of this high com-
plexity there have been early warnings as to the reproducabili-
ty, especially under different gel conditions.

Fig. 4) Examples
of 3 different
classes of
HumACTBP2 alle-
les.

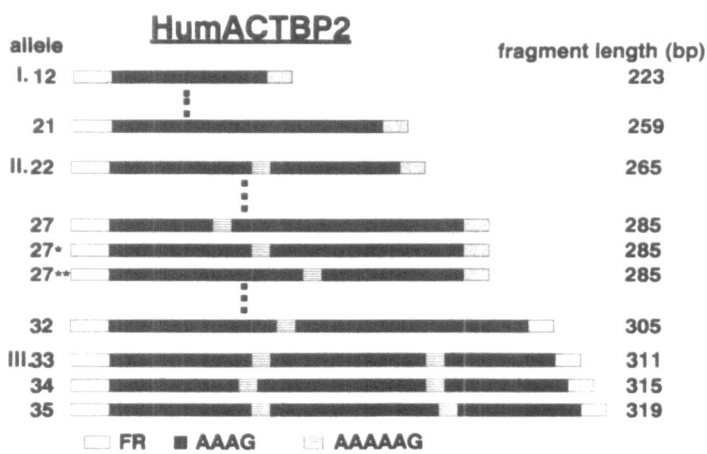

Sequencing of 250 randomly selected alleles lead to approximately 100 structure and length variants while typing of 1200 was
associated with about 30 electrophorecticly detectable alleles
only. - The DI of 99.8% is equivalent to the combined DI of VWA,
TH01, CD4 (Table 2).
The mean phenotype frequency between the old and the new nomenclature was even decreased by the factor 10. Apart from this
extreme efficiency, sequencing would also lead to a high level
of accuracy and specificity. The aforementioned systems are only
selected examples. Further examples are HumTH01 for group (1)
and D21S11 for group (3).

Table 1) ACTBP2: Increase of forensic efficiency values including sequencing data. MEC = mean exclusion chance.

HumACTBP2

n sequenced alleles:	250
n defined alleles:	98

Discrimination power:	99.8 %
	(≙VWA, TH01, CD4)
MEC:	94.0 %

x̄ phenotype (f) old:	1.0 %
x̄ phenotype (f) new:	0.1 %

STR microvariation is caused by point mutations, repeat insertions/deletions and gross changes (Möller et al. 1994, Meyer et al. 1995, Brinkmann et al. 1995). The highest new mutation rate observed so far is associated with ACTBP but still lies under 0.8% which is approximately equivalent to some RFLPs. This figure seems to be extremely small in the low microvariation systems (Table 3). We have predominantly observed either insertions or deletions of single repeats (Brinkmann et al. 1995).

Table 2) Overview of forensically relevant parameters of STRs with low, intermediate and high microvariation.
MEC = mean exclusion chance; HWE = Hardy-Weinberg equilibrium.

STR Genetics

	system	meioses (n=)	mutations n	mutations %	MEC (%) Caucasian data	HWE	homozyg excess
low	CD4	278	0		41		
	FES	525	0	< 0.1%	44	yes	no
	F13B	509	0		44		
	TH01	725	0		59		
inter-med	VWA	741	2	< 0.3%	63	yes	no
high	D21	529	1	< 1.0%	65	yes	no
	ACTBP2	508	4		89		

comb. 99.9 %

Differences of phenotype frequencies

Based on the observed differences of allele frequencies in major ethnic groups we calculated the combined phenotype frequencies comparing different populations using 50 individuals randomly taken from each population sample (basic population). Their individual frequencies were calculated using 6 STRs. In the population to be compared, the frequency of each phenotype was calculated as well and also the ratio between both populations. Ratios greater than 1 indicate that the profile occurs more often in the basic population; e. g. 100 would indicate a frequency difference of 100-fold. Ratios smaller than 1 indicate that the profile is more common in the population compared. – Example (Table 4): The first Japanese individual – J1 – has a frequency of 10^{-8} and the German equivalent 10^{-11} leading to a ratio of 10^3. The mean value in this group is also ca. 10^3. In other words, the mean difference is ca. 1000. The other way around, i. e. starting with the Germans (basic population), the average ratio is 10^6.

Table 3) Example of combined phenotype frequency differences between Japanese and Germans. Ind. = Individual; J = Japanese; G = German; MV = mean value. Further explanation see text.

Phenotype (f)

(n = 6 systems)

Ind.	Jap.	Ger.	ratio	Ind.	Ger.	Jap.	ratio
J 1	10^{-8}	10^{-11}	10^3	G 1	10^{-9}	10^{-14}	10^5
J 2	10^{-9}	10^{-9}	10^0	G 2	10^{-6}	10^{-11}	10^5
J 3	10^{-7}	10^{-12}	10^5	G 3	10^{-8}	10^{-16}	10^8
.	.	.	.	.	.	.	.
.	.	.	.	.	.	.	.
J 50	10^{-8}	10^{-10}	10^2	G 50	10^{-7}	10^{-13}	10^6
		MV = 10^3				MV = 10^6	

Between German Caucasians and two other Caucasian populations this difference is less than one order of magnitude (Fig. 5). Compared to other major ethnic groups, the mean differences range between 10^3 and 10^8.

Fig. 5) Graphi-
cal presenta-
tion of com-
bined phenotype
frequency dif-
ferences between
Germans and oth-
er populations
using 3-6 STRs.
3 systems = THO1,
VWA, FES; 4 sys-
tems = THO1, VWA,
FES, F13B;
5 systems = THO1,
VWA, FES, F13B,
CD4; 6 systems = THO1, VWA, FES, F13B, CD4, D21S11.

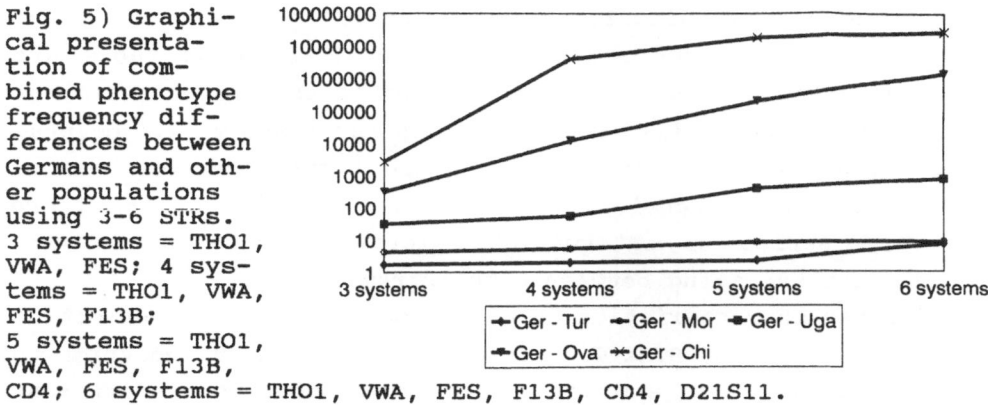

The reconstruction of phylogenetic trees involving 9 populations
using the UPGMA method (average linkage analysis; Nei 1987)
(DISPAN software kindly provided by Dr. Nei, Pennsylvania) leads
to a phylogenetic tree grouping closely related populations
(Fig. 6). They form a first category of pairwise relationships:
Turks-Germans, Papuans-Aborigines, Japanese-Chinese, Ovambos-
Ugandas. In the second category the Moroccans are grouped together with Turks and Germans and also, the Chinese-Japanese on the
one side and the Papuans-Aborigines on the other side.

Fig. 6) Phylogenetic
tree reconstructed
using average link-
age analysis (UPGMA).
The numbers represent
the bootstrap values.

TH01, VWA, FES, F13B

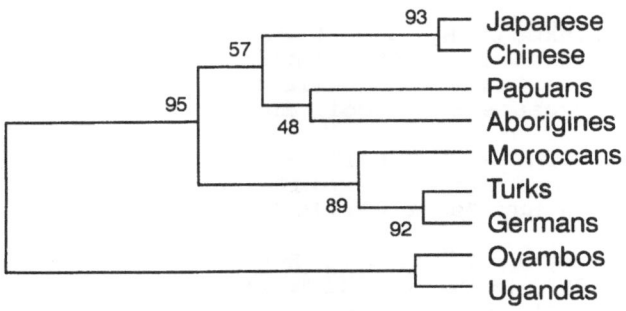

To summarize: STRs seem to have some reciprocal properties:
1. There exist robust systems with a low microvariation which
are usually easily typeable and associated with low mutation

rates and a high discrimination power between populations of different major ethnic groups. On the other hand there are highly variable systems. The definition of the respective alleles necessitates skill. Their mutation rates are still acceptable. Their possibility to distinguish between populations is low, but their forensic efficiency values are high. And there exist a series of intermediate microvariation systems with properties averaging between both extremes.

From these characteristics it can be derived that the selection of an ideal set of STRs will strongly depend on the question to be solved, i. e. in a mixed population consisting of different major ethnic groups, STRs with high microvariation could be useful in order to keep the resulting phenotype frequency differences low. Other parameters will be the through-put of labour, the machines available and the composition of the populations involved and of course the sample quality.

Literature

Alper B, Meyer E, Schürenkamp M, Brinkmann B (1995) HumFES/FPS and HumF13B: Turkish and German population data. Int J Legal Med (in the press)

Barber MD, Piercy RC, Anderson JF, Parkin BH (1995) Structural variation of novel alleles at the Hum vWA and HumFES/FPS short tandem repeat loci. Int J Legal Med 108:31-35

Brinkmann B, Möller A, Wiegand P (1995) Structure of new mutations in 2 STR systems. Int J Legal Med 107:201-203

Brinkmann B, Sajantila A, Goedde HW, Matsumoto H, Nishi K, Wiegand P (1995) Population genetic comparisons among eight populations using allele frequency and sequence data from three microsatellite loci. Eur J Hum Genet (in the press)

Edwards A, Civitello A, Hammond HA, Caskey CT (1991) DNA typing and genetic mapping with trimeric and tetrameric tandem repeats. Am J Hum Genet 49:746-756

Meyer E, Wiegand P, Rand SP, Kuhlmann D, Brack M, Brinkmann B (1995) Microsatellite polymorphisms reveal phylogenetic relationships in primates. J Mol Evol 41:10-14

Möller A, Meyer E, Brinkmann B (1994) Different types of structural variation in STRs: HumFES/FPS, HumVWA and HumD21S11. Int J Legal Med 106:319-323

Polymeropoulos MH, Rath DS, Xiao H, Merril CR (1992) Tetranucleotide repeat polymorphism at the human beta-actin related pseudogene H-beta-Ac-psi-2 (ACTBP2). Nucleic Acids Res 20:1432

Tautz D (1993) Notes on the definition and nomenclature of
tandemly repetitive DNA sequences. In: Pena SDJ, Chakraborty R,
Epplen JT, Jeffreys AJ (eds) DNA fingerprinting: state of the
science. Birkhäuser, Basel, pp 21-28

Tautz D, Renz M (1984) Simple sequences are ubiquitous repetitive components of eukaryotic genomes. Nucleic Acids Res 12:4127-
4138

Weber JL, May PE (1989) Abundant class of human DNA polymorphisms which can be typed using the polymerase chain reaction.
Am J Hum Genet 44:388-396

Analysis of sequence variations in the alleles from three STR loci.

L. Perlee, J. Neuweiler, I. Balazs

Lifecodes Corp., 550 West Ave., Stamford Ct 06902, USA

INTRODUCTION

DNA polymorphic loci resulting from variations in the number of short tandem repeats (STR), especially tetranucleotide repeats, are finding increased application in human identification. The main advantage of these loci are the small size of their alleles and their ability to be detected by PCR based DNA amplification. We have developed a multiplex system composed of 3 loci. The alleles from each locus fall within discreet size ranges and do not overlap. Although in theory the alleles from these loci differ by changes in the number of tetranucleotide repeats, additional variants may exist due to sequence variations between similar size alleles. Sequence studies, by Adams et al. (1993), of the alleles of the locus D11S554 have shown the occurrence of sequence variants among the same size alleles. The objective of this study was to report our initial findings on the primary sequence of multiple alleles from the 3 polymorphic STR loci.

MATERIALS AND METHODS

The alleles analyzed belong to the loci D3S1744, D12S1090 and D18S849.

DNA samples, from individuals possessing the allele(s) to be sequenced, were amplified with the locus specific primers (Lifecodes Corp.) using the conditions described by Neuweiler et al. (1995). The amplified alleles were fractionated by electrophoresis in an agarose gel. A portion of the gel containing the allele to be sequenced was sampled using a Pasteur pipette and the DNA re-amplified using one of the primer pairs 5'-labeled with biotin. DNA sequence was generated in both orientations by amplification with biotin-labeled primer for the 5' and 3' ends of the DNA fragment. The amplified product was purified by absorption to Streptavidin coated magnetic beads (Dynal, Inc) and sequenced using the Taq Dye-deoxy Terminator Cycle Sequencing kit (Perkin-Elmer) in an ABI Model 373A automated sequencer.

RESULTS AND DISCUSSION

DNA sequence analysis of alleles from the loci D3S1744, D12S1090 and D18S849 reveals that the main source of the size polymorphisms is the result of variations in the number of GATA repeat units.

Locus D18S849, consisted of alleles having from 9 to 19 tetranucleotide repeats. Alleles containing 10 and 13 repeats were not detected in the 200 individuals examined to date. In all allele sizes, the third repeat was a TATA followed by GAATA instead of GATAGATA. To determine if we could detect sequence differences between alleles of the same size, we selected the most common allele for locus D18S849. Alleles of the same size, from 8 unrelated individuals were sequenced. The results did not reveal differences in DNA sequence, however, a larger number of allele samples, from different populations, may have to be examined to determine the possible level of sequence variation at this locus,

Locus D3S1744 contained from 14 to 22 GATA repeats and was flanked by short dinucleotide repeats with the sequence TC and TA respectively. In addition, all the allele sizes contained the sequence GAT, instead of the third GATA repeat.

Locus D12S1090 was the locus with the largest number of alleles. The number of GATA repeats varied from 9 to 33 in the different size alleles. These repeats were flanked by stretches containing TA repeats. Some alleles contained changes in the sequence such as G to C in the second repeat of many alleles. Some alleles also had one or two base insertions of T or TA or deletions of GA in the region of the repeats. A summary of the sequence of the STR region of these alleles have been summarized in Table 1. The number of different size alleles identified by gel electrophoresis was more than 25. Because of the large number of alleles at this locus, the allelic ladder made for the analysis of this locus was prepared using only every other allele. From approximately 400 alleles examined, 3 alleles could be classified as rare variants. These alleles had a 1 or 2 base difference with the common allele with allele sizes of 251, 255, and 285 bases (Table 1). Sequence analysis of same size allele from a limited number of unrelated individuals has not yet revealed sequence differences. A larger survey, however, may reveal sequence differences. The internal sequence variations observed between different size alleles suggest that this marker may be useful in studies of population diversity.

REFERENCES

Adams M, Urquhart A, Kimpton C, Gill P (1993) The human D11S554 locus: four distinct families of repeat pattern alleles at one locus. Human Molecular Genetics 2:1373-1376

Neuweiler J, Perlee L, Venturini J, Balazs I (1995) Properties of an STR multiplex marker system suitable for paternity and forensic determinations. this proceeding.

Table 1. Sequence of the STR region for alleles from the D12S1090 locus

ALLELE SIZE								
306	TATATATATATATATA	GATAGATA 15x(GATA)	GAT	2x(GATA)	2x(GATT) GATTA 10x(GATA)			GATGTTATAGATATATATTATAT
302	TATATATATATATATA	GATACATA 14x(GATA)	GAT	2x(GATA)	2x(GATT) GATTA 10x(GATA)			GATGTTATAGATATATATATAAT
298	TATATATATTATATA	GATACATA 13x(GATA)	GAT	3x(GATA)	2x(GATT) GATTA 9x(GATA)			GATGTTATAGATATATATT AT
294	TATATATATTATATA	GATACATA 13x(GATA)	GAT	2x(GATA)	2x(GATT) GATTA 9x(GATA)			GATGTTATAGATATATATT AT
290	TATATATATTATATA	GATACATA 12x(GATA)	GAT	3x(GATA)	GATT GATTA 9x(GATA)			GATGTTATAGATATATATA AT
288	TATATATATATATATA	GATAGATA 13x(GATA)	GATTA	5x(GATA)TA	2x(GATA) GATTA 3x(GATA)			GATGTTATAGATATATATAAT
285	TATATATATATATATA	GATACATA 13x(GATA)	GATTA	10x(GATA)				GATGTTATAGATATATATAAT
284	TATATATATATATATA	GATAGATA 11x(GATA)	GATTA	5x(GATA)TA	2x(GATA)GATCAG 3x(GATA)			GATGTTATAGATATATATATAAT
277	TATATATATTATATA	GATACATA 13x(GATA)	GATTA	8x(GATA)				GATGTTATAGATATATATATAAT
269	TATATATATATATATA	GATACATA 12x(GATA)	GATTA	7x(GATA)				GATGTTATAGATATATATATAAT
261	TATATATATATATATA	GATAGATA 11x(GATA)	GATTA	6x(GATA)				GATGTTATAGATATATATATAT
257	TATATATATATATATA	GATAGATA 10x(GATA)	GATTA	6x(GATA)				GATGTTATAGATATATATATTAT
255	TATATATATTATATA	GATAGATA 10x(GATA)TA	GATTA	5x(GATA)				GATGTTATAGATATATATATTAT
253	TATATATATTATATA	GATAGATA 10x(GATA)	GATTA	5x(GATA)				GATGTTATAGATATATATATTAT
251	TATATATATATATATA	GATAGATA 9x(GATA) TA 2x(GATA)	GATTA	3x(GATA)				GATGTTATAGATATATATATAAT
244	TATATATATTATATA	GATAGATA 14x(GATA)						GATGTTATAGATATATATATTAT
236	TATATATATTATATA	GATACATA 12x(GATA)						GATGTTATAGATATATATATAAT
228	TATATATATTATATA	GATACATA 10x(GATA)						GATGTTATAGATATATATATTAT
220	TATATATATTATATA	GATAGATA 8x(GATA)						GATGTTATAGATATATATATTAT
212	TATATATATTATATA	GATAGATA 6x(GATA)						GATGNTATAGATATATATATTAT

Underlined numbers, represent alleles used for the allelic ladder.
Numbers in bold, represent common alleles not present in the allelic ladder.
Numbers in italic, represent rare allelic variants

AMPFLP-TYPING FOR THE HUMCD4 STR POLYMORPHISM IN AN AUSTRIAN CAUCASOID POPULATION SAMPLE: SEQUENCE DATA AND ALLELE DISTRIBUTION

B.Glock, D.W.M.Schwartz, E.M.Dauber, E.M.Schwartz-Jungl, W.R.Mayr

Clinical Institute for Blood Group Serology and Transfusion Medicine, University of Vienna

Waehringer Guertel 18-20/4I A-1090 Vienna, Austria

INTRODUCTION

Short tandem repeat (STR) polymorphisms are microsatellite loci containing repeat motifs 2 to 7 nucleotides long. Several hundred STR marker systems have been described until now. They are widely spread throughout the human genome and most of them show high levels of heterozygosity. Since STR sequences may even be amplified from small amounts of highly degraded template DNA, they have become very useful in human identification e.g. for forensic casework and paternity testing.
Application of allelic ladders as standard size markers is a reliable and precise method of allele designation in test samples and has been described for several VNTR and STR loci before (e.g. Puers et al.1993).
We used this procedure to evaluate the HUMCD4 (AAAAG) pentanucleotide polymorphism in the CD4 gene (Edwards M.C. et al. 1991; Wall et al. 1993) at 12pter-p12 (GenBank M86525) in an Austrian Caucasoid population sample of 300 healthy, unrelated individuals.

MATERIAL AND METHODS

Samples

Genomic DNA was extracted from peripheral blood of 300 healthy, unrelated Austrian individuals by standard techniques.

Primers

5`TTG GAG TCG CAA GCT GAA CTA GC-3` (forward primer, CTTTT strand)
5`-GCC TGA GTG ACA GAG TGA GAA CC-3` (reverse primer, AAAAG strand)
(Edwards M.C. et al. 1991).

PCR

PCR amplifications of the population samples were performed in 50µl volume with 8ng template, 0.4µM of each primer, 1U polymerase (Dynazyme™, Finn Zymes Oy), 0.8x PCR buffer (1x: 50mM KCl, 10mM TrisCl pH=9.0 at 25°C, 0,1% Triton-X-100 and 1.5mM MgCl2) and 200µM of each dNTP, overlaid with 50µl paraffine oil using a Hybaid Omnigene thermocycler.
A modified PCR-protocol (based upon Wall et al. 1993) was used for all amplifications: 10 min 98°C, without polymerase,1 cycle; then 10 min 58.5°C, 1 cycle adding the polymerase; followed by 1 min 94°C and 45 seconds 58.5°C for 10 cycles; then 1 min 90°C and 45 sec 58.5°C for 20 cycles; final annealing 58.5°C, 10 min, 1 cycle.

Electrophoretical Methods

Electrophoresis on 9% native polyacrylamide gels in 112mM Tris-Acetic Acid rehydration buffer and 200mM Tris-Tricine electrode buffer and subsequent silver staining was carried out as described by Schwartz at al. (1994). Typing was done by side by side comparison with the allelic ladder.

Allelic Ladder

Single bands of heterozygous population samples corresponding to distinct alleles were eluted from the gel, DNA was purified using Wizard PCR Preps, DNA Purification System (Promega, technical bulletin), diluted and reamplified. Equal concentrations of the amplification products were pooled to build up an allelic ladder.

Sequencing

Single stranded sequence determination of the different alleles took place on an automatic DNA-Sequencer (ALF™ Pharmacia LKB Technology AB) according to the protocol of Pharmacia AutoRead™ Sequencing Kit.

For each allele the strand and anti-sense strand were sequenced. Preceding strand separation was performed with support of Streptavidin attached magnetic beads.

Statistics

In a χ^2 test alleles 6,7,8,10 and 11 were grouped.

RESULTS AND DISCUSSION

DNA samples of healthy, unrelated Austrian Caucasian individuals were amplified revealing 8 individual alleles, which were used to construct an allelic ladder by pooling amplification products of the purified allele DNAs.

Sequencing of both strands of 35 alleles including the ladder alleles (six alleles 4, six alleles 5, one allele 6 and one 7, two alleles 8, four alleles 8`, seven alleles 9, five alleles 10 and three alleles 11) showed a regular repeat structure with only one polymorphic repeat motif (table 1). The five shorter alleles 4-8 contain 4 to 8 iterations of the (AAAAG) repeat unit. The three longer alleles show 6 to 8 regular repeat units, then one repeat unit with an A to G transition changing AAAAG to AAAGG, and subsequently two copies of the core repeat, which led us to designate them 9,10 and 11 following the rule of the first four alleles and counting the AAAGG unit for a AAAAG. (Allele designations were done following the recommendations of the DNA commission of the International Society of Forensic Haemogenetics 1994).

Table 1 Repeat Structures and Frequencies of the HUMCD4 Alleles

Allele designation	Sequence structure	Length (bp)	Allele frequency $\pm SE^a$ (%)
4	$-(AAAAG)_4 -$	86	36.3 ± 2.0
5	$-(AAAAG)_5 -$	91	31.6 ± 1.9
6	$-(AAAAG)_6 -$	96	0.2 ± 0.2
7	$-(AAAAG)_7 -$	101	0.2 ± 0.2
8	$-(AAAAG)_8 -$	106	1.2 ± 0.4^b
8`	$-(AAAAG)_5 \, AAAGG \, (AAAAG)_2 -$	106	-
9	$-(AAAAG)_6 \, AAAGG \, (AAAAG)_2 -$	111	27.5 ± 1.8
10	$-(AAAAG)_7 \, AAAGG \, (AAAAG)_2 -$	116	2.5 ± 0.6
11	$-(AAAAG)_8 \, AAAGG \, (AAAAG)_2 -$	121	0.5 ± 0.3

$\chi^2=8.18; \; 6df; \; p=0.23$
Heterozygosity observed = 0.73
Heterozygosity expected = 0.69

Mean exclusion chance (Krueger et al.1968) :W= 0.44
Power of discrimination (Kloosterman et al. 1993)=0.85
Discrimination index (Wong et al. 1987)=0.13

[a] SE indicates standard error calculated according to Edwards et al. 1992
[b] Common frequency of the electrophoretically indistinguishable alleles 8 and 8´

In addition we encountered a variant form of allel 8, which doesn`t show 8 continous copies of the repeat motif, but contains the A to G transition. This variant allele 8` appeared with a frequency of 4 out of 6 sequenced alleles. It was not included in the allelic ladder because it was indistinguishable from allele 8 in population sample testing on native polyacrylamid gels. Side by side comparison of the sequences revealed absolute length and sequence conformities of the 5`and 3` flanking regions of all sequenced alleles. No other microheterogenities were found. Allele sizes ranging from 86 to 121 basepairs were correlated with the sequence provided in GenBank (Accession No.M86525), which corresponds to our allel 9.
The sequenced ladder was employed to characterize 600 chromosomes from unrelated Austrian Caucasoids by AMPFLP-typing on native polyacrylamide gels (fig. 1). A total of eight distinguishable alleles appearing with frequencies between 0.2% to 36.3% were observed within our population sample. There are three common alleles

57

4, 5 and 9, two rare alleles 8 (and 8`) and 10 and three very rare alleles 6, 7 and 11. No deviations from Hardy-Weinberg eqilibrium could be observed (table 1).

Fig.1 AMPFLP-typing of Austrian Caucasoid population
samples employing the sequenced allelic ladder for the
HUMCD4 STR locus containing alleles 4 to 11.

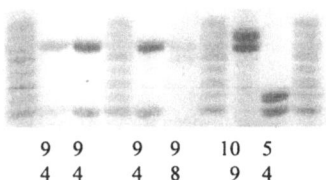

```
9  9      9  9      10  5
4  4      4  8      9   4
```

The data obtained in this study suggest that the HUMCD4 pentanucleotide polymorphism is a potential marker for personal identification applications. The assignment of alleles using a well characterized allelic ladder is a simple, precise and reliable method independent of the used electrophoresis systems. Further advances should be made to obtain such ladders for all practicable STR loci, especially for those applied in forensic cases and paternity testing.

REFERENCES

Bassam BJ, Caetano Anolles G, Gresshoff PM (1991) Fast and sensitive silver staining of DNA in polyacrylamide gels. Anal Biochem 196:80-83

DNA comission of the ISFH (1994) DNA recommendations- 1994 report concerning further recommendations of the DNA comission of the ISFH regarding PCR-based polymorphisms in STR (short tandem repeat) systems. Int J Leg Med 107:159-160

Edwards A, Hammond HA, Jin L, Caskey CT, Chakraborty R (1992) Genetic variation at five trimeric and tetrameric tandem repeat loci in four human population groups. Genomics 12:241-253

Edwards MC, Clemens PR, Tristan M, Pizzuti A, Gibbs RA (1991) Pentanucleotide repeat length polymorphism at the human CD4 locus. Nucleic Acids Res 19:4791

Kloosterman AD, Budowle B, Daselaar P (1993) PCR-amplification and detection of the human D1S80 VNTR locus. Int J Leg Med 105:257-264

Krueger J, Fuhrmann W, Lichte KH, Steffens C (1968) Zur Verwendung des Polymorphismus der sauren Erythrozytenphosphatase bei der Vaterschaftsbegutachtung. Deutsch Z Gerichtl Med 64:127-146

Puers C, Hammond HA, Jin L, Caskey CT, Schumm JW (1993) Identification of repeat sequence heterogeneity at the polymorphic short tandem repeat locus HUMTH01[AATG]n and reassignment of alleles in population analysis by using a locus-specific allelic ladder. Am J Hum Genet 53:953-958

Schwartz DWM, Jungl EM, Krenek OR, Mayr WR (1994) Simple and rapid typing for VNTR polymorphisms using high resolution electrophoresis of PCR products on rehydratable polyacrylamide gels. Advances in Forensic Haemogenetics 5:170-172, Springer, Berlin, FRG

Wall WJ, Williamson R, Petrou M, Papaioannou D, Parkin BH (1993) Variation of short tandem repeats within and between populations. Hum Mol Genet 2:1023-1029

Wong Z, Wilson V, Patel I, Povey S, Jeffreys AJ (1987) Characterization of a panel of highly variable minisatellites cloned from human DNA. Ann Hum Genet 51:269-288

Zuliani G, Hobbs HH (1990) Tetranucleotide repeat polymorphism in the LPL gene. Nucleic Acids Res 18:4958

ACKNOWLEDGEMENTS

The authors are grateful to B.Brinkmann for providing an allelic ladder for comparison and to H.Gnauer for his excellent technical assistance.

TYPING OF THE HUMVWA MICROSATELLITE POLYMORPHISM: ALLELE FREQUENCIES AND SEQUENCING DATA

D.W.M.Schwartz, E.M.Dauber, B.Glock, W.R.Mayr

Clinical Department for Blood Group Serology

University of Vienna

Waehringer Guertel 18-20/4I, A-1090 Vienna, Austria

SYSTEM AND LOCUS

tetranucleotide polymorphism in intron 40 of the human von Willebrand factor gene 12p12-12pter; Genbank Acession No.25858 [Kimpton 1992]

POPULATION AND SAMPLE SIZE: Vienna region (Austria). N=354

METHODS

PCR

0.4µM primer VWA1   5'-ccc tag tgg atg ata aga ata atc-3'
0.4µM primer VWA2   5'-gga cag atg ata aat aca tag gat gga tgg-3' [Kimpton 1992]
40ng template DNA, 2U polymerase (Dynazyme™, Finn Zymes Oy), 200µM each dNTP, 1x PCR buffer, final reaction volume 50µl, layer with 50µl paraffine oil

amplification:	1.cycle:	98°C 5min	58°C 10 min	
	30 cycles:	94°C 1min	50°C 1min	72°C 110sec
	last cycle:	72°C 10min		

thermocycler: Hybaid OmniGene

AMPFLP Typing

PAGE and silver staining was carried out on 7% native polyacrylamide gels in 120mM Tris/Acetic Acid and 200mM Tris/Tricine in horizontal mode (ramp: 1200V/7mA/30W; final: 1200V/15mA/30W) as previously described [Schwartz 1994]. Typing was performed by side-to-side comparison with a sequenced allelic ladder, composed of distinct alleles as described elsewhere in this issue.

Sequencing

Automated single strand sequence determination of alleles corresponding to the ladder alleles was performed on an automatic DNA-Sequencer (ALF™, Pharmacia LKB Technology) according to the protocol of the Pharmacia AutoRead™ Sequencing Kit (dye primers, T7 polymerase) on a 6% sequencing gel. For each sample, the sense and the antisense strand were sequenced.

RESULTS AND COMMENTS

A total of 12 alleles could be resolved by AMPFLP. At this level, one new allele (11) and two interalleles (14s and 15 f) could clearly be identified. Allele 13 and 22, that have been described by other workers [Moeller1994, Sajantila 1994] were not detected in our population. Frequencies, together with the forensic statistical efficiency values are listed in Tab.1. The phenotype distribution showed no significant deviation from Hardy-Weinberg expectations.
Sequencing showed the allele 11 to conform with the basic repeat structure that has been described by Moeller[1994]. Allele 14s showed a variation in the core repeat region (c→t transition in the third of 9 tcta repeats). In allele 15f the same variation of the core repeat region as in allele 14 [Moeller 1994] could be detected and an additional variation in the 3'-constant region.
In conclusion, HUMVWA shows a complex sequence polymorphism as already described [Moeller 1994]. Comparison of phaenotype distribution shows significant differences between different populations. AMPFLP typing is usually without ambiguities and with good forensic efficiency. HUMVWA can be recommended for the use in forensic applications.

Table 1: HUMVWA allele frequencies (n=354)

allele designation	frequency (%)
11	0.1
13	---
14	8.3
14s	0.1
15f	0.1
15	12.6
16	20.5
17	24.9
18	21.2
19	10.5
20	1.6
21	0.1
22	---

$\chi 2=33.13$; df=55; $0.990<p<0.995$
mean paternity exclusion chance (MEC)   0.64646
mean exclusion probability (MEP)   0.63402
polymorphism information content (PIC)   0.79214

Table 2: HUMVWA microsatellite sequence polymorphism

```
allele  size  5'constant                                                                3'constant region
        (bp)  region                                                                        (39bp)
              (43bp)

C11²    126 .......... tcta          (tctg)3     (tcta)7         ...........................
 13¹    134 .......... tcta          (tctg)4     (tcta)8         ...........................
C14₂    138 .......... tcta(tctg)(tcta)(tctg)4 (tcta)3 (tcca) (tcta)3  .......................c....
 14₂    138 .......... tcta          (tctg)4 (tcta)2 (ttta) (tcta)6    ...........................
 15²    142 .......... tcta(tctg)(tcta)(tctg)4 (tcta)3 (tcca) (tcta)3  (tcca)3    t  ............
C15₁    142 .......... tcta          (tctg)3     (tcta)11        ...........................
 15¹    142 .......... tcta          (tctg)4     (tcta)10        ...........................
 161    146 .......... tcta          (tctg)3     (tcta)12        ...........................
C16     146 .......... tcta          (tctg)4     (tcta)11        ...........................
C17₃    150 .......... tcta          (tctg)4     (tcta)12        ...........................
C18³    154 .......... tcta          (tctg)4     (tcta)13   (tcca) (tcta) t  .......t....
C19     158 .......... tcta          (tctg)4     (tcta)14        ...........................
C20     162 .......... tcta          (tctg)4     (tcta)15        ...........................
C21₁    162 .......... tcta          (tctg)4     (tcta)16        ...........................
 22¹    170 .......... tcta          (tctg)4     (tcta)17        ...........................
```

5' constant region: 5'- [ccc tag tgg atg ata aga ata atc] agt atg tga ctt gga ttg a -3'
3' constant region: 5'- tcca tcta t [cca tcc atc cta tgt att tat cat ctg tcc] - 3'
C11,14,... Alleles included in allelic cocktail for AMPFLP typing
[] denotes primer target sequences
[1] alleles and variants described by Moeller [1994]
[2] alleles and variants described by Schwartz [this study]
[3] EMBL M25858 sequence

REFERENCES

Kimpton C, Walton A, Gill P: A further tetranucleotide repeat polymorphism in the vWF gene. Hum.Mol.Genet. 1: 287 (1992)

Moeller A, Meyer E, Brinkmann B: Different types of structural variation in STRs: HumFES/FPS, HumVWA and HumDS21S11. Int.J.Leg.Med. 106: 319-323 (1994)

Sajantila A, Pacek P, Lukka M, Syvaenen AC, Nokelainen P., Sistonen P, Peltonen L, Budowle B: A microsatellite polymorphism in the von Willebrand factor gene: comparison of allele frequencies in different population samples and evaluation for forensic medicine. Forensic Sci.Int. 65: 169-175 (1994)

Schwartz DWM, Jungl EM, Krenek OR, Mayr WR: Simple and rapid typing for VNTR polymorphisms using high resolution electrophoresis of PCR products on rehydratable polyacrylamide gels. Advances in Forensic Haemogenetics 5: 170-172, Springer, Berlin, FRG (1994)

ACKNOWLEDGEMENTS

The authors are grateful to B.Brinkmann for providing an allelic ladder for standardisation and to H.Gnauer for his excellent technical assistance.

SEQUENCING AND SIZE DETERMINATION OF THE D1S80 INTERALLELE

H.Fukushima, N.Harashima, Y.Katsuyama, M.Ota, CY.Liu and Y.Hama

Department of Legal Medicine, Shinshu University School of Medicine, 3-1-1 Asahi, Matsumoto, 390 JAPAN

As a useful VNTR locus, the D1S80 system has been applied in forensic practice by laboratories worldwide . The D1S80 allele variants are valuable for paternity testing and individual identification. However, there are few reports concerning these variants[1] and their sequencing.   In this paper, we report on the variant of allele 27 and its sequencing, based on our previous investigation of the D1S80 polymorphism in the Japanese population.

Materials and Methods

DNA Extraction

Genomic DNA from unrelated Japanese individuals was isolated from blood using proteinase K/SDS lysis and phenol extraction.

PCR Amplification

PCR was performed according to our previous method[2], with the exception that one of the primers was labeled with a fluorescent dye HEX or FAM. For fragment size determination, the amplified samples were run on a 6% denaturing polyacrylamide gel and automatically analyzed by an ABI 373A sequencer using Genescan software.

DNA Extraction from PAG

Amplified products were electrophoresed on a 6% polyacrylamide gel. After electrophoresis, the target alleles which were stained with ethidium bromide were excised from the gel and extracted through GENE CAPSULE. Some extracted DNA was diluted with water and used as template for the next PCR.

Cloning

DNA fragments were isolated from PAG and cloned in pBluescript. Recombinant clones were randomly selected.

Sequence Analysis

Sequencing was performed with a 6% denaturing polyacrylamide gel on an ABI 372A sequencer using the dideoxy chain termination method.

Results and Discussion

On a 6% polyacrylamide nondenaturing gel, the variant showed a different migration rate compared with allele 27 (Fig. 1).

Allele 27 has a higher frequency in Japanese and other Oriental populations compared with Caucasians, Hispanics and African Americans (Tab. 1). In our 121 samples of Japanese individuals, sixteen had allele 27, among which 4 alleles were found to be the variants.

On a denaturing sequencing gel, allele 27 and its variant showed the same migration rate. Fig. 2 shows a Genescan electropherogram, in which the peaks of allele 27 and its variant match closely. This suggests that allele 27 and its variant have the same fragment size.

After treatment with Msp I, allele 27 and its variant showed different electrophoretic band patterns (Fig. 3). Changes in the Msp I cleavage sites were found in the sequence of the repeating units of the variant. As a result, allele 27 had 8 Msp I cleavage sites in the repeating units, while the variant had 9 cleavage sites.

```
             195                             226
Allele 27 :  GAAGACCACAGGCAAG  GAGGACCACCGGAAAG
Variant :    - - G - - - - -C- -A- - -  - -A - - - - - - - C- - -
```

As shown above, the region of repeating units of the variant from position 195 (counting from the upstream primer combination site) to position 226 showed five base changes. Altogether 18 such base changes were found in the sequence of the repeating units of the variant. The sequences of the upstream flanking regions of allele 27 and its variant were compared and no changes were found. The sequence changes in the repeating units may lead to a conformational change of the variant, which would account for its faster migration rate.

Reference

1. K. Skowasch, P. Wiegand, and B. Brinkmann. pMCT 118 (D1S80) : a new allelic ladder and an improved electrophoretic separation lead to the demonstration of 28 alleles. Int J Leg Med : 105, 165 - 168, 1992.
2. E. Sugiyama, K. Honda, Y. Katsuyama, A. Tsuchikane, M. Ota and H. Fukushima. Allele frequency distribution of the D1S80 (pMCT118) locus polymorphism in the Japanese population by the polymerase

chain reaction. Int J Leg Med : 106, 111-114, 1993.

3. S. Y. Chuah, W. F. Tan, K. H. Yap, H. E. Tai and S. T. Chow. Analysis of the D1S80 locus by amplified fragment length polymorphism technique in the Chinese, Malays, and Indians in Singapore. Forens Sci Int : 68, 169-180. 1994.

4. B. Budowle, F. S. Baechtel, J. B. Smerick, K. W. Presley, A. M. Giusti, G. Parsons, M. C. Alevy and R. Chakraborty. D1S80 population data in African Americans, Caucasians, southeastern Hispanics, southwestern Hispanics, and Orientals. J Forens Sci : 40, 38 - 44. 1995.

Table 1   Distribution of allele 27 in different populations

Population	frequency (%)
Japanese[2]	6.6
	5.0(allele 27)
	1.6 (variant)
Chinese[3]	4.4
Malays[3]	5.5
Indians[3]	1.2
Caucasian[4]	0.7
Hispanic[4]	1.6
African American[4]	0.8

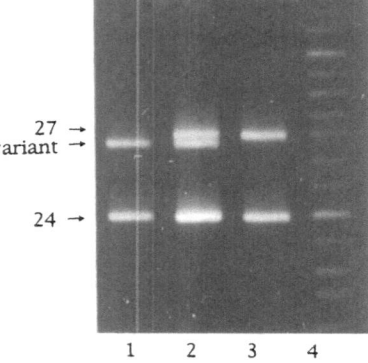

Fig. 1. Electrophoretic band patterns of allele 27 and the variant on a 6% polyacrylamide gel. Lane 1:24 / variant ; lane 2 ; a mixture of the sample 24/27 and the sample 24/variant; lane 3: 24/27; lane 4 : D1S80 allelic ladder.

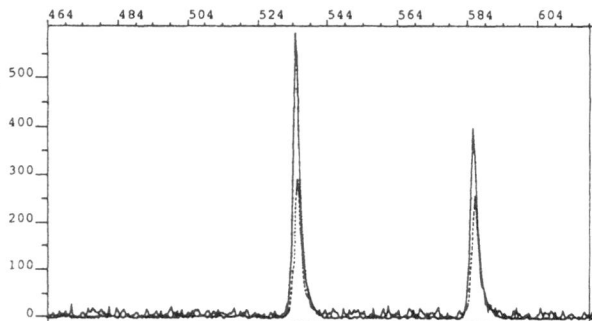

Fig. 2. A Genescan electropherogram. Two samples, 24/27 and 24/variant, were labeled with HEX and FAM respectively and were applied in the same lane. Bold line : 24/27; dotted line : 24/variant.

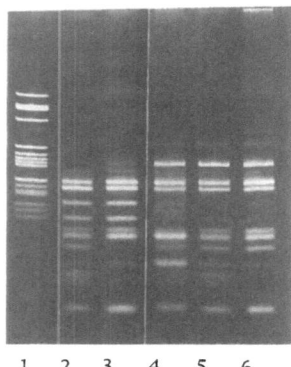

Fig 3. Electrophoretic band patterns of allele 27 and the variant after the treatment with Msp I. Lane 1 : pBR322 - Hae III ; lane 2-3, variant ; lane 4-5, allele 27; lane 6, RMS

ANALYSIS OF THE SHORT TANDEM REPEAT POLYMORPHISM D18S51: ALLELE FREQUENCIES AND SEQUENCE STUDIES

P. Berschick, * J. Reinhold

Institut fuer Zoophysiologie, Duesseldorf, Germany, *Institut fuer Labormedizin, Wuerzburg, Germany

INTRODUCTION

The analysis of Short Tandem Repeat polymorphisms is widely used as a method for human identification. There is a demand to combine several STR loci with high discrimination power for multiplex analysis. STR polymorphisms with few alleles (e.g.: TC11, F13A) do not have the discrimination power compared to STR-systems like SE33 (ACTBP2). SE33 has more than 30 alleles and thus the space for the combination with other STR loci in multiplex analysis is reduced. Therefore STR polymorphisms like FGA (HUMFIBRA) and D18S51 with about 15-20 alleles seem to be a good compromise.

The aim of the study was to get information about allele frequencies of the STR loci D18S51 in the German population. For typing these alleles correctly in size we started to sequence some alleles on the GATC Direct Blotting System (MWG-Biotech, Germany).

MATERIAL AND METHODS

DNA was extracted from whole blood according to standard procedures. Amplification of the STR locus D18S51 was carried out with the primers:
D18S51/1:   5'-CAAACCCGACTACCAGCAAC-3'
D18S51/2:   5'-Dig-GAGCCATGTTCATGCCACTG-3'

Amplification conditions:
10 mM Tris/HCl , 50 mM KCl (pH 8,3), 1.0 mM $MgCl_2$, 0.2 mM each dNTP, 0.5 µM each primer, 0.1 U Taq DNA polymerase (Boehringer) and 2.5 ng DNA. The reaction volume was 12.5 µl. Samples were amplified after an initial step of 1 min at 93°C for 30 cycles of 1 min at 93°C,1 min at 60°C and 1 min at 72°C. PCR products were diluted 1:20 in water and an aliquot was further diluted 1:5 in formamide dye mix. 1.5 µl of this dilution was loaded on a 30 cm long, 0.2 mm thick, 4% DBE sequencing gel (Direct Blotting Electrophoresis GATC 1500 sequencer, MWG, Germany) and run at constant 30 W (about 1700 V, 17 mA). As described previously (Berschick et al., 1994) the samples run through the gel and were blotted onto a nylon membrane (Macherey-Nagel, Germany). DNA was fixed onto the membrane by exposure to UV light for 2 min and the products visualized with the DIG Nucleic Acid detection kit. Some of the samples were analysed with an ABI sequencer.

Sequencing of the PCR products
Homozygous DNA samples, purified after amplification with Nucleotrap kit (Macherey-Nagel), were used as a template for sequencing. About 1/5th of the purified

PCR product was used for sequencing with the Sequitherm Cycle Sequencing kit (Biozym, Germany). We add 3% DMSO to the sequencing reaction to prevent unspecific stops. After 45 cycles of 30 sec at 93°C and 5 min at 55°C the reaction was stopped by adding 3 µl of formamide dye mix. 1.5 µl of the sample was loaded on a sequencing gel and run at constant 30W. After 50 min prerun the blotting membrane was started with a speed of 20 cm/h for 1h 30 min. Fixation of DNA and colorimetric detection was done as described above.

RESULTS AND DISCUSSION

To identify the alleles of D18S51 and for sequencing, DIG labelled samples were separated with direct blotting electrophoresis. With this quick and easy method it is possible to analyse a one basepair difference and therefore it is easy to type alleles of STR loci.

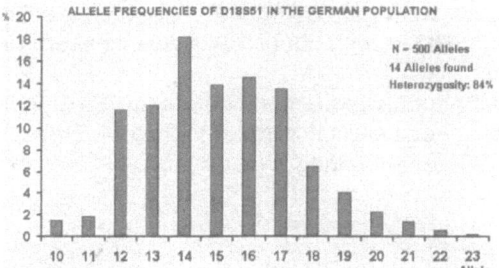

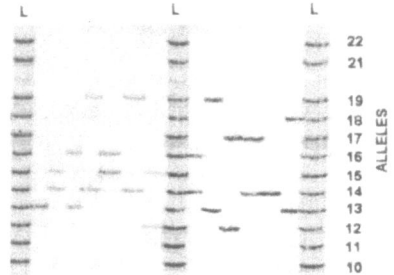

Fig. 1: Allele frequencies at the STR-locus D18S51 in the German population. Allele typing is based on the number of repeats.

Fig. 2: Examples of blotting D18S51 samples of unrelated individuals. L = allelic ladder.

Fig.1 shows the allelic distribution for D18S51 calculated from analysing 250 unrelated German individuals. For this STR loci we could not detect any interalleles so the repeat units were always 4 bp in length. On the blot (Fig. 2) D18S51 shows one distinct band for each allele.The heterozygosity index is 0. 84. The distribution found is according to Hardy-Weinberg eqilibrium. Analysing 130 meiosis we could not detect any de novo mutation.
For typing the allleles we sequenced 3 different alleles. With the use of DMSO we could reduce background of unspecific stops and could read through the sequence. The whole sequence for allele 16 is shown in table 1. The differences between the alleles was the number of GAAA repeats as shown in Table 2. The length of the products differ by 2 basepairs compared to the published data (Straub et al., 1993; Urquhart et al., 1995) but the published allele lengths are not based on sequencing.

Tab. 1: Sequence of allele 16 locus D18S51 amplified from DNA .The length variabl site is shown in bold letters. Primers are underlined.

```
----------------------------------------------------------------------------------------
GAGCCATGTT CATGCCACTG CACTTCACTC TGAGTGACAA ATTGAGACCT        50
GTCTCAGAAA GAAAGAAAGA AAGAAAGAAA GAAAGAAAGA AAGAAAGAAA       100
GAAAGAAAGA AAGAAAGAAA AAGAGAGAGG AAAGAAAGAG AAAAAGAAAA       150
GAAATAGTAG CAACTGTTAT TGTAAGACAT CTCCACACAC CAGAGAAGTT       200
AATTTTAATT TTAACATGTT AAGAACAGAG AGAAGCCAAC ATGTCCACCT       250
TAGGCTGACG GTTTGTTTAT TTGTGTTGTT GCTGGTAGTC GGGTTTG         297
```

Tab 2: DNA sequences of three D18S51 alleles. Only the varying repeat units are shown.

Allele	Length (bp)	Sequence
12	281	...GTCTCA **(GAAA)**$_{12}$ A (AG)$_4$...
13	284	...GTCTCA **(GAAA)**$_{13}$ A (AG)$_4$...
16	297	...GTCTCA **(GAAA)**$_{16}$ A (AG)$_4$...

The sequences determined in this study are perhaps 1 bp shorter than the putative allele length of the allele typing because of the addition of one nucleotide to the end of the PCR product. This is due to the tranferase activity of the Taq polymerase (Clark et al., 1988; Kimpton et al, 1993).

References

Berschick P, Henke J, Henke L (1995) Analysis of the Short Tandem Repeat polymorphism SE33: A new high resolution separation of SE33 by means of direct blotting electrophoresis. In: Bär W, Fiori A, Rossi U (eds) Advances in Forensic Haemogenetics 5, Springer, Berlion Heidelberg, New York, p 323-325

Clark JM (1988) Novel non-template addition reactions catalyzed by procaryotic and eucaryotic DNA polymerases. NAR 16, 9677-9686.

Kimpton CP, Gill P, Walton A, Urquhart A, Millican ES, Adams M (1993) Automated DNA profiling employing multiplex amplification of short tandem repeat loci. PCR Methods Appl. 3, 13-22.

Straub RE, Speer MC, Luo Y, Rojas K, Overhauser J, Ott J Gilliam C (1993) A microsatellite genetic linkage map of human chromosome 18. Genomics 15, 48-56.

Urquhart A, Oldroyd NJ, Kimpton CP, Gill P (1995) Highly discriminating heptaplex short tandem repeat PCR system for forensic identification. BioTechniques 18, 116-121.

INVESTIGATION OF THE STR HUMLIPOL IN AUSTRIAN CAUCASOID INDIVIDUALS: SEQUENCE DATA AND ALLELE FREQUENCIES

B.Glock, D.W.M.Schwartz, E.M.Dauber, E.M.Schwartz-Jungl, W.R.Mayr

Clinical Institute for Blood Group Serology and Transfusion Medicine, University of Vienna

Waehringer Guertel 18-20/41 A-1090 Vienna, Austria

INTRODUCTION

Short tandem repeat polymorphisms (STR′s) are tracts of di- to hexa- or heptanucleotides, which are tandemly repeated. They are highly polymorphic in respect to the number of repeats and widely spread throughout the human genome (Tautz 1989; Edwards 1992).
Since the introduction of PCR amplification techniques these microsatellite markers have become useful tools for forensic casework including paternity testing, but they are also employed in genomic mapping linkage analysis and anthropology.
Application of sequenced allelic ladders as internal size standards is a very precise and reliable method of allele assignment in test samples, which allows allele designation according to the number of repeats.

In this work we present the sequence data of a ladder of the STR polymorphism in intron 6 of the lipoprotein lipase gene (Hammond et al. 1994; Zuliani and Hobbs 1990), designated HumLIPOL, and allele frequencies obtained in an Austrian Caucasian population sample using the AMPFLP-technique (N=550).

MATERIALS AND METHODS

Samples

Genomic DNA was extracted from peripheral blood of 550 healthy, unrelated Austrian individuals by the „salting out method" described by Miller et al. (1988).

Primers

5′-ATC TGA CCA AGG ATA GTG GGA TAT A-3′   (forward primer, TTTA strand)
5′-CCT GGG TAA CTG AGC GAG ACT GTG TC-3′   (reverse primer, TAAA strand)
(Zuliani and Hobbs 1990).

PCR

Amplifications of the population samples were performed with 20ng template, 0.6μM each primer, 2U polymerase (Dynazyme™, Finn Zymes Oy), 1x PCR buffer (50mM KCl, 10mM TrisCl pH=9.0 at 25°C, 0,1% Triton-X-100 and 1.5mM MgCl2) and 200μM of each dNTP, overlaid with 50μl paraffine oil, using a Hybaid Omnigene thermocycler.
A modified PCR protocol (based on Zuliani and Hobbs 1990) was used in all amplifications:
first denaturing 10 min 98°C, 1 cycle; 10 min 68°C, 1 cycle, adding the polymerase; followed by 1 min 94°C and 6 min 68°C, 10 cycles; 1 min 90°C and 6 min 68°C, 18 cycles; final annealing 10 min 68°C, 1 cycle.

Electrophoretical Methods

PAGE was carried out as described by Schwartz et. al. (1994) on 7% native polyacrylamide gels in 120mM Tris-Acetic Acid rehydration buffer and 200mM Tris-Tricine electrode buffer.
Subsequent silver staining was applied to visualize DNA (Bassam et al. 1991).
Typing was done by side by side comparison with the allelic ladder.

Allelic Ladder

Single bands of heterozygous population samples, corresponding to distinct alleles, were eluted from the gel. DNA was purified using Wizard PCR Preps, DNA Purification System (Promega, technical bulletin), diluted and reamplified. Equal concentrations of the amplification products were pooled to construct an allelic ladder.

67

Sequencing

Single stranded sequence determination of the different alleles took place on an automatic DNA-Sequencer (ALF™ Pharmacia LKB Technology AB) according to the protocol of the Pharmacia AutoRead™ Sequencing Kit (dye primers) on a 6% sequencing gel. For each allele both strands were sequenced.

Statistics

In a χ^2 test, performed to confirm the Hardy-Weinberg expectations, genotypes beyond expected values of 5 were grouped together.

RESULTS AND DISCUSSION

AMPFLP-typing of healthy, unrelated Caucasian individuals of Austria revealed 7 distinct alleles. One sample of each allele was used to construct the allelic ladder as decribed above.

Sequencing of 22 alleles (three alleles 7, four alleles 9, five alleles 10, three alleles each 11, 12, 13 and one allele 14) ,including the ladder alleles, showed a simple repeat structure, with 7 and 9 to 14 iterations of the [TTTA] repeat motif (table 1). Allele designation was in accordance with the repeat number following the recommendations of the International Society for Forensic Haemogenetics 1994.
In contrast to other STR loci (e.g. D21S11), which show a more complex structure and microheterogenities, side by side comparison of the sequencing pattern proved absolute length and sequence conformities of the 25 basepair 5` flanking regions and the 7 basepair 3`flanking regions.

Allele sizes, which were determined by comparing the sequence pattern of the sense and antisense strand, range from 111 to 139 basepairs (Table 1). They were correlated with the sequence provided in Genbank (Accession No. X15736), which corresponds to our allele 11.

Table 1 Sequencing data of the HumLIPOL alleles

Allele designation	Repeat structure	Length (bp)	Number of sequenced alleles
7	$(TTTA)_7$	111	3
10	$(TTTA)_{10}$	123	5
11	$(TTTA)_{11}$	127	3
12	$(TTTA)_{12}$	131	3
13	$(TTTA)_{13}$	135	3
14	$(TTTA)_{14}$	139	1

The sequenced ladder was employed in testing 550 DNA samples (1100 chromosomes) of healthy, unrelated Austrian individuals on 7% native polyacrylamide gels (Fig. 1).
We found three common alleles 10, 11 and 12, two rare alleles 9 and 13 and two very rare alleles 7 and 14 (Table 2).
Observed heterozygosity is 72.9 %, not significantly deviating from the expected value of 70.8 %. Population data met the Hardy-Weinberg expectations (p=0.195).
Power of discrimination is 0.86, mean exclusion chance is 0.52 and discrimination index is 0.13.

Fig. 1 AMPFLP-typing for HUMLIPOL alleles employing
the allelic ladder containing alleles 7 and 9 to 14

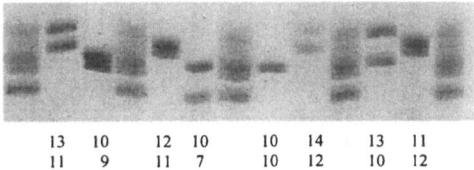

Table 2 Allele frequencies at the HumLIPOL STR locus in an Austrian Caucasoid population sample (N=550)

Allele Designation	Observed Alleles	Allele Frequency ±SE (%)[a]
7	3	0.3 ± 0.2
9	22	5.3 ± 0.7
10	190	38.5 ± 1.5
11	143	27.8 ± 1.4
12	126	25.1 ± 1.3
13	17	2.6 ± 0.5
14	2	0.4 ± 0.2

$$\chi^2 = 10.56;\ 6\ df;\ p = 0.195$$

Mean exclusion chance (Krueger et al. 1968) W = 0.52
Power of discrimination (Kloosterman et al. 1993) PD = 0.86
Discrimination index (Wong et al. 1987) DI = 0.13

[a] Standard error was calculated according to Edwards et al. (1992)

The application of the allelic ladder described in this paper allows a clear designation of alleles in unknown test samples in a precise and reliable way and there is no need for an additional size marker. The results of this study suggest that the HumLIPOL polymorphism could be suitable for forensics and other application fields as well.

REFERENCES

DNA comission of the ISFH (1994) DNA recommendations- 1994 report concerning further recommendations of the DNA comission of the ISFH regarding PCR-based polymorphisms in STR (short tandem repeat) systems. Int J Leg Med 107:159-160

Bassam BJ, Caetano Anolles G, Gresshoff PM (1991) Fast and sensitive silver staining of DNA in polyacrylamide gels. Anal Biochem 196:80-83

Edwards A, Hammond HA, Jin L, Caskey CT, Chakraborty R (1992) Genetic variation at five trimeric and tetrameric tandem repeat loci in four human population groups. Genomics 12:241-253

Hammond HA, Jin L, Zhong Y, Caskey CT, Chakraborty R (1994) Evaluation of 13 short tandem repeat loci for use in personal identification applications. Am J Hum Genet 55:175-189

Kloosterman AD, Budowle B, Daselaar P (1993) PCR-amplification and detection of the human D1S80 VNTR locus. Int J Leg Med 105:257-264

Krueger J, Fuhrmann W, Lichte KH, Steffens C (1968) Zur Verwendung des Polymorphismus der sauren Erythrozytenphosphatase bei der Vaterschaftsbegutachtung. Deutsch Z Gerichtl Med 64:127-146

Miller SA, Dykes DD, Polesky HF (1988) A simple salting out procedure for extracting DNA from human nucleated cells. Nucleic Acids Res 16:1215

Schwartz DWM, Jungl EM, Krenek OR, Mayr WR (1994) Simple and rapid typing for VNTR polymorphisms using high resolution electrophoresis of PCR products on rehydratable polyacrylamide gels. Advances in Forensic Haemogenetics 5:170-172, Springer, Berlin, FRG

Tautz D (1989) Hypervariability of simple sequences as a general source for polymorphic DNA markers. Nucleic Acids Res 17:6463-6471

Wong Z, Wilson V, Patel I, Povey S, Jeffreys AJ (1987) Characterization of a panel of highly variable minisatellites cloned from human DNA. Ann Hum Genet 51:269-288

Zuliani G, Hobbs HH (1990) Tetranucleotide repeat polymorphism in the LPL gene. Nucleic Acids Res 18:4958

ACKNOWLEDGEMENT

The authors are grateful to H.Gnauer for his excellent technical assistance

D12S391: A HIGHLY USEFUL STR FOR FORENSIC PURPOSES

M.V. Lareu, F. Barros, A. Salas, C. Pestoni, I. Muñoz, M.S. Rodriguez-Calvo and A. Carracedo.

Institute of Legal Medicine. Faculty of Medicine. Santiago.de Compostela Spain

SYSTEM: CHLC. GATA 11 HO8.
LOCUS: D12S391
POPULATION: GALICIA (NW SPAIN)
SAMPLE SIZE: N= 130

METHODS

PRIMERS:

FORWARD PRIMER: 5' AACAGGATCAATGGATGCAT 3'

REVERSE PRIMER: * 5' TGGCTTTTAGACCTGGACTG 3'
(* primer 5' end labelled with fluorescent dye)

AMPLIFICATION CONDITIONS

PCR Singleplex reaction

5-10 ng of genomic DNA in a 50 μM reaction volume.
10mM TRIS-HCL (pH8.3), 50mM Kcl, 0.01% Gelatin, 1.5mM MgCl2, 200μM each dNTP,
0.25μM each primer and 1.25 U AmpliTaq DNA Polymerase (Cetus, Emervylle, Calif).

PCR Triplex reaction

Identical buffer, dNTPs and enzyme concentration.
Primers concentration:
        HUMCD4: 0.10μM each primer
        HUMTHO1: 0.15μM each primer
        D12S391: 0.25μM each primer

PCR CYCLING (Individual and triplex reaction)

        94°C - 45 sec.
        60°C - 60 sec.   30 CYCLES
        72°C - 60 sec.

SEQUENCING

Sequencing from templates derived from PCR products were carried out using the fmol TM DNA
Sequencing System Sample (Promega).

ALLELIC LADDER

It was obtained after combination of 12 sequenced alleles (Fig. 1).

DETECTION SYSTEM

A.L.F. DNA Sequencer (Pharmacia)

Analysis of fragment: 6% Polyacrylamide denaturig gels.
      Electrophoresis conditions: 1600V, 42mA, 45W at 40°C for 4 h.

Sequencing: 6% Polyacrylamide denaturig gels.
      Electrophoresis conditions: 1600V, 38mA, 45W at 50°C for 5 h.

RESULTS

POPULATION STUDY

12 alleles ranging from 210 to 254 bp were found.
Allelic designation of the STR D12S391 was made according the number of repeats.

Observed genotypes of D12S391 in the Galician population.

Gen.	Obs.	Gen.	Obs.	Gen.	Obs.	Gen.	Obs.
15-15	1	17-17	1	18-21	6	20-21	4
15-17	2	17-18	2	18-22	9	20-22	3
15-18	1	17-19	1	18-23	4	20-23	1
15-19	3	17-20	1	18-24	5	21-21	2
15-20	1	17-21	2	18-25	1	21-22	5
15-21	1	17-22	5	19-20	5	21-23	2
15-23	1	17-23	4	19-21	1	22-22	1
16-17	1	17-24	1	19-22	6	22-23	2
16-18	2	17-26	1	19-23	5	22-24	4
16-20	1	18-18	6	19-24	1	23-24	2
16-21	1	18-19	11	19-25	1	23-25	1
16-25	1	18-20	6	20-20	2	24-26	1

Allele frequencies of D12S391 in the Galician population.

Allele	Frequency	allele	frequency	allele	frequency	allele	frequency
15	0.0420	18	0.2252	21	0.0992	24	0.0534
16	0.0229	19	0.1298	22	0.1374	25	0.0153
17	0.0840	20	0.0992	23	0.0840	26	0.0076

The system is in Hardy-Weinberg equilibrium (Exact test: $p = 0.54132$).
Heterozigosity: 90.08%
Discrimination power: 98.04%

SEQUENCE STRUCTURE

The 12 alleles showed a common repeat structure with a core sequence:
$$(AGAT)_{8-16}(AGAC)_{6-10}(AGAT)_{0-1}$$

TRIPLEX

Triplex amplification of the HUMCD4, HUMTH01 and D12S391 has proved that it gives good results.

CONCLUSION

The characteristics of the system, including the high polymorphism, normal electrophoretic behaviour, easy amplification and easy multiplexing makes this STR considerably interesting for forensic purposes

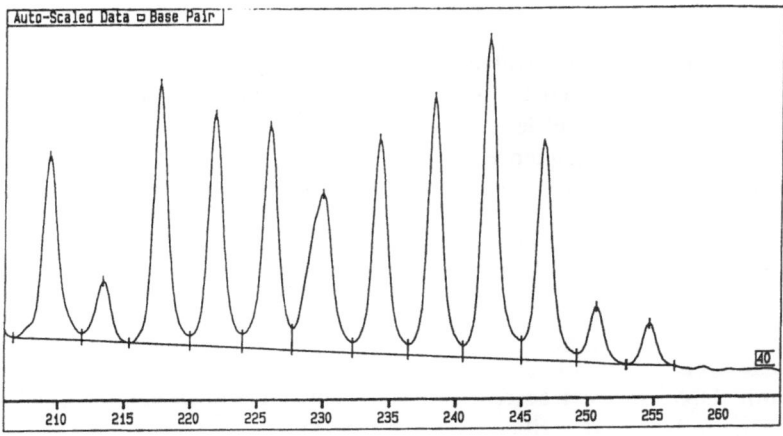

Figure 1. D12S391 allelic ladder. The allelic ladder was obtained after combination of 12 sequenced alleles.

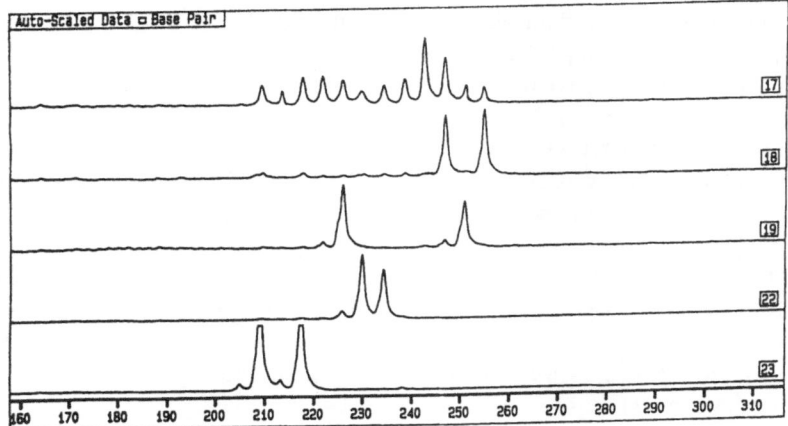

Figure 2. Electropherogram from the STR D12S391 from a 6% denaturing polyacrylamide gel. Lane 17 (allelic ladder), lane 18 (24-26), lane 19 (19-25), lane 22 (20-21) and lane 23 (15-17).

DNA Sequence analysis of the PCR Products of the MCT118 locus in Japanese DNA Samples

Kazumasa Sekiguchi, Ikuko Sakai, Natsuko Mizuno, Kanako Yoshida, Kentaro Kasai, Hajime Sato, and Sueshige Seta

National Research Institute of Police Science
6 Sanbancho, Chiyoda-ku, Tokyo, JAPAN

INTRODUCTION

MCT118 (D1S80) locus is widely used for forensic DNA typing. Many population studies have been reported by using allelic ladder marker. However, the whole DNA sequences of each allele of MCT118 locus have not been reported. In this report the whole DNA sequence of MCT118 locus including both flanking regions and repeat regions has been revealed and the difference between different alleles has been analyzed.

METHOD

DNA extraction:
Genomic DNA was extracted from the human blood or bloodstain by phenol-chloroform method as described by Sakai (1991).
PCR amplification and purification:
PCR amplification of MCT118 locus was performed as follows:
10ng of genomic DNA was in 40ul of PCR buffer (66.7mM Tris-Cl (pH 8.3), 1.7mM $(NH_4)_2SO_4$, 1mM each dNTP, 2 mM each primer for MCT118 primer (Kasai 1990), 3mM $MgCl_2$, 0.17mg/ml BSA, 10mM 2-mercapto-ethanol, 10% DMSO, and 2U of AmpliTaq polymerase), and amplified as described by Kasai 1990.

PCR products were separated by agarose gel electrophoresis. Bands of PCR products were visualized with ethidium bromide under UV transilluminator, and then excised and purified as described by Heery 1990. Purified PCR products were cloned into the pCRII™ vector (*invitrogen*) followed with the protocol of TA cloning kit. Each cloned allele was confirmed with PCR amplification and electrophoresis, and then performed further sequencing analysis.
DNA Typing:
Amplified PCR products were separated with 5% native polyacrylamide gel electrophoresis along with allelic ladder markers precipitated with ethanol before loading (Sekiguchi 1994). Then, the gel visualized with ethidium bromide under UV transilluminator was photographed and analyzed by FragmeNT Software (Molecular Dynamics).
DNA Sequencing:
Cloned plasmids were sequenced with the reagents from the Taq DyeDeoxy Terminator Cycle Sequencing Kit and Taq Dye-primer Cycle Sequencing Kit (ABI), and analyzed with ABI 373A DNA sequencer. To confirm the sequence of each

allele, another sequencing reaction was performed with SequiTherm Long Read Kit with labeled (-29) forward primer and RV primers as the sequencing primers, and analyzed with LiCOR dNA sequencer.

RESULTS

Eleven alleles of MCT118 locus were succeeded in cloning and sequencing. PCR fragments of the cloned alleles were typed as the same repeat number with the threshold value of ±0.3 repeat, and they were appeared to be the same size.

```
allele
   14 : ABCDDE--GHI------------------I-IILG      A: TCAGC CCAA GGAAG
   16 : ABCDDE-CGHI------------------IHIILG      B: ACAGA CCACA GGCAAG
   18 : ABCDDE-CGHI---------------IHIKIILG       C: GAGGA CCACC GGAAAG
   18 : ABCDDE-CHHI---------------IHIKIILG       D: GAAGA CCACC GGAAAG
   23 : ABCD-E-CGHI---JJIIH-------IIHIKIILG      E: GAAGA CCACA GGCAAG
   24 : ABCDDE-CGHI---JJIIH-------IIHIKIILG      F: GAGGA CCACA GGCAAG
   25 : ABCDDE-CGHI---JJIIH------IIIHIKIILG      G: GAAGA CCACC GGCAAG
   27 : ABCD-E-CGHI---JJIIHIIH---IIIHIKIILG      H: GAGGA CCACC GGCAAG
   28 : ABCDDE-CGHI---JJIIJIIH---IIIHIKIILG      I: GAGGA CCACC AGGAAG
   28 : ABCDDE-CGHI---HHIIHIIH---IIIHIKIILG      J: GAAGA CCACC GGCAAG
   28 : ABCDDE-CGHI---JJIIJIIJ---IIIJIKIILG      K: GAGAA CCACC AGGAAG
   28 : ABCDDE-CGHI---JJIIHIIHIK---IHIKIILG      L: GAGGA CCACT GGAAAG
   31 : ABCDDEFCGHI--IHJIJHJIJIJIIH--IKIILG
   32 : ABCDDE-CGHI-H-HIIHIJJIIHIIHIIIKIILG
   35 : ABCDDEFCGHIIHIHIHJIJIJIKIIHKIIIHIKIILG
   5' flanking region sequence (116 bp)
      GAAAC TGGCC TCCAA ACACT GCCCG CCGTC CACGG CCGGC CGGTC CTGCG
      TGTGA ATGAC TCAGG AGCGT ATTCC CCACG CGCCA GCACT GCATT CAGAT
      AAGCG CTGGC TCAGT G
   3' flanking region sequence (32 bp)
    CCTGC AAGGG GCACG TGCAT CTCCA ACAAG AC
```
Fig. 1 The composition of the sequence of repeat units in the MCT118 locus. The repeat units are shown with the proposed nomenclature shown above.

Characterization of the MCT118 locus by nucleotide sequences revealed a fixed order of 16 bp core repeat units except 1st repeat, which is 14 bp. Figure 1 shows the first 6 repeats units from 5' end and the last 4 units from 3' end are the same stable region among alleles. However, the sequences of the core repeat units between 7th repeat from 5' end and 5th repeat from 3' end seemed to be variable among alleles, and so this region was named variable region (Fig. 1). The 16 bp sequences of core units in variable region consist of 4 kinds of core repeat units (H, I, J, K) and the arrangements of these units were seemed to have some order. Almost every same allele has same mobility in

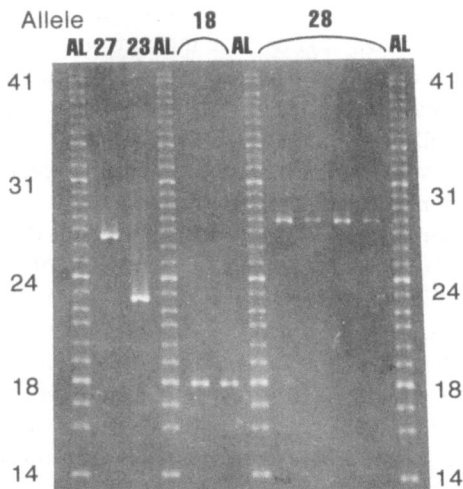

Fig. 2 The electrophoresis of cloned alleles Each 18 and 28 repeats allele is different each other. Their sequences are shown in Fig. 1

native-PAGE regardless of their different sequences in variable region (Fig. 2). However, two alleles, 23 repeat and 27 alleles, have differences in the first 6 repeats, and have slightly fast mobility in native PAGE (Fig. 2). The sequences of the 5' and 3' flanking region of the MCT118 locus were completely same among alleles. Because the ambiguity region was found in 5' flanking region, allele specific PCR was applied and determined the complete sequence. These results showed the correct length of the PCR product was 146 + 16 x N (N: number of repeat units).

DISCUSSION

At the first time, MCT118 typing had been made by calculating the repeat numbers with DNA size marker (e.g. 123 bp marker). Recently, however, allelic ladder marker of MCT118 (D1S80) locus has been available (Baechtel 1993; Perkin Elmer 1993), and it showed fast migration with its calculated molecular weight in native-PAGE (Kasai 1992; Sugiyama 1993). These results indicate the sequence of MCT118 locus may affect its migration in native-PAGE. Twenty-eight and more alleles in MCT118 locus have been already reported (Budowle 1995). Every allele was found almost the same migration with allelic ladder marker, but a few alleles that show slightly fast or slow migration with allelic marker were also found. It has been thought these different migrations might be caused by the sequence deletion within repeat units and/or the unequal sequence composition (Skowasch 1992; Sugiyama 1993; Kloosterman 1993). Several deletions were found within the core repeat units in Col2A1 VNTR (Berg 1993) and ApoB VNTR (Boerwinkle 1989). In MCT118 locus, however, no deletion was found within the core repeat units, and only replacements were found within them. This indicates abnormal migrations in MCT118 locus might be caused not by the deletion of core units but by the substitution of base in the core units. In this study, cloned 23 repeat and 27 repeat alleles have slightly fast mobility from allelic markers. No deletions were found in both alleles but the order of repeat units in stable region was different from other alleles. This implies the possibility that the difference of stable region makes mobility difference. However, some alleles like 28 repeats, which have the same repeat numbers but have different sequences in core repeat units in variable region, had no apparent different mobility in native-PAGE (Fig. 2). So, this implies the order of core units in variable region does not affect the mobility in native-PAGE. Probably, the changes of the order of core units in stable region may affect the mobility in native-PAGE.

Comparing the order of the core repeat units in each allele, the changes of the order have found only in variable region, while there is no change in stable region. The variable region consisted of only 4 kinds of core repeat units in every allele, and the increase or decrease of the repeat numbers in MCT118 locus seemed to happen not by randomly adding or deleting the core units but by concurrently adding or deleting a couple of core units. This implication may cause the discontinuous repeat numbers and the unequal distribution of allele frequency in inter- or intra-population.

REFERENCE

Baechtel F S, Smerick J B, Presley K W, Budowle B (1993) Multigenerational amplification of a reference ladder for alleles at locus D1S80. J Forens Sci 38:1176-1182

Berg ES, Olaisen B (1993) Characterization of the Col2A1 VNTR polymorphism. Genomics 16: 350-354

Boerwinkle E, Xiong W, Fourest E, Chan L (1989) Rapid typing of tandemly repeat hypervariable loci by the polymerase chain reaction : Application to the apolipoprotein B 3' hypervariable region. Proc Natl Acad Sci USA 86: 212-216

Budowle B, Baechtel F S, Smerick J B, Presley K W, Giusti A M, Parsons G, Alevy M C, Chakraborty R (1995) D1S80 Population Data in African Americans, Caucasians, Southeastern Hispanics, Southwestern Hispanics, and Orientals. J Forens Sci 40: 38-44

Heery D M, Gannon F, Powell R (1990) A simple method for subcloning DNA fragments from gel slices. Trend Genet 6: 173

Kasai K, Nakamura Y, White R (1990) Amplification of a variable number of tandem repeats (VNTR) locus (pMCT118) by the polymerase chain reaction (PCR) and its application to forensic science. J Forens Sci 35: 1196-1200

Kloosterman A D, Budowle B, Daselaar P (1993) PCR-amplification and detection of the human D1S80 VNTR locus. Amplification conditions, population genetics and application in forensic analysis. Int J Leg Med 105:257-264

Perkin Elmer (1993) AmpliFLP D1S80 PCR Amplification Kit, 1-20

Sakai I, Kasai K, Yoshida K, Mukoyama H (1991) An Improved Method for DNA isolation From Human Bloodstains and Typing of the Isolated DNA Using Single Locus VNTR Probes. Reports Nat Res Inst Pol Sci 44: 36-49

Sekiguchi K, Ikuko S, Mizuno N, Yoshida K, Kasai K, Sato H, Sueshige S (1994) Sequence analysis and characterization of allelic ladder on MCT118 locus. DNA polymorphism 2: 77-81

Skowasch K, Wiegand P, Brinkmann B (1992) pMCT118 (D1S80): a new allelic ladder and an improved electrophoretic separation lead to the demonstration of 28 alleles. Int J Leg Med 105:165-168

Sugiyama E, Honda K, Katsuyama Y, Uchiyama S, Tsuchikane A, Ota M, Fukushima H (1993) Allele frequency distribution of the D1S80 (pMCT118) locus polymorphism in the Japanese population by the polymerase chain reaction. Int J Leg Med 106: 111-114

3 Statistics

Statistical analysis of STR data

I.W.Evett[1] and J.S.Buckleton[2]

1. Forensic Science Service, Gooch St North, Birmingham, B5 6QQ, UK

2. ESR: Forensic, Mt. Albert, Private Bag 92-021, Auckland, New Zealand.

INTRODUCTION

The debate on the statistics of forensic DNA profiling has been dominated by restriction fragment length polymorphism (RFLP) data. However, conventional population genetic analyses require unequivocal identification of homozygotes and that is not, in general, possible with RFLP profiles. This has added to the air of confusion which has characterised the debate.

Fortunately, with short tandem repeat (STR) data the problem of identifying true homozygotes is minimised and this means that it has been easier to apply conventional methods of statistical analysis. This, in turn, has brought into sharper focus an issue that has troubled the authors for some time and which we discuss. In short, we question the relevance of conventional independence testing to the forensic use of profiling systems.

Classical wisdom would have it that the multiplication inherent in most methods of interpretation is only valid if the assumptions of independence are proved. We maintain that, not only is it not possible to prove the assumptions true, but they are certainly false. The essential issue is not to determine whether independence exists (it does not) but rather to assess the practical consequences of the departure from independence.

INDEPENDENCE TESTING

The basic forensic evidence transfer problem is as follows. A crime has been committed by a man who left a body fluid stain at the scene. The investigator has arrested a man whom he suspects of being the offender. A DNA profile of the crime sample is found to be indistinguishable from that of a sample provided by the suspect. How is this result to be interpreted?

Assuming - as is generally the case - that there is no question of a close relative of the suspect being involved then it is necessary to consider two competing explanations for the evidence:

C: the stain was left by the suspect
$\overline{C}$: the stain was left by an unknown man

Then it is necessary to consider the probability of the evidence given each of these hypotheses and the ratio of these two probabilities - the *likelihood ratio* (LR) - can in this situation be shown to reduce to $1/f$, where f is the frequency of the observed genotype among members of the population to which the 'unknown man' credibly belongs. This must be estimated using data from a sample of people from the relevant population.

The STR profile is a multilocus genotype and the simplest way to estimate its frequency is to multiply together the constituent allele frequency estimates both within and between loci: the recent debate has been dominated by questions about this procedure. The issue, of course, is independence and conventional wisdom calls for tests of independence. Within locus this is a test for Hardy-Weinberg proportions - often called Hardy-Weinberg equilibrium (HWE). Between locus it is a test for linkage equilibrium (LE) proportions.

Classical independence testing revolves around the concept of a *null hypothesis*. This is the postulation of a state of affairs sufficiently simple for a test statistic to be devised with a known sampling distribution. For the within-locus test, the null hypothesis will be that the genotype frequencies are identical to the Hardy-Weinberg proportions. Put another way, it is that perfect independence exists in the population under consideration. The expectations under this hypothesis are then compared with functions of the sample data by means of a test statistic which itself is compared with a probability distribution. The area underneath the probability distribution corresponding to values of the statistic more extreme than that actually observed is called a *p*-value. Small *p*-values cast doubt on the validity of the null hypothesis. The word *significant* has been associated with the *p*-value 0.05 and the idea of "statistical significance" is something which has been included in training of most scientists.

There are various problems with this approach. Not least of these is that we are testing a hypothesis which is *certainly not true*: the conditions for HWE and LE cannot exist in real human populations. The alternative hypothesis, which is given scant attention, is that the null hypothesis is false. This is hardly an interesting hypothesis for two reasons. First, we know that it is true. Second it is so vague that, although it is true, it does not tell us how to proceed with forensic casework. The null hypothesis is a precise state of independence. The alternative hypothesis is everything else!

So the essence of this is that we are testing the truth of a precise hypothesis which we know to be false against a vague hypothesis which we know to be true. Scientists believe this to be the right way because their statistical education has taught them that it is necessary for scientists to look at their problems as classical statisticians do. It's not necessary at all - indeed, forcing practical scientific problems into an artificial theoretical framework inevitably causes confusion. This is one of the reasons why most scientists hate Statistics.

Let's see what happens when we do play the significance testers' game. We carry out a test and let us assume that we accept that a particular *p*-value - typically 0.05 -is "significant". Then one of two things can happen: either the result is significant or it isn't. If it is significant then we reject the null hypothesis - hardly a surprising result because we knew it wasn't true anyway. If it's not significant then we are told - correctly - that we haven't proved the null hypothesis (but then we didn't want to prove something that we knew was false) and if we'd taken a bigger sample, or used a different test then we might have seen a "significant" result. It is a game that we can't win.

This last argument invokes the concept of "power" which says, basically, that the more powerful the test (or the bigger the database), the more likely it is to detect departures from independence. The detection comes through the *p*-value which, whatever the power of the test, tends to be used as a measure of the extent of the departure from independence: a small *p*-value is taken to imply an appreciable departure from independence.

Directing attention to possible meanings of "appreciable" is a fruitless pursuit. Our concern is with the use of the typing system in forensic casework and our question is "if we use this system in casework then to what extent may the results mislead a court?". The *p*-value is of no use here because in no case is it designed to provide any sort of measure of the practical consequences of using the independence model.

A DNA analysis is undertaken for the purpose assisting a criminal justice system in its objectives of excluding the innocent and incriminating the guilty. The greater the power of the analysis to assist the achievement of these ends, the greater the utility of the technique. But there are two possibilities which have negative utility: excluding the guilty and incriminating the innocent. The latter is rightly regarded with abhorrence and for this reason it has come to dominate the DNA debate.

If we set aside any discussion of laboratory error then an STR comparison has a theoretically zero chance of excluding the true offender. The chance of incriminating an innocent person is that of a chance match between two people. With any new technique, forensic scientists know that it is necessary to estimate PM - the probability of a match between two unrelated people - or (1-PM) (Jones, 1972), called the discriminating power. For the STR quadruplex of VWA, THO1, F13A1 and FES, PM is about 1 in 10,000 in Caucasians. Here is our first measure which contributes to an assessment of forensic utility.

CONSERVATISM

It has become accepted, and the authors must accept some of the blame, that wherever there is some doubt the 'most conservative' answer should be given in the sense that the most conservative answer is that which most favours the defendant. We now maintain that this principle is wrong and that its application leads to serious misconceptions.

There appear to be three main ideas underlying the wish to be conservative. The first, which is laudable, is an attempt to save the falsely accused suspect from conviction. The second is a search for some kind of "comfort factor" for the forensic scientist. The third is that the assumptions underlying the calculation may not be correct in the case at hand. We consider these three in turn.

Falsely accused suspect

The first of these ideas has strong intuitive appeal but appears to have no foundation in logic. It says, effectively, "we know that our technique can lead to false inclusions so we will revise our LR's downward". This is a matter of policy rather than science and adopting a deliberately conservative policy means that in every case in which the suspect is truly the offender we will understate the strength of the DNA evidence. But the policy has only negligible impact on cases in which the suspect is not the offender because in 99.99% of such cases the suspect is excluded and the LR is at its absolute minimum of zero. Safety for innocent suspects lies in very discriminating techniques, both technological and inferential.

It must be recognised that a policy of understating the evidence applies equally to the truly culpable and the truly innocent. What do we really think we have achieved? Moderate understatement of the evidence will provide only a small effect in assisting the falsely accused suspect. Perhaps we intend a massive understatement of the evidence. This renders DNA evidence essentially useless to the courts. Is this useful?

Comfort factor

The principle of conservatism, though we are not aware of its having been formally stated anywhere, seems to take the form "any plausible explanation of the evidence that most favours the defendant is to be preferred". It is a fallacy to believe that this line can make it more comfortable in court. There is a never ending line of "could be's" for creating less and less plausible situations that favour the defendant still more. Whatever the scientist does to be conservative it will always be possible for defence, perfectly legitimately, to find another scientist who will argue for a more conservative interpretation. The only way to be uniformly conservative is to report an exclusion in every case, a LR of zero is unequivocally the lowest LR that can be reported.

For a scientist to claim in evidence that his LR is conservative in that it is in some sense a lower limit of some "true LR" is to invite a cross-examination along the lines "could the true answer be as small as ...." or "how can you be sure that your LR is smaller than the true value". There is no true LR - every calculation exists within a framework of assumptions.

Validity of the assumptions

It is not possible to make any assessment of evidence without making assumptions and, as far as possible these should be made clear to the court. We suggest the following.

"The LR is my best assessment of the strength of the evidence. In making my calculations I have made assumptions and approximations in ways which I do not believe to be prejudicial to the defendant. My methods have been tested in experiments on actual data and these have included simulations of cases in which the offender and the defendant are different unrelated people. These experiments indicate that there is a small chance of my quoting a LR as big as the one I have given if the defendant is not the offender. From such experiments I estimate that on average this chance is about 1 in ...." The experiments described later shows how such an answer may be given.

TWO PRACTICAL ILLUSTRATIONS

First we consider the recent paper by Drozd et al (1994) which reports a survey of the VWA genotypes in 200 British Caucasians. The authors say "Before such a polymorphic system is used, checks are made to ensure that the chosen system is in Hardy-Weinberg equilibrium.." They duly carried out a goodness of fit test which compared the observed genotype frequencies with those expected from Hardy-Weinberg proportions. They found the result to be: "very significant (P<0.01), suggesting that the sampled population may not be in Hardy-Weinberg equilibrium." That's an unduly cautious statement - the population is most certainly not in Hardy-Weinberg equilibrium - it couldn't possibly be, because the required conditions cannot be met in real human populations.

The authors showed that the high value of the goodness of fit test statistic was caused by differences between observed and expected frequencies for the 17/17 and 16/17 genotypes. They saw 22 17/17's against an expected number of 14 and 8 16/17's against an expected 19. Is this cause for concern?

We have taken a file of 1660 British Caucasians typed at four loci which is an amalgamation of data collected by the FSS, MPFSL and Strathclyde laboratories. We have calculated the four locus genotype frequency for each sample in the combined database using the allele frequencies multiplied together for three of the loci (THO1, F13A1 and FES) but using two different methods for VWA: (a) multiplying allele frequencies and (b) using the actual observed genotype frequency. Figure 1 compares the LR's based on the two methods.

It would be difficult to expect better correspondence. The vigilant observer will point to the extreme right point which shows a two order of magnitude difference between the two calculations. This point corresponds to a single observation of genotype (12,20) and has nothing to do with the 16/17 'problem'. The independence model for VWA represents no practical disadvantage.

Figure 1.

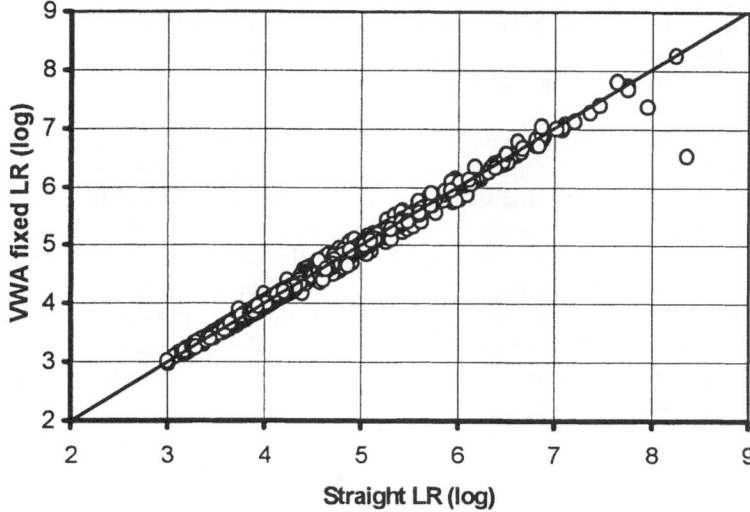

Next, here is an example from the analysis of quadruplex data on 1400 Caucasians as described in Evett, Gill, Scranage and Weir (1995). The exact test was used, determining *p*-values by shuffling the databases. The single locus tests for F13A1 and FES gave moderate *p*-values, but the two locus composite test gave a *p*-value of 0.001 - "highly significant" according to conventional wisdom. Does this result mean that we must abandon our independence model?

One way of looking deeper at the effect is to consider the individual allele specific disequilibria Weir (1990). This can be done by comparing the observed frequency of the co-occurrence of each two locus allele combination with that expected from the assumption of between-locus independence. When this is done it is found that the effect can be localised to three specific combinations as shown in the following table.

F13A1	FES	Observed	Expected
3	11	88	78.8
3	12	26.5	38.1
15	11	13.5	19.7

These are the observed and expected numbers of times that individuals carry the given pair of alleles. For two of the combinations the observed number is *smaller* than expected so, using the expected number from multiplying across the two loci is actually in the defendant's favour. For the first combination of the three the observed frequency is 12% larger than that expected: is this cause for concern? We do not believe that such a difference would make any discernible impact on the impression created on a jury.

TIPPETT EXPERIMENTS

It is not normally recognised by those who have recently entered the DNA debate that the forensic community has been thinking about issues of discrimination and evidential value for many years. In particular, an imaginative experiment was carried out by a team headed by Tippett (1968) to study the power of paint comparisons and similar methods were later used by Gaudette and Keeping (1974) for hair examination. These researchers introduced the concept of between-source comparisons as a way of investigating the forensic utility of a technique and their methods form the basis of our preferred means for evaluating DNA techniques as already described in papers such as Evett, Scranage and Pinchin (1992).

Given a file of STR data for a combination of loci, the following experiments can contribute to assessing the forensic utility of the method. For illustration we use the file of 1660 Caucasians that we described earlier. The first step is to estimate the performance of the method in cases in which the suspect is truly the person who left the crime stain. For STR's, where the matching stage is trivial (RFLP's require duplicate analyses for this stage) this is simply done by going through the file and calculating the LR for each individual using the chosen method of calculation. In this instance we have simply used allele frequencies estimated from the file itself and multiplied within and between loci. Our one concession to allowing for sampling effects is to use a default minimum frequency of 0.01. The distribution of LR's from this experiment are summarised as shown in the Figure 2.

Figure 2

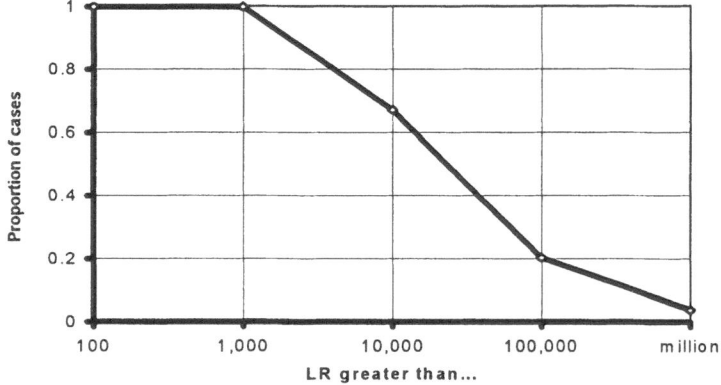

It has an unusual design so it is worth explaining it carefully. The *x* axis is in terms of LR and it is decremental in that the *y* co-ordinate is the proportion of those cases (in which the suspect truly is the person who left the crime sample) in which the LR can be expected to *exceed* the value on the *x* axis. See, for example, that in all cases the LR will be greater than 100 and that in nearly all cases it will exceed 1,000. In slightly over 65% of cases the LR will exceed 10,000 and in 20% of cases it will exceed 100,000.

But the concerns, such as they are, seem never to be about cases in which the suspect truly is the offender. They relate to cases in which the suspect is truly *not* the offender. The between-person experiment is carried out to assess the performance of the method in cases in which the suspect is not the person who left the crime stain. A file of 1660 gives us 1660.1659/2 = 1,376,970 comparisons; put another way, the simulation of about 1.4 million cases in which the offender and suspect are different people. Figure 3 summarises the output from that experiment. Note that the horizontal axis is the same as that in the previous figure. The *y* axis is now, however, in cases per 100,000. So, a fortuitous match will occur in about 1 case in 10,000, which tells us the average discriminating power of the technique. Further, we can see that a fortuitous match and a LR of

10,000 can be expected in about 1 case in 50,000. It is our view that this diagram sets the
forensic value of this technique in context.

Figure 3

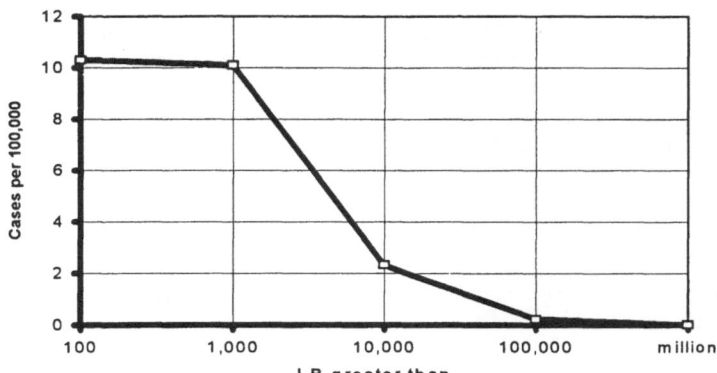

It can be shown that the number of large LR's in the between-person experiment is robust to
dependence, whether artificially induced by mixing of populations or by creating populations with
known disequilibria. It would appear that some substantial departure from the model is required
before the performance of the independence model starts to produce a large excess of big LR's.
So it might be argued by proponents of the significance testing that this analysis has low power to
detect dependence effects. This is true: but this is entirely the point - small or moderate
departures from independence have negligible impact on the forensic value of the technique.

Other methods - such as the exact test - will detect the departures from perfect independence
long before these departures have any practical consequence. The Tippett style experiment leads
to an estimate of the magnitude of the *effect* of the departure.

It has been the custom for forensic scientists to tell courts about the length of their experience,
how many cases they have done, how many comparisons they have made. The between-person
comparison experiment is an extension of this tradition. One of the authors is a firearms examiner
and one is a former document examiner: each of us can cite the hundreds of comparisons we have
made within our respective evidence types. Most of these comparisons were in cases so the true
state of affairs was unknown. With the between-person comparisons we can go much further -
we can cite millions of comparisons (Lambert et al, 1995), not made personally, of course, but on
our behalf using the power of modern computers. In these instances we know the true state of
affairs - we set the experiment up this way. We can assess our model really quite rigorously. Yet
the DNA evidence we give is no stronger in essence than the qualitative opinions we would offer
in our other fields.

DISCUSSION

We maintain that the model of perfect independence performs adequately in the context we have
been discussing though we accept that it is for each court to judge its reliability. This judgement
can be usefully informed by a description of the results of Tippett experiments.

We further maintain that classical hypothesis testing has only a small part to play in assessing reliability. We do not advocate the abandonment of testing for disequilibria but contend that the results do not address the questions of practical impact, and provide no guidance on how to proceed after testing.

We also maintain that comfort in the witness box should be based, not on deliberately diluting the evidence, but on the strength which comes from depth of understanding of the underlying issues, full experimentation, and comprehensive training. It is the function of the scientist to aim for the best assessment of the evidential strength within the circumstances of the case, supported with a plausible explanation of the reliability of that assessment.

REFERENCES

Brookfield JFY (1995) The effect of relatedness on likelihood ratios and the use of conservative estimates. Genetica: 13-19.

Drozd MA, Archard L, Lincoln PJ, Morling N, Nelleman LJ, Phillips C, Soteriou B, Syndercombe Court D (1994) An investigation of the HUMVWA31A locus in British Caucasians. For Sci Int 69: 161-170.

Evett IW, Gill PD, Scranage JK and Weir BS (1995) Establishing the robustness of STR statistics for forensic applications. Am J Hum Gen (Submitted)

Evett IW, Scranage JK and Pinchin R (1992) An illustration of the advantages of efficient statistical methods for RFLP analysis in forensic science. Am J Hum Gen 52: 498-505.

Gaudette BD and Keeping ES (1974) An attempt at determining probabilities in human scalp hair comparison. J For Sci 19: 599-606.

Jones DA (1972) Blood samples: probability of discrimination. J For Sci Soc 12: 355-359.

Lambert JA, Scranage JK and Evett IW (1995). Large scale database experiments to assess the significance of matching DNA profiles. Int J Leg Med (In press).

Tippett CF, Emerson VJ, Fereday MJ, Lawton F and Lampert SM (1968) The evidential value of the comparison of paint flakes from sources other than vehicles. J For Sci Soc 8: 61-65.

Weir BS (1990) Genetic Data Analysis, 1st edn. Sinauer, Sunderland, MA.

The Use of Likelihood Ratios in Reporting Difficult Forensic
Cases

D.L. Monahan*, S.J. Cordiner and J.S. Buckleton

Institute of Environmental Science and Research Limited (ESR),
Wellington Science Centre, PO Box 30-547, Lower Hutt, New
Zealand

INTRODUCTION

The advantages of using a likelihood ratio for forensic
evidence interpretation has long been recognised by Ian
Evett[1]. This approach has gained increasing support especially
in the areas of DNA and glass evidence interpretation.

When using a likelihood ratio approach, the probability of the
evidence is evaluated under two alternative hypotheses.

The ratio of the probabilities of the DNA evidence under each of
these two hypotheses is a measure of the weight of the
scientific evidence and is known as the likelihood ratio (LR).

$$LR = \frac{P(E|C)}{P(E|\bar{C})} = \frac{\text{probability of the DNA evidence given the semen originated from suspect}}{\text{probability of the DNA evidence given the semen originated from a random male}}$$

In this simple case the LR numerator $P(E|C)=1$.

The LR denominator, $P(E|C)$, will depend on the particular
alternative hypothesis. In the absence of any particular
defence, we use random man i.e. the suspect is innocent and the
match occurred by chance. Thus, the frequency of the profile
bands in a relevant database is used to estimate the frequency
of the profile in the population.

Unfortunately, not all forensic DNA cases are as simple as this
and often there are situations where the LR numerator $\neq$ 1. It is
these cases where reporting a "frequentist" number becomes
difficult. The following three cases illustrate this point.

1 Missing Person

Police believed a missing woman had been murdered but could find
no body. A T-shirt was found which was identified as being
similar to hers. The T-shirt had a bullet hole in the back and
was heavily blood-stained. The missing woman had a father and
brother still alive. Her mother was deceased. Reference blood
samples from her brother(B) and father(F) were provided to
compare with the blood stain from the T-shirt.

The DNA profile obtained from the blood stain on the T-shirt had
two bands. One of these bands matched a band in the victim's
father's profile(c). The other band matched what was determined
to be the maternal band of the brother's profile(a). Therefore,
the blood stain is either from a child of F and sibling of B or

alternatively the blood is from some unrelated person and the observed match has occurred by chance. The LR allows us to weight these two alternatives.

LR = probability of the DNA evidence if the blood stain is from
<u>a child of F and a sibling of B</u>
probability of the DNA evidence if the blood stain is from a random person.

It can be shown that LR = $\frac{½a + ¼(1-a)}{2ac}$ where a&c = frequency of the bands.

This equation is derived from a form of Bayes Theorem for multiple hypotheses and takes the prior probability into account:

$$P(M|B) = \frac{P(B|M)P(M)}{\sum P(B|M)P(M)}$$

Overall, it was 114 times more likely that the blood was from a child of F and sibling of B rather than from some unrelated individual.

2   Family Relationships

The accused in a rape trial was the victim's natural father, though she could not identify him. She had been raped on a hay bale in a barn. A DNA match was found between the accused's blood and the semen stain on the hay bale. At each of five loci a band in the semen stain profile matched that of the victim as well as the accused.

The reference blood sample from the accused had previously been ruled inadmissible by the court due to a consent issue. Therefore it was necessary to interpret the results without reference to that sample. The relatedness identified in the matches was used. A blood sample was obtained from the victim's mother. This showed that each of the crime bands which matched that from the victim was the paternal band.

The hypotheses for this case

LR = probability of the DNA evidence if the semen originated
<u>from the victim's natural father</u>
probability of the DNA evidence if the semen originated from another random male

The numerator is the probability that the father will pass on the paternal band (q). There is a 50% chance (probability = 0.5) he will pass on q. (Unless it is a homozygote in which case probability =1; however assuming the true father is heterozygote is conservative, i.e. favours defendant.)

The denominator is the frequency of q in the database, i.e. an estimate of the frequency with which the paternal band occurs in the population.

Over five probes the likelihood ratio was 10,000 i.e. the DNA evidence is at least 10,000 times more likely if the semen on the hay originated from the victim's natural father rather than if it originated from a man chosen at random from the New Zealand population.

3 Mixture of DNA Profiles

A woman was found raped and murdered. Blood samples were obtained from three suspects and their DNA profiles compared to the DNA profile from the victim's swabs which showed a mixture present.

The four bands in the crime samples could all be accounted for between two of the suspects tested. Therefore the possibilities are:

C1 the semen on the swabs is a mixture of semen from suspect 1 and suspect 2
C2 the semen on the swabs is a mixture of semen from suspect 1 and some other random male
C3 the semen on the swabs is a mixture of semen from suspect 2 and some other random male
C4 the semen on the swabs is a mixture of semen from two random males unrelated to the suspects

To take all four of these possibilities into account in a single LR would require estimation of prior probabilities. This can be avoided however with the following conservative approach:

For example consider suspect 1

The strongest evidence would be $LR = \dfrac{P(E|C1)}{P(E|C3)}$
This would be 1/2ab.

The most conservative evidence would be $\dfrac{P(E|C2)}{P(E|C4)}$

The numerator $P(E|C2) = 1 \times 2cd$ with cd being the frequency of suspect 2's bands in the population.

For bands with frequencies abcd, the denominator $P(E|C4) = 24$ abcd. This the calculation for mixture of two random males according to Evett[2]:

This gives $LR = {}^{2cd}/24abcd$

For this case for 5 loci it was reported as the DNA evidence was as least 113,000 times more likely if the semen from the swabs is a mixture of semen from suspect 1 and some other male rather than if it is from two other men selected at random from the racially-mixed New Zealand population.

REFERENCES:

[1] Evett, I.W., Buffery, C., Willot, G. and Stoney, D. (1991) J. For. Sci. Soc., 31(1):31-40.

[2] Evett, I.W.(1990) Forensic Science Progress 4. Springer, Berlin , pp141-179,

Identification of biological stains: probability of identity or of kinship

K. Hummel*), W. Bär**), and N. Fukshansky*)

*) Institute for Blood-Group Serology and Genetics. D-79008 Freiburg. Germany
**) Institute of Legal Medicine. CH-8057 Zürich. Switzerland

In cases of disputed identity, one should use probability values instead of only phenotypical frequencies in the population: $W_{id} = 1/[1+f(Ph)]$; W_{id} = probability of identity; $f(Ph)$ = frequencies of the stain's phenotype in the adequate population. It is sufficient to report to the court probabilities because from these the judge like anyone else can appreciate the weight connected with a decision for or against identity in the actual case.

If $W_{id} \geq 99$ % the identity is "highly probable", if $W_{id} \geq 99,73$ % identity would be "practically proven". It must be mentioned, that *Bayes' probabilities*, as W_{id} values are, can only be valid if they include a *prior probability*. According to *Bayes' Postulate*, introduced 200 years ago, an expert should hold a neutral position with respect to the pros and cons and should therefore use **a neutral prior** of 0.5 which says that the suspect "*a priori*" - that is, for the first time - has an **equal** chance of being the producer of the stain or not. In reality real producers of stains are more frequently found among the suspected people than non-producers; therefore W_{id} values, based on a prior value of 0.5, are underrated. In court this may be considered as a "factor of caution".

The formula $W_{id} = 1/[1+f(Ph)]$ is only valid for cases with only **one** suspect and only if the stain is not a "mixed" one; i.e.: deriving from only **one** individual. Most forensic cases belong to this "standard type". In the other ones the simple formula can **not** be applied.

The **special** cases can be divided into different groups, depending on which mathematical method one has to apply.

One group might include cases, in which $f(X)$ and $f(Y)$ in the formula $W_{id} = f(X)/[f(X) + f(Y)]$ are frequencies of **pedigrees**, for example in cases in which the suspect claimed that not he but his brother produced the stain (= cases of "brother objection"). In other cases it is asked, if a certain individual is the sibling of the stain's producer. In this cases $f(X)$ means the frequency of the pedigree in which the two persons are siblings, $f(Y)$ the frequency of the two persons as not related with one another. W_K is the probability of kinship. In cases of "reverse paternity" it may be asked, if a couple will be the parents of a stain's producer. Then $f(X)$ will be the frequency of the parent-child combination, and $f(Y)$ the frequency of the 3 individuals, not related with one another.

The next group of special cases are "mixed-stain" cases. These have to be divided into two subgroups: The one without participation of the victim (= the stain does not show any band of the victim), the other one **with** findings of the victim (= the stain shows DNA bands deriving from the victim).

Let us assume that in a certain case of mixed stain two individuals are the producers of the stain, but only one suspect was arrested. The judge's question is: What is the probability that the suspect is one of the producers? The frequencies approach will never enable to give a reasonable answer because there are two *hypotheses* to consider: "The suspected and an unknown produced the stain (=X)" and "Two unknown individuals are the producers of the stain (=Y)".

In another case arised the question, if two suspects (A;B) could be the producers of a stain. Then there exist four possible *hypotheses*:
1. A and B are the producers of the stain;
2. A and an unknown are the producers of the stain;
3. B and an unknown are the producers of the stain;
4. Two unknowns are the producers of the stain.

One has to calculate frequencies for all the four *hypotheses* - system for system. The final frequencies are reached by addition of the partial frequencies. Plausibilities for each *hypothesis* are found by comparison: $f(1) + f(2) + f(3) + f(4) = 1$. Calculations which have to be made by head are time consuming. A computer program does not exist as yet.

In the group of **mixed stains in which bands from the victim were found** one has to distinguish 4 different possibilities (also in combinations)
cases with one suspect;
cases with more then one suspect;
cases with one victim;
cases with more than one victim.

Table 1 shows the formulas of W_{id} for 5 different categories of band constellations found in mixed stains, this for cases with **one** suspect and **one** victim. Cases which are more complex (**more** than one suspect or/and **more** than one victim) need proper formulas, which are to be constructed depending on the special situation of the actual case.

Table 1: Formulas for calculate W_{id} in cases with mixed stains in which the victim participates

constell.	bands	frequencies	mixed stain	victim	suspect	formula
No.1	A	a	+	+	-	$W_{id} = 1/(1+2cd)$
	B	b	+	+	-	
	C	c	+	-	+	
	D	d	+	-	+	
No.2	A	a	+	+	-	$W_{id} = 1/(1+2bc)$
	B	b	+	-	+	
	C	c	+	-	+	
					or or	
No.3	A	a	+	+	- - +	$W_{id} = 1/\{1+2c[c+2(a+b)]\}$
	B	b	+	+	- + -	
	C	c	+	-	+ + +	
					or or	
No.4	A	a	+	+	+ + -	$W_{id} = 1/[1+(a+b)^2]$
	B	b	+	+	- + +	
					or	
No.5	A	a	+	+	- +	$W_{id} = 1/[1+(b^2+2ab)]$
	B	b	+	-	+ +	

It has to be emphasized, that W_{id} values were always **lower** when taking into account the victim's bands found in the stain. It is therefore indispensable to include the victim's bands in any biostatistical evaluation of stain results with regard to statements about their identity with possible producers.

Summary: In usual cases of disputed identity, one should use probability values instead of only phenotypical frequencies in the population.

If the case is more complicated, such as one with blood relationship between the involved persons or with mixed stains (with or without bands from the victim), then the probability of the *null hypothesis* will be defined by $f(X)/[f(X)+f(Y)]$ and the probability of the *counter hypothesis* by $f(Y)/[f(X)+f(Y)]$.

The frequencies $f(X)$ and $f(Y)$ can be calculated by head or by computer using an appropriate program (like the *kinship program* of Ihm and Hummel 1975). A further possibility is to allow our Institute in Freiburg to conduct the biostatistical evaluation of the findings in such an unusual case.

Reference:
Ihm P, Hummel K (1975) Ein Verfahren zur Ermittlung der Vaterschaftswahrscheinlichkeit aus Blutgruppenbefunden unter beliebiger Einbeziehung von Verwandten. Z ImmunForsch 149: 406-416

Decision-making in paternity diagnostics using SLPs

Evaluation based on a three-year material

B. Olaisen and M. Stenersen

Institute of Forensic Medicine, University of Oslo, Noway

INTRODUCTION

A number of factors represent a challenge to the establishment of a sound theoretical statistical basis for decision-making in paternity diagnostics with hyperpolymorphic minisatellite loci; for example the degree of variation itself, the "pseudo-continous" allele distribution, the choice of matching criteria, the influence of kinship, and the presence of considerable mutation rates (see e.g. Cohen 1990, Chakraborty 1991, Lewontin and Hartl 1991, Morton 1992, Roeder 1994).

We wanted to use empirical data to test if the product rule, applied on match/nonmatch typing results obtained with hyperpolymorphic SLPs, is invalidated. If it is not, and if a sufficient number of extremely informative markers is chosen, the power of this typing approach could pave the way for considerable reductions in the tedious casework evaluation procedures in common use.

MATERIAL AND METHODS

Material: Blood samples from 3431 (mother)/child/man pairs or triplets in consecutive paternity cases in Norway (1992, 1993, and 1994). Cases where case information indicated cosanguinity between the man and the true father (6 cases) were excluded.

Genetic markers: 5 SLPs: D2S44 (probe YNH24), D7S21 (g3), D7S22 (MS31), D12S11 (MS43A), and D14S13 (CMM101).

Methodology: DNA extraction (Miller 1988), Southern technique using EDNAP standards, HinfI and chemiluminescence/p32 detection.

Typing procedure: Typing as match (M) or nonmatch (NM) was performed independently by two experienced persons, by a manual procedure. Visual comparison between fragments in adjacent lanes was employed, using fragment gel positions within 0.5 mm as match criterion.

Subdivision of material: The material described was divided into one of nonfathers (921 men), and one of fathers (2510 men) by the following procedure: Cases with the type combinations 4M1MN, 3M2MN, and 2M3MN were analysed with three more SLPs (probes MS1, B6.7 and MS205) and/ or a battery of STRs), whereby an unambigous establishment of the paternity state was obtained in each of these 103 cases. Having experienced no nonfathers among 82 men with the 4M1MN combination, we assumed that there were no nonfathers among the 2424 men with 5M either. Similarly, since there were no fathers among 16 men with 2M3NM, we ascertained all 175 with 1M4NM and all 729 with 5NM to the group of fathers.

RESULTS AND DISCUSSION

In table 1 is shown the typing results with each of the SLPs in the 2510 fathers. Studies indicate that the probability that a true match is typed a nonmatch by the present procedure is less than one in one thousand, and more than 80 of the 89 nonmatches in fathers have been shown to represent true mutations (data not given here). The narrow limits for a match is therefore not to a noticeable degree influenced by such "false nonmatches". They do, however, leed to a relative high number of nonmatches caused by small mutations.

Table 1	TYPING RESULTS OF EACH SLP IN 2510 FATHERS					
SLP	D2S44	D7S21	D7S22	D12S11	D14S13	AVG.
NONMATCH	10	22	32	5	20	18
NM RATE	0,004	0,009	0,013	0,002	0,008	0,007

Table 2 demonstrates the results in the 921 nonfathers. Applying the present matching criteria yields a high power of detecting allele differences. The probability that a nonfather has at least one SLP with a NM result is extremely high (0.99999984).

Table 2	TYPING RESULTS OF EACH SLP IN 921 NONFATHERS					
SLP	D2S44	D7S21	D7S22	D12S11	D14S13	AVG.
NONMATCH	884	885	879	856	891	879
NM RATE	0,960	0,961	0,954	0,929	0,967	0,954

Combined typing results in the total material of 3431 man/child pairs as well as in each of the two subgroups of fathers and nonfathers are given in Table 3. For the latter two groups are also given the expected distribution of type combinations, applying the product rule on average match-/nonmatch rates in each of the five loci applied.

MATCH/NONMATCH COMBINATION	NO. OF PAIRS	FATHERS		NONFATHERS	
		obs.	exp.	obs.	exp.
5 M, 0 NM	2424	2424	2422	0	10^{-4}
4 M, 1 NM	82	82	87	0	10^{-2}
3 M, 2 NM	5	4	1.15	1	0.75
2 M, 3 NM	16	0	10^{-2}	16	16
1 M, 4 NM	175	0	10^{-5}	175	175
0 M, 5 NM	729	0	10^{-8}	729	729

Table 3   TYPING RESULTS IN 3431 MAN/CHILD PAIRS WITH 5 SLPs: D2S44, D7S21, D7S22, D12S11, AND D14S13

In the group of fathers, there is a statistically not significant surplus og 3M2NM pairs. The typing of the 82 4M1NM pairs in three additional SLPs, however, did not give indication of any tendencies towards multiple mutation (independence in mutation rate between these loci) (data not shown). Expected numbers in each type group in nonfathers are in very good accordance with expectations.

The present evaluation indicates that the use of the product rule is not grossly invalidated when applied to SLP locus specific average match- and nonmatch rates in fathers and nonfathers. This may allow for a simple decision-making procedure in paternity casework. In Table 4, paternity indices are based on the theoretical frequency of each match/nonmatch combination in the present groups of fathers and nonfathers, and by applying the product rule. Nothing else known about the typing results, the paternity index of a 5M combination is about 6 millions. Observations of the distribution of individually calculated paternity indices (based on allele frequencies) indicate that the individual paternity index of a 5M type practically never will be less than 10^5 (data not shown). In our opinion, this type combination - occuring in 71% of the man/child pairs - could ordinarily make a sound basis for establishing paternity. Similarly, the nonpaternity indices in the 1M4NM and 5NM combinations could make the basis for a decision of nonpaternity. This means that 97% of the cases is solved by employing the match/nonmatch combination of the five SLPs. For the 4M1NM (2% of the cases) and 2M3NM (0.5% of the cases) combination the addition of for instance the STR triplex analysis with a combined nonmatch rate in nonfathers of 99.77% (Dupuy and Olaisen, this conference), would raise indices to the level found in the former combinations. The 2M3NM combination is obviously practically noninformative as to the paternity status of the man, and must be solved using additional genetic markers (about 2 cases a year in the present material) .

Table 4 PATERNITY INDEX AND "NON-PATERNITY INDEX" WITH 5 SLPs: D2S44 D7S21 D7S22 D12S11 D14S13			
MATCH/NONMATCH COMBINATION	PATERNITY INDEX	NON-PATERNITY INDEX	PERCENT OF MEN
5 M, 0 NM	$6*10^6$		71
4 M, 1 NM	$2*10^3$		2
3 M, 2 NM	0,6	1,8	0,2
2 M, 3 NM		$6*10^3$	0,5
1 M, 4 NM		$3*10^7$	5
0 M, 5 NM		10^{11}	21

CONCLUSIONS

The present evaluation of a large paternity case material shows that the distribution of match/nonmatch combinations in 5 SLP is in good accordance with expectations based on match/nonmatch typing rates of each SLP and the use of the product rule. We argue that paternity diagnostics could be performed without any fragment sizing, allele frequency determinations or further individual case statistics.

REFERENCES

Chakraborty R (1991) Statistical interpretation of DNA typing data. Am J Hum Genet 49: 895-897
Cohen JE (1990) DNA fingerprinting for forensic identification. Am J Hum Genet 49: 358-368
Lewontin RC, Hartl DL (1991) Population genetics in forensic DNA typing. Science 254:1745-1750
Miller SA (1988) A simple salting out procedure for extracting DNA from human nucleated cells. Nucleic Acid Res 16(3): 1215-1217
Morton NE (1992) Genetic structure of forensic populations. Proc Natl Acad Sci USA 89: 2556-2560
Roeder K (1994) DNA fingerprinting: A review of the controversy. Statistical Science 222-278

Hardy-Weinberg Equilibrium in RFLP Databases

Charles H. Brenner
DNA·VIEW
2486 Hilgard Avenue, Berkeley, California 94709, USA
email: cbrenner@ccnet.com

INTRODUCTION

Population data of RFLP fragment sizes often shows an excess of homozygosity compared to the expectation based on Hardy-Weinberg equilibrium, a fact that has potential repercussions on the use of DNA for identification in criminal work. Three explanations have been suggested:

(i)   binning error due to band coalescence (Brenner & Morris 1990),
(ii)   bands run off the gel (Chakraborty et al, 1994) or are overlooked, and of course
(iii)   disequilibrium in nature (Green & Lander 1991, Giesser & Johnson 1993).

The principal results this paper are these:

A.   The mechanism of (i) is explained, and a method of analysis (which eluded us in 1990) is given to get around it.

B.   Analysis of a very large collection of data permits a fair perspective on the overall situation. No single explanation is adequate to explain apparent excess homozygosity, but mostly it is explained by (i).

MATERIALS & METHODS

Databases were accumulated over a six year period from laboratories in the United States and Europe. Most of the data was collected using the DNA·VIEW™ software. In all 228 databases from 20 laboratories were analyzed for the study, covering 13 racial and ethnic groups, 27 probes, and three restriction enzymes. A total of 247,000 people/probe combinations are represented.

Testing whether the rate of homozygosity in a gel -analyzed RFLP system conforms to the Hardy-Weinberg condition of random assortment is confounded by several factors. The first difficulty is the effectively continuous nature of the fragment size spectrum, which precludes a direct computation of $\sum p^2$. The problem thus arises how to define homozygosity for purposes of a test. One natural way is to call a person homozygous whenever the person's two bands are sufficiently close as to merge (or "coalesce"). This approach has been tried (Brenner & Morris 1990, Lander 1990) but coalescence is so difficult to predict that the method is useless in practice. Finally, in desperation, one considers the distasteful possibility of forcing the round peg of continuous fragment sizes into the square hole of size classes called "bins." Therefore for each database a set of up to 20 bins were determined such that they would have roughly equal numbers of fragments, subject to the proviso that no bin should be too narrow. However a subtle but serious difficulty arises.

DISCUSSION & RESULTS

Binning error due to band coalescence

To see the problem, suppose that in some RFLP system a population of four people have the fragment lengths, in bases, as shown in **Table 1**. The initial digit is emphasized to suggest binning by 1000's. From the point of view of the implied allele categories the four people thus have genotypes *1,1*, *1,2*, *1,2*, and *2,2*. Insofar as only four genotypes can suggest Hardy-Weinberg equilibrium, these do.

Table 1

*1*331,*1*728
*1*995,*2*001
*2*222,*1*111
*2*468,*2*345

However, if the data is measured by gel electrophoresis the genotypic categories will not be correctly inferred. The two bands for the second person will coalesce into a single band (perhaps a bit fat), and will therefore be typed either as *1,1* or as *2,2*, but certainly not as *1,2*. The collection of phenotypes thus may be *1,1*, *1,1*, *1,2*, and *2,2*. In any case the number of pseudo-homozygotes[1] rises from two to three in the transition from nature to observation.

It is worth being clear that the effect is unlike measurement error, which misclassifies as many bands in one direction as in the other. The binning error from coalescence creates a bias in collecting data: when two bands are near each other on opposite sides of a bin boundary one band in effect sucks the other across, whereas there is no compensating mechanism in the opposite direction that would tend to separate two bands that are really in the same bin.

It seems likely that the simple mechanism just explained has not been widely understood. Giesser & Johnson (1993) and Green (1992) guessed that the effect would be insignificant when the bins are large, which is false. Pseudo-homozygosity still can easily be inflated by 15-30%. Lander (1990) said that he had allowed for "the effect of coalescence" but he didn't. Chakraborty et al (1994) tried to explain away all the apparent excess as due to missing bands, which is impossible. Only Devlin et al (1990) correctly, albeit indirectly, circumvent the problem.

In any event the consequence is that Wahlund's (1928) test -- comparing the observed to expected number of people with two bands in the same bin -- is useless for RFLP data.

A Modification of the Wahlund Test

Another way to look at the difficulty with the Wahlund test is depicted in **Figure 1**. Under the classification of fragment sizes into bins 1, 2, ... discussed above, each person has a binned phenotype like *i,j*, represented by a square or, if *i=j*, a triangle. Band coalescence causes some *i+1,i* and *i,i-1* genotypes to cross a heavy black boundary line and turn into an *i,i* phenotypes. Therefore the binned data is biased toward triangles, i.e. pseudo-homozgotes. Moreover the extent of the misclassification bias is unpredictable, so there is no adequate way to estimate the number of measurements expected to fall into the triangular regions under the hypothesis of Hardy-Weinberg equilibrium.

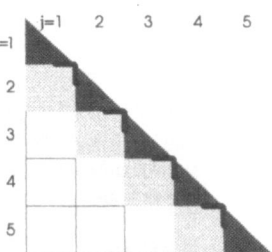

Figure 1 Modified Wahlund Test

However, the augmented shaded area, obtained by also including the sub-diagonal, *can* be estimated, because there is no systematic misclassification around the new boundary. Therefore, a *Modified Wahlund Test* can be performed using the straightforward procedure that fails for a Wahlund test. In order to compare the results, we'll perform both tests at once.

Let n_{ij} be the number of people counted in bin *i,j*, N be the total number of people, and p_i=band frequency in bin *i*. Then $O = \sum_{0 \le i-j \le \theta} n_{ij}$ and $E = N \sum_{|i-j| \le \theta} p_i p_j$ represent the observed and expected (assuming HWE and

neglecting any bias in binning) numbers to fall in a shaded area, where $\theta=1$ for the modified Wahlund test, and putting $\theta=0$ would give the Wahlund test. **Table 2** compares O vs. E using a binomial model and 1-tailed significance test, for some representative databases.

The new test is successful in showing that in some (but not in all) databases any appearance of excess homozygosity is definitely just factitious -- that is, not reflecting nature (iii) nor even laboratory procedures (ii) but is only an artifact (i) that arises from introducing bins for analysis and using them carelessly.

---

1   homozygote relative to the binning scheme -- i.e. having two fragments in the same bin

Table 2 Analysis of homozygote excess for typical databases

	Database	people N	Wahlund test, $\theta=0$			modified test, $\theta=1$		
			O=obs homoz	% excess	signif level	O=near homoz	% excess	signif level
g3	Hin Caucasian	300	44	140%	<0.001	71	40%	0.001
pYNH24	Hin Black	146	23	190	<0.001	37	59	0.001
EFD52	Hae Black	16523	1045	22%	<0.001	2484	0%	0.4
EFD52	Hae Caucasian	12779	1111	31	<0.001	2251	-2	0.8
pH30	Hae Chinese	276	25	79	0.002	47	15	0.2
g3	Hin Caucasian	1220	77	7%	0.3	191	0%	0.5
pH30	Hae Black	2240	116	4	0.4	319	-2	0.7
TBQ7	Hae Chinese	120	6	-6	0.6	17	-9	0.7
EFD52	Hae Hispanic	466	26	-3	0.6	62	-14	0.9

Significance level = likelihood to observe so much homozygosity by chance if HWE obtains.
% excess = (O-E)/E.

SUMMARY AND CONCLUSIONS

i. A quarter of the 228 databases, represented by the middle group in Table 1, have an apparently significant (using $\theta=0$) excess of homozygosity that can persuasively be explained away (significance level using $\theta=1$) as binning error. There is no reason to be suspicious of these databases from a forensic point of view.

ii. One sixth, like the first two in Table 1, have an excess beyond binning error. For many of them it is reasonable to suspect running off the gel. For example most of the databases for the g3 probe, which is well-known for missing bands (Niels Morling, personal communication), fall into this category. However, case-by-case followup and careful analysis will be necessary.

iii. The remaining 50+% of the databases both individually and as a group show no statistically significant excess of homozygotes even under the incorrect, Wahlund, test. This is an interesting fact that also requires followup analysis.

Acknowledgments

Thanks to Amanda Soser, Niels Morling, and other members of the DNA·VIEW Users' Group, to Lotte Henke, Theresa Aulinskas, and to the FBI, for friendly collaboration and sharing of data.

REFERENCES

Brenner CH, Morris JW (1990) Paternity Index Calculations in Single Locus Hypervariable DNA Probes: Validation and Other Studies. In: Promega Corporation (pubs) Proc for the International Symposium on Human Identification 1989, Madison, Wisconsin, pp21-53

Chakraborty R, Zhong Y, Jin L, Budowle B (1994) Nondetectability of Restriction Fragments and Independence of DNA Fragment Sizes Within and Between Loci in RFLP Typing of DNA. Am J Hum Genet 55:391-401

Devlin B, Risch N, Roeder K (1990) No Excess of Homozygosity at Loci Used for DNA Fingerprinting. Science 249:1416-1420

Geisser S, Johnson W (1993) Testing Independence of Fragment Lengths within VNTR Loci. Am J Hum Genet 53:1103-1106

Green P (1992) Population Genetic Issues in DNA Fingerprinting. Am J Hum Genet 50:440-441

Green P, Lander ES (1991) Forensic DNA Tests and HW Equilibrium. Science 253:1038-1039

Lander ES (1991) Lander Reply. Am J Hum Genet 49:899-903

Wahlund S (1928) Zusammensetzung von Populationen usw. Hereditas 11:65-106

SEDNA: A computer program for semiparametric estimation of densities and match probabilities in DNA forensic identification and paternity cases

D. Alonso[1], R. Cao[1], A. Carracedo[2] and E. Valverde[3]
[1]Dept. of Mathematics, Faculty of Computing Sciences, University of A Coruña, Spain
[2]Institute of Legal Medicine, Faculty of Medicine, University of Santiago de Compostela, Spain
[3]PharmaGen, S.A., C/ Calera, 3, Tres Cantos, Madrid, Spain

Recent approaches to estimate match probabilities in VNTR loci (Devlin et al. 1992; Berry et al. 1992; Evett et al. 1992) have made use of density functions. In this communication we present a computer program, based on a model previously reported, which shows very good practical results. This model relies on a semiparametric estimation of density functions (Valverde et al. 1992) and a subsequent calculation of the probability of a match between 2 bands by means of a reformulation of the Bayes theorem in terms of the conditional density function. The model has been further extended to the comparison of two-banded profiles, taking account of the correlation observed in the measurement errors of each pair of bands. This method has been implemented in C language, resulting in the so-called SEDNA program.

SEDNA uses an initial database containing information with measured fragment lengths and their correspondent true values to calibrate the experimental error. This adjustment can also be made from data of allelic controls analyzed repeatedly. A variety of databases pertaining to different loci, different restriction enzymes or different populations can be handled by SEDNA. This allows computation of the semiparametric density estimation of the fragment length as well as match probabilities. The program facilitates the use of information about relatives in paternity cases and also produces graphical outputs.

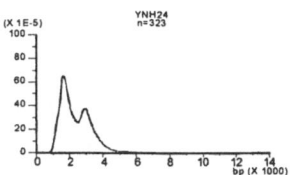

Figure 1. Plot of the density function of fragment lengths for the VNTR polymorphism HaeIII/YNH24 in the Spanish population.

To assess the practical performance of this method we carried out an experiment, similar to that described by Evett et al. (1992), using a data set of 229 individuals analyzed in duplicate. From this experiment we extracted information about comparisons both between persons and within persons. In the total of 26335 comparisons made using three probes (MS31, MS43a and YNH24) we didn't find any incorrect matches or non- matches. It is worth noting in this setting that previous calibration of the experimental error has a remarkable influence on the probability values, however this effect does not lead to an incorrect assignment of matches or non-matches (Figure 2).

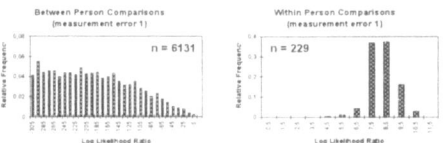

Figure 2A. Measurement error = 0.92 %. In the between person comparisons, 19975 (76.5 %) of 26106 values tested were outwith log likelihood ratio capacity of computer, therefore assumed = 0.

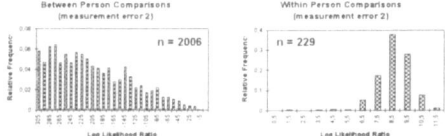

Figure 2B. Measurement error = 0.745 %. In the between person comparisons, 24100 (92.3 %) of 26106 values tested were outwith log likelihood ratio capacity of computer, therefore assumed = 0.

PROGRAM FUNCTION

SEDNA is a computer software package (programmed in C language) that carries out several calculations concerning the estimation of the experimental error, as well as the density function of the fragment length (which is also plotted) and match probabilities in either one-allele (disputed paternity) or two-allele (forensic identification) cases.

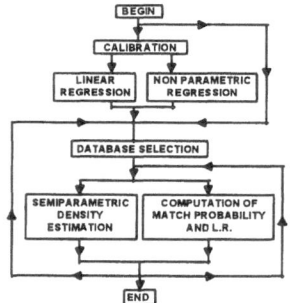

Figure 3. Flow diagram of SEDNA.

A number of different methods are available in the program to compute the estimated variance of the experimental error. Among them we emphasize the non parametric regression and the linear regression approximations to address that problem. This calibration for the program is only executed whenever the data concerning true and observed fragment lengths are updated for a particular laboratory.

The second part of the program is devoted to the estimation itself. A semiparametric estimation of the density function is computed and plotted for the user's selected database. Furthermore, given the observed fragment lengths the match probability is computed by the program in either one-allele or two-allele situations. An important technical problem in this part of the program relates to the achievement of fast computation by the kernel method for estimating the density function. This has been addressed by using the fast Fourier transform algorithm.

REFERENCES

Berry, DA; Evett, IW and Pinchin, R (1992) Statistical inference in crime investigations using deoxyribonucleic acid profiling. Appl Statist 41:499-531

Devlin, B; Risch, N and Roeder K (1992) Forensic inference from DNA fingerprints, J Am Stat Assoc 87:337-350

Evett, IW; Scranage, JK and Pinchin R (1992) An efficient statistical procedure for interpreting DNA single locus profiling data in crime cases. J Forensic Sci Soc 32:307-326

Valverde, E; Cabrero, C; Cao, R; Rodríguez-Calvo, MS; Díez, A; Barros, F; Alemany, J and Carracedo, A (1993) Population genetics of three VNTR polymorphisms in two different Spanish populations. Int J Leg Med 105:251-256

DNA PCR POLYMORPHISMS IN PATERNITY TEST PROTOCOLS.
A BIOSTATISTICAL APPROACH

Domenici R, Fornaciari S, Nardone M, Rocchi A, Spinetti I, Venturi M, Bargagna M

Department of Biomedicine, Section of Legal Medicine, University of Pisa, Italy

INTRODUCTION

Over the years there has been a continuous increase of the number of genetic polymorphisms which have become available for paternity testing. The range has extended from the red blood cell groups, through serum proteins and erythrocyte enzymes polymorphisms to white cells antigens of the HLA system. With these "classical" markers, the use of several laboratory techniques is needed to achieve a sufficiently high standard of efficiency both in paternity exclusion and inclusion.

In the last few years the analysis of DNA polymorphisms has been routinely introduced into the forensic haemogenetics laboratories. Due to the very high level of variability and to the great number of these novel polymorphisms, just one well defined technique (e.g.: Southern blot hybridisation of multilocus minisatellites, single locus profiling, PCR essay) could be regarded as an exhaustive way to investigate a paternity relationship. As a consequence, also the variability among protocols adopted in different laboratories is considerably increased .

Until 1991, the Forensic Haemogenetics Laboratory of the University of Pisa used, in disputed parentage cases, six blood cell groups (AB0, RH, MNS, K, FY and JK), nine serum protein systems (HP, GC, TF, PI, C3, BF, PLG, IGHG and IGK) and eight red cell enzyme polymorphisms (ACP1, PGM1, AK, ADA, 6PGD, GPT, ESD and GLO). Since then, we included PCR essay. Currently, we use seven DNA polymorphisms: DQA1, D1S80, YNZ22, APOB, TH01, VWA and FES. Shortage of manpower resources and cost-benefit considerations discourage us, a small laboratory, from the routinary typing of 30 different systems for every paternity case.

In this paper our criteria of choice of polymorphisms are discussed. The biostatistical evaluation of efficiency in paternity exclusion plays a predominant role.

MATERIALS AND METHODS

Allele frequencies of DQA1, APOB, D1S80, YNZ22, TH01, VWA and FES polymorphisms were estimated from adequate population samples (n=110-165) of healthy individuals born in Tuscany (APOB: see Domenici *et al* 1994a, TH01: see Domenici *et al* 1994b, FES: see Tagliabracci *et al* 1995; other polymorphisms: unpublished data). The average power of exclusion (A) for the PCR-based systems has been calculated according to Garber and Morris (1983).

The data about allele frequencies of the 23 classical polymorphisms in Italy and their average power of exclusion were found in Piazza *et al* (1989) and in Bargagna and Domenici (1988).

Statistical parameters of the 7 PCR-based polymorphisms have been compared to those of the 23 traditional genetic markers. In this regard three parameters were taken into account:

cum A≥1 = cumulative chance of finding at least a single incompatibility
cum A≥2 = cumulative chance of finding at least two incompatibilities
cum A≥3 = cumulative chance of finding at least three incompatibilities

The last two indexes have been obtained by an iterative calculation, using the equations:

$$\Delta cum\ A{\geq}2 = A\ (cum\ A{\geq}1 - cum\ {\geq}A2)$$

$$\Delta cum\ A{\geq}3 = A\ (cum\ A{\geq}2 - cum{\geq}A3)$$

where $\Delta cum A{\geq}2$ and $\Delta cum A{\geq}3$ are the increase of power of exclusion for each new system that is added to the analysis, and A in the power of exclusion of the new system.

RESULTS AND DISCUSSION

Table 1 shows the allelic frequencies of DQA1, D1S80, APOB, YNZ22, TH01, VWA and FES in Tuscany, and their average power of exclusion (A). The mean value of A, in these polymorphisms, is about 60%. Only in FES system A is less than 50%. In contrast, the higher A value in classical systems is 33% of PGM1 and HP subtypes. Moreover, only 7 out of 23 traditional systems (RH, MNS, HP, GC, PI, ACP1, PGM1) have A higher than 25%.

Table 1: Allelic frequencies and average power of exclusion of seven PCR-based systems

DQA1	n = 110	TH01	n = 165	VWA	n = 110	FES	= 162
1.1	.154	6	.239	14	.091	10	.287
1.2	.186	7	.182	15	.105	11	.358
1.3	.082	8	.136	16	.209	12	.278
2	.146	9	.155	17	.282	13	.068
3	.086	9.3	.261	18	.241	14	.009
4	.345	Rare	.027	19	.064	Rare	.000
				Rare	.008		
A =	.595	A =	.599	A =	.599	A =	.445

APO B	n = 128	YNZ22	n=165			D1S80	n = 148
31	.074	1	.061	14	.007	28	.044
33	.070	2	.164	16	.003	29	.057
35	.266	3	.118	18	.162	30	.014
36	.008	4	.270	19	.003	31	.078
37	.363	5	.061	20	.020	32	.014
39	.070	6	.030	21	.034	34	.007
41	.012	7	.021	22	.037	35	.007
43	.004	8	.033	23	.010	36	.007
45	.012	9	.103	24	.429	37	.007
47	.047	10	.073	25	.027	40	.003
49	.066	11	.021	26	.020	>41	.010
51	.008	12	.039				
		13	.003				
		14	.003				
A =	.583	A =	.775			A =	.596

Table 2: The cumulative power of exclusion of different combinations of systems

# Systems	cum A≥1	cum A≥2	cum A≥3
23 (Traditional)	99.10%	94.22%	81.79%
7 (PCR-based)	99.87%	98.30%	90.77%
30 (Overall)	99.999%	99.98%	99.82%
20 (Selected)	99.996%	99.93%	99.48%
14 (Selected)	99.99%	99.82%	98.75%

Table 2 shows individual an overall values of cumA≥1, cumA≥2 and cumA≥3 in the traditional and PCR-based polymorphisms. Even if the 7 DNA polymorphisms appear to be more informative than the 23 traditional ones, either the first ones or the second ones alone could be regarded as a self-sufficient way to investigate a paternity relationship, on the ground of cumA≥1 values. Nevertheless, its as been a hallmark of paternity testing that in any situation scientists have always preferred to obtain evidence of non-paternity on more than one test system (for a recent review on criteria for paternity investigations, see: Mayr and Rossi 1993). So, cumA≥2 seems to be a better parameter than cumA≥1 for assessing the efficiency of conventional systems to provide evidence of non-paternity. By using our combination of traditional systems, it is expected that in about 6% of parentage cases involving non-fathers further investigation is needed.

As far as DNA systems are concerned, we feel that - in the present state of insufficient knowledge about their mutation rates - at least three incompatibilities should be obtained as a solid proof of paternity exclusion.

Table 2 shows that in about 10% of cases of non-paternity it is not possible to achieve three incompatibilities by using only the 7 PCR-based systems.

The whole repertoire of 30 test systems (both conventional and DNA) would satisfy our rather conservative standards (see table 2), albeit with an unfavourable cost-benefit rate. Comparable figures can be obtained through our present protocol, including 20 selected systems (ABO, RH, MNS, HP, GC, TF, PI, C3, ACP1, PGM1, ESD, GLO, GPT, DQA1, D1S80, APOB, YNZ22, TH01, VWA and FES). Also a more time and money saving protocol, based on 14 systems only - exclusively chosen on the ground of biostatistical criteria (A>25% as a threshold: RH, MNS, HP, GC, PI, ACP1, PGM1, DQA1, D1S80, APOB, YNZ22, TH01, VWA and FES) - would be appropriate. But we prefer to keep some redundancy in the number of conventional polymorphisms. This allows to obtain in the large majority of non-paternity cases (97%, in our protocol) incompatibilities in both traditional and DNA systems, and also to preserve the technical abilities acquired by laboratory staff over many years.

The goal of any forensic haemogenetics laboratory is to produce results that could not to be reasonably questioned in court trials. In our opinion, this means that we should reach either a probability of paternity higher than 99,8-99,9% or 2-3 genetic incompatibilities. $CumA{\geq}1$ is the key biostatistical parameter to evaluate the efficiency of test systems used both in exclusion and in inclusion (the mean value of probability of paternity [W] is mathematically related to $cumA{\geq}1$: see Nijenhuis 1979 and Morris 1983), but in our experience also $cumA{\geq}2$ and $cumA{\geq}3$ proved to be useful in choosing the more convenient protocol.

REFERENCES

Bargagna M, Domenici R (1988) L'esclusione di paternità. In: Bargagna M, Domenici R, Giari A (eds) Applicazioni medico-legali della immunoematologia. Masson, Milano pp 89-103

Domenici R, Fornaciari S, Nardone M, Ricciardi MF, Spinetti I, Venturi M, Bargagna M (1994a) Study of the Apo B Polymorphism in Tuscany (Italy). Adv Forens Haemogenet 5:493-495

Domenici R, Nardone M, Spinetti I, Venturi M, Bargagna M, Cucurachi N, Buscemi L, Regazzi E, Ferrara D, Previderè C, Peloso G, Tagliabracci A, Mencarelli R (1994b) The distribution of HumTH01 Polymorphism in Northern and Central Italy. Adv Forens Haemogenet 5:496-498

Garber RA, Morris JW (1983) General equations for the average power of exclusion for genetic systems of n codominant alleles in one-parent and no-parent cases of disputed parentage. In: Walker RH (ed) Inclusion probabilities in parentage testing. AABB, Arlington, VA, pp 277-280

Mayr WR, Rossi U, eds (1993) Basic methods and criteria for paternity investigations. Proceedings Educational Course following 15th Int Congr Int Soc Forens Haemogenet

Morris JW (1983) Relationships between power of exclusion and probability of paternity. In: Walker RH (ed) Inclusion probabilities in parentage testing. AABB, Arlington, VA, pp 267-275

Nijenhuis LE (1979) Some mathematical aspects of the paternity index (I=X/Y) and their application in a statistical material. Proceedings 8th Int Congr Soc Forens Haemogenet pp 584-589

Piazza A, Olivetti E, Barbanti M, Reali G, Domenici R, Giari A, Benciolini P, Caenazzo L, Cortivo P, Bestetti A, Bonavita V, Crinò C, Pascali VL, Fiori A, Bargagna M (1989) The distribution of some polymorphisms in Italy. Gene Geography 3:69-139

Tagliabracci A, Paoli M, Rodriguez D, Buscemi L, Cucurachi N, Ferrara SD, Previderè C, Peloso G, Riva A, Pierucci G, Domenici R, Fornaciari S, Spinetti I, Nardone M, Bargagna M. (1995) Allele frequencies of the HUMFES/FPS system in Northern and Central Italy. Abstracts 16th Int Congr Int Soc Forens Haemogenet

4 DNA Polymorphisms

Methods for Typing the STR Triplex CSF1PO, TPOX, and HUMTHO1
That Enable Compatibility Among DNA Typing Laboratories

B. Budowle, B.W. Koons, K.M. Keys, and J.B. Smerick

Forensic Science Research Unit, Laboratory Division, FBI
Academy, Quantico, Virginia 22135, USA

INTRODUCTION

Typing polymorphic loci at the DNA level has become a routine
procedure in the paternity and identity testing fields.
Originally, highly polymorphic variable number of tandem
repeats (VNTR) loci were characterized by restriction fragment
length polymorphism (RFLP) analysis (Wyman and White 1980;
Jeffreys et al. 1985a; Jeffreys et al. 1985b). A subgroup of
these VNTR loci is the short tandem repeats (STR) loci. These
loci are highly polymorphic and are abundant in the human
genome (Edwards et al. 1991; Edwards et al. 1992). The STR
loci are composed of tandemly repeated sequences of 2-7 base
pairs in length. Because the allele size of STRs is generally
less than 350 base pairs, they are amenable to amplification
by the polymerase chain reaction (PCR) (Saiki et al. 1985;
Edwards et al. 1991). Therefore, STRs can be typed with a
high degree of specificity and sensitivity, in a relatively
short time period, and without the need for isotopic detection
methods. Moreover, the amplified products of STRs can be
resolved at least to a single repeat unit by separation on
denatured polyacrylamide gels (Edwards et al. 1991;
Hochmeister et al 1995; Huang et al. 1995). Thus, more
discretized allelic data can be obtained for the loci than was
possible with VNTRs typed by RFLP analysis.

The typing of STR loci for human identity testing has been
facilitated by the ability to amplify two or more STR loci
simultaneously in one PCR by a procedure known as multiplex
PCR (Edwards et al. 1991; Edwards et al. 1992; Gill et al.
1992; Sullivan et al. 1992). The advantages of a multiplex
system are that less sample DNA is consumed than when
analyzing each locus independently, less reagents are
required, and the time needed to perform population studies on
several loci is greatly reduced. The amplified STR products
of a multiplex PCR can be separated by polyacrylamide gel
electrophoresis, and the amplicons are detected by silver
staining or by laser excitation of a fluor attached to the 5'
end of one primer of each of the primer sets. The fluor-
labeled PCR products can be detected in real time (using the
ABI 373A or ABI 310, Perkin-Elmer) or using a decoupled
detection system after gel electrophoresis (FluorImager SI or
Hitachi FM BIO). Both detection schemes - manual silver
staining and automated fluor detection - can be used to obtain
reliable data for STR typing. The silver staining approach is
simple and does not require expensive equipment for detecting
the amplified STR products. However, in order to obtain
unequivocal typing of the various loci in the multiplex their

sizes cannot overlap. In contrast, because of the advent of different colored fluors, the loci in the fluor-labeled multiplex need not be of different size.

The loci CSF1PO, TPOX, and HUMTHO1 are STRs containing tetranucleotide repeat sequences. The tetranucleotide STR loci were selected for analysis because the alleles, based on the repeat sequence, generally can be resolved by polyacrylamide gel electrophoresis (Hochmeister et al 1995; Huang et al. 1995), and these loci generally exhibit less stutter (or shadow) bands than STR loci containing smaller repeat size sequences. Also, the size of the largest allele in the triplex (allele 15 in the CSF1PO locus allelic ladder) is less than 300 bp in size (GenePrint Technical Manual 1994). Thus, forensic biospecimens that contain substantially degraded DNA may be more readily typed than when analyzing VNTR loci by RFLP typing or by typing loci such as D1S80. Some characteristics of the CSF1PO, TPOX, and HUMTHO1 loci are displayed in Table 1 (GenePrint Technical Manual 1994).

Table 1. Information on CSF1PO, TPOX, and HUMTHO1 loci.

Locus	Chromosome Location	Repeat Sequence	Non-Four Base Repeat alleles	K562 Types
CSF1PO	5q33.3-34	AGAT	NA	10,9
TPOX	2p13	AATG	NA	9,8
HUMTHO1	11p15.5	AATG	9.3	9.3,9.3

This paper describes procedures for typing a commercially-available STR triplex - CSF1PO, TPOX, and HUMTHO1 - that can be performed using either silver staining or automated laser fluorescence detection. Thus, the multiplex STR typing can be implemented into most human identity testing laboratories, enabling greater compatibility among laboratories for sharing casework results and population data.

MATERIALS AND METHODS

Sample Preparation

Whole blood was obtained in EDTA vacutainer tubes by venipuncture or by fingerprick and placed on cotton cloth and air-dried. The DNA was extracted by the phenol-chloroform method and washed using microcon 100 filters (Amicon) according to the method of Comey, et al. (1994). The quantity of extracted DNA was estimated using the slot-blot procedure described by Waye, et al. (1989) using chemiluminescent detection (Budowle et al. 1995).

Multiplex PCR

The coamplification of HUMTHO1, TPOX, and CSF1PO was performed using the GenePrint kit (Promega Corporation, Madison, WI) according to the following conditions. The PCR was carried out in 25 or 50μl reaction volumes containing 0.1-5 ng template DNA and 1.5 units of Taq DNA polymerase per 50μl reaction. The primers for the STRs were described previously (Huang et al. 1995). The reactions were placed into a Perkin Elmer 9600 thermal cycler and were subjected to denaturation at 95°C for 30 seconds, primer annealing at 67°C for 30 seconds, and primer extension at 70°C for 30 seconds, for a total of 28 or 30 cycles, depending on the initial quantity of template DNA.

Typing

Three different methods were used to type the STR triplex. Method I: Three μl of loading dye (10 mM NaOH, 95% formamide, 0.05% bromophenol blue, and 0.05% xylene cyanol FF) were mixed with 3 μl of PCR product. The samples were denatured for 2 minutes in a Perkin Elmer Model 480 DNA thermal cycler and 5 μl were loaded onto the cathodal end of the gel. A discontinuous denaturing polyacrylamide gel was used to separate the STR amplicons. These polyacrylamide gels (6%T, 2.%C; cross-linker was piperazine diacrylamide; 31 cm long and 0.4 mm thick) contained 7M urea and 60 mM Tris-formate, pH 9.0 (with respect to the formate ion). The gel was permitted to polymerize for a minimum of one hour at ambient temperature. The gel was placed in a SA 32 apparatus (GIBCO-BRL, Gaithersburg, MD) and the electrode buffer was 90 mM Tris-borate, pH 8.3 (90 mM with respect to the borate ion). Electrophoresis was performed initially at 80 W for approximately five minutes and then continued with settings of 25 W at ambient temperature. The run was allowed to continue until the xylene cyanol tracking dye migrated to the top of the lower reservoir buffer (approximately three hours). The gels were stained with silver according to the method of Budowle et al. (1991).

Method II: Two μl of loading dye (10 mM NaOH, 95% formamide, 0.05% bromophenol blue, and 0.05% xylene cyanol FF) were mixed with 4 μl of PCR product. The samples were denatured for 2 minutes in a Perkin Elmer Model 480 DNA thermal cycler and 5.5 μl were loaded onto the cathodal end of the gel. The denaturing polyacrylamide gels (4%T, 5%C; cross-linker was bisacrylamide; 31 cm long and 0.4 mm thick) contained 7 M urea and 0.5X (or 90 mM) Tris-Borate-EDTA buffer, pH 8.3 (TBE). The electrode reservoir also was 0.5X TBE buffer. Electrophoresis was carried out on an SA 32 Electrophoresis Apparatus (BRL, Gaithersburg, MD). The conditions for electrophoresis were set at a constant power of 40 watts at ambient temperature. Electrophoresis was stopped when the xylene cyanol dye migrated 6 cm from the anode (approximately 75 minutes). After electrophoresis, the fluor labeled amplicons were detected using the FluorImager SI with the PMT set at 1000 (Molecular Dynamics).

Method III: With this method only 1 ng of DNA template was used in the PCR, and the PCR was for 25 cycles. Four μl of loading dye (10 mM NaOH, 95% formamide, 0.05% bromophenol blue, and 0.05% xylene cyanol FF) and 0.5 μl of the GS 500 internal standard were mixed with 1.5 μl of PCR product. The samples were denatured for 2 minutes in a Perkin Elmer Model 480 DNA thermal cycler and 5.5 μl were loaded onto the cathodal end of the gel. The denaturing polyacrylamide gels

(6%T, 5%C; cross-linker was bisacrylamide; 28.5 cm long and 0.4 mm thick; 12 cm well to read distance) contained 7.5 M urea and 1X Tris-Borate-EDTA buffer, pH 8.3 (TBE). The electrode reservoir was 0.5X TBE buffer. Electrophoresis was carried out on an ABI 373A. The conditions for electrophoresis were set at 50W, 1200V, and 50mA at ambient temperature. During electrophoresis, the fluor labeled amplicons were detected in real time with the PMT set at 585.

Allele designations were determined by comparison of the sample fragments with those of the allelic ladders supplied with the GenePrint kit. Allele designations were made according to recommendations of the DNA Commission of the International Society of Forensic Haemogenetics (1994).

RESULTS AND DISCUSSION

This study demonstrates that the STR triplex CSF1PO, TPOX, and HUMTHO1 can be typed using several different electrophoretic separation and detection strategies. Figs. 1-3 show that typing results for the multiplex were obtained using discontinuous formate-borate denaturing gels and silver staining, discontinuous formate-borate denaturing gels and automated fluor detection (using the FluorImager SI), and continuous TBE denaturing gels and automated fluor detection (using the ABI 373A), respectively.

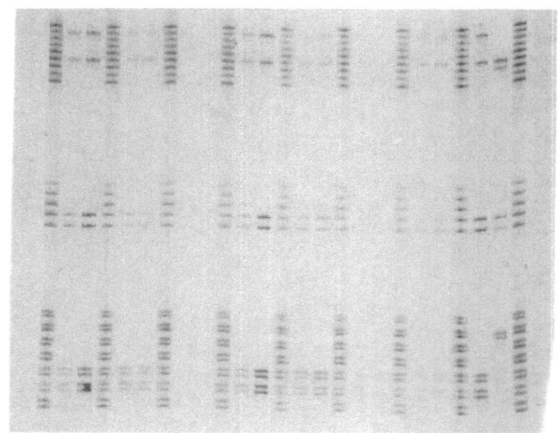

Figure 1. A silver stained discontinuous gel displaying STR triplex types from semen stains that have resided in sunlight or shade up to 10 weeks.

PCR Conditions

The PCR conditions used in this study differ from those recommended by the manufacturer. The temperatures and times for each step of the PCR cycle are designed for the Perkin-Elmer 9600 thermal cycler, while those advocated by the manufacturer are designed for the Perkin-Elmer 480 thermal cycler. Sensitivity of detection of DNA samples was increased using the PCR conditions described in this study. Samples containing template DNA from 4 ng to as little as 125 pg can be typed readily.

In addition, for the triplex kit, where amplicons are detected
by silver staining, the annealing temperature was raised from
64°C to 67°C. The higher annealing temperature did not
compromise typing, and it could be anticipated, with a higher
stringency, that artifact bands would be reduced. Since the
introduction of the silver staining triplex kit, a
fluorescently-tagged quadplex kit has been developed. The
quadplex contains the same three loci as the triplex, and the
locus VWF has been added. In order to obtain amplification of
all four STR loci, the annealing temperature for the PCR was
reduced to 60°C. This was done to accommodate the VWF locus.
Currently, we have decided to maintain the annealing
temperature at 67°C, which will not enable typing at the VWF
locus. If another locus is to be added to the triplex, the
PCR annealing temperature for that locus could be similar to
that of the other triplex loci.

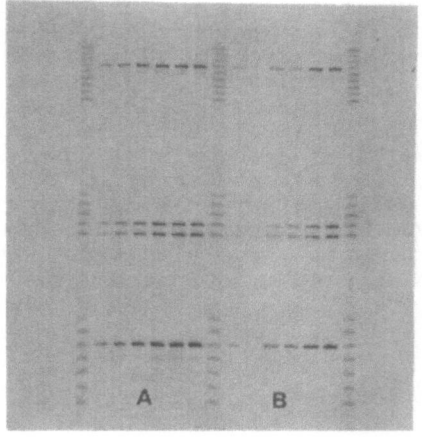

Figure 2. A FluorImager SI generated discontinuous gel image
displaying the STR triplex. The samples in Region A were
amplified for 30 cycles and contained template DNA (from left-
to-right) of 125 pg, 250 pg, 500 pg, 1 ng, 2 ng and 5 ng and
in Region B were amplified for 28 cycles and contained
template DNA (from left-to-right) of 125 pg, 250 pg (failed
amplification), 500 pg, 1 ng, 2 ng and 5 ng.

Size of STR Loci

The feature of this STR triplex that enables compatibility
among laboratories is that the loci CSF1PO (295-327 bp), TPOX
(232-248 bp), and HMUTHO1 (179-203 bp) do not overlap in size.
Thus, this triplex can be used in DNA typing laboratories that
are equipped with high-technology apparatuses, as well as in
laboratories with limited resources.

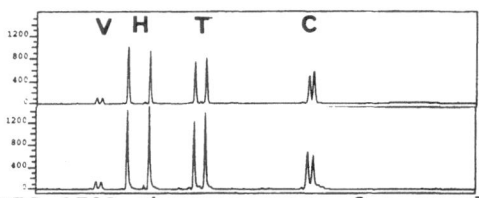

Figure 3. An ABI 373A chromatogram of a sample run on a continuous gel displaying an STR triplex profile. The top chromatogram is a sample amplified for 25 cycles and the bottom was amplified at 26 cycles. The template DNA was at 1ng. V = VWA (note that their is low level VWA detected even though the annealing temperature was at 67°C); H = HUMTHO1; T = TPOX; C = CSF1P0.

Separation of Alleles

All samples were separated electrophoretically in a denatured environment. The separation distances between fragments differing by one repeat unit were augmented under denaturing conditions compared with native gel conditions (data not shown). With the formate-borate system, the distance between CSF1PO alleles 7 and 15 was approximately 1.5 cm, between TPOX alleles 8 and 12 was approximately 1.2 cm, and between HUMTHO1 alleles 5 and 11 was approximately 2.5 cm. All alleles in the triplex were resolved to one repeat unit (i.e., four base pairs). Moreover, the HUMTHO1 9.3 allele, which is a relatively common allele in Caucasians (Edwards et al. 1992; Hochmeister et al. 1995; Lorente et al. 1994, Puers et al. 1993), is one base pair smaller in size than the 10 allele, and could be resolved. The ability to type unequivocally the 9.3 allele demonstrates the resolving capacity of the electrophoretic system used in our study for typing HUMTHO1.

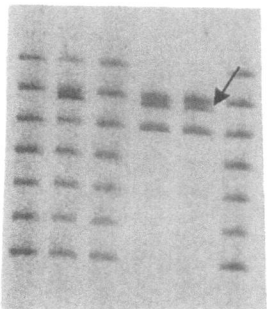

Figure 4. A FluorImager SI generated image of a discontinuous gel displaying resolved 9.3 and 10 alleles (indicated by arrow).

Differences Between Silver Staining and Fluor Detection

There were some notable differences between the silver stain detection approach and the fluor detection method using, for example, the FluorImager SI. With fluor detection only one of the two strands from the denatured duplex can be observed; in contrast, silver staining will enable detection of both strands. With the denatured gel systems used in this study only the denatured strands at the HUMTHO1 locus are resolved. Detection of STR amplicons as single bands or as separated double bands does not compromise typing. The use of the FluorImager SI was less laborious than silver staining. There was no need to separate the glass plates after electrophoresis for fluor detection. Thus, there were no additional steps for

staining. In addition, there was no requirement for photography to record the image; the image can be printed on an inexpensive paper medium. The advantage of silver staining is that there is no requirement for expensive equipment. Finally, the most sensitive detection system was fluor detection using the ABI 373A; it generally provided at least an order of magnitude more sensitivity than the FluorImager SI or silver staining.

CONCLUSION

Using multiplex PCR, separation of the PCR products on denaturing polyacrylamide gels, and silver staining or fluor detection, rapid typing with high resolution of the loci CSF1PO, TPOX, and HUMTHO1 can be obtained. The multiplex analytical procedures described above are relatively simple and can be implemented into most application-oriented laboratories.

This is publication number 95-14 of the Laboratory Division of the Federal Bureau of Investigation. Names of commercial manufacturers are provided for identification only, and inclusion does not imply endorsement by the Federal Bureau of Investigation.

REFERENCES

Budowle B, Chakraborty R, Giusti AM, Eisenberg AJ, Allen RC (1991) Analysis of the variable number of tandem repeats locus D1S80 by the polymerase chain reaction followed by high resolution polyacrylamide gel electrophoresis. Amer J Hum Genet 48:137-144

Budowle B, Baechtel FS, Comey CT, Giusti AM, Klevan L (1995) Simple protocols for typing forensic biological evidence: chemiluminescent detection for human DNA quantitation and RFLP analyses and manual typing of PCR amplified polymorphisms. Electrophoresis (in press)

Comey CT, Koons BW, Presley KW, Smerick JB, Sobieralski CA, Stanley DM, Baechtel FS (1994) DNA extraction strategies for amplified fragment length polymorphism analysis. J Forens Sci 39:1254-1269

DNA recommendations - 1994 report concerning further recommendations of the DNA Commission of the ISFH regarding PCR-based polymorphisms in STR (short tandem repeat) systems. Int J Leg Med 107:159-160

Edwards A, Civitello A, Hammond HA, Caskey CT (1991) DNA typing and genetic mapping with trimeric and tetrameric tandem repeats. Amer J Hum Genet 49:746-756

Edwards A, Hammond H, Jin L, Caskey CT, Chakraborty R (1992) Genetic variation at five trimeric and tetrameric repeat loci in four human population groups. Genomics 12:241-253.

GenePrint Fluorescent STR Systems - Technical Manual (1994) Promega Corporation, USA, pp 26-27

Gill P, Kimpton CP, Sullivan K (1992) A rapid method for identifying fixed specimens by DNA profiling. Electrophoresis 13:173-175

Hochmeister MN, Budowle B, Borer UV, Dirnhofer R (1995) Swiss population data on three tetrameric short tandem repeat loci - HUMTHO1, TPOX, CSF1PO - derived using the GenePrint Triplex PCR Amplification Kit. Int J Leg Med 107:246-249

Huang NE, Schumm J, Budowle B (1995) Chinese Population Data on Three Tetrameric Short Tandem Repeat Loci - HUMTHO1, TPOX, AND CSF1PO - Derived Using Multiplex PCR and Manual Typing. Forens Sci. Int 71:131-136

Jeffreys AJ, Wilson V, Thein SL (1985a) Hypervariable minisatellite regions in human DNA. Nature 314:67-73

Jeffreys AJ, Wilson V, Thein SL (1985b) Individual-specific fingerprints of human DNA. Nature 316:76-79

Lorente JA, Lorente M, Budowle B, Wilson MR, Villanueva E (1994) Analysis of the HUMTH01 (TC11) allele frequencies in the Spanish population. Forens Sci Int 39:1270-1274

Puers C, Hammond HA, Jin L, Caskey CT, Schumm JW (1993) Identification of repeat sequence heterogeneity at the polymorphic short tandem repeat locus HUMTHO1 $[AATG]_n$ and reassignment of alleles in population analysis by using a locus-specific allelic ladder. Am J Hum Genet 53:953-958

Saiki RK, Scharf S, Faloona T, Mullis KB, Horn GT, Erlich HA, Arnheim N (1985) Enzymatic amplification of beta-globin genomic sequences and restriction analysis for diagnosis of sickle cell anemia. Science 230:1350-1354

Sullivan KM, Pope S, Gill P, Robertson JM (1992) Automated DNA profiling by fluorescent labeling of PCR products. PCR Meth Appl 2:34-40

Waye JS, Presley L, Budowle B, Shutler GG, Fourney RM (9189) A simple method for quantifying human genomic DNA in forensic specimen extracts. Biotechniques 7:852-855

Wyman AR, White R (1980) A highly polymorphic locus in human DNA. Proc Natl Acad Sci USA 77:6754-6758

Selection of STR loci for forensic identification systems.

Urquhart, A.J., Oldroyd, N.J., Downes, T., *Barber, M., Alliston-Greiner, R., Kimpton, C.P. and Gill, P.D.

The Forensic Science Service, Birmingham, UK
*Metropolitan Police Forensic Science Laboratory, London, UK

INTRODUCTION

Short Tandem Repeat (STR) profiling is rapidly growing as a method of individual identification for forensic and other purposes. Several multiplex STR systems are available (e.g. Kimpton et al, 1993), offering matching probabilities of about 10^{-4}. The quadruplex STR system developed in our laboratory and presently in use in forensic casework gives a matching probability of this order in three British populations (Kimpton et al, 1993). We have investigated numerous STR loci for use in further multiplex STR systems. Here we discuss the criteria for locus selection, with particular reference to the repeat sequence at the loci under investigation.

SELECTION CRITERIA

STR loci were initially selected on the basis of their reported heterozygosity (over 70%, or a Discriminating Power of >0.8). The next considerations are their size range, optimal annealing temperature and ability to co-amplify with other selected loci. Once a prototype multiplex has been designed, we investigate the propensity to form stutter bands, the ratio of n to n+1 peaks (Robertson et al., 1995).

SEQUENCE VARIATION

We have divided STR loci into 3 categories on the basis of their variable sequence (Urquhart et al, 1994). *Simple repeats* comprise an invariant unit of 3, 4 or 5 base pairs repeated a variable number of times; *compound repeats* contain 2 or more adjacent simple repeats; *complex repeats* consist of several repeat blocks of variable unit length along with more or less variable intervening sequence (Urquhart et al, 1994). Each type of repeat may exhibit alleles which differ from the consensus sequence at that locus, such as the well-characterised 9.3 allele at HUMTHO1 (Puers et al, 1993). Some loci exhibit alleles which show sequence variation between alleles of the same size, e.g. HUMVWFA31/A, HUMACTBP2 and D11S554 (Urquhart et al, 1993 and 1994; Adams et al, 1993).

NEW STR SEQUENCE DATA

The most comprehensively investigated tetranucleotide repeat loci are those which comprise TCTA/TAGA and AAAG/CTTT repeat units. This may reflect the primers used to search for repeats rather than their relative frequency in the genome. A search of GenBank for loci containing $(TCTA)_5$ or its complement revealed several loci in which the majority repeat unit TCTA had apparently mutated (Urquhart et al, 1994). The most common variant repeat unit was TCTG, but TCCA, TCA and TA were also found. We have recently sequenced 3 more TCTA loci (Fig. 1). TCTG repeats are seen at D6S502, TCA at D3S1359 and TA at D19S253. In addition, we find a TGTA unit at D3S1358 and a CA unit at D19S253.

D6S502 $(TCTA)_{8-12}$
          $(TCTA)_{1-2}(TCTG)_{1-2}(TCTA)_{9-15}$

D19S253 $TCTA.TA.TCTA.CA.TA(TCTA)_{5-14}$

D3S1359 $(TCTA)_{11-18}$
          $(TCTA)_{7-9}TGTA(TCTA)_{5-12}$
          $(TCTA)_{7-9}TGTA.TCTA.TCA(TCTA)_{8-17}$

Figure 1. Sequences found at the D6S502, D19S253 and D3S1359 loci.

We have also sequenced the primarily AAAG repeats at the D18S51, HUMFIBRA and HUMAPOAI1 loci (Barber et al, to be published) (Fig. 2). D18S51 is a compound repeat of AAAG and AG. Most alleles contain an AG dinucleotide followed by 4 AG dinucleotides immediately 3' to the AAAG tract. A minority of alleles contain 6 AG dinucleotides in this position. This difference causes the occurrence of intermediate alleles (designated X.2). The repeat at the HUMFIBRA locus is complex, comprising polymorphic GAAG and AAAG tracts as well as other variants on the AAAG basic unit. The difference between X and X.2 alleles is the absence in the X.2 alleles of one AG dinucleotide immediately 3' to the large AAAG tract. One X allele and 2 X.2 alleles contain insertions immediately 5' to the large AAAG tract. One (shown on the left in Fig. 2) comprises $(AAAG)_5GAAG$. Of the other two (on the right in Fig. 2), one has a sequece of $(AAAG)_3(GAAG)_3$, while the other has this sequence followed by $(AAAG)_{13}(ACAG)_5$. Other alleles close in size to the latter have been seen, bit not yet sequenced. The alleles containing these

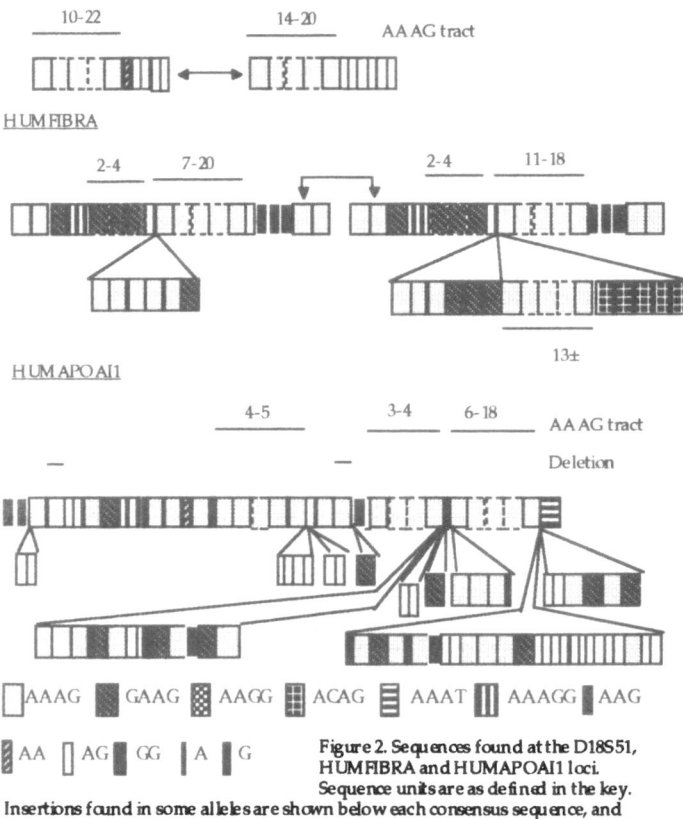

Figure 2. Sequences found at the D18S51, HUMFIBRA and HUMAPOAI1 loci. Sequence units are as defined in the key. Insertions found in some alleles are shown below each consensus sequence, and deletions and variable-length polymorphic tracts are above. Arrows show possible mutations between two types of allele at a locus.

insertions are the largest seen at the locus. We speculate that these insertions are stabilized by the presence of variant (non-AAAG) sequence within the repeat area, as has been proposed at other repeat loci. Alleles at HUMAPOAI1 are extemely complex both by our narrow definition and in the general sense of the word. Insertions containing odd numbers of base pairs are common, leading to alleles differing by 1 bp accross almost the entire alllelic size range.

STR EVOLUTION

Inspetion of the sequence within and adjacent to repeat sequences suggests some mechanisms that may be involved in STR evolution. The most common repeat units associated with AAAG repeats are AG and AAGG, while those at TCTA repeats are TCTG, TA and TCA (Urquhart et al, 1994). As might be expected, substitutions normally retain purine or pyrimidine at the affected positon, while the commonest deletions preserve adjacent bases. Mutations to di- or tetranucleotides, particularly AAGG, AG and TCTG appear prone to further expansion. Interestingly, both AAAG and TCTA appear to mutate to ACAG or its complement TCTG (AAAG at one HUMFIBRA allele, TCTA at many loci).

ALLELES DIFFERING BY ONE BASE PAIR

There is a well-chracterised 1 bp allele difference at the HUMTHO1 locus (Puers et al, 1993). We have recently seen an 8.3 allele at this locus. Since the launch of the UK's National DNA Database, we have typed a huge number of individuals at six STR loci. We have found two apparent instances of 1 bp allele differences at other loci. The alleles concerned are a 64.1 allele at D21S11 and a 16.1 allele at HUMFIBRA. We have developed an interpretation system which will reliably type alleles differing by 1 bp (Gill et al, to be published). Sequencing of these alleles is under way.

REFERENCES

Adams M, Urquhart A, Kimpton C, Gill P (1993) The human D11S554 locus: four distinct families of repeat pattern alleles at one locus. Hum. Molec. Genet. 2: 1373-1376

Barber M, McKeown B, Parkin B (to be published) Structural variation in the alleles of a short tandem repeat system at the human alpha fibrinogen locus (HumFGA). Forensic Sci. Int.

Gill P, Urquhart A, Millican E, Oldroyd N, Watson S, Kimpton C (to be published) Criminal intelligence databases and interpretation of STRs. Adv. Forensic Haemogenetics

Kimpton CP, Gill P, Walton A, Urquhart A, Millican ES, Adams M (1993) Automated DNA profiling employing multiplex amplification of short tandem repeat loci. PCR Methods Applications 3: 13-22

Puers C, Hammond HA, Jin L, Caskey CT, Schumm JW (1993) Identification of repeat sequece homogeneity at the polymorphic short tandem repeat locus HUMTHO1[AATG]n and reassignment of alleles in population analysis by using a locis-specific allelic ladder. Am. J. Hum. Genet. 53: 953-958

Robertson JM, Badger CA, Buoncristiani MR (1995) Design of short tandem repeat systems suitable for human identification. Proc. 5th Intl. Symposium on Human Identification 1994. Promega Corp.

Urquhart A, Kimpton CP, Doownes TJ, Gill P (1994) Variation in short tandem repeat sequences: a survey of twelve microsatellite loci for use as forensic identification markers. Int. J. Leg. Med. 107: 13-20

Urquhart A, Kimpton CP, Gill P (1993) Sequence variability of the tetranucleotide repeat of the human beta-actin related pseudogene H-beta-Ac-psi-2 (ACTBP2) locus. Hum. Genet. 92: 637-638

PCR TYPING OF ALU ELEMENTS - MOLECULAR GENETICS AND FORENSIC APPLICATION

Peter M. Schneider, Lin Zhang, Christina Esdar, Gabriele Rittner, Mark A. Batzer*, and Christian Rittner

Institute of Legal Medicine, Johannes Gutenberg University, Am Pulverturm 3, 55131 Mainz, Germany; *Dept. of Pathology, Stanley S. Scott Cancer Center, Louisiana State University Medical Center, New Orleans, LA 70112, USA.

Introduction

Alu repeats belong to the family of short interspersed elements (SINEs) and are among the most abundant repetitive DNA sequences in the mammalian genome. They represent mobile genetic elements ancestrally derived from the 7SL RNA gene and have presumably spread within the genome by retroposition (reviewed in [1]). A particular group of Alu repeats appears to be human-specific (HS subfamily) and has expanded only recently within the human genome as indicated by distinct dimorphisms at various loci due to the presence or absence of an Alu repeat. In recent extensive studies, the frequency distributions of Alu insertions at selected loci in various human racial groups and populations were determined. Significant differences in frequency distribution between these populations were observed which could be used to determine the evolutionary origin as well as the phylogenetic relationship between racial groups [2,3]. These genetic markers should therefore be useful to obtain clues on the race of an unknown stain donor in forensic casework. In the present study, we have determined the frequency and segregation behaviour of Alu insertions at six loci in the German population.

Material and Methods

In the population study, DNA samples from 49 unrelated individuals as well as 23 children from South-Western Germany were tested. All individuals were obtained from consecutive routine paternity cases, whereby family relationships had been been determined using conventional blood group as well as DNA VNTR systems.

Table 1: Primer sequences for amplification of Alu insertions

Repeat	Chromosomal location	5'-primer (5'->3')	3'-primer (5'->3')
D1	3	TGCTGATGCCCAGGGTTAGTAAA	TTTCTGCTATGCTCTTCCCTCTC
ACE	17	CTGGAGACCACTCCCATCCTTTCT	GATGTCGCCATCACATTCGTCAGAT
TPA25	8	GTAAGAGTTCCGTAACAGGACAGCT	CCCCACCCTAGGAGAACTTCTCTTT
APO	11	AAGTGCTGTAGGCCATTTAGATTAG	AGTCTTCGATGACAGCGTATACAGA
FXIIIB	1	TCAACTCCATGAGATTTTCAGAAGT	CTGGAAAAAATGTATTCAGGTGAGT
PV92	16	AACTGGGAAAATTTGAAGAGAAAGT	TGAGTTCTCAACTCCTGTGTGTTAG

The six Alu repeat loci D1, ACE, TPA25, APO, FXIIIB, and PV92 were typed using the polmerase chain reaction (PCR) with locus-specific primers flanking the Alu insertion site. The PCR primer sequences as well as the chromosomal locations of the six systems are given in Tab. 1 [3]. Standard PCR amplification was carried out using 100 ng template DNA, 0.5 µM of each primer, 200 µM dNTP's, 1.5 mM $MgCl_2$, and 2U of Taq polymerase (Gibco Life Technologies GmbH) in a 1x PCR buffer (provided by the

Table 2: Observed and expected genotypes of six Alu loci in the German population (n=49)

Locus	Genotype	Observed (n)	Observed (%)	Expected (n)	Expected (%)	p (exact test)
D1	+ +	7	14.3	6.6	13.5	
	+ –	22	44.9	22.8	46.5	0.64
	– –	20	40.8	19.6	40.0	
ACE	+ +	13	26.5	13.8	28.2	
	+ –	26	53.1	24.4	49.8	0.66
	– –	10	20.4	10.8	22.0	
TPA25	+ +	6	12.2	5.9	12.0	
	+ –	22	44.9	22.2	45.3	0.87
	– –	21	42.9	20.9	42.6	
APO	+ +	46	93.9	46.0	94.0	
	+ –	3	6.1	2.9	5.9	0.52
	– –	0	0.0	0.1	0.1	
FXIIIB	+ +	14	28.6	11.3	23.0	
	+ –	19	38.8	24.5	49.9	0.12
	– –	16	32.7	13.3	27.1	
PV92	+ +	1	2.0	1	2.0	
	+ –	12	24.5	12	24.5	0.78
	– –	36	73.5	36	73.5	

+ + homozygous with insertion, + – heterozygous, – – homozygous without insertion

The observed and expected genotype frequencies as well as the p values of the exact test are shown in Tab. 2. No significant deviations from Hardy-Weinberg equilibrium were found. Also, no mutation or aberrant segregation behaviour was observed in the family study comparing the genotypes of parents and offspring in 46 meioses. Except for the APO locus, heterozygosity is between 24 and 53 % in the German population.

By comparing Alu insertion frequencies from different racial groups, significant differences were observed by comparing the results from the present study with frequencies of the African-American population [3] for the loci APO and FXIIIB (see Fig. 2). The combined exclusion chances for all six loci are 61.2 % in paternity tsting and 98.8 % in identification cases for Germans and 66.8 % and 99.4 % for African-Americans, respectively. Thus the Alu insertion polymorphisms provide another useful tool in forensic DNA analysis with the potential to obtain information on the possible race of an unknown stain donor.

References

1. Deininger PL, Batzer MA (1993) Evolution of retroposons. Evolutionary Biol 27:157-196

2. Batzer MA, Stoneking M, Alegria-Hartman M, Bazan H, Kass DH et al. (1994) African origin of human-specific Alu insertions. Proc Natl Acad Sci USA 91:12288-

3. Batzer MA, Arcot SS, Phinney JW, Alegria-Hartman M, Kass DH, et al. (1996) Genetic variation of recent Alu insertions in human populations. J Mol Evol (in press)

4. Guo SW, Thompson EA (1992) Performing the exact test of Hardy-Weinberg proportion for multiple alleles. Biometrics 48:361-372

polymerase manufacturer). Routinely, 32 cycles of a three-step PCR were performed in a TC-1 thermocycler (Perkin-Elmer GmbH) using the following protocol: denaturation for 1' at 94°C, annealing for 1' at various temperatures (55°C for APO and PV92, 56°C for FXIIIB, 58°C for ACE and TPA25, 61-58°C touchdown PCR for D1), extension for 1' at 72°C with a final extension of 7' at 72°C. Ten µl of each PCR reaction were separated by electrophoresis in a 1.2 % agarose gel. A size difference of approx. 300 bp indicated the presence or absence of the Alu insertion at a given locus. The observed homozygous and heterozygous genotypes were counted and possible deviations from the Hardy-Weinberg equilibrium was analysed using an exact test [4]. Exact test and exclusion chances were calculated using the paternity analysis software PATER (C. Brenner, Berkeley, CA).

Results and Discussion

The typical DNA fragment patterns of heterozygous genotypes (from individuals with and without Alu insertions) from all six loci are depicted in Fig. 1. The PCR fragments are easy to discriminate and vary in size between 100 bp for the alleles without insertion (APO and TPA25) and approx. 800 bp for the allele with insertion (FXIIIB). In a series of dilution experiments to test the sensitivity, amplification of the FXIIIB-specific fragments and detection by ethidium bromide staining could be achieved with 2-5 ng of template DNA (not shown).

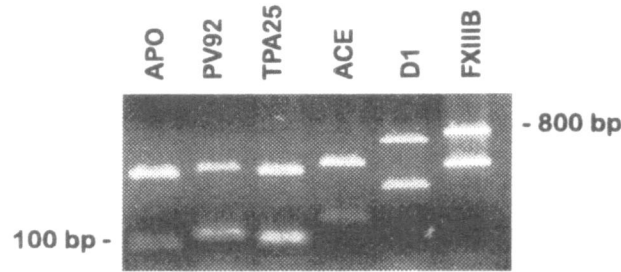

Fig. 1:   Heterozygous genotypes of the six Alu insertion loci analysed. The fragments were visualized after separation in a 1.2% agarose gel by ethidium bromide staining.

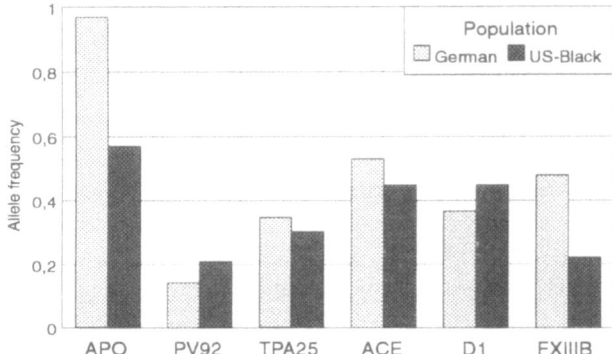

Fig. 2:   Comparison of Alu insertion allele frequencies in the German (n=49) and the US-African-American populations (n=46, from ref. [3]).

AN INVESTIGATION OF VARIATION IN THE SIZING OF SHORT TANDEM REPEAT LOCI

D Syndercombe Court, C Phillips, J Thomson, P Lincoln

Department of Haematology, The London Hospital Medical College, London, UK

INTRODUCTION

Forensic identity testing has been transformed by the development of PCR-based systems to investigate polymorphic short tandem repeat (STR) loci, offering greatly increased sensitivity over DNA single locus probe testing while providing discrete allelic types (Lygo et al 1993). The use of automated DNA sequence apparatus to measure the size of STR alleles in DNA amplified with fluorescently labelled primers has increased the sensitivity of this system further. Alleles are sized with reference to an internal lane standard and types designated according to the number of repeat units present (DNA Commission of the International Society for Forensic Haemogenetics, 1992). Variation in the size measurement of alleles in an allelic ladder has been examined by Kimpton et al (1993); Lygo et al (1994) have extended this work to validate their forensic casework samples. The current study was performed to investigate, within our own laboratory, the reproducibility of STR sizes within and between gels. The same allelic types in different individuals were also examined to investigate whether variability was greater than when repeated measurements were made on the same sample.

MATERIALS AND METHODS

Samples: DNA, extracted using a 5% chelating resin, from blood samples of 90 mother-child pairs was used to examine within gel reproducibility. Each mother was run in a lane adjacent to her child and also separated from her child by half a gel. Five DNA extracts from individuals, selected to represent a range of allelic types for the STR alleles examined, were amplified both in bulk and stored frozen, and amplified freshly, for each analysis. Samples were analysed over ten gels, arranged in a Latin Square design to eliminate possible position bias, to examine the between gel reproducibility. To examine the variability of size measurement within STR alleles across a large number of unrelated people, amplified samples from 110 individuals were run over 15 gels.

PCR: PCR was carried out in a 5μl reaction volume with 2μl of DNA extract, 200mM dNTP, 0.25μM of primer for HUMVWA and HUMFES/FPS and 0.1U of Taq polymerase. PCR conditions were 94°C x 45s, 54°C x 60s, 72°C x 60s for 26 cycles

Automated fluorescent detection: 1μl of PCR product was mixed together with 2μl of formamide/dextran blue and 0.3μl of internal size standard GS2500. Samples were denatured at 95°C for 5 min before loading into a 36 well 6% polyacrylamide, 8M urea denaturing gel (Sequagel-6, National Diagnostics). Electrophoresis was carried out in an ABI 373 DNA Sequencer at 30W for 3 hours. Fragment sizes were analysed with 672 GeneScan software using a local Elder and Southern fit.

RESULTS

Within gel variation: Repeat measurements of STR alleles from the same person, or between common alleles in mother-child pairs, lay within a range of around 0.8 - 1bp for mother-child samples in adjacent lanes (n=87), and for samples separated by a half gel distance, whether mother-child pairs (n=87) or samples from the same person (n=87). The variation observed in HUMFES/FPS was similar to that in HUMVWA. However this excludes six HUMFES/FPS alleles which showed greater variation (up to 2.4 bp total range).

Between gel variation: The total size variation (minimum to maximum), observed in alleles from the five individuals and measured over ten gels, was also around 1bp, regardless of whether the amplified sample had been stored frozen for use, or prepared fresh for each gel. Eight outliers, around 1bp away from the bulk of the measurements, were observed with HUMFES/FPS. This phenomenon was associated with the observation of a split peak in the GS2500 internal 233bp size standard giving a shoulder at 232bp with a main peak at 233bp. The 233bp peak had been selected as the appropriate standard in these cases and this standard would have been used for the HUMFES/FPS allele sizing. This phenomenon was not seen with HUMVWA sizes which are smaller and do not involve the 233bp standard in their measurement.

Allele size variation in different individuals: Measurements of alleles (n=178) were made for HUMVWA and plotted in a histogram (Fig. 1). Seven alleles were observed with a maximum size variation of around 1.5bp, thus producing distinct allelic types. Windows from Lygo et al (1994) are shown superimposed over the data, illustrating the bunching of data towards the higher end of each window. Some data begins to fall outside the window towards the higher molecular weights, but generally the modes lie at a 4bp separation. Figure 2 shows the data for HUMFES/FPS (n=220 alleles). Seven allele types were observed but the spread of size measurements within any allele was greater (2-4bp). Superimposing appropriate windows, as described above, makes it clear that the modes of the data no longer lay 4bp apart and some appear to fall into the next allelic class.

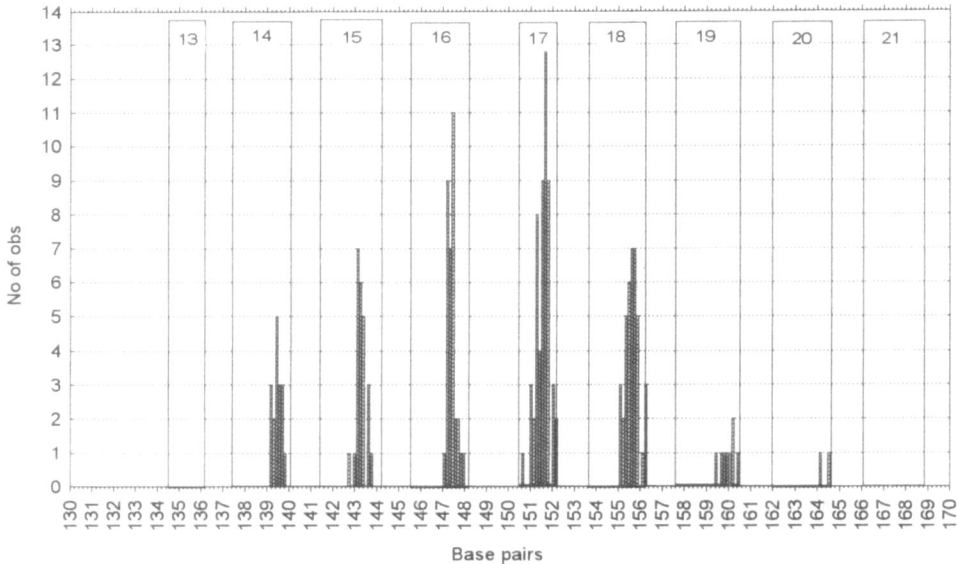

Figure 1: Histogram of molecular distribution of HUMVWA alleles with windows from Lygo et al (1994) superimposed

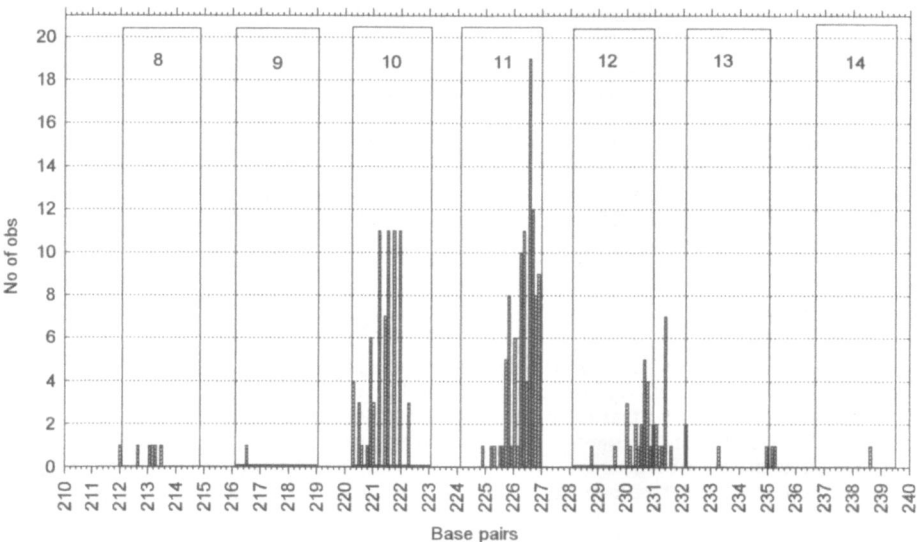

Figure 2: Histogram of molecular distribution of HUMFES/FPS alleles with windows from Lygo et al (1994) superimposed

DISCUSSION

Using allelic ladders Kimpton et al (1993) have reported within gel standard deviation for automated STR detection using the ABIs using an ABI 373 DNA Sequencer as between 0.07 and 0.12 bp, increasing to 0.31 bp between gels which is consistent with the 1bp maximum to minimum range we have observed between gels. We have not, however, observed a smaller variation within a gel, although possibly the variation in adjacent lanes is less. Lygo et al (1994) report a range of results from their analysis of allelic ladders and 24 case samples. Our samples mirror their results for HUMVWA, although the mode appears shifted by around 1bp. For HUMFES/FPS the modes of our data appear considerable shifted, with the spacing increasing towards the higher molecular weight. We are investigating whether this is associated with the observation of an occasional split peak on the GS2500 size standard. The designation of supposedly discrete allelic types thus depends on knowledge of the variation within any one system. Individual laboratories should fully validate their own windows before assigning type to avoid misclassification.

REFERENCES

Recommendations of the DNA Commission of the International Society for Forensic Haemogenetics relating to the use of PCR-based polymorphisms (editorial) (1992) Forensic Sci Int 55:1-3
Gill P, Sullivan KM, Werrett DJ (1990) The analysis of hypervariable DNA profiles: problems associated with the objective determination of the probability of a match. Hum Genet 85:75-79
Kimpton CP, Gill P, Walton A, Urquhart A, Millican ES, Adams M (1993) Automated DNA profiling employing 'multiplex' amplification of short tandem repeat loci. PCR Methods Appl 3:13-22
Lygo JE, Johnson PE, Holdaway DJ, Woodroffe S, Whitaker JP, Clayton TM, Kimpton CP, Gill P (1994) The validations of short tandem repeat (STR) loci for use in forensic casework. Int J Leg Med 107: 77-89

Male identification using Y-chromosomal STR polymorphisms

L.Roewer*, M.Kayser*, M.Nagy* and P.de Knijff**

* Institut für Gerichtliche Medizin, Humboldt University,
   D-10115 Berlin, Germany
** Forensic Laboratory for DNA Research, MGC-Department of
   Human Genetics, Leiden University, 2300 RA Leiden,
   The Netherlands

INTRODUCTION

The overall paucity of Y chromosome polymorphisms (Malaspina
et al. 1990) refers also to a widely used class of sequence
variants, the short tandem repeat (STR) polymorphisms (Tautz
1989). STR polymorphisms appear to occur less frequently on
the Y chromosome compared with autosomes (Spurdle and Jenkins
1992). Only one tetrameric simple repeat polymorphism mapped
to Yp (27H39/DYS19: Roewer et al. 1992) and three dimeric
(YCAI, YCAII, YCAIII: Mathias et al. 1994) have been described
so far. These STRs show moderate levels of polymorphism and
are used for routine forensic as well as for anthropological
applications (Roewer and Epplen 1992; Roewer et. al. 1993;
Gomolka et al. 1994; Mathias et al. 1992).
We now demonstrate that these four together with four other
polymorphic Y-chromosomal STRs (DYS385, DYS389I/II, DYS390,
DYS391) can be used to construct highly discriminative Y
haplotypes. As a result most of the unrelated males in a population can now be distinguished using eight different STRs.
Since the non-pseudoautosomal (male-specific) part of the Y
chromosome is -like mt DNA- uniparental inherited, Y
chromosomes actually represent ancient patrilineages. Provided
a low mutation rate at the respective Y loci these paternal
lineages trace back to the male ancestors of a recent local
population. Our study includes the STR-based Y-haplotyping of
father/son pairs to give a rough estimation of the mutation
rate of the applied STR systems.

MATERIALS AND METHODS

DNA was extracted from blood samples of 70 randomly chosen
male individuals of German ancestry according to standard
procedures. The eight STR loci were additionally studied in 41
father/son pairs, whose paternity had been positively
confirmed by conventional and DNA analysis.
The amplification primers of the eight Y-chromosomal STR

- 27H39LR/DYS19   (Roewer et al. 1992)
- YCAI, YCAII, YCAIII   (Mathias et al. 1994)
- DYS385   (GDB Id. G00-316-257)
- DYS389   (GDB Id. G00-367-936)
- DYS390   (GDB Id. G00-367-957)
- DYS391   (GDB Id. G00-367-966)

applied in this study are designated according to the Genome Data Base (GDB) entries or to the published sequences. PCR conditions and primer sequences were optimized to allow co-amplification (multiplexing) of up to four loci in one PCR. Amplifications were carried out using one fluorescently labeled primer which enables laser-induced detection of the PCR products after electrophoretic separation. For allele-sizing the fluorescent labeled PCR products were run together with in-lane size standards on an ALF™ DNA Sequencer (Pharmacia Biotech, Freiburg, Germany). The allele lengths were ascertained with the ALF Fragment Manager™ 1.1 Software. To designate the STR-based Y haplotypes the consecutive locus-specific alleles are temporarily named according to their length with the shortest allele found at each locus defined as allele 1.

RESULTS AND DISCUSSION

To establish an efficient male identification system using STR-based Y-chromosomal haplotypes we have analysed in detail four published and four other tetrameric Y-chromosomal STR polymorphisms recently entered into the Genome Data Base. Analysis of male and female DNA confirmed that the latter STR polymorphisms (DYS385, DYS389, DYS390, DYS391) are exclusively male specific. The systems DYS385, DYS389, YCAI, YCAII, YCAIII are supposed to consist of two homologous male specific loci with different repeat lengths. For these duplicated loci we choose a simple designation of the two male-specific alleles according to their lengths ignoring their origin from either of the two loci. This proposal appears favourable for practical reasons, as long as the exact localisation and structure of these homologous loci is still unknown. The lengths of the co-amplified repeat units at the locus DYS389 differ by more than 100 base pairs which allow a definite allocation of the alleles to a locus DYS389I and a locus DYS389II.
The number of alleles/allele pairs detected at the eight STR loci varied between 2 (YCAI) and 24 (DYS385). At the loci YCAI, YCAII and YCAIII described by Mathias et al. (1994) several new alleles were found in this study, whereas for the locus 27H39/DYS19 the number of alleles and their distribution published earlier for a German population sample (Gomolka et al. 1994) was confirmed. The allele lengths at the loci differ between 124 bp (YCAI/allele 1) and 405 bp (DYS385/allele 13). After sequential PCR-typing of the whole set of eight STR systems simply encoded Y-chromosomal compound haplotypes were constructed. With the exclusion of two males which both carry the same haplotype all Y chromosomes of the unrelated 70 German males assembled in this study can be differentiated by the eight STR loci.
For all STRs applied in this study holandric transmission was confirmed. For 41 father/son pairs which were typed for the respective loci we established full-size haplotypes. All Y haplotypes were found to be inherited regularly with the exception of one father/son pair with slippage mutations occured at DYS389II and DYS390.

CONCLUSION

The main fields of application of the proposed Y chromosome STR-based haplotyping are:

1. the forensic identification of male DNA (Roewer and Epplen 1992) preferably in rape cases with male/female stain mixtures (combined gender/identity testing)
2. paternity analysis preferably for deficiency cases with a male offspring (Chakraborty 1985) and
3. the analysis of migration, settlement or mating structure of human populations in historic (rather than evolutionary) time spans (Roewer et al. 1993).

For those applications the proposed sequential multilocus PCR typing of eight different Y-chromosomal STRs provides a simple, reproducible and sensitive method.

REFERENCES

Chakraborty R (1985) Paternity testing with genetic markers: are Y-linked genes more efficient than autosomal ones? Am J Med Genet 21: 298-305
Gomolka M, Hundrieser J, Nürnberg P, Roewer L, Epplen JT, Epplen C (1994) Selected di- and tetranucleotide microsatellites from chromosomes 7, 12, 14, and Y in various Eurasian populations. Hum Genet 93: 592-596
Malaspina P, Persichetti F, Noveletto A, Iodice C, Terrenato L, Wolfe J, Ferraro M, Prantera G (1990) The human Y chromosome shows a low level of DNA polymorhism. Ann Hum Genet 54: 297-305
Mathias N, Bayes M, Tyler-Smith C (1994) Highly informative compound haplotypes for the human Y chromosome. Hum Mol Genet 3: 115-123
Roewer L, Arnemann J, Spurr NK, Grzeschik KH and Epplen JT (1992) Simple repeat sequences on the human Y chromosome are equally polymorphic as their autosomal counterparts. Hum Genet 89: 389-394
Roewer L, Epplen JT (1992) Rapid and sensitive typing of forensic stains by PCR amplification of polymorphic simple repeat sequences in case work. Forensic Sci Int 53: 163-171
Roewer L, Nagy M, Schmidt P, Epplen JT, Herzog-Schröder G (1993) Microsatellite and HLA class II oligonucleotide typing in a population of Yanomami Indians. In: Pena SDJ, Chakraborty R, Epplen JT, Jeffreys AJ (eds) DNA Fingerprinting: State of the Science. Birkhäuser, Basel Boston Berlin, p 221
Spurdle AB, Jenkins T (1992) The Y chromosome as a tool for studying human evolution. Current Opinion in Genetics and Development 2: 487-491
Tautz D (1989) Hypervariability of simple sequences as a general source for polymorphic DNA markers. Nucleic Acids Res 17: 6463-6471

This work was supported by the Deutsche Forschungsgemeinschaft (Ro-1040/2-1).

CORRESPONDING REPEATS IN STRs AND THE INTERNAL STANDARD IN FRAGMENT ANALYSIS
REPRODUCIBILITY WITH THREE HYPERPOLYMORPHIC STRs

B. Myhre Dupuy and Bjørnar Olaisen

Institute of Forensic Medicine, University of Oslo

Introduction: Automated fragment analysis with ABI Sequencer using the internal standard GS2500 or GS500 gives sufficient reproducibility to allow typing of regular tetrameric STR´s. It is, however, a general experience that it does not allow fool-proof typing of alleles differing in size by one basepair only.
The main purpose of this study was to evaluate whether the use of internal standards composed of the same repeats as those of the STR to be analysed could overcome this obstacle. Here we show that this is indeed the case. The principle is then applied on the AAAG repeat STRs ACTBP2, APOAI1 and D11S554, and with fragment measurements using an internal standard composed of AAAG repeats. It is demonstrated that each of the three STRs are highly efficient, and that together (for instance in triplex runs) they constitute a powerful tool in forensic diagnostics.

Population and sample size: The material consists of blood samples from 300 Norwegians (150 of each sex), involved in consecutive paternity cases from all over Norway. Selected samples from the same population were also used for construction of the internal standard and in tests for intergel fragment sizing reproducibility.

Methods: Primers (Polymeropoulos 1992, Phromchotikul 1992): ACTBP2, APOAI1 and D11S554 were labelled with TAMRA, FAM, and JOE respectively.

PCR amplification condition: 500 mM Kcl, 100 mM Tris-HCl,10% TritonX-100, 2mM MgCl, 6 pmol of each primer in 25 ul reaction volume. Denaturation 2 min. 94°C, 28 cycles: 94° 20 sec., 58°C 45 sec., 72°C 1 min, followed by 10 min. elongation. ACTBP2 was run singleplex while APOAI1 and D11S554 were run duplex.

Electroforetic methods: 6% PAGE, 26W, 9 hours, on the ABI373A Sequencer. Software: 672 Genescan. Typing was performed by internal allelic ladder in each lane.

Internal standard: An internal standard was composed of DNA fragments containing mainly AAAG repeats. The standard includes 25 ROX labelled fragments with a relatively even size distribution from 174 to 327 bp. It is composed of four alleles from D11S554 (the smallest ones), while the rest are ACTBP2 alleles. The fragments were once and for all sized against a GS2500 standard. The samples applied to tests for intergel sizing reproducibility were also run with the GS500 internal standard.

Table 2:ALLELE MEASUREMENTS IN 300 UNRELATED NORWEGIANS

ACTBP2:

Average	SD	Tot.obs	Average	SD	Tot.obs	Average	SD	Tot.obs
231.15 [1]	0.14	4	259.57	0.02	2	290.48 [9]	0.09	55
234.66 *	0.04	4	260.46	0.00	1	294.31 [10]	0.12	51
236.47	0.00	1	261.45 [5]	0.05	24	298.28 [11]	0.06	43
238.24	0.05	17	263.52	0.05	6	302.09 [12]	0.21	29
240.03	0.07	3	265.47 [6]	0.07	15	304.15	0.00	1
241.88 [2]	0.05	24	267.45	0.07	9	306.10 *	0.06	17
243.62	0.00	1	269.34 *	0.10	7	309.98	0.12	6
245.70	0.07	28	270.58	0.00	1	311.68 *	0.25	3
246.73	0.00	1	271.37	0.08	14	313.81	0.07	3
247.59	0.00	1	273.34 *	0.04	4	315.62 *	0.00	1
248.79	0.04	2	275.13	0.10	23	319.77 *	0.00	1
249.67 [3]	0.05	38	278.93 *	0.12	18	327.52 [13]	0.00	1
253.52	0.09	33	282.75 [7]	0.04	27			
257.47 [4]	0.06	53	286.60 [8]	0.14	28			

APOAI1:

Average	SD	Tot.obs	Average	SD	Tot.obs	Average	SD	Tot.obs
251.22	0.04	15	271.86	0.06	13	283.34	0.07	20
256.08	0.00	1	272.96	0.00	1	284.32	0.07	22
258.08	0.00	1	273.79	0.07	57	285.19	0.07	66
260.02	0.00	1	275.70	0.06	21	287.09	0.04	16
262.03	0.06	34	276.59	0.11	4	288.05	0.07	8
264.02	0.01	2	277.51	0.07	63	289.03	0.06	17
265.10	0.00	1	278.50	0.05	6	291.02	0.03	4
266.02	0.07	77	279.45	0.05	9	292.05	0.06	4
267.98	0.04	7	280.46	0.06	18	292.08	0.06	2
269.81	0.08	14	281.36	0.08	85	296.78	0.04	3
270.85	0.02	3	282.36	0.04	4	302.44	0.00	1

D11S554:

Average	SD	Tot.obs	Average	SD	Tot.obs	Average	SD	Tot.obs
174.42*	0.12	8	217.10	0.07	37	235.98	0.00	1
193,49*	0.10	3	218.26	0.12	19	236.62	0.00	1
197.32	0.04	24	221.38	0.11	23	237.78	0.13	6
199.26	0.05	4	222.52	0.10	42	239.59	0.04	6
200.10	0.00	1	224.49	0.00	1	241.47	0.06	4
201.12	0.07	33	225.55	0.09	7	243.31	0.11	25
203.09	0.01	2	226.65	0.10	51	245.31	0.00	1
204.95*	0.08	55	229.63	0.10	5	247.25	0.15	17
208.80	0.06	62	230.73	0.10	66	251.29	0.12	13
209.85	0.11	4	232.57	0.00	1	255.05	0.12	2
212.71*	0.10	49	233.16	0.00	1	261.13	0.00	1
213.99	0.07	4	234.30	0.10	19	282.59	0.05	2

*;used as internal standard fragments

Alleles marked [1-13] correspond to sequenced alleles (Anke Möller, pers.comm.) with the following lengths
1:223bp, 2:235bp, 3:243bp, 4:251bp, 5:255bp, 6:259bp, 7:277bp, 8:281bp, 9:285bp, 10:289bp, 11:293bp,
12:297bp, 13:321bp.

Results:

Table 1: Standard deviation in repeated intergel fragment sizing using different internal standards.

Internal Standard	ACTBP2 (AAAG) SD	APOAI1 (AAAG) SD	APOAI1 (TTTC) SD
AAAG repeat fragments	0.04	0.04-0.11	1.49-1.67
GS500	0.28-0.83	0.31-0.72	0.24-0.42

Fragment sizing reproducibility was tested in each system by rerunning 1-10 individuals on 8-10 successive gels. Table 1 demonstrates the dramatic effect the choice of internal standards has on the fragment sizing reproducibility. Repeated measurements of the same AAAG STR fragment whether in ACTBP2 or APOAI1 reveal remarkably good results, with 3 SDs being well below 0.5bp. This is a reasonable limit for allowing automated allele typing in STRs with one-bp-differences between alleles. The results with the synthetic GS500 fragment standard are significantly poorer and insufficient for our purpose, while choosing «opposite» base composition (AAAG versus TTTC) in the standard as compared to the fragments measured, clearly makes any allele typing based on fragment sizing impossible.

Having shown that the present internal standards meets our demands in terms of sizing reproducibility of identical alleles, we typed the 300 individuals of our population material in ACTBP2 (singleplex) as well as APOAI1 and D11S554 (duplex). The samples were run on 30 different gels. The results are given in Table 2 where allele sizes as well as SDs of each allele are indicated. There are discrete alleles, and with practically no exception the SDs are within acceptable limits for each allele in all three systems.

Table 3 gives some basic data concerning the efficiency of the three STRs. The probability that two unrelated individuals have the same type in all three STRs is 5×10^{-7}, and the combined paternity exclusion capacity is **99.77%**. We are currently applying these STRs (singleplex and duplex PCR, triplex run) in paternity casework and will probably introduce them for forensic casework and intelligence databases in the near future.

Table 3: Number of alleles, discrimination power (DP), and paternity exclusion power (EP) of ACTBP2, APOAI1, and D11S554.

LOCUS	NO. ALLELES	DP %	EP %
ACTBP2	40	99.45	89.19
APOAI1	33	98.81	83.85
D11S554	36	99.18	86.72

References: Phromchotikul, Hum. Mol. Gen. Vol. 1, No. 3 :214, 1992
Polymeropoulos, Nuc. Acid Res. Vol. 20, NO. 6 : 1432, 1992

Construction And Calibration Of Allelic Ladders For The PCR-Based Systems D8S320 and AR

P. Huber[1], W. Schmidt[2] and J. Holtz[1]

[1]Inst. of Forensic Medicine, University of Bonn, Germany
[2]IHF, Hamburg, Germany

Introduction

Amplified fragments of STRs and AmpFlps were analyzed after electrophoretic separation and staining with ethidium bromide or silver. Exact allele determination requires comparison with allelic ladders. We construct such ladders for the tetrameric STR D8S320 and the trimeric X-linked polymorphism in the Androgen receptor gene (AR). Calibration of the ladders was performed by comparing the results of conventional separation on PAGE and subsequent silver staining with those of the ABI Sequencer in connection with the GeneScan Software 672.
Based on these ladders we conducted population studies for both systems.

Material and Methods

Systems:
D8S320 (8q); Primers: Riley et al., 1993
AR (Xq 11-12); Primers: Sleddens et al., 1992

PCR amplification conditions:
Hot start: 5 min 94 °C, 5 min 80 °C; denaturation: 1 min 94 °C, annealing: 45 s 60 °C, extension: 45 s 72 °C, cycles: 13, denaturation: 1 min 94 °C, annealing: 45 s 62 °C, extension: 45 s 72 °C (3 s elongation each cycle), cycles: 17, final extension: 10 min 72 °C

Electrophoretic separation:
native, vertical PAA gels: AR (8% T), D8S320 (7% T); detection method: silver staining

Construction and calibration of the allelic ladders:
1-3 µl of the selected PCR products were pooled and diluted 10^6-fold with water. 20 µl of the dilution were reamplified in a 100 µl reaction volume using the described conditions above .
For calibration the same dilutions were amplified with dye labelled primers (D8S320: labelled with „Fam", AR: labelled with „Rox") under the same conditions except the cycle number (D8S320, total cycle number: 25; AR, total cycle number: 32).
Fragment size was determined by running on the ABI Sequencer 373 A with an internal standard (GenScan 350, labelled with „Tamra") using the GenScan Software 672.

Results

Allelic ladders
The AR - allelic ladder contains the alleles 16-32 (Fig. 1). The fragment sizes range from 190 bp to 238 bp (Fig. 3). The determined sizes are 1 bp bigger than the sizes calculated according to the sequence published by Lubahn et al. (1989).
The D8S320 - allelic ladder includes 5 alleles (in bp): 394, 398, 402, 410, 418 (Fig. 2+4).

131

Allele-No.

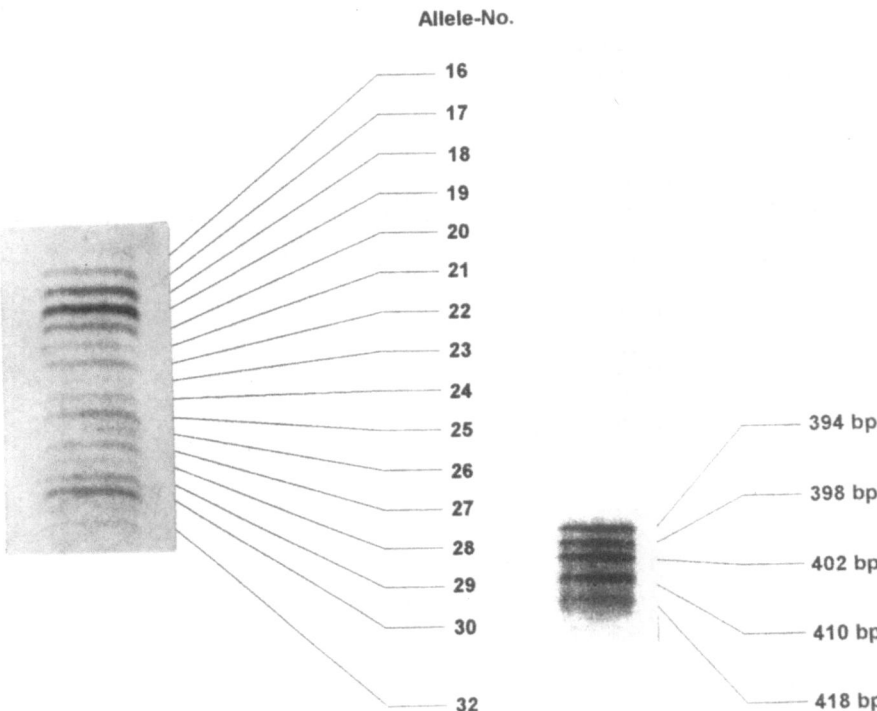

Fig. 1 AR - allelic laddder
The ladder contains the alleles between 16 and 32.
(nomenclature according to Edwards et al., 1992)

Fig. 2 D8S320 - allelic ladder
The ladder includes 5 alleles

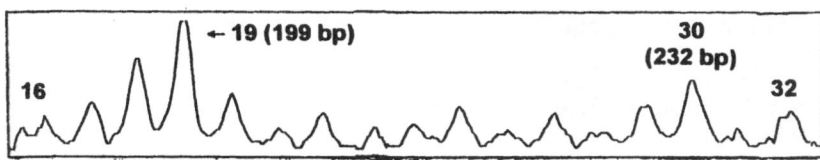

Fig. 3 AR - allelic ladder: fragment size determination
The fragment sizes were determined using the ABI sequencer 373 A and the GeneScan software 672.
The determined sizes are 1 bp bigger than the calulated sizes according to the sequence published by
Lubahn et al. (1989).

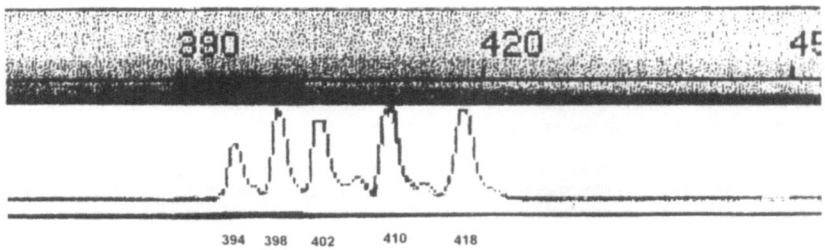

Fig. 4 D8S320 - allelic ladder: fragment size determination
The length (in bp) of the 5 alleles in the ladder are: 394, 398, 402, 410, 418

Population studies

The studies were conducted on samples of unrelated individuals selected from the north-west German population (area of Bonn); AR: n=153 (female: 77, male: 76), D8S320: n=128

Table 1: AR allele distribution (n=230)

allele-no[1]	% ,female (n = 154)	% ,male (n = 76)	%, pooled (n = 230)
16	1,3	1,3	1,3
17	9,1	5,3	7,8
18	7,1	6,6	7,0
19	14,9	17,1	15,2
20	17,5	19,7	18,3
21	6,5	11,8	8,3
22	9,7	7,9	9,1
23	5,8	11,8	7,8
24	8,4	4	7
25	5,8	5,3	5,7
26	3,9	0	2,6
27	3,3	4	3,5
28	3,3	1,3	2,6
29	2	1,3	1,7
30	1,3	1,3	1,7
31	0	0	0
32		1,3	0,4

Table 2: D8S320 allele distribution (n=256)

allele (bp)	%
386	0,4
390	0
394	3,1
398	14,5
402	14,8
406	19,1
410	13,7
414	16,4
418	17,6
422	0,4

1) nomenclature according to Edwards et al., 1992

Hardy-Weinberg equilibrium and forensic efficiency data

Table 3

Locus	Hardy-Weinberg equilibrium	power of exclusion	discrimination power	heterozygosity [%]
AR	no significant deviation (p>0,05) (5-allele model; χ^2=17,91; df=14; 0,2<p<0,3	0,81[2]	0,98[2]	77,9[2]
D8S320	no significant deviation (p>0,05) (7-allele model; χ^2=34,94; df=27; 0,1<p<0,2	0,70	0,95	73,4

2) for female individuals

References

Edwards A, Hammond HA, Jin L, Caskey CT, Chakraborty R (1992): Genetic variation at five trimeric and tetrameric repeat loci in four human population groups. Genomics **12**: 241-253

Lubahn DB, Brown TR, Simental, JA, Higgs, HN, Migeon CJ, Wilson EM, French SF (1989): Sequence of the intron/exon junctions of the coding region of the human androgen receptor gene and identification of a point mutation in a family with complete androgen insensitivity. Proc Natl Acad Sci USA **86**: 9534-9538

Riley R, Nelson L, Lu J, Robertson M, Ballard L, Connoly J, Ward K (1993): Tetranucleotide polymorphism at the D8S320 locus. Hum Mol Genet **2**: 1512

Sleddens HFBM, Oostra BA, Brinkmann AO, Trapman J (1992): Trinucleotide repeat polymorphism in the androgen receptor gene (AR). Nucleic Acids Res **20**: 1427

ESTABLISHMENT OF A HIGHLY DISCRIMINATING PENTAPLEX-PCR-SYSTEM FOR DETECTION OF PCR-FRAGMENTS IN SILVERSTAINED POLYACRYLAMIDE GELS

HAAS, H., WEILER, G.

Institut für Rechtsmedizin, Justus-Liebig-Universität Giessen,
Frankfurter Str.58, D-35392 Giessen, GERMANY

Introduction

Multiplex-PCR is defined as the simultaneous amplification of multiple sequences in a single reaction. It was first indroduced by CHAMBERLAIN et al. in 1988 for the amplification of nine segments of the human dystrophin gene [1]. This method was transferred to routine forensic work for simultaneous amplification of VNTR and/or STR-systems [3, 5, 7, 8, 9, 10]. Most of the systems introduced so far are based on automated fluorescent detection. Because the necessary equipment is not easily acquired for many laboratories, different detection methods have to be used. Therefore we use the sensitive silverstain method from BUDOWLE et al. to detect the DNA-fragments after polyacryamide gel electrophoresis, a method which is already employed for singleplex-PCR [4].

We have evaluated a sensitive multiplex-PCR-system with five different STR-regions. The fragments were detected by silverstaining, and the results were highly discriminative. We employed the STR-loci HUMFIBRA, D18S21, D21S11, HUMVWFA31 and HUMTH01 listed in table 1 for our pentaplex-system. These five STR-systems are all of tetrameric nature and are located on different chromosomes. The repeat sequence structure was already described in 1994 by URQUHART et al. [10].

Table 1: Data of the 5 Loci

STR-loci	GenBank Access. No.	Chromosomal localisation	Repeat motif
HUMFIBRA (Fibra)	M64982	4q28	TTCT
D18S51	L18333	18q21.3	AAAG
D21S11	M84567	21	TCT[AvG]
HUMTH01 (TH01)	D00269	11p15-15.5	AATG
HUMVWFA 31 (vWF)	M25858 M25716	12p12-pter	[AvG]TCT

Since a successful multiplex-PCR involves the design of appropriate primers, the primer specifications of the 5 loci are listed in table 2. The primer length, the sequence, the %GC content and the calculated melting temperature for the forward and reverse strand are listed. The fragment range and the alleles of each STR-region of this pentaplex-system, which can be expected after electrophoretic separation are also listed in table 2.

Table 2: Primer sequences, length , % GC-content, melting temperature (Tm) and corresponding fragment length

STR-Locus	Primer sequences	Length [bp]	% GC	Tm [°C]	Fragment Range (Alleles)
HumFibra	Forward: AAGGCTGCAGGGCATAACATTATC	24	45.8	63.9	455 (32) to
	Reverse: CAGCCACATACTTACCTCCAGTCG	24	54.2	62.5	401(5)
D18S51	Forward: CAAACCCGACTACCAGCAAC	20	55.0	57.9	323(29) to
	Reverse: GAGCCATGTTCATGCCACTG	20	55.0	57.0	275(5)
D21S11	Forward: ATATGTGAGTCAATTCCCCAAG	22	40.9	55.3	249(76) to
	Reverse: TGTATTAGTCAATGTTCTCCAG	22	36.4	49.0	205(54)
HumTH01	Forward: GTGGGCTGAAAAGCTCCCGATTAT	24	50.0	64.8	202(11) to
	Reverse: ATTCAAAGGGTATCTGGGCTCTGG	24	50.0	66.9	179(5)
HumVWFA31	Forward: CCCTAGTGGATGATAAGAATAATCAGTATG	30	36,7	62.9	167(21) to
	Reverse: GGACAGATGATAAATACATAGGATGGATGG	30	40.0	66.4	135(11)

Materials and Methods:

Amplifications were carried out in a 50 µl total reaction volume. 0,5 to 10 ng template-K562 DNA, 1x Perkin Elmer PCR-buffer, 200 µM of each dNTP, 1.25 Units Taq-polymerase and primersets in concentrations from 0,04 to 04 µM were tested. The PCR conditions started with a single denaturation for 5 minutes at 94°C, then a three step PCR of 95, 60 and 72 °C each for 1 min. and a post-PCR extension for 10 minutes at 72 °C. To establish the multiplex-PCR-conditions, different reaction parameters described by CHAMBERLAIN et al. 1994 were tested [2].

Results and Discussion:

Figure 1 shows a native 7.5%T, 5%C-PDA and 60 mM formate polyarylamide gel after variation of primer concentrations and annealing temperature of all 5 loci using K562 template-DNA. In lanes 1, 8 and 15 different visual markers are visible. Lanes 2 to 7 show the result of 0.1 µM final primer concentration and lanes 9 to 14 show the result of 0.2 µM primer concentration, both with K562 DNA-concentrations in descending order from 10 to 0.5 ng. On the left side the result of a 0,1 µM primer concentration for all loci is shown at an annealing temperature of 56 °C. At this temperature many unspecific bands are visible at high and low template concentrations. The vWF bands are more intense and the alleles of D21S11 don't show up. At an annealing temperature of 62°C (figure 2) with the same primer concentrations, there are many artefacts at high DNA-concentrations, too. A three banded pattern of K562 for the locus D21S11 is visible and the signal of vWF is weak again. This 3 banded pattern is a suggestion of the presence of an additional chromosome. Since K562 is derived from a tumor cell line and the DNA is purified from a subculture of human chronic leukemia cell line, this aneuploidy of chromosome 21 can occur [6]. Doubling the total primer concentration from 0.1 to 0.2 µM of the primersets results in a lower signal intensitiy for all loci. This is visible on the right side in figure 1a and 1b. The reaction mix with a final primer concentrations of 0,08 µM for FIBRA, 0,04 µM for D18S51, 0,1 µM for D21S11, TH01 and vWF gave the best results (see figure 2). It is visible that all specific alleles of the cell line K562 are detectable with 4 ng template-DNA (lane 4 in figure 2). Lower amounts of template DNA yielded no interpretable results for vWF.

This may be compared to the quadruplex-system based on silverstaining presented by SCHUMM et al. 1993 [8] as being more sensitive. Based on the Pm values that OLDROYD et al. 1995 [7] determined by typing 50 Caucasians, this pentaplex-system would give a combined Pm value of 3,6 x 10-7, meaning that for a randomly selected sample we would expect to find one match in 2,7 billion individuals. This is approximately equivalent to the power of 4 single locus probes.

Conclusions:

A pentaplex system is established for use in routine work in a forensic laboratory. A prerequisite, therefore was, that all the STR loci should be on different chromosomes, which is the case here. With this system it is possible to detect the alleles of each STR-system in distinct separate areas after silverstaining of polyacrylamide gels. It is possible to detect 4 ng of template DNA. This is very sensitive in comparison to the quadruplex-system presented by SCHUMM et al. [8], who obtained the best results with 5 ng of template DNA. The alleles of the loci are shown with nearly the same signal intensity, and the sensitivity of this system is comparable to the multiplex-PCR-system based on fluorescent detection. The combined Pm-value of this Pentaplex-system of with 3,6 x 10-7 for caucasians is very good. Because there is still space between some STR-regions, an integration of other STR-systems and/or sex-typing system like amelogenin is possible.

Literature:

1. CHAMBERLAIN, J.S., GIBBS, R.A., RANIER, J.E., NGUYEN, P.N., CASKEY, C.T.:
   Nucl. Acids Res. 16, 11141-11156 (1988)
2. CHAMBERLAIN, J.S., CHAMBERLAIN, J.R.: In: MULLIS, K., FERRE, F., GIBBS, R.A.:
   The polymerase chain reaction. Birkhäuser: Berlin, 38-46 (1994)
3. FREGEAU, C.J., FOURNEY, R.:
   BioTechniques 15 (1), 100-119 (1993)
4. HAAS, H., BUDOWLE, B., WEILER, G.:
   Electrophoresis 15, 153-158 (1994).
5. LYGO, J.E., JOHNSON, P.E., HOLDAWAY, D.J., WOODROFFE,S., WHITAKER, J.P., CLAYTON, T.M., KIMPTON, C.P., GILL, P.:
   Int. J. Legal. Med. 107, 77-89 (1994)
6. MANSFIELD, E.S.:
   Hum.Mol.Genetics 2 (1), 43-50, (1993)
7. OLDROYD, N., URQUHART, A.J., KIMPTON, C.P., MILLICAN, E.S., WATSON, ST.K., DOWNES, T., GILL, P.:
   Electrophoresis 16, 334-337 (1995).
8. SCHUMM, J., LINS, A., PUERS, C., SPRECHER, C.:
   In: The Fourth International Symposium on Human Identification, Promega Corporation: Madison, WI., 177-187 (1993).
9. SULLIVAN, K.M., MANNUCCI, A., KIMPTON, C., GILL, P.:
   BioTechniques 15, 636-641 (1993)
10. URQUHART, A., OLDROYD, N.J., KIMPTON, C.P., GILL, P.:
    BioTechniques 18, 11-121 (1995)

Figure 1a:
Horizontal 7.5 % T, 5%C(PDA), 60 mM formate polyacrylamide gel of PCR-products after pentaplex PCR at an annealing temperature of 56°C. Lanes 1, 8 and 15 visual markers (1 kb, pGEM and 123 bp-ladder). Lanes 2 to 7 and 9 to 14 different yields of K562 template DNA in descending order (10, 5, 4, 2, 1 to 0.05 ng). Lanes 2 to 7 all primers at 0.1 μM primer concentrations. Lanes 9 to 14 all primers at 0.2 μM primer concentrations.

Figure 1a

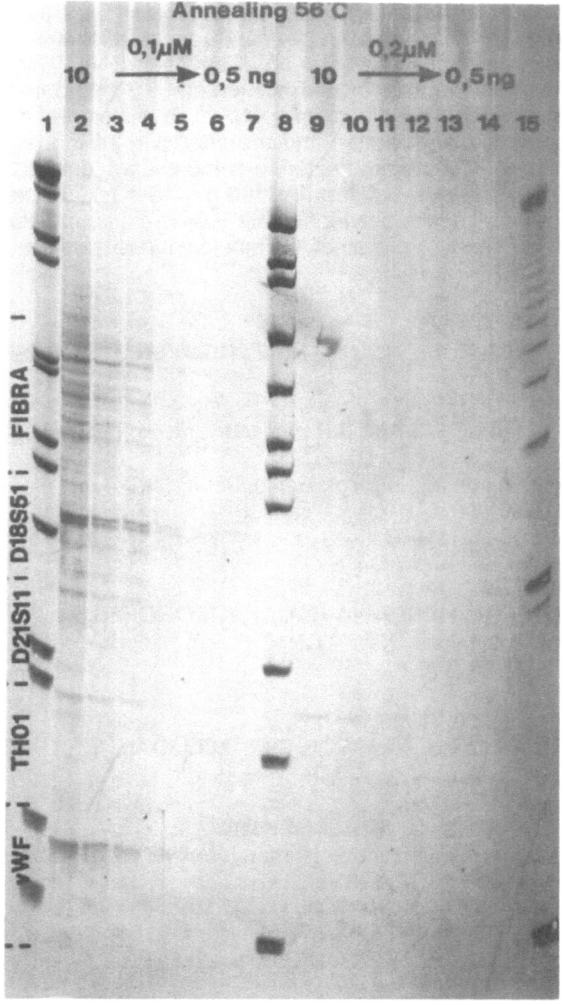

Figure 1b:
Horizontal 7.5 % T, 5%C(PDA), 60 mM formate polyacrylamide gel of PCR-products after pentaplex PCR at an annealing temperature of 62°C. Lanes 1, 8 and 15 visual markers (1 kb, pGEM and 123 bp-ladder). Lanes 2 to 7 and 9 to 14 different yields of K562 template DNA in descending order (10, 5, 4, 2, 1 to 0.05 ng). Lanes 2 to 7 all primers at 0.1 µM primer concentrations. Lanes 9 to 14 all primers at 0.2 µM primer concentrations.

Figure 1b

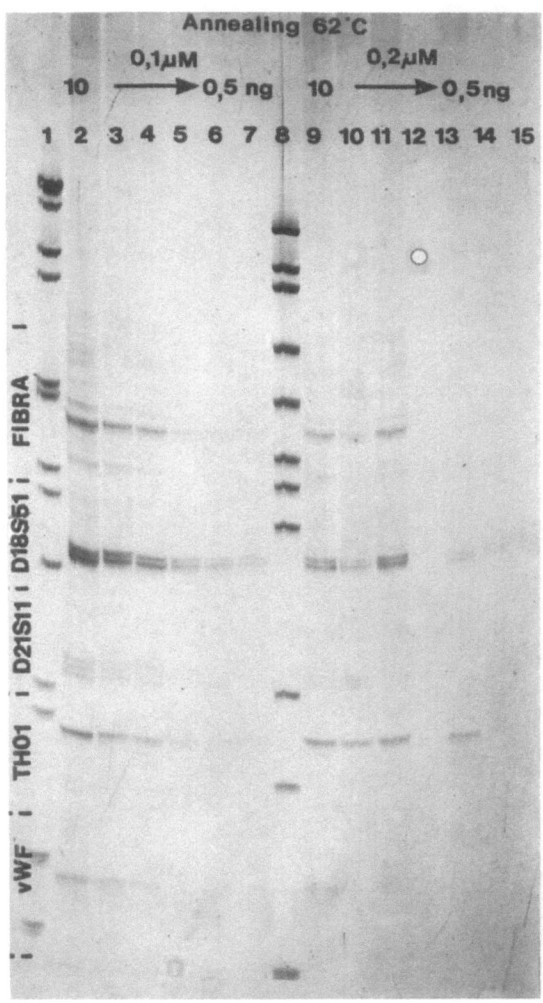

138

Figure 2:
Horizontal 7.5 % T, 5%C(PDA), 60 mM formate polyacrylamide gel of PCR-products after pentaplex PCR (optimal PCR-conditions see text) at an annealing temperature of 60°C. Lanes 1 and 8 visual markers (1 kb and pGEM). Lanes 2 to 7 different yields of K562 template DNA in descending order (10, 5, 4, 2, 1 to 0.05 ng).

Figure 2

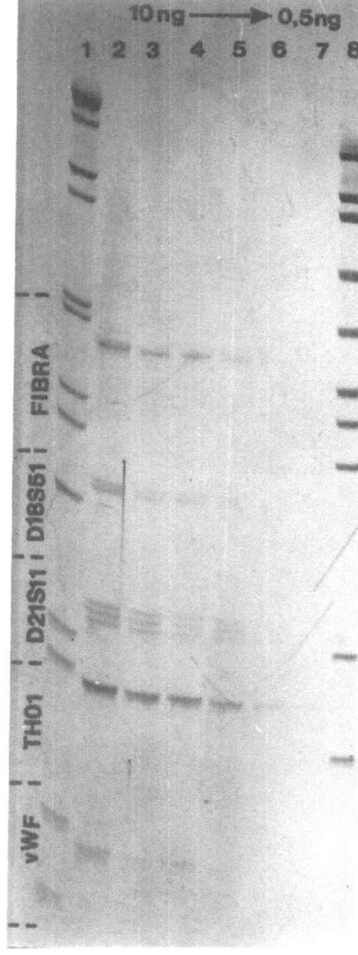

MULTIPLEX AMPLIFICATION AND AUTOMATED FLUORESCENT TYPING OF SHORT TANDEM REPEAT (STR) LOCI : THE FRENCH EXPERIENCE.

F. ROUSSELET, H. PFITZINGER and P. MANGIN

Institut de médecine légale, 11 rue Humann, 67085 Strasbourg Cedex, FRANCE

INTRODUCTION
The great majority of the biological samples available in forensic investigations for DNA identification purposes are severely degraded or present in minute amounts and can not be analysed by conventional RFLP (Restriction Fragment Length Polymorphism) methods using single locus probing. The polymerase Chain Reaction (PCR) amplification of short tandem repeat (STR) loci appears to be an efficient, sensitive and rapid DNA identification system for highly degraded samples. In order to use STR-PCR for forensic purposes or parental testing in routine analyses, a significant number of individuals (>100) has to be typed to determine accurately the allelic frequencies in the population of interest. Allele frequencies for the HUMTH01 (TH01) and HUMFESFPS (FES) STR loci were obtained through singleplex PCR and manual silver staining detection. The purchase of the automated ABI 373A sequencer allowed us to establish the allelic distributions for HUMVWA31A (VWA) and HUMF13A1 (F13) STR loci by duplex amplification and automated fluorescence-based detection. The quadruplex PCR of these four STR loci was then developped and performed on biological samples of various origins and appear to be robust. Furthermore, we studied a pentaplex-PCR, including 4 STR loci (D6S502, D18S51, D21S11 and HUMFIBRA) and the X-Y homologous gene amelogenin for sex determination : allelic frequencies were also determined.

MATERIALS AND METHODS

PRIMER SEQUENCES
The primer sequences for the HUMTH01, HUMFESFPS, HUMVWA31A, HUMF13A1, D18S51, D21S11 and HUMFIBRA STR loci and the X-Y amelogenin gene have already been described (Kimpton 1993 ; Urquhart 1995). Primer sequences for the D6S502 locus, selected from the Co-operative Human Linkage Centre (CHLC) data base, were kindly provided by the Forensic Science Service (FSS, UK).

QUADRUPLEX PCR
The amplification was performed in a final volume of 25 µl containing 10 to 20 ng of DNA, 1X PARR buffer, 1U Taq DNA polymerase (Gibco BRL), 200 µM dNTPs, 0.2 µM VWA and TH01 primers, 0.25 µM F13 primers and 0.5 µM FES primers. The TH01-1 and FES-1 primers were labeled with the FAM dye and the VWA-1 and F13-1 primers were labeled with the JOE dye. The cycling conditions were as follows : 45s-94°C, 30s-54°C and 30s-72°C for 28 cycles in a 9600 thermalcycler (Perkin Elmer). After amplification, a mixture of 2 µl PCR product, 4 µl formamide and 0.5 µl standard Genescan ROX 2500 (ABI) is loaded on a 6% denaturing polyacrylamide gel and run for 6 hours at 30 W. Alleles were identified using the corresponding allelic ladders and the genescan 2500 ROX internal molecular weight marker.

PENTAPLEX PCR
The pentaplex PCR was performed in the buffer described before for the quadruplex, on 5 ng of DNA, with the following primer concentrations : 0.05 µM HUMAMGXA and HUMAMGY, 0.1 µM D18S51, 0.25 µM D21S11, 0.4 µM HUMFIBRA and 0.9 µM D6S502. The cycling conditions were : 30s-93°C, 75s-58°C and 15s-72°C for 30 cycles. The amel-1, D18-1 and D21-2 primers were labelled with the 6-FAM dye, the D6-1 primer with the TET dye and the FGA-2 primer with the HEX dye. The PCR product was loaded on the gel as described previously in the presence of the Genescan 2500 TAMRA (ABI) molecular weight marker and run for 8 hours.

The allelic ladders for the 8 STR systems were kindly provided by the FSS (UK).

RESULTS AND DISCUSSION

The genotype distributions for the eight STR loci described in materials and methods, were in Hardy-Weinberg Equilibrium : no significant deviations were found in either system. The allelic distributions are shown in the following figure (fig 1).

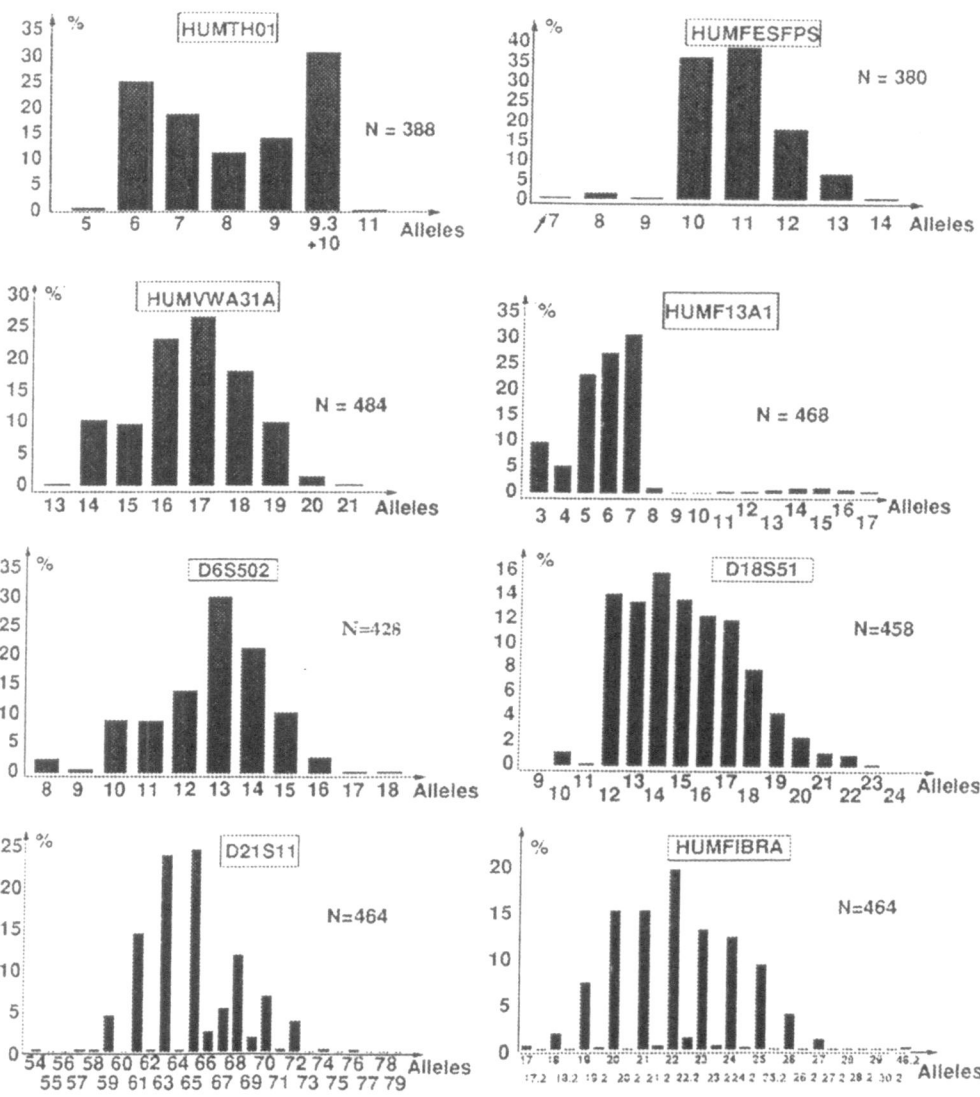

Figure 1 : Allele frequency distributions of the 8 STR loci studied, obtained from a minimum of 190 french caucasian individuals (N). At the HUMFIBRA locus, alleles ranged from 17 to 46.2 with possible stutter alleles designated as ".2" alleles.

The allelic distributions at the 4 loci (TH01, FES, VWA and F13), analized through quadruplex PCR, were compared to already published caucasian data and appeared to be similar to most of the samples studied. Differences were only noticed when comparing F13 frequencies in very small population samples (N≈50) where rare allele frequencies were overestimated. For D18S51, D21S11 and HUMFIBRA loci, the french and english population samples revealed to be homogeneous.

For each locus we determined the observed heterozygosity (Obs h), the allelic diversity (h) and the discrimination power (Pd) :

	TH01	FES	VWA	F13	D6S502	D18S51	D21S11	FGA
Obs h	0.77	0.73	0.81	0.76	0.77	0.89	0.82	0.86
h	0.77	0.70	0.81	0.77	0.82	0.88	0.84	0.87
Pd	0.91	0.80	0.94	0.90	0.94	0.97	0.95	0.97

QUADRUPLEX PCR : it was first performed on blood DNA samples, showing an efficient co-amplification of TH01, FES, VWA and F13 STR loci. When amplifying various DNA samples (blood stains on different types of tissues or support, mixed blood and sperm stains, sperm stains, vaginal swabs, cigarette buds and organs), the four STR loci rarely co-amplified as efficiently as with blood DNA samples. Most of the time, only three, two or only one STR loci could be detected at once, but the problem can, in some cases, be resolved by performing several PCR on different amounts of DNA. Furthermore, we amplified DNAs extracted from 7 different organs taken from the same body and animal DNAs, and showed the good reliability and human specificity of the system.
From a general point of view, the fluorescent JOE and FAM dyes, used to label the primers in the quadruplex PCR, will be replaced by HEX and 6-FAM dyes, which are much more sensitive.

PENTAPLEX PCR : in a first step, it was performed on blood DNA samples and on DNAs extracted from different organs of the same individual, and showed an efficient and reliable co-amplification of all loci. Validation tests are presently realized.

CONCLUSION
The multiplex amplification and automated fluorescent typing of STR and X-Y loci show to be very convenient. The multiplex PCR is robust and reproducible.
The co-amplification is very successful for DNAs extracted from blood samples or biological samples of good quality, but it can be more problematic for degraded or contaminated DNAs. The absence of amplification at some loci may be overcome by repeating the amplification on a series of different DNA concentrations. The use of different fluorescent dyes and the ranges of sizes of the chosen STRs allow the inclusion of additional loci to further increase the discrimination power of our multiplex systems, although the combination of the 8 polymorphic STRs described herein, including sex determination, is already a highly discriminating PCR for human individual identification (Pm for the 8 STR loci : 1.5×10^{-10}).

BIBLIOGRAPHY
-Kimpton et al. (1993) Automated DNA profiling employing "multiplex" amplification of short tandem repeat loci. PCR Methods & Applications 3:13-22
-Urquhart et al (1995) Highly discriminating heptaplex short tandem repeat PCR system for forensic identification. Biotechniques 18:116-121

ACKNOLEDGMENTS
We wish to thank Estelle Carniel for helpful technical assistance, as well as Colin Kimpton, Peter Gill and Andy Greenfield, from the FSS, for their great help and their kindness.

A Tetraplex PCR system for the analysis of paternity cases

C.Seidl, O.Jäger, E.Seifried

Institute for Transfusion Medicine and Immunohematology, Red Cross Blood Donor Service Hesse, Sandhofstrasse 1, 60528 Frankfurt, Germany

INTRODUCTION

Short tandem repeat loci (STR) with repeat unit lenght between 2-6 bp represent highly polymorphic markers in the human genome, that are ideal markers for genomic mapping and genetic linkage analysis and can be used for forensic and paternity applications. In contrast to the highly polymorphic VNTR loci, STR loci exhibit a limited polymorphism resulting in a reduced discrimination power. Feasability of amplification of STR loci using the polymerase chain reaction allows to multiplex several STR loci in a single PCR reaction. In combination with the use of fluorescence labelled primers employing different fluorescence dyes STR loci with overlapping or identical allele size ranges can be analyzed together in the same lane of a polyacryamid gel thus providing a rapid and sensitive method for human identification.

We have established a tetraplex PCR-STR sytem to combine the discrimination power of four tetrarepeat STR polymorphism at locus HUMTH01, HUMCYP19, HUMD8S639 and HUMACPP.

METHODS AND MATERIALS

STR-loci and PCR conditions. The STR Loci and corresponding primer sequences are summarized in table 1.

Table 1: Primersequences and fluorescence dye labels of the tetraplex PCR system

STR-Loci	Primersequences 5'- 3'	Dye-label	Ref.
HUMTH01 locus:11p15.5-p15 repeat:AATG	P5 GTGGGCTGAAAAGCTCCCGATTAT P3 GTGATTCCCATTGGCCTGTTCCTC	HEX	Polymeropoulos 1991
HUMCYP19 locus:15q21.1 repeat:TTTA	P5 GCAGGTACTTAGTTAGCTAC P3 TTACAGTGAGCCAAGGTCGT	FAM	Polymeropoulos 1992
HUMACPP locus:3q21-qter repeat:AAAT	P5 GGGCAACATGGTGAAACCTT P3 CCTAGCCTATACTTCCTTTC	TAMRA	Polymeropoulos 1991
HUMD8S639 locus: 8p21-p11 repeat: AGAT	P5 GAGTGATGGAAGAAAACAAGTAGC P3 CTCAACCAAAAAATGTAAAGTCAGG	HEX	Nelson 1994

All oligonucleotides were commercially synthesized and the 5'Primers were labeled with fluorescence dye markers (ABI DNA Facility, Weiterstadt, Germany). Following the allelic size distribution of the different STR-Systems, HUMCYP19 was labelled with FAM (5-carboxylfluorescein), HUMTH01 was labelled with HEX (6-carboxy-2',4',7',4,7-Hexachlorofluorescein), HUMACPP was labelled with TAMRA (N,N,N',N'-tetramethyl-6-carboxyrhodamine) and HUMD8S639 with HEX. Tetraplex PCR amplification was performed using 10-100ng genomic DNA in a 50µl reaction volume comprising 0,5 Units Taq DNA polymerase (Appligene), 1x PCR buffer (Appligen) , 200 mM each deoxyrinucleoside triphosphate (dNTP) (Boehringer Mannheim, Germany). Samples were amplified for 29 cycles of 30 sec at 94 C, 40 sec at 54 C and 30 sec at 72 C followed by a 5 min extension period at 72 C on a Perkin Elmer 9600 DNA Thermal Cycler. Primer concentrations were 10 pmol D8S639/P5 and P3, 5 pmol ACPP/P5 and P3, 5 pmol TH01/P5 and P3 and 5pmol CYP19/P5 and P3.

Allele size analysis. PCR products were analysed together with an internal standard in the same lane of a standard 6% polyacrylamid denaturing sequencing gel. The internal standard fragments were generated by PCR amplification using various primer combinations from the vector pGL2-basic (Promega). Internal standard fragments were labelled with the dye ROX (6-carboxy-X-rhodamine). A 2,5 µl aliquot of each amplification reaction was combined with 6 fmoles of the internal standard. Subsequently, samples were heat denatured before being loaded. Fragment separation was performed by gel electrophoresis at 30 W for 8 hours on an Applied Biosystems automated DNA sequencer model 373A. Relative position of fragments were calculated by measuring the laserlight induced fluorescence emission of the DNA fragments. Fragment sizes were determined automatically using GENESCAN 672 software (Perkin Elmer-ABI) employing the SOUTHERN local method for local reziproc calculation of fragment sizes utilising standard fragments of known size. Alleles were assigned according to the number of repeat unit of the individual allel. Alleles of HUMTH01 were assigned according to published sequences (Edwards 1992) whereas for allele assignment of HUMCYP19, D8S639 and HUMACPP individual alleles that we observed in our population study were sequenced.

Statistical analysis. Allele and genotype frequencies were collected from a minimum of 100 unrelated caucasian individuals for each STR loci. The polymorphic information content (PIC) was calculated using the formula of Botstein (1980). The discrimination index (DI) and the matching probability (pM) were calculated by the method of Jones (1972). The sample gene diversity (frequency of heterozygotes expected under Hardy-Weinberg equilibrium) was calculated as discribed by Kimpton (1993). Hardy-Weinberg-Equilibrium was calculated using the Chi squared goodness of fit test.

RESULTS

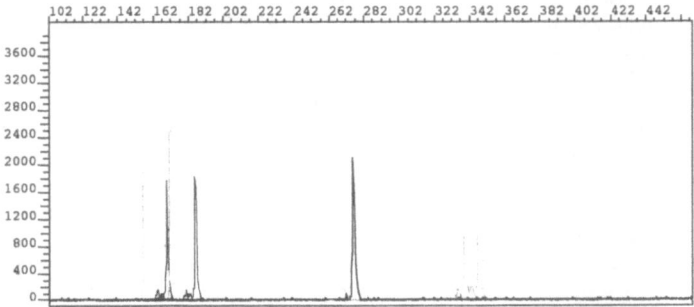

Fig.1: Fluorescence based analysis of the tetraplex STR system on a 6% polacryamid gel.

Table 2: Heterozygosity rate (HR), polymorphic information content (PIC), discrimination index (DI) and matching probability (pM) of the tetraplex PCR system.

STR loci	Alleles	Size range (bp)	HR	PIC	DI	pM
HUMTH01	6	154 - 174	0,746	0,727	0,91	0,09
HUMCYP19	7	168 - 191	0,727	0,719	0,88	0,12
HUMD8S639	14	317 - 373	0,857	0,819	0,95	0,05
HUMACPP	6	263 - 283	0,630	0,591	0,81	0,19
Combined					0,99	$1,0 \times 10^{-4}$

DISCUSSSION

In the present study we describe a tetraplex PCR system that combines STR loci with heterozygosity rates between 0,63 to 0,86 from four different chromosomes. All STR loci are easily amplified using the PCR conditions described giving distinct fragment sizes. Locus ACPP, however, is sensible to generate unspecific amplification products. Thus we would recommend to use an individual fluorescence dye label for this locus in a multiplex PCR system. Sequence analysis of the loci HUMCYP19, HUMD8S639 and HUMACPP reveals a basic tetranucleotide repeat unit structure of the individual alleles. In the present population sample, we observed 7 alleles for Locus HUMCYP19, 6 alleles for the loci HUMTH01 and HUMACPP and 14 alleles for locus D8S639. Locus D8S639, however comprises alleles that have structural differences but identical fragment sizes. Analysis of these alleles can only be performed using allele groups.

The combined discrimination index of all four STR loci is 0,99 with a propability of match of $1,0 \times 10^{-4}$. Combined pM values of all analysed loci below 10^{-8} may not be sufficient to determine paternity cases. The combination of this tetraplex system with additional STR loci and / or multiplex systems should however increase pM values and thus will contribute to improve the analysis of paternity or forensic cases.

REFERENCES

Botstein D., White R.L.,Skolnick M., Davis R.W (1980) Construction of a genetic linkage map in man using restriction fragment lenght polymorphisms. Am.J.Hum.Genet. Vol 32: 182-190

Edwards A, Hammond HA, Jin L, Caskey CT, Chakraborty R (1992). Genetic variation at five trimeric and tetrameric tandem repeat loci in four human population groups. Genomics 12: 241-253

Jones DA (1972) Blood samples: Probability of discrimination. J.Forens.Sci.Soc., Vol 12: 355-359

Kimpton CP, Gill P, Walton A, Urquhart A, Millican ES, Adams M (1993) Automated DNA profiling employing multiplex amplification of short tandem repeat loci. PCR methods and applications, Vol 3: 13-22

Nelson L, Lu J, Petterson M, Riley R, Ward K (1994) Tetranucleotide repeat polymorphism at the D8S639 locus. Human Molecular Genetics, Vol. 3, No 7: 1209

Polymeropoulos MH, Xiao H, Rath DS, Merril CR (1991) Tetranucleotide repeat polymorphism at the human tyrosine hydroxylase gene (TH). Nucleid Acids Research, Vol. 19: 3753

Polymeropoulos MH, Xiao H, Rath DS, Merril CR (1992) Tetranucleotide repeat polymorphism at the human aromatase cytochrome P-450 gene (CYP19). Nucleic Acids Research, Vol.19, No.1: 195

Polymeropoulos MH, Xiao H, Rath DS, Merril CR (1991) Tetranucleotide repeat polymorphism at the human prostatic acid phosphatase (ACPP) gene. Nucleid Acids Research, Vol. 19, No. 17: 4792

Puers C, Hammond HA, Jin L, Caskey CT, Schumm JW (1993) Identification of repeat sequence heterogeneity at the polymorphic short tandem repeat locus HUMTH01 [AATG]n and reassignement of alleles in population analysis by using a locus specific allelic ladder. Am.J.Hum.Genet. Vol 53: 953-958

DEVELOPMENT AND APPLICATIONS OF HIGH THROUGHPUT MULTIPLEX STR SYSTEMS

J. Schumm, C. Sprecher, A. Lins, and K. Micka

Promega Corporation, 2800 Woods Hollow Road, Madison, WI 53711, U.S.A.

INTRODUCTION

This chapter describes nine polymorphic tetrameric short tandem repeat (STR) loci (Edwards et al, 1991, 1992, Polymeropoulos et al., 1991) and the development of methods which are compatible with both silver and fluorescent detection, providing a pwerful set of markers for universal application. The creation of allelic ladders and multiplex sets involving these systems accelerates and simplifies analysis providing for rapid, efficient, and precise application to allele identification.

CHOICE OF STR SYSTEMS AND CONSTRUCTION OF ALLELIC LADDERS

Following an initial screening of over 35 STR loci, we selected 9 loci for additional applications development. These nine systems carry tetranucleotide repeats and display fewer artifacts than the rejected loci whether detected using silver stain analysis (Bassam et al, 1991) or fluorescence. Table 1 displays the chromosome location and the known allele size range for each of the 9 STR systems and the amelogenin locus (Sullivan et al, 1993). The amelogenin locus, which is not a true STR, generates a 212 bp fragment from the X chromosome and a 218 bp fragment from the Y chromosome, thus allowing its application to sex identification.

For each of the nine STR loci and the amelogenin locus, we constructed an allelic ladder, i.e. a mixture of many or all of the possible amplified alleles for the individual locus. Allelic ladders serve as size standards allowing rapid and precise comparison of amplified sample DNAs with well-characterized allelic ladder components (Puers et al, 1994). Using these size standards, there is no need for measurement of migration distance or calculation to determine the size of each allele. The components of the allelic ladder for each locus and the size ranges for these fragments are listed in Table 1.

MULTIPLEX STR SYSTEMS

To achieve high throughput with the STR systems, we have developed two triplex sets for use with silver stain (See Figure 1 for silver stain of the CTT triplex) or other post-electrophoresis staining technologies and two related quadriplex systems which

Table 1.

Locus	Chromosome Location	Size Range of Known Alleles (bases)	Size Range of Allelic Ladder (bases)	Allelic Ladder Component Names[1]
Amelogenin	X:Y	212, 218	212, 218	212, 218
CSF1PO	5q33.5-34	295 - 327	299 - 323	7 through 15
F13A01	6p24-25	281 -331	283 - 331	4 through 9, 11 through16
F13B	1q31-q32.1	169 - 189	169 - 185	6 through 10
FESFPS	15q25-qter	222 - 250	226 - 246	8 through 13
HPRTB	Xq26	259 - 303	259 - 303	6 through 17
LPL	8p22	105-133	105 - 133	7 through 14
TH01	11p15.5	179 - 203	179 - 203	5 through 11
TPOX	2p23-2pter	224 - 252	232 - 248	6 through13
vWF	12p12-pter	131 - 171	143 - 167	14 through 20

[1] Names of alleles represent the number of repeats within the alleles. The TH01 allele 9.3 (198 bases), F13A01 allele 10 (307 bases) and allele 3.2 (281 bases), F13B allele 11, FESFPS alleles 7 and 14, and vWF alleles 11, 13, and 21 are not currently included in these allelic ladders.

can be used in conjunction with fluorescence detection equipment such as the Hitachi FMBIO100, Molecular Dynamics FluorImager, or Applied Biosystems DNA Sequencer 373 or 377 instruments (Table 2). The combined use of the two quadriplexes provides matching probabilities ranging from 1 in 17.000.000 to 1 in 430.000.000 depending on the population being studied (Table 2). Either the CTT triplex or the CTTv quadriplex can be used in co-amplification with the sex identification locus, amelogenin, to generate a quadriplex or pentaplex, respectively, known as CTAT and CTATv.

Table 2.

	Matching Probability[1]		
	Caucasian-American	African-American	Hispanic-American
Multiplexes for Silver Detection			
CTT Triplex (CSF1PO,TPOX,TH01)	1 in 424	1 in 1639	1 in546
FFv Triplex (F13A01,FESFPS,vWF)	1 in 909	1 in 2785	1 in 1342
Both Triplexes (6 loci, above)	1 in 385000	1 in 4565000	1 in 733000
Multiplexes for Fluorescent Detection			
CTTv Quadriplex (CSF1PO,TPOX,TH01,vWF)	1 in 6623	1 in 25575	1 in 7194
FFFL Quadriplex (F13A01,FESFPS,F13B,LPL)	1 in 2632	1 in 16807	1 in 3279
Both Quadriplexes (8 loci, above)	1 in 17400000	1 in 430000000	1 in 23600000

[1] Matching probabilities have been determined as part of an unpublished collaborative study among S Creacy and RA Bever of Genetic Design (Greensboro, NC) and authors CJ Sprecher and JW Schumm.

The most efficient use of these systems is achieved by simultaneous detection of both quadriplexes in a single gel lane using the Hitachi FMBIO instrument. This can be performed with the CTTv quadriplex labeled with one fluorescent dye and the FFFL quadriplex with a second fluorescent label. This machine takes as little as 10 minutes to scan the gel following electrophoresis of the amplified products of both quadriplexes in the same gel lane using a standard gel rig. The resulting scans can be cleanly separated into individual black and white images for ease of interpretation as seen in Figure 2.

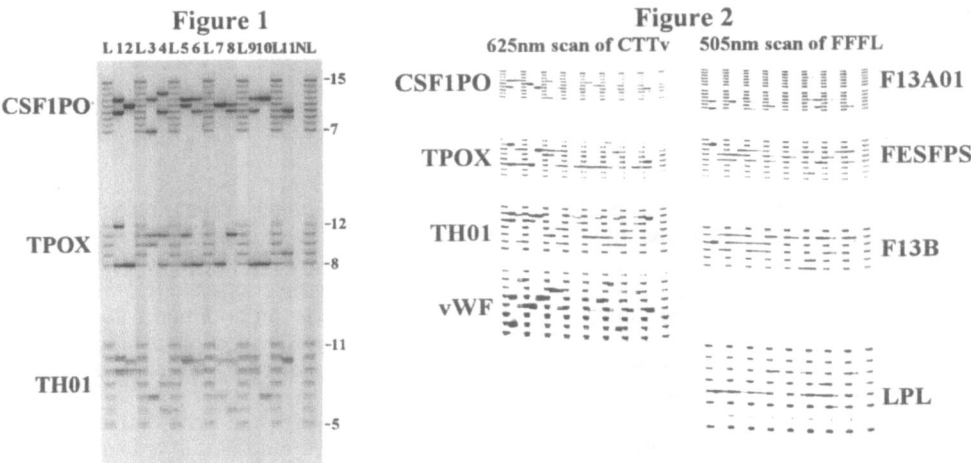

Figure 1 displays silver stain visualization of 11 samples (Lanes 1-11) amplified simultaneously at the three STR loci the CTT triplex. Allelic ladders for each locus have been included (Lanes L) to simplify interpretation of unknown samples. The numbers to the right of each locus indicate the number of tetranucleotide repeats present in each component of the allelic ladders.

Figure 2 shows simultaneous fluorescent detection of two STR quadriplex systems using the Hitachi FMBIO machine. The CTTv and FFFL quadriplexes were labeled with different fluorescent dyes and detected with 625nm and 505nm scans, respectively. Each STR locus is labeled. Allelic ladders for each locus have been included to simplify interpretation of unknown samples.

REFERENCES

Bassam BJ, Caetano-Anolles G, and Gresshoff PM (1991) Fast and sensitive silver staining of DNA in polyacrylamide gels. Anal. Biochem. 196:80-83.

Edwards A, Civitello A, Hammond HA, and Caskey CT (1991) DNA typing and genetic mapping with trimeric and tetrameric tandem repeats, Am. J. Hum. Genet. 49:746-756

Edwards A, Hammond HA, Jin, L, Caskey CT, and Chakraborty R (1992) Genetic variation at five trimeric and tetrameric tandem repeat loci in four human population groups, Genomics 12:241-253

Polymeropoulos, MH,Xiao H, Rath DS, and Merril CR (1991) Tetranucleotide repeat polymorphism at the human tyrosine hydroxylase gene (TH), Nucl. Acids Res. 19:3753

Puers, C, Lins AM, Sprecher CJ, Brinkmann B, and Schumm JW (1994) Analysis of polymorphic short tandem repeat loci using well-characterized allelic ladders. In: Proceedings from the Fourth International Symposium on Human Identification 1993. Promega Corporation, pp 161-172

Sullivan K, et al (1993) A rapid and quantitative DNA sex test: Fluorescence-based PCR analysis of X-Y homologous gene amelogenin, Biotechniques 15:636-641

Properties of an STR multiplex marker system suitable for paternity and forensic determinations.

J. Neuweiler, L. Perlee, J. Venturini, I. Balazs

Lifecodes Corp., 550 West Ave., Stamford Ct 06902, USA

INTRODUCTION

Simple sequence repeat polymorphisms composed of tandem di-,tri- or tetranucleotide repeats (STR) are highly abundant in the human genome (Williamson et al. 1990) and are particularly suitable for detection by PCR amplification. These type of loci have been used for population genetic studies, determination of paternity or forensic analysis (Edwards et al. 1991, Kimpton et al. 1993). Analysis of these markers has been performed either by individual amplification of single loci or by the simultaneous amplification of several loci (i.e. multiplexing). Alleles can be detected by gel electrophoresis followed by radioactive labeling, silver staining or fluorescence detection.
We developed a combination of 3 polymorphic loci containing GATA repeats that is highly informative for paternity and forensic determinations and can be amplified in a single PCR reaction.

MATERIALS AND METHODS

DNA was isolated from blood samples of unrelated individuals by either phenol/chloroform extraction or by a non-organic procedure. The amount of DNA in each sample was determined with the use of a yield gel.

The amplification reaction was assembled using the components of the Multiplex I Kit (Lifecodes Corp.) consisting of 5 ul Primer Mix , 5 ul of 10 x PCR buffer, 5 ul of dNTPs. The mixture was combined with 1.25 U Taq polymerase and 10 ng of human DNA. Final volume was 50 ul. The Multiplex-I Primer Mix contained primers specific for the amplification of D3S1744, D12S1090 and D18S849 loci. Samples were amplified in a Perkin-Elmer 480 Thermo-cycler with 30 cycles of 1 min at 95°C, 1 min at 65°C and 1 min at 72°C.

The amplified material was denatured and fractionated by electrophoresis in 4% acrylamide/8M urea gel (0.4 mm x 17 cm x 32 cm) for 1 hour at 2000 volts. Following electrophoresis, the gel was fixed in acetic acid, stained with silver nitrate and developed with sodium carbonate/thiosulfate. A photograph of the results was obtained by placing the gel on a light box and exposing it to an X-ray duplicating film (Kodak).

For each sample, the size of alleles was measured by comparison to size standards made by mixing the individual alleles of these loci (i.e. allelic ladder). The allelic ladder was loaded in lanes flanking the sample(s). The exact size of each rung in the ladder was determined by DNA sequence analysis of individual alleles (Perlee et al. 1995)

RESULTS AND DISCUSSION

Analysis of DNA samples from random individuals resulted in the identification of 9 alleles for D3S1744 and D18S849 and more than 25 alleles for D12S1090. Sequence analysis of the alleles indicate that these polymorphisms are the result of variations in the number of tetranucleotide repeats present in these loci (Perlee et al. 1995).

The primers used to amplify these loci were designed to produce allele sizes that did not overlap between loci. As a result, these loci can be amplified simultaneously in a single amplification reaction and their respective alleles separated by gel electrophoresis. Locus D18S849 has alleles that vary in size from 93 to 133 bases, D3S1744 has alleles from 150 to 182 bases and D12S1090, from 212 to 306. A summary of the general properties of the loci composing the Multiplex are summarized in Table 1.

The analysis of DNA from random individuals from North American Black and Caucasoid populations was used to generate a table of allele frequencies. An analysis of the frequency of the observed genotypes versus those calculated from the frequency of the alleles indicate that the loci are in H-W equilibrium. A summary of the frequency of alleles in these two populations are shown in Table 2. A large number of alleles have been observed in both populations with a sightly higher heterogeneity observed in the Black population.

The ability of this multiplex system to resolve cases of disputed paternity and for human identification was calculated for these loci. The results indicate that for paternity determinations the combined power of exclusion of the 3 loci is about 98% and the combined power of discrimination is 1 in 5600. Therefore, this multiplex , is a useful combination of genetic markers for application in human identification.

Table 1. General properties of the Multiplex loci.

Locus:	D3S1744	D12S1090	D18S849
Chromosome:	3q24	12q12	18q12-q21
Size range of alleles:	150 to 182 bases	212 to 306 bases	93 to 133 bases
Number of alleles:	9	>25	9
Heterozygosity: Black	87%	96%	75%
Cauc.	83%	95%	75%
P. E. for Paternity: Black	63%	87%	51%
Cauc.	63%	84%	51%
Power of Discrimination: Black	1 in 15	1 in 98	1 in 4
Cauc.	1 in 16	1 in 88	1 in 4

Populations analyzed (number of individuals):   North American Blacks (103);
North American Caucasoids (110)

Table 2. Allele frequency in North American Black and Caucasoid populations.

D3S1744			D12S1090			D18S849		
Allele size	Black	Cauc.	Allele size	Black	Cauc.	Allele size	Black	Cauc.
150	0.005	0.005	212	0.010	0.009	93	0.068	0.005
154	0.053	0.109	216	0.005	0.009	97	0.000	0.000
158	0.121	0.095	220	0.034	0.045	101	0.019	0.000
162	0.146	0.109	224	0.112	0.036	105	0.015	0.000
166	0.325	0.286	228	0.049	0.036	109	0.000	0.000
170	0.141	0.227	232	0.029	0.027	113	0.010	0.068
174	0.160	0.141	236	0.019	0.005	117	0.136	0.136
178	0.044	0.023	240	0.010	0.014	121	0.417	0.395
182	0.005	0.005	244	0.005	0.009	125	0.262	0.268
			248	0.039	0.018	129	0.058	0.123
			253	0.053	0.073	133	0.015	0.005
			257	0.121	0.100			
			261	0.063	0.105			
			265	0.068	0.091			
			269	0.053	0.114			
			273	0.049	0.068			
			277	0.044	0.068			
			281	0.053	0.114			
			284	0.063	0.045			
			288	0.034	0.009			
			290	0.005	0.005			
			294	0.039	0.000			
			298	0.024	0.000			
			302	0.015	0.000			
			306	0.005	0.000			

REFERENCES

Edwards A, Civitello A, Hammond HA, Caskey CT (1991) DNA typing and genetic mapping with trimeric and tetrameric tandem repeats. Am J Hum Genet 49:746-756

Kimpton CP, Gill P, Walton A, Urquhart A, Millican ES, Adams M (1993) Automated DNA profiling employing multiplex amplification of short tandem repeat loci. PCR Methods and Applications 3:13-22

Perlee L, Neuweiler J, Balazs I (1995) Analysis of sequence variations in the alleles from three STR loci. this proceeding.

Williams R, Bowcock A, Kidd K, Pearson P, Schmidtke J, Chan HS et al. (1990) Report of the committee and catalogues of cloned and mapped genes and DNA polymorphisms. Cytogenet Cell Genet 55:457-778

ANALYSIS OF D1S80 VNTR ALLELE POLYMORPHISM AND ASSOCIATION WITH A NEARBY FLANKING SEQUENCE POLYMORPHISM IN TWO SPANISH POPULATIONS

C. Albarrán[1], O. García[2], R. Deka[3], A. Alonso[1], P. Martín[1], M. Sancho[1], D.N. Stivers[4] and R. Chakraborty[4].

[1] Sección de Biología. Instituto de Toxicología. M° de Justicia e Interior. Madrid. SPAIN
[2] Laboratorio UTAP. Departamento de Interior. Gobierno Vasco. Bilbao. SPAIN
[3] Department of Human Genetics, University of Pittsburgh. Pittsburgh. USA
[4] Human Genetics Center, University of Texas, Health Science Center, Houston. Texas. USA

INTRODUCTION

Variable number of tandem repeats (VNTR) loci are highly informative markers for linkage analysis and identity testing. In addition to the variation in the number of repeats, some VNTR loci display variabilty of the repeat sequence so that an additional polymorphism level can be observed analyzing the interspersion pattern of variant repeats along the tandem repeat array (Jeffreys et al. 1991; Neil and Jeffreys 1993). For the majority of VNTR loci, however, the extent of polymorphism of the flanking sequences is not known, despite some early studies showing linkage between VNTR specific-alleles and nearby RFLPs (Higgs et al. 1986; Cox et al. 1988; Renges et al. 1992; Martinson et al. 1994).

We have recently described a polymorphic Hinf I restriction site in the flanking region of the VNTR locus D1S80 (Alonso et al. 1995). In this study, we have determined the RFLP/VNTR D1S80 haplotype frequencies in a cosmopolitan population of individuals living in Madrid (Central-Spain) and in a population of autochthonous individuals from the Basque Country (North-Spain) in order to evaluate the magnitude of linkage between VNTR specific-alleles and the biallellic RFLP polymorphism.

MATERIALS AND METHODS

Population Sample and Sample Preparation

EDTA blood samples were collected from two different spanish population samples: a cosmopolitan population sample of 205 unrelated individuals living in Madrid and a population sample of 201 autochthonous individuals from the Basque Country. The DNA was extracted by the standard phenol/chloroform extraction procedure.

PCR, Digestion and Typing

PCR amplification of D1S80 was performed according to the manufacturer´s recomendations using the AmpliFLP D1S80 Kit (Perkin-Elmer Corporation, Norwalk, CT). Restriction of the PCR products was performed as previously described (Alonso et al. 1995). Undigested PCR products and Hinf I restricted ones were typed by vertical polyacrylamide gel electrophoresis followed by silver stain (Alonso et al. 1995).

Statistical Analysis

The allele frequencies at individual loci were computed by the gene count method (Li CC, 1976). The haplotype frequencies in the two Spanish populations were estimated based on a maximum likelihood approach following an E-M algorithm of haplotype frequency estimation from two-locus genotype data (Long et al. 1995).

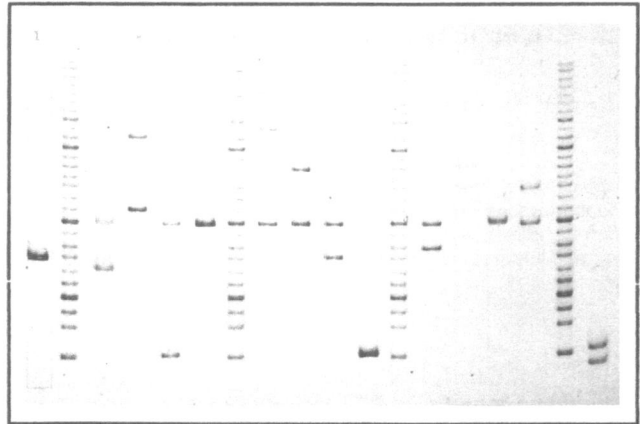

Fig 1. Representative D1S80 profiles as analyzed by restriction of the PCR products with *Hinf* I and subsequent polyacrylamide gel electrophoresis followed by silver stain. All samples were previously typed before *Hinf* I restriction. **Samples** (from left to right): 21-21-; ladder; 24+24-; 29+36+; 18+24-; 24-24-; ladder; 24-37+; 24-29-; 24-25+; 18+18+; ladder; 22-24-; 31+33+; 24-28+; 24-31+; ladder; 17+18+.

Table 1. Haplotype frequencies estimated using (Long 1995)´s haplotype estimation program. Figures in parentheses are expected haplotype frequencies when an absence of linkage disequilibrium is assumed. The G statistic, twice the negative log of likelihood ratios (which is roughly distributed as a χ^2 statistic) was 236.23 for the Madrid sample and 294.34 for the Basque sample; the null hypothesis is no disequilibrium between the two loci. Both are significant (p < 0.001), based on 1000 Monte Carlo simulations. Gene frequency totals were estimated directly from the sample, not by adding haplotype frequenies, and hence may differ slightly due to rounding error .

| D1S80 | Basque Country | | | | | Madrid | | | | |
	Hinf I -		*Hinf* I +		Totals	*Hinf* I -		*Hinf* I +		Totals
17	--	(--)	--	(--)	-	.0024	(.0025)	.0024	(.0024)	.005
18	--	(.1442)	.2637	(.1194)	.264	--	(.1263)	.2488	(.1226)	.25
20	.0368	(.0245)	.008	(.0203)	.045	.0122	(.0062)	--	(.006)	.012
21	.0547	(.0327)	.005	(.027)	.06	.0395	(.0223)	.0045	(.0216)	.044
22	.0327	(.0272)	.017	(.0225)	.05	.025	(.0235)	.0209	(.0228)	.046
23	.0075	(.0041)	--	(.0034)	.007	.0073	(.0037)	--	(.0036)	.007
24	.3279	(.1811)	.0029	(.1498)	.331	.3294	(.1794)	.0243	(.1742)	.354
25	.0373	(.0204)	--	(.0169)	.037	.0272	(.0272)	.0264	(.0264)	.054
26	.0050	(.0027)	--	(.0023)	.005	.0132	(.0074)	.0015	(.0073)	.015
27	--	(.0095)	.0174	(.0079)	.017	--	(.0025)	.0049	(.0024)	.005
28	--	(.0191)	.0348	(.0158)	.035	.0027	(.0223)	.0412	(.0216)	.044
29	.0324	(.0286)	.0198	(.0237)	.052	.033	(.0297)	.0255	(.0288)	.06
30	.0078	(.0109)	.0121	(.009)	.02	--	(.0037)	.0073	(.0036)	.007
31	.0026	(.0381)	.0671	(.0315)	.07	.0025	(.0247)	.0462	(.0240)	.05
32	.0025	(.0027)	.0025	(.0023)	.005	.0076	(.0062)	.0046	(.0060)	.012
33	--	(--)	--	(--)	-	--	(.0025)	.0049	(.0024)	.005
34	--	(--)	--	(--)	-	--	(.0025)	.0049	(.0024)	.005
35	--	(--)	--	(--)	-	--	(.0025)	.0049	(.0024)	.005
36	--	(--)	--	(--)	-	--	(.005)	.0098	(.0048)	.01
37	--	(.0013)	.0025	(.0011)	.002	--	(.005)	.0098	(.0048)	.01
40	--	(--)	--	(-)	-	.0049	(.0025)	--	(.0024)	.005
Total	.547	(.547)	.453	(.453)		.51	(.51)	.49	(.49)	

RESULTS AND DISCUSSION

Fig 1. shows some representative D1S80 profiles as analyzed by restriction of the PCR products with *Hinf* I and subsequent polyacrylamide gel electrophoresis followed by silver stain. A total of 21 VNTR-alleles and 31 RFLP/VNTR haplotypes were observed in the population sample of individuals living in Madrid while a total of 15 VNTR alleles and 23 RFLP/VNTR haplotypes were observed in the population of autochthonous individuals from the Basque Country.

Table 1 shows the estimated haplotype frequencies and allele frequencies in the two Spanish populations. Also shown are the expected haplotype frequencies in the two samples under the assumption of linkage equilibrium between the two sites (i.e., computed by multiplying the respective allele frequencies). As can be seen, the haplotype frequencies determined in both population samples show an extreme association between the *Hinf* I + allele and the VNTR allele of 18 repeats and between the *Hinf* I - allele and VNTR allele of 24 repeats, while the remaining VNTR allele associate more randomly with the two flanking *Hinf* I alleles. The linkage disequilibrium observed between the flanking polymorphism and the two high frequency modal VNTR alleles (18 and 24) that is share by the two different populations analyzed, together with the fact that mutation at minisatellite occurs without exchange of flanking regions (Jeffreys et al. 1994), suggest that the 18 and 24 alleles could be the original VNTR alleles at this locus and the rest of VNTR alleles associated with the *Hinf* I + mutation would arise from the 18 allele, while the VNTR allele associated with the *Hinf* I - mutation would arise from the allele of 24 repeats.

Data gathered in this work also indicates the utility of polymorphisms at these two sites for identity testing and parentage analysis. First, the genotype frequencies in these two samples are in general conformity with their respective Hardy-Weinverg expectations. This is checked by the likelihood ratio test and exact test, as performed in Edwards et al. (1992), Hammond et al. (1994), and Deka et al. (1995), particulary when the rare alleles of frequencies of 0.05 or less at the D1S80 site are merged with their adjacent alleles (data not shown). Second, at the level of the allele frequencies at individual loci, as well as at the level of haplotypes these two Spanish populations are not significantly different (haplotype frequency heterogeneity $\chi^2 = 56.7$ with 41 df, p ~ 0.06), suggesting that these two populations are not genetically very dissimilar. Third, with heterozygosity of nerly 50% at the *Hinf* I site and approximately 80% at the D1S80 VNTR loci in these samples, these two polymorphisms offer an average probability of discrimination between genotypes of two unrelated individuals exceeding 94%. In other words, these two polymorphism can constitute important elements of forensic and parentage analysis based on PCR-based DNA typing protocols.

REFERENCES

Alonso A, Martín P, Albarrán C, Sancho M (1995) Int J Legal Med 107: 216-218
Cox NJ, Bell GI, Xiang K-S (1988) Am J Hum Genet 43: 495-501
Deka R, Jin L, Shriver MD, Yu LM, DeCroo S, Hundrieser J, Bunker CH, Ferrell RE, Chakraborty R (1995) Am J Hum Genet 56: 461-474
Edwards A, Hammond HA, Jin L, Caskey CT, Chakraborty (1992) Genomics 12: 241-253
Hammond HA, Jin L, Zhong Y, Caskey CT, Chakraborty R (1994) Am J Hum Genet 55: 175-189
Higgs DR, Wainscoat JS, Flint J, Hill AVS, Thein SL, Nicholls RD, Teal H, et al. (1986) Proc Natl Acad Sci USA 83: 5165-5169
Jeffreys AJ, MacLeod A, Tamaki K, Neil DL, Monckton DG (1991) Nature 354: 204-209
Jeffreys AJ, Tamaki K, MacLeod A, Monckton DG, Neil DL, Armour JAL (1994) Nature Genetics 6: 136-145
Li CC (1976) First Course in Population Genetics, Pacific Grove, California, p.16
Long JC, Williams RC, Urbanek M (1995) Am J Hum Genet 56: 799-810
Martinson JJ, Boyce AJ, Clegg JB (1994) Am J Hum Genet 55: 513-525
Neil DL, Jeffreys AJ (1993)Hum Mol Genet 2: 1129-1135
Renges H-H, Peacock R, Dunning AM, Talmud P, Humphries SE (1992) Ann Hum Genet 56: 11-13

SOMATIC INSTABILITY IN CANCER AT SEVEN TETRAMERIC STR LOCI USED IN FORENSIC GENETICS

A. Alonso*, P. Martín*, C. Albarrán*, A. Guzman***, B. Aguilera**, H. Oliva*** and M. Sancho*

* Sección de Biología ** Sección de Anatomía Patológica. Instituto de Toxicología. Mº de Justicia e Interior. Madrid. SPAIN.
*** Fundación Jimenez Díaz. Departamento de Anatomía Patológica. Madrid. SPAIN.

INTRODUCTION

Microsatellite repeats have been reported to be unstable in some inhereted diseases (Caskey et al. 1992; Richards et al. 1992) and in several human cancers (Aaltonen et al. 1993; Thibodeau et al. 1993; Ionov et al. 1993). Abnormalities in the DNA mismatch-repair pathway have been proposed as being responsible for microsatellite instability in some type of cancers (Fishel et al. 1993; Leach et al. 1993).

In an attemp to evaluate the impact that the microsatellite instability observed in human cancers could have in some forensic DNA studies (i.e. genetic identification of fixed tumor specimens that were thought to have been mis-paired, paternity testing from fixed tumor biopsies in cases involving deceased parents,...) we have analyzed seven polymorphic STR loci (TH01, TPOX, CSF1PO, VWA, FES/FPS, F13A1, and F13B) in DNAs extracted from paired normal and colorectal or gastric tumor tissue samples corresponding to 21 individuals.

Our preliminary results show a high incidence of allele gain in gastric tumors that affects multiple STR loci concurrently, and a relatively low incidence of genetic instability in colorectal tumors restricted to allelic imbalance at the CSF1PO locus.

MATERIALS AND METHODS

The DNA was extracted by the standard phenol/chloroform extraction procedure from fresh-frozen tumor (13 colorectal adenocarcinomas and 8 gastric adenocarcinomas) and normal tissues corresponding to 21 individuals. The amplification of STR loci was performed by single-locus PCR reactions in the case of VWA, FES/FPS, F13A1, and F13B loci or by a multiplex PCR reaction in the case of TH01, TPOX, and CSF1PO loci according to the manufacturer's recommendations using the GenePrint STR System (Promega Corporation, Madison, WI, USA). PCR products were analyzed by denaturing polyacrylamide gel electrophoresis and subsequent detection by silver stain (Budowle et al. 1991; Martín et al. 1995). Alleles were designed according to the number of the repeat units using sequenced allelic ladders. Samples that showed differences in the STR profiles between tumor and normal DNAs were reanalyzed from a second DNA extract.

RESULTS AND DISCUSSION

Instability at one or more loci was observed in 75% (6/8) of gastric tumors and 15% (2/13) of colorectal tumors (Table 1).

Instabilities were apparent for the majority of gastric tumors as partial allelic losses as well as extra-alleles of different size in the tumor that were not present in the normal DNA (Fig. 1). 17 out of 21 STR instabilities observed in gastric tumors were extra-alleles, while only 4 were partial allelic losses. The difference in size between the extrabands observed in the tumors and the closest allele detected in the paired normal DNAs varied from one to six repeat units (Fig. 1). The only instability observed in 2 out of 13 colorectal tumors analyzed was a partial allelic loss at the CSF1PO locus (chromosome 5p). The loci that presented higher numbers of instabilities were CSF1PO (4 cases of allele imbalance and 3 cases of extra-alleles out of 21 cases) and VWA (5 cases of extra-alleles out of 21 cases).

Our results support previous studies which showed a high incidence of STR instability in gastric tumors (Han 1993) and also allow to confirm two patterns of genetic instability in sporadic cancers: allele gain which is the most frequent pattern of instability observed in the present study in gastric adenocarcinoma and allele loss which is the only STR instability (restricted to the CSF1PO locus) observed in colorrectal adenocarcinoma. Apart from cancer type, other factors that could influence the pattern of instability (tumor stage, sequence of the STR repeat unit, chromosomal location,...) should be further investigated.

In conclusion, although the incidence of instability in tetrameric STR loci depends on the type of cancer and other factors, this kind of genetic alterations should be taken into account as a potencial source of error when interpreting STR profiles obtained from neoplasic tissues in identity testing studies.

Table 1. Abnormalities of microsatellite repeats found in tumors.

MICROSATELLITE MARKER			TUMOR TYPE				TOTAL MARKER
Chromosome Location	Name	Repeat unit sequence	Colon		Stomach		
			Pattern of Instability				
			Loss	Gain	Loss	Gain	
1q31-q32.1	HUMF13B	AAAT	--	--	--	2	2 (9.5%)
2p13	HUMTPOX	AATG	--	--	--	2	2 (9.5%)
5q33	HUMCSF1PO	AGAT	2	--	2	3	7 (33.3%)
6p24-6p25	HUMF13A1	AAAG	--	--	1	1	2 (9.5%)
11p15.5	HUMTH01	AATG	--	--	1	1	2 (9.5%)
12p12-pter	HUMVWA	AGAT	--	--	--	5	5 (23.8%)
15q25-qter	HUMFES/FPS	AAAT	--	--	--	3	3 (14.3%)
TOTAL (tumor type)			2 (15.4%)		6 * (75%)		

(*) Total number of gastric tumors showing instabilities (three gastric tumors showed instability for 5 STR loci and the other three showed instability for two STR loci.

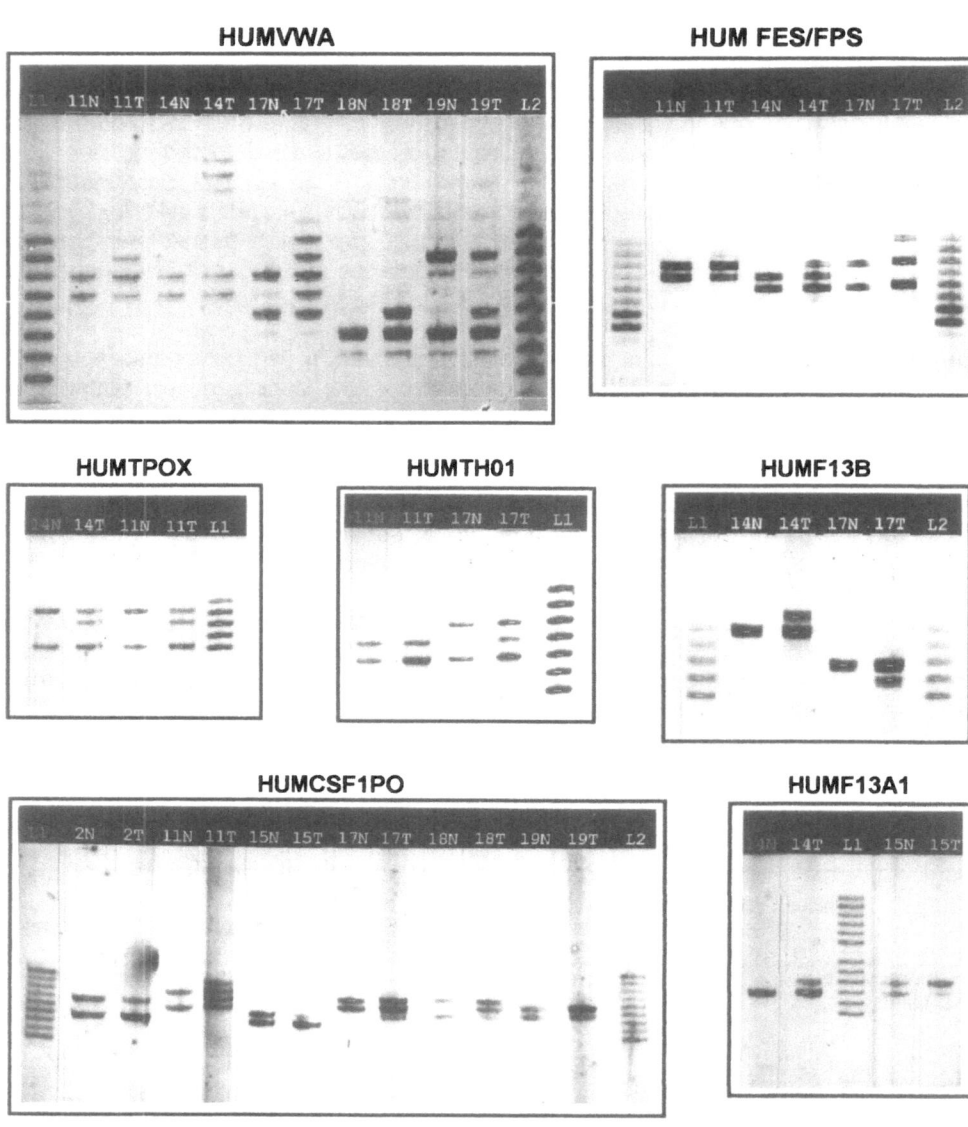

Fig. 1. Abnormalities of STR profiles in tumor DNA compared to constitucional STR profiles in normal DNA from the same patient. (L): allelic ladder.

REFERENCES

Aaltonen LA, Peltomaki P, Leach FS, Sistonen P, Pylkkanen L, Meckline JP, Jarvinen PJ, Powell SM, Jen J,
Budowle B, Chakraborty R, Giusti AM, Eisenberg AJ, Allen RC (1991) Am J Hum Genet 48: 137-144
Caskey CT, Pizzuti A, Fu YM, Fenwick RG, Nelson DL (1992) Science 256: 784-788
Fishel R, Lescoe MK, Rao MRS, Copeland NG, Jenkins NA, Garber J, Kane M, Kolodner R (1993) Cell 75: 1027-1038
Hamilton SR, Petersen GM, Kiuzler KW, Vogelstein B, De la Chapelle A (1993) Science 260: 812-816
Han MJ, Yanagisawa A, Kalo Y, Park J-G, Nakamura Y (1993) Cancer research 53: 5087-5089
Ionov Y, Peinado MA, Malkshosyan S, Shibata D, Perucho M (1993) Nature 363: 558-561
Leach FS, Nocolaides NC, Papadopoulus N et al. (1993) Cell 75: 1215-1225
Martín P, Alonso A, Budowle B, Albarrán C, García O, Sancho M (1995) Int J Leg Med (in press)
Richards RF, Sutherland GR (1992) Cell 70: 709-712
Thibodeau SN, Bien G, Schaid D (1993) Science 266: 816-819

NULL ALLELES DETECTION IN LOCI D1S7, D7S21 AND D12S11 BY PCR

Alonso S[1], Castro A[1], Fernández-Fernández I[1], García-Orad A[1], Tamayo G[2], Martínez de Pancorbo M[1,2].

[1]Servicio de Diagnóstico de la Paternidad Biológica e Identificación Genética. Fac. Medicina. [2]Instituto Vasco de Criminología. Universidad del País Vasco. SPAIN.

INTRODUCTION

The assumption of HWE is essential to estimate the genotype frequencies, particularly in systems with a large number of alleles, as it is the case of VNTR loci. HWE can be checked by comparing the observed and expected number of homocygotes and heterozygotes. Some authors claim that VNTR loci show an excess of homocygotes due mainly to population heterogeneity (Lander, 1989), that is, the existence of two or more groups within the population whose individuals show limited intergroup mating and different allele frequencies (Devlin et al., 1990).

Devlin et al (1990) proposed a mathematical test to demonstrate that this excess of homozygotes is not necessarily real, because many heterozygotes with similar allele sizes are misclassified as homozygotes. Similarly, Chakraborty et al. (1992) mathematically demostrate that non-detected alleles can explain this defect of heterozygosity. Small sized alleles, with few repeat units, can run off the gel during the electrophoresis or simple pass undetected due to their characteristic low hybridization efficiency. In this sense, Budowle (1991) demonstrated that single banded profiles were heterozygotes when digested with another restriction enzyme, but up to now, no study on population databases has been performed to reveal these pseudo-homozygotes.

With this aim, based on previous experience of Jeffreys et al. (1988), Armour et al (1989) and Gray and Jeffreys (1991), we propose a method employing PCR amplification (Mullis *et al.,* 1986) of homozygous individuals for loci D1S7, D7S21 and D12S11 for the screening of population databases in search of null-alleles that can explain the possible departure of HWE.

MATERIALS AND METHODS

The population analized consisted of those individuals detected as homozygotes with probes MS1, MS31 or MS43A and restriction enzyme Hinf I in our databases of about 350 individuals for each locus. 16 individuals were analyzed for locus D1S7, 20 for D7S21 and 23 for D12S11.

Reaction mixes

D1S7: 50 mM KCl, 10 mM Tris-HCl pH 9, 0.1% Triton X-100, 0.5 mg/ml BSA, 1.5 mM MgCl$_2$, 0.25 mM dNTPs, 0.3 µM each primer, and 1.5 U Taq polimerase in 20 µl final Volume.

D7S21: 50 mM KCl, 10 mM Tris-HCl pH 9, 0.5 mg/ml BSA, 1.5 mM MgCl$_2$, 0.25 mM dNTPs, 0.15 μM each primer , and 1.5 U Taq polimerase in 20 μl final Volume.

D12S11: 50 mM KCl, 10 mM Tris-HCl pH 9, 0.1% Triton X-100. 0.5 mg/ml BSA, 1.5 mM MgCl$_2$, 0.25 mM dNTPs, 0.1 μM each primer, and 1.5 U Taq polimerase in 20 μl final Volume.

Ten ng of DNA were amplified for D1S7 and D7S21 whilst 100ng were employed for D12S11.

Primers' sequences

locus D1S7	primer A (24 mer)	5'-GCTTTTCTGTGATGAGCCTTGATG-3'
	primer B (24 mer)	5'-AAGAAGCATATGCAACCCATGAGG-3'
locus D7S21	primer A (24 mer)	5'-CCCTTTGCACGCTGGACGGTGGCG-3'
	primer B (24 mer)	5'-ACACCGTCCCCACACGCCCATCCG-3'
locus D12S11	primer A (23 mer)	5'-CTATACATGTTTACACACATGCC-3'
	primer B (23 mer)	5'-GCGGGAGAAATAGAAATAGAACT-3'

Amplification parameteres

Samples were amplified using a capillary thermocycler (Linus) using the following parameters

	1X		4X		20X		1X	
D1S7	96°C	20"	97°C	20"	95°C	20"	50°C	5"
			58°C	5"	50°C	5"	70°C	5'
			70°C	2'	70°C	2'		

	1X		5X		31X		1X	
D7S21	96°C	20"	97°C	15"	95°C	15"	57°C	5"
			61°C	5"	57°C	5"	70°C	5'
			70°C	1'30"	70°C	1'30"		

	1X		3X		22X		1X	
D12S11	96°C	20"	96°C	20"	94°C	10"	48°C	5"
			50°C	5"	48°C	5"	70°C	5'
			70°C	2'	70°C	2'		

After amplification, 10 μl were loaded in an 1% agarose gel and run in similar conditions as conventional VNTR agarose typing gels, until the 2.3 Kb λ Hind III fragment reached 10 cm from the origin. After Southern transfer, membranes were hybridized with NICE probes MS1, MS31 and MS43A respectively following the manufacturer´s protocol.

RESULTS AND DISCUSSION

Ten out 16 individuals presented a second short-sized D1S7 allele, non detected previously with restriction enzyme Hinf I. Only one individual presented positive amplification of a D7S21 null-allele, and no individual showed amplification of null alleles by PCR for D12S11. In all systems, Hinf I alleles shorter than 4-6 Kb could also be amplified. The high number of pseudohomozygotes observed with D1S7 is in concordance with the deviation found previously with only Hinf I alleles, from HWE proportions in favor to a excess of homocygotes, while the systems with no significant deviation from HWE, D7S21 and D12S11 show only one or none null alleles. Colalescence of similar size alleles seems not to be a major cause in deviations from HWE given the grouping of alleles necessary to estimate allele frequencies in these systems. Instead, the lack of signal of short alleles appears to be a problem for the detection of these alleles, particularly with re-hybridized membranes and non-isotopically labeled probes. These results also suggest that care should be taken specially when establishing exclusions of paternity by Landsteiner's second rule with these systems.

REFERENCES

Armour JAL, Wong Z, Wilson V, Royle NJ, Jeffreys AJ. (1989) Sequences flanking the repeats arrays of human minisatellites: association with tandem and dispersed repeat elements. Nucleic Acids Research 13:4925-4935.

Budowle B, Giusti AM, Wayne JS, Baetchel FS, Fourney RM, Adams DE, Presley LA, Deadman HA and Monsosn KL. (1991) Fixed-bin analysis for statistical evaluation of continuos distributions of allelic data from VNTR loci, for use in forensic comparisons. Am J Hum Genet 48:137-144.

Chakraborty R, De Andrade M, Daiger SP, Budowle B. (1992) Apparent heterozygote deficiencies observed in DNA typing data and their implications in forensic applications. Ann Hum Genet 56:45-57

Devlin B, Risch N, Roeder K. (1990) No excess of homozygosity at loci used for DNA fingerprinting. Science 249:1416-1420.

Gray IC, Jeffreys AJ. (1991) Evolutionary transience of hypervariable minisatellites in man and the primates. Proc R Soc Lond 243-253.

Jeffreys AJ, Wilson V, Neumann R, Keyte J. (1988) Amplification of human minisatellites by the polimerase chain reaction; towards DNA fingerprinting of single cells. Nucleic Acids Research 16: 10953-10971.

Lander ES. (1989) DNA fingerprinting on trial. Nature 339:501-505.

Mullis K, Faloona F, Scharf S, Saiki R, Horn G, Erlich H. (1986) Specific enzymatic amplification of DNA in vitro: the polimerase chain reaction. Cold Spring Harbor Symp Quant Biol 51:915-924.

Mutation rate variation in the hypervariable VNTR g3 (D7S22) is associated with a flanking DNA sequence polymorphism near the repeat array.

Rune Andreassen and Bjørnar Olaisen
Institute of Forensic Medicine, University of Oslo.
0027 Oslo, Norway.

INTRODUCTION

The human minisatellite D7S22 (probe g3) is extremely polymorphic (heteroz. freq. 97%) with a paternal mutation rate estimated at 1.4% (Stenersen et al.1994).The size distribution of g3 alleles (fig. 1) reveals some size clustering of alleles. The smallest alleles (0-2 kb) show comparably reduced allelic diversity with one common small allele (14 repeats, freq 12.5%, Andreassen and Olaisen, 1994). No mutated 14 repeat alleles were found in a material with 2808 father-child observations, indicating that this allele has a reduced mutation rate.

A recent study of MS32 (locus D1S8, Moncton et al. 1994) has indicated that minisatellite stability is regulated by elements in the flanking DNA. A polymorphism in such a sequence could affect its abilities to act as mutagenic initiator. VNTR alleles with a suppression variant of such a flanking polymorphism would be more stable and be allowed to drift to relatively high population frequencies.

Fig. 1.

The reduced allelic diversity among small alleles in g3 could possibly reflect such a mechanism.To test this hypothesis, we have nucleotide sequenced the flanking DNA 3' to the tandem repeat array in 40 small family groups with de novo germline mutants as well as in 50 small alleles, in an attempt to reveal if there is any association between flanking polymorphism(s) and mutation rate.

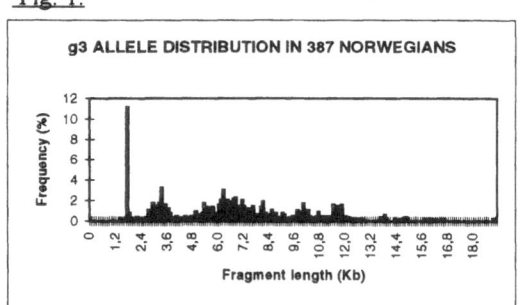

MATERIAL AND METHODS

Sothern blots consisting of 6388 consecutive parent-child triplets were screened for mutations in the VNTR g3. 40 de novo germline mutants were identified using 0.5 mm. as the largest difference in band migration accepted for a band match. The progenitor band was chosen as the parental band most similar in size to the mutant allele (Wolff et al. 1989).The paternity (or maternity) was confirmed by typing in six other VNTR loci.

All mutations were found to be changes in the repeat array rather than a change in the HinfI restriction site when digested with PstI. Thus, a total of 101 individuals were further analysed, aiming at an unambigous haplotyping of all 40 progenitor and mutated alleles as well as the 80 accompanying ones.

12 homozygous and 10 heterozygous individuals with the 14 repeat allele as well as 16 samples with rare small alleles (1.5-2.0 Kb on HinfI blots) were also chosen for further studies.

PCR-amplification:

The primers A (5'TGTAAAACGACGGCCAGTGGAACAGACATTGCTGTAAG3') with a -21M13 tail and B (5'TCTGTGAGACGCTGCGTATC 3') with a biotinylated 5' end were choosen for amplification of the flanking sequence 3' to the repeat array (236 bp).

If necessary, allele specific PCR was performed in individuals with small alleles (<2Kb) using primer C (5'AGGCTGCCTGCAGATTGCCT 3') located on the other side of the repeat array and primer B, followed by a semi-nested PCR reaction (primer A and B) to amplify the flanking sequence.

When haplotyping longer alleles, samples were HinfI digested and separated on a 0.7% agarose gel. The area containing the alleles was excised from the gel and the DNA was then recovered from the gel slice using the Geneclean II kit (BIO 101 Inc.) and then used as template in a PCR amplification using primer A and B as described.

DNA sequencing

An improved DNA sequencing method using streptavidin coated magnetic beads (Dynabeads M280, Dynal AS) was used to generate single stranded, purified and consentrated template (Leren et al. 1993). DNA sequencing was performed using Sequenase® version 2.0, -21M13 sequencing primers and sequenase dye primer sequencing kit (Applied Biosystems inc.) as described by the manufacturer. The DNA sequence analyses were performed using the ABI 373 sequencing system software version 1. 2. 0. (Applied Biosystem inc.) followed by visual examination of the chromatograms.

The haplotypes were determined by family typing. When both parental samples were heterozygous, an allele specific PCR was performed followed by a DNA sequencing of this haplotype.

RESULTS AND DISCUSSION

Two base substitution polymorphisms were found: a C/G transversion and a A/G transition 54 and 173 bp upstream of the repeat array, respectively. The frequencies of 54G or C alleles were 36% and 64%, and those of 173A or G alleles were 71% and 29%, respectively, when estimated from the accompanying alleles (nonmutated alleles in offspring and non progenitor alleles in progenitor). All combinations of haplotypes were found.

All the 50 selected small alleles were 54G and 173A, indicating a common origin of the 14 repeat alleles.

Using the Chi-square test with the accompanying alleles as "matched controls", there was a significant association (x^2= 9.6, p= 0.002) between mutation rate and the alleles at the 54C/G polymorphic site. Haplotypes with 54C tend to mutate more frequently than those with 54G. Most of the mutations in g3 were of paternal origin (85%) and they tend to be gain mutations. However, among the four mutated 54G alleles, two were of maternal origin and three represent losses. Variants of the 173A/G polymorphism did not reveal any significant association to mutation rate.

There was a higher mutation rate in the 4-9 Kb allele size cluster than those with smaller or larger size (fig. 2). Thus , the mutation rate is probably not directly related to allele size.

The 54G variant, associated with a relatively low mutation rate and present in all small alleles, could be responsible for the low diversity in this allele size group. The 173A variant, also found in most of the mutating alleles, could not. These findings migth indicate that the mutation rate variation is primarily associated with the 54C/G polymorphic site.

The 54C/G polymorphism is located in one of three basepairs that interrupts a sequence (ATGCACAC/GAATAA) that otherwise would have been a perfect match with the octamer motif (ATGCAAAT, Parslow et al. 1984). Previous studies have shown that there excist both degenerated variants (Baumruker T. et al. 1988) and variants extending the sequence by having basepairs that interrupt the motif (ATGCATAAAT, Castrillo et al.1989).

One variant of the octamer motif (ATGATAAT) located in the adenovirus 2 inverted terminal repeat is involved in adenovirus DNA replication (Pruijn et al. 1986). Another study (Iguchi-Ariga and Ogawa 1993) suggests that the octamer sequence (ATGCAAATNA) might serve as part of a replication origin in mammalian cells. Furthermore, using the GCG computer software, a 100% fit with the octamer like sequence (ATGCACACAAT) was found within a 983 bp human sequence with autonomously replicating activity (Wu et al. 1993), suggesting that this sequence contains a replication origin.

One could speculate that the octamer like sequence found in this study could act as a regulatory element binding a factor essential for a possible origin of replication. The variation in stability might then be related to the ability of the two variants of the octamer like sequence to act as a component in an origin of DNA replication. The main mutational mechanism responsible for the repeat array instability could then be replication slippage during DNA replication. This would be consistent with an excess of small size changes (Levison et al. 1987), and could also account for the difference in mutation rate between the sexes found in this VNTR.

In the MS32 study the mutation rate associated polymorphism was found in a 16 bp palindrome sequence. The octamer motif like sequence is located almost in the same position relative to the repeat array, but it shows no sequence similarity with this palindrome sequence. Nevertheless, our findings support the hypothesis that there exist elements in the flanking DNA affecting the repeat array stability.

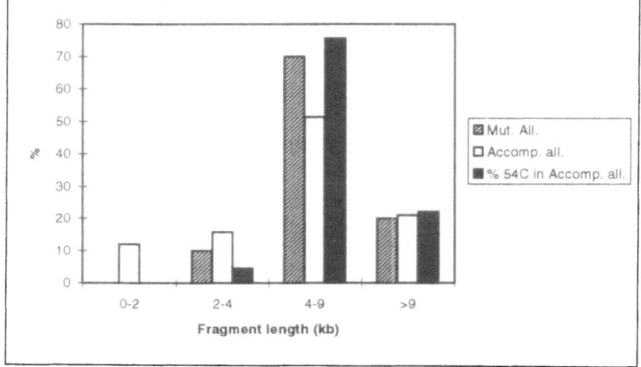

Fig.2. Fragment size distribution of 40 mutated g3 alleles compared with 76 accompanying alleles

REFERENCES

Andreassen R, Olaisen B (1994) Study of short alleles in the VNTR locus D7S22 (λg3). Paper presented at the twelwth nordic meeting of forensic medicine, Lillehammer, Norway August 10-13.

Baumruker T, Sturm R, Herr W (1988) OBP100 binds remarkably degenerate octamermotifs through spesific interaction with flanking sequences. Genes Dev. 2: 1400-1413.

Castrillo JL, Bodner M, Karin M (1989) Purification of growth hormone-spesific transcription factor GHF-1 containing homeobox. Science 243:814-817

Igushi-Ariga SM, Ogawa N (1993) Identification of the initiation region of DNA replication in the murine immunoglobulin heavy chain gene and possible function of the octamer motif as a putative DNA replication origin in mammalian cells. Biochimica et biophysica Acta 1172(1-2):73-81.

Leren TP, Rødingen OK, Røsby O, Solberg K, Berg K (1993) Screening for point mutations by semi-automated DNA sequencing using Sequenase and magnetic beads. Bio techniques 14:618-623.

Levison G, Gutman GA (1987) Slipped strand mispairing: a major mechanism for DNA sequence evolution. Mol. Biol. Evol. 4:203-221.

Moncton DG, Neumann R, Guram T, Fretwell N, Tamaki K, Macleod A, Jeffreys AJ (1994) minisatellite mutation rate variation associated with a flanking DNA sequence polymorphism. Nature genet. 8: 162-170.

Parslow TG, Blair DL, Murphy WJ, Granner DK (1984) Strukture of the 5' ends of immunoglobulin genes: a novel conserved sequence. Proceed. of the Nat. Acad of Science, USA 81: 2650-2654.

Pruijn GJM, van Driel W, van der Vliet PC (1986) Nuclear factor III, a novel sequence- spesific DNA-binding protein from HeLa cells stimulating adenovirus DNA replication. Nature 322: 656-659.

Stenersen M, Hoff-Olsen P, Olaisen B (1994) Paternity investigations experiences using single locus probes. Paper presented at the twelwth nordic meeting of forensic medicine, Lillehammer, Norway August 10-13.

Wolff RK, Plaetke R, Jeffreys AJ, White R (1989) Unequal crossingover between homologous chromosomes is not the major mechanism involved in the generation of new alleles at VNTR loci. Genomics 5: 382-384.

Wu C, Friedlander PA, Lamoreux C, Zannis-Hadjopoulus M, Price GB. cDNA clones contain autonomous replication activity. AC L08438 EM.Unpublished.

The approach of using random priming for small forensic DNA-samples

A. Baasner, M. Prinz, C. Schmitt

Institute of Forensic Medicine, University of Cologne, Melatenguertel 60-62, 50823 Koeln, FRG

Introduction

We are investigating the applicability of a new method called primer-extension-preamplification (PEP; Zhang et al., 1992) for forensic casework. Using standard PCR procedures the sensitivity for STR`s lies between 50-100 pg, and for AmpFLP`s between 500 pg - 1ng of genomic DNA. In the past DNA-samples containing very small amounts of template DNA could only be analyzed once. Employing PEP prior to the regular PCR we have been able to type several VNTR-loci from one PEP-sample. In order to systematically study the advantages and disadvantages of the PEP procedure, we amplified DNA-solutions in varying degrees of magnitude using random primers and analyzed aliquots of the PEP-reaction for various VNTR`s.

Materials and Methods

Several DNA-dilutions were amplified by multiple rounds of primer extension using a collection of 15-base oligonucleotides in which any one of the four possible bases could be present at each position.

Each PEP amplification sample contained:
1µl template (100pg, 50pg, 10pg), 1,5 µl of a 400µM solution of random primers (Operon Technologies, Alameda, CA), 3µl 10xPCR buffer, 1,5µl of a mixture of the 4 dNTPs (each at 2mM), 0,4µl Taq polymerase (5U/µl, Promega), brought to 30µl with water

Temperature cycle: denaturation for 1 min at 92°C, annealing for 2 min at 37°C, extension for 4 min at 55°C, a total of 40 or 50 cycles was carried out in a Trio-Thermoblock (Biometra)

Aliquots of the PEP were tested for specific DNA sequences.
Nested Apo B analysis was performed as described previously (Schmitt et al., 1994).

VWA/F13A1
Amplification conditions
2 U Taq polymerase (Promega), 0,25 µM each primer, 150 µM dNTPs, 2,5 µl 10x PCR buffer, 1,5 mM $MgCl_2$
Temperature cycle (VWA): 1 min 94°C, 1 min 50°C, 2 min 72°C, 29 cycles
Temperature cycle (F13A1): 1 min 94°C, 1 min 55°C, 2 min 72°C, 27 cycles

Primer sequences (VWA; Kimpton et al., 1992)

Primer sequences (F13A1, Polymeropoulos et al., 1991)

Electrophoresis

Apo B electrophoresis was performed as described previously (Schmitt et al., 1994).

For VWA: Polyacrylamid gels (8% T, 3% C) were 0,8 mm thick with 1x TBE. The vertical electrophoresis was run for 26 cm (1200 V, 65 W, 90 mA) at 50°C - 60°C on the Gibco BRL Model S2 Electrophoresis Apparatus. The DNA fragments were detected by silver staining.

For F13A1: Long Ranger (5%), Urea (7M), gels were 0,35 mm thick with 1xTBE. The electrophoresis was run for 240 min (1500 V, 38 mA, 34W, 3 W Laser, at 40°C). The DNA fragments were visualized by fluorescence detection using the A.L.F. sequencer (Pharmacia).

Results

Our first experiment was designed to estimate the efficiency of the PEP procedure. DNA of three different individuals was diluted to achieve varied concentrations which were verified using the dot blot procedure.

Table 1: VWA typing results with and without the PEP procedure

Lane	Sample	Genotype	DNA amount	PEP	Results
2	215	17/19	100 pg	yes	17/19
3	215	17/19	100 pg	no	no result
4	215	17/19	10 pg	yes	19
5	215	17/19	10 pg	no	no result
7	216	16/17	10 pg	yes	16/17
8	216	16/17	10 pg	no	no result
9	217	14/15	10 pg	yes	14/15
10	217	14/15	10 pg	no	no result

The PEP procedure increased the sensitivity of VWA typing. Two 10 pg samples that couldn't be typed without PEP yielded correct results. A strong preferential amplification of the longer allelic product could be observed.
In order to find out if the PEP reaction produces fragments of at least 600 bp in length or more the AmpFLP Apo B (allele range 590 - 900 bp) was typed for the PEP samples.

Correct ApoB genotypes were identified for 17 out of 36 reactions, which means that the PEP generates fragments >590 bp. The typing results shows a high incidence of no result or allelic drop out. Increasing the PEP aliquot input for ApoB PCR (5 µl, 10 µl, 20 µl; data not shown) did not improve the success rate.

Table 2: ApoB typing results after PEP reaction for different individuals and DNA concentrations

Sample	Geno-type	DNA amount for PEP	input after PEP for nested ApoB analysis	Total no. of investi-gations	Results
215	33/37	100 pg	1 µl	3	2x 33/37 1x 33
216	37/37	100 pg	1 µl	3	3x 37
217	35/37	100 pg	1 µl	3	3x 35/37
215	33/37	50 pg	1 µl	3	2x 33 1x arti-ficial band
216	37/37	50 pg	1 µl	3	3x 37
217	35/37	50 pg	1 µl	3	2x 35/37 1x no result
215	33/37	10 pg	1 µl	6	1x 33 5x no result
216	37/37	10 pg	1 µl	6	4x 37 2x no result
217	35/37	10 pg	1 µl	6	6x no result

Table 3: F13A1 typing results after PEP procedure for different individuals and DNA concentrations

Probe	Genotype	DNA-amount for PEP	input after PEP for F13A1 ana-lysis	Results
215 (lane 1)	6/7	50 pg	1 µl	no result
215 (lane 2)	6/7	50 pg	5 µl	6/7
216 (lane 3)	5/5	50 pg	1 µl	no result
216 (lane 4)	5/5	50 pg	5 µl	5
217	5/7	50 pg	1 µl	5/7
217	5/7	50 pg	1 µl	5/7
215 (lane 29)	6/7	100 pg	1 µl	6/(7)
215 (lane 30)	6/7	100 pg	5 µl	6/7
216 (lane 32)	5/5	100 pg	1 µl	5
216 (lane 33)	5/5	100 pg	5 µl	5
217	5/7	100 pg	1 µl	5/7
217	5/7	100 pg	5 µl	5/7

Since the detection limit for F13A1 in our hands lies between 50 pg - 100 pg the approach of PEP increased the sensitivity for this locus too. Here, increasing the DNA input after PEP from 1 µl to 5 µl improved the results, so that both alleles for each person could be reproducibly identified.

Discussion

Our results show that the PEP procedure enhances the sensitivity of PCR DNA typing. The most reproducible results could be obtained by using 100 pg amounts of DNA. Since only 1µl aliquots are amplified further, in optimal cases a 30µl PEP sample allows the typing of 30 loci, a number that even with multiplexing of primer pairs would be difficult to achieve otherwise. Aside from the results that are shown here, the loci HumTHO1 and SE33 could also be correctly typed after PEP, so that so far we were able to get results from five loci for one PEP sample starting with 100 pg of DNA.

The PEP results were influenced by allelic drop out, not only of the larger, but also of the smaller alleles. The occurence of allelic drop out was theoretically expected; allelic drop out of the smaller alleles was only observed for 10 pg amounts of DNA. DNA dilutions this low are affected by stochastic effects and random fluctuation of alleles. Parallel to specific PCR amplification the random primer extension is expected to be less effective for longer stretches of DNA. This expectation is verified by our ApoB results: the longer alleles were the first drop out; compared to the STR`s the necessary DNA input was higher. Since nested PCR has a single cell detection limit, the fact that even the amplification of PEP aliquots of 20µl didn`t improve the results, means that the ApoB alleles were not present in the PEP sample. The size distribution of PEP products is not known, and will be difficult to establish since the amount of DNA present after PEP is still to low to be detected by conventional means. Furthermore using haploid single cells, Zhang et al. (1992) showed that only 80% of the genomic DNA are amplified by the random primers, which leads to a statistical incidence of drop out of genetic loci.

Huber and Holtz (1994) described the succesful application of PEP for several forensic samples. Our study was designed to generate data regarding the reliability of PCR typing results after PEP. The occurence of preferential amplification and allelic drop out pose a major problem, because it could lead to the incorrect typing of a heterozygote sample as homozygote. PCR typing following PEP should therefore be limited to STR loci with short alleles. Even though results can be obtained with less DNA, for forensic case work, the PEP DNA input should not be lower than 100 pg to avoid any stochastic effects. Following these precautions, PEP offers the possibility to achieve reliable typing results for several loci with very small amounts of DNA.

References

1. Huber P, Holtz J (1994). Random priming and multiplex PCR with three short tandem repeats in forensic caseworks. Adv for Haemogenetics 94: 363 - 365
2. Kimpton C, Walton A, Gill P (1992). A further tetranucleotide repeat polymorphism in the vWF gene. Hum Mol Gen 1: 287
3. Miller S, Dykes D, Polesky H (1988). A simple salting out procedure for extracting DNA from human nucleated cells. Nucleic Acids Res 16: 1215
4. Polymeropoulos M, Raths D, Xiao H, Merril C (1991). Tetranucleotide repeat polymorphism at human coagulation factor XIII A subunit gene (F13A1). Nucleic Acids Res 19: 4036
5. Schmitt C, Schmutzler A, Prinz M, Staak M (1994). High sensitive DNA typing approaches for the analysis of forensic evidence: comparison of nested variable number of tandem repeats (VNTR) amplification and a short tandem repeat (STR) polymorphism. For Sci Int 66: 129 - 141
6. Zhang L, Cui X, Schmitt K, Hubert R, Navidi W, Arnheim N (1992). Whole genome amplification from a single cell: Implications for genetic analysis. Proc Natl Sci USA 92: 5847 - 5851

Use of a PCR Triplex System for DNA Typing of Forensic Samples

M. L. Baird, L. Perlee, J. Neuweiler, L. Galbreath and I. Balazs

Lifecodes Corporation, 550 West Avenue, Stamford, Connecticut 06902.

Introduction

Identification testing based on DNA composition has been applied to forensic (Baird et al., 1986) and paternity (Balazs et al., 1986) analysis since the mid 1980's. Because each person's DNA is unique (except for identical twins) and inherited from their biological parents, methods of examining DNA for differences are highly informative in establishing identity and lineage. Differences resulting from insertions, deletions, or sequence changes in the DNA molecule were first detected by RFLP analysis. Since RFLP analysis requires high molecular weight DNA and can take several weeks to perform, PCR analysis (Mullis et al., 1986) has gained increasing use in routine forensic analysis, specially for samples containing degraded or very small quantity of DNA. Several systems have been developed using PCR analysis including the reverse dot blot used to detect HLA DQalpha alleles (Erlich et al., 1990), analysis of AmpFLPs like D1S80 (Budowle et al., 1991), and more recently the analysis of STRs (Edwards et al., 1991). In this report, PCR analysis was applied to the analysis of forensic and paternity samples using a multiplex system of three independent STR loci. Each locus is composed of fragments which differ by four nucleotide repeats. Allele detection was accomplished by silver staining and allelic ladders used for allele assignment.

Materials and Methods

DNA was isolated from reference blood samples and evidentiary blood and semen stains by organic extraction and dialysis using standard procedures. The amount of human DNA available for analysis was determined by hybridization with Alu repeat sequences (Jelinek et al., 1980) using NANO-BLOT (Lifecodes Corp.). A total of 5 to 10 nanograms of DNA was removed from each sample and placed into an appropriately labeled 0.5 microliter thin walled tube designed for PCR amplification. The following reagents were added to each tube to be amplified: 5 microliter of a 10X PCR buffer; 5 microliter of 10X dNTPs; 5 microliter of MultiPlex I Primer mix (Lifecodes Corp.); 0.25 microliter (1.25 units) of Taq I Polymerase; and nuclease free distilled water to 50 microliter. Two drops of mineral oil were added to each tube to be amplified and the tubes placed in a Perkin-Elmer 480 Thermo Cyclers. The following conditions were used for 30 cycles: denature at 95°C for 1 minute; anneal at 65°C for 1 minute; and elongate at 72°C for 1 minute. At the end of the cycling time, the samples were removed from the thermocycler and store at 4°C separate from pre-PCR samples and reagents.

The amplified DNA fragments were separated by polyacrylamide electrophoresis in denaturing gels. The glass plates used for the gel separation were treated as follows. The larger plate was treated with Sigmacote™ to prevent the gel from sticking to it. The smaller plates were treated with methacryloxpropyltarimethoxysilane to bind the gel. Gel molds were assembled using treated plates and 0.4 millimeter spacers along the edges.

The acrylamide required for a 200 X 310 X 0.4 mm 4.0% denaturing gel was prepared by adding: 24 grams of urea; 5 ml of a 40% acrylamide (19:1) solution; 5 ml of 5X TBE buffer; and deionized water to 50 ml. After stirring to dissolve the urea, the solution was filtered through an 0.2 micron filter into a 100 ml beaker. Next, 25 microliter of TEMED and 250 microliter of freshly prepared 10% ammonium persulfate were added and mixed. This solution was poured between glass plates and a comb placed into gel at the top. The gel was allowed to polymerize at least 1 hour.

The gel was pre-run at 2000 volts for 30 minutes in 0.5 X TBE buffer. The urea in the wells was flushed with buffer and samples were loaded as follows: Three microliters of amplified product was placed into a microcentrifuge tube and 3 microliters of formamide loading buffer (95% formamide, 0.005% bromphenol blue) added. The tubes were placed in a 95°C water bath for 10 minutes then removed and placed on ice. Samples and size markers were loaded into the wells on the gel and electrophoresed at 2000 volts for 1 hour.

The separated DNA fragments were visualized by silver staining. The allele designation was established by comparing the DNA fragments in the amplified samples with the alleles of the marker lanes.

Results and Discussion

The PCR triplex system utilized for analysis of samples permits the simultaneous detection of three polymorphic loci: D18S849, D3S1744, and D12S1090. Since alleles from each locus are differentiated by size, the products of the simultaneous amplification of these three loci can be resolved in a single gel. Allele differences at each locus are due to variations in the number of tetranucleotide repeats. The alleles at the D12S1090 locus range from 212 to 306 bases (>25 alleles), at the D3S1744 locus from 150 to 182 bases (9 alleles), and at the D18S849 locus from 93 to 133 bases (9 alleles). Based on the allele frequency distribution at these three loci, the power of exclusion of this triplex is about 1 in 6,000.

Figure 1 shows the results of forensic and paternity analyses. A and B contains samples from rape cases. The lanes labeled V contain DNA from a blood sample of the victim. The lanes labeled S contain DNA from the suspect. The lane labeled E contains DNA isolated from vaginal swabs. In both cases, A and B, the evidentiary DNA pattern matched the DNA pattern obtained from the suspect. In Case A, the alleles detected at D12S1090 in the evidence and suspect are 19, 26. The size standards for this locus contain every other allele to allow for adequate resolution. Thus, the largest allele is between markers alleles 27 and 25. The allelic ladder for the D3S1744 and D18S849 loci contain all the observed alleles to date. The close doublet nature of the bands is due to the mobility differences of the two strands of DNA in the denaturing gel. Using standard population genetics and the allele frequencies, the frequency of occurrence of the STR profile in the suspect in Case A is 1 in 37,200 and in Case B 1 in 50,336.

Case C contains the results of a paternity analysis with two alleged fathers. The lane labeled M contains DNA from the mother, C from the child, AF1 from alleged father 1, and AF2 from alleged father 2. The results indicate that alleged father 1 is not excluded as the biological father while alleged father 2 is excluded by the result at D12S1090. This exclusion was confirmed by additional genetic analysis using VNTR loci. The paternity index for alleged father 1 was 3,330 for the North American Caucasoid population.

In conclusion, the use of PCR analysis of a triplex system of three loci which detect STRs can provide useful information to help resolve issues involving identification or parentage.

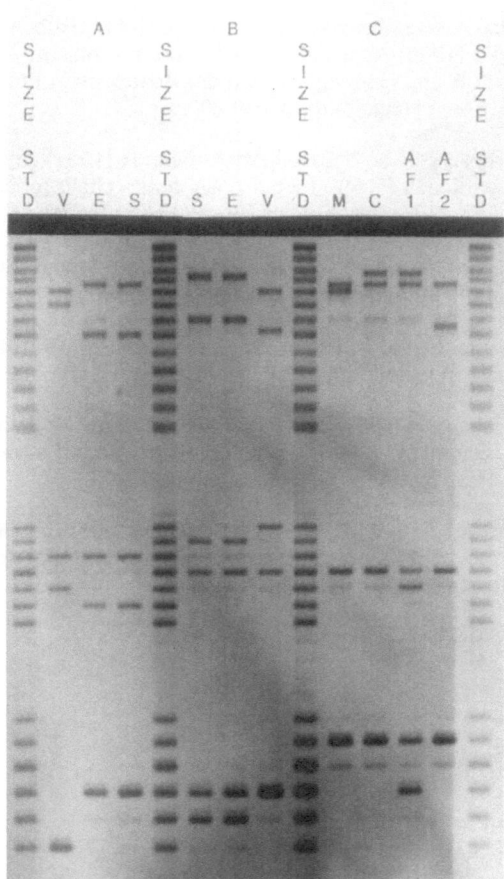

References

Baird M, Giusti A, Balazs I, Glassberg J (1986) Application of DNA polymorphisms to forensic examination of semen. In: Brinkmann B and Henningsen K (eds) Advances in Forensic Haemogenetics, vol 1. Springer-Verlag, Berlin Heidelberg, p 356-360.

Balazs I, Wexler K, Nicholas L, Miyazaki L, Giusti A, Baird M, Rubinstein P, Allen F, Sussman L, Glassberg J (1986) Application of DNA polymorphisms to the determination of paternity. In: Brinkmann B and Henningsen K (eds) Advances in Forensic Haemogenetics, vol 1. Springer-Verlag, Berlin Heidelberg, p 196-200.

Budowle B, Chakraborty R, Giusti A, Eisenberg A, Allen R (1991) Analysis of the variable number of tandem repeat locus D1S80 by the polymerase chain reaction followed by high resolution polyacrylamide gel electrophoresis. Amer J Hum Genet 48:137-144.

Edwards A, Civitello A, Hammond H, Caskey T (1991) DNA typing and genetic mapping with trimeric and tetrameric tandem repeats. Amer J Hum Genet 49:746-756.

Erlich H, Higuchi R, Lichtenwalter K, Reynolds R, Sensabaugh G (1990) Reliability of HLA-DQalpha PCR-based oligonucleotide typing system. J Forn Sci 35:1017-1018.

Jelinek W, Tomey T, Leinwand L, Duncan C, Biro P, Choudary P, Weisman S, Rubin C, Houck C, Deininger P, Schmid C (1980) Ubiquitous interspersed repeated sequences in mammalian genomes. Proc Nat Acac Sci 77:1398-1402.

Mullis K, Faloona F, Scharf S, Saiki R, Horn G, Erlich H (1986) Specific enzymatic amplification of DNA in vitro: The polymerase chain reaction. Cold Spring Harbor Symposium on Quantitative Biology 51:263-273.

Evaluation of New STR Loci for Forensic DNA Typing

Raphaël Coquoz

Institut de Police Scientifique et de Criminologie, University of Lausanne, Bâtiment de Chimie, 1015 Lausanne-Dorigny, Switzerland

Introduction

STR DNA typing has become the method of choice for the identification of the source of human biological material. The main reasons are its sensitivity and its ability to analyse degraded material. The main drawback of most of the STR loci presently in use in forensic science is their very limited polymorphism which contrasts with the extraordinary polymorphism of the VNTR loci used in RFLP typing. A few STRs are very polymorphic, but they are also rich in microheterogeneities (for example locus HUMACTBP2) which makes the identification of alleles difficult and the comparison of results between laboratories uncertain.

Table 1: Polymorphism of STR loci commonly used in forensic science

Locus		Heterozygosity (caucasian)	Ref.	Matching probability	Ref.
THO1	① ②	0.74	[6]	0.09	[4]
VWA	① ②	0.75	[6]	0.07	[6]
D21S11	①	0.83	[6]	0.05	[6]
FIBRA (FGA)	①		[6]	0.04	[6]
D19S253	①	0.76	[6]	0.08	[6]
D18S51	①	0.88	[6]	0.03	[6]
TPOX	②	0.66	[1]		
HPRTB	②	0.77	[3]	0.08	[3]
CSF1PO	②	0.74	[3]	0.11	[3]
FES/FPS	②	0.67	[4]	0.19	[4]
ACTBP2		0.94	[4]	0.02	[4]
F13A1		0.72	[4]	0.13	[4]
F13B		0.66	[5]		
LPL		0.68	[3]	0.16	[3]
CD4		0.68	[3]	0.16	[4]

① belongs to the heptaplex of the British DNA database
② belongs to the Promega multiplex STR systems

Recent advances in genetics have allowed the discovery of hundreds or even thousands of STR loci each year. All these new loci are stored in large databases which are then a potential rich source of STR loci. Although most of the stored STR loci display a limited polymorphism, it is certain that STR loci should be found which would bring substantial improvements compared to the current set of loci.

A set of 6 loci have been chosen for this study. The goal was to do a crude evaluation to sort out the best loci deserving a future more thorough examination. This first step was essentially an allele frequency determination.

Material/Methods

Database   : The Human Genome Data Base (GDB), at Johns Hopkins University in Baltimore, has been searched (http://gdbwww.gdb.org/.). GDB is a database created for gene mapping purposes. In early 1995, it contained more than 7000 STR loci, among which more than 2000 tetranucleotide repeats. When questionned for tetranucleotide repeat STRs, with a heterozygosity greater than 0.85, the database brought about 200 hits. Most of these loci are, in fact, poorly described with only an estimate of the true polymorphism in the form of a "maximum heterozygosity" based on a very limited sample. A few of these loci have been chosen for more detailed examination.

Samples : The DNA samples were extracted from blood given by anonymous donors from the local blood transfusion center.

PCR   : The amplification conditions were essentially those described in the files from the Human Genome Data Base (GDB). The amplifications were done on either a Thermocycler TC480 (Perkin-Elmer) or Crocodile (Appligene), in 25μl of a solution containing 10mM Tris-HCl pH 9, 50mM KCl, 0.2mM dNTP, 1.5mM MgCl$_2$, 0.25μM primers, 0.01% gelatine and 0.25U Taq polymerase. After 3 min incubation at 94°C, the samples went through 30 cycles (45"/94°C ; 45"/annealing temperature ; 1'/72°C), followed by a final 5' incubation at 72°C. The annealing temperature was adjusted to the requirements of each locus, as described in the files from the database.

Electrophoresis   [2]: The samples were separated on discontinuous horizontal polyacrylamide gel electrophoresis (acrylamide / piperazine diacrylamide : 6 - 8.5% T, 5% C ; 60mM formate-Tris), on 12 - 28 cm long gels. The electrode buffer (0.75M borate-Tris pH 9) was absorbed in 6 sheets of 1.5 cm wide blotting paper. The PCR products were revealed by silver staining.

Results

Table 2 : Description of the STR loci tested and their polymorphism

STR locus	max. het.①	primer sequence	anneal. temp.	chrom. nb.②	allele nb.	obs. het.③	Pm④
D20S85	0.86	5'-ATTACAGTGTGAGACCCTG-3' 5'-GAGTATCCAGAGAGCTATTA-3'	55°C	108	8	0.74	0.06
D7S1517	1.00	5'-AGCCTGATCATTACCAGGT-3' 5'-CTATTGGGGCCATCTTGC-3'	50°C	94	12	0.87	0.03
D7S1520	0.94	5'-AGATGACATACGGATGAATGG-3' 5'-GTCTCCTCTATCATCTTTCGA-3'	50°C	120	6	0.75	0.08
D6S965	1.00	5'-GTCACCTGCGTGAAGGAAA-3' 5'-GGTTGTGGGTTTTGTAGGC-3'	54°C	94	15	0.87	0.02
D1S1171	0.94	5'-GGGCAACAAAGTAAGACCC-3' 5'-TTTCCCATAGCCCCTGTGC-3'	65°C	118	9	0.78	0.07
D2S1242	0.94	5'-TGACATAGCGAGACCCTGTC-3' 5'-CCATTCTCATCCAGCAGGA-3'	55°C	92	10	0.83	0.06

① Heterozygosity displayed in the corresponding file in the Human Genome Data Base
② Number of chromosome tested
③ Percentage of heterozygotes in the sample tested
④ Matching probability ($\sum p_i^2$)

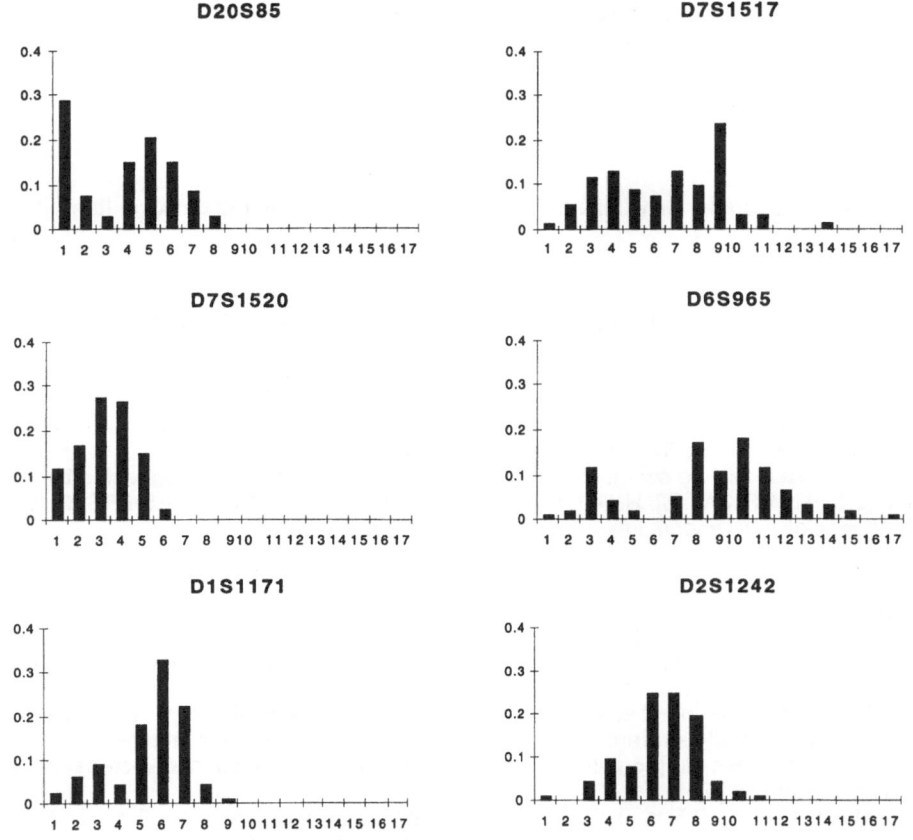

Conclusion

From this small-scale screening of new STR loci, it is evident that sets of STR loci can be found which are more powerful than those already used in forensics. We intend to screen many other loci until we find some which have the capacity to improve substantially the present power of identification. It is worth remembering that a set of 4 loci with a matching probability of 0.05 (discrimination power : 0.95) are more powerful than a set of 6 loci with a matching probability of 0.15 (discrimination power : 0.85).

References

[1] Anker R, Steinbrueck T, Donis-Keller H (1992) Tetranucleotide repeat polymorphism at the human thyroid peroxidase (hTPO) locus. Hum. Mol. Genet. 1(2) 137
[2] Budowle B, Chakraborty R, Giusti AM, Eisenberg AJ, Allen RC (1991) Analysis of VNTR locus D1S80 by the PCR followed by high-resolution PAGE. Am. J. Hum. Genet. 48, 137-144
[3] Hammond HA, Jin L, Zhong Y, Caskey CT, Chakraborty R (1994) Evaluation of 13 short tandem repeat loci for use in personal identification applications. Am. J. Hum. Genet. 55, 175-189
[4] Kimpton CP, Gill P, Walton A, Urquhart A, Millican ES, Adams M (1993) Automated DNA profiling employing multiplex amplification of short tandem repeat loci. PCR Methods & Applications 3, 13-22
[5] Nishimura DY, Murray JC (1992) A tetranucleotide repeat for the F13B locus. Nucleic Acids Res. 20(5) 1167
[6] Urquhart A, Oldroyd NJ, Kimpton CP, Gill P (1995) Highly discriminating heptaplex short tandem repeat PCR system for forensic identification. BioTechniques 18(1) 116-121

Automated Profiling of Multiplexed DNA Markers. An Italian Database of Four Coamplified STR Loci.

F. De Stefano, L. Casarino, M.G. Costa, A. Mannucci, G. Bruni

Istituto di Medicina Legale, Università di Genova, via De Toni 12, 16132 Genova, Italy

Introduction

Automated DNA profiling by fluorescent-based technology and its application on multiplex amplified polymerase chain reaction (PCR) products have been studied and validated for use in forensic laboratory routine [1-5]. The most diffused protocol provides coamplification of 4 short tandem repeat (STR) loci labelled by 2 different fluorescent dye markers and separation of PCR products by electrophoresis on an automated DNA sequencer 373A Leon (Applied Biosystems).

To define a database we coamplified 4 STR loci in a single reaction as suggested by literature [3,5]: HUMF13A1 [6], HUMTH01 [7], HUMVWA31/A [8] and HUMFES/FPS [9]. Allele frequencies in a random Italian population is here described.

Materials and methods

Samples. DNA was extracted by common phenol/chloroform protocols from 202 unrelated blood donors, and controlled on a 0.8 % agarose gel. Estimation of DNA quantity was made by minifluorometer TKO 100 (Hoefer Instruments).

Amplification. From 1 to 5 ng of extracted DNA was amplified in 0.5 ml thin-walled tubes in a total volume of 50 μl as referenced [3, 5]. Mineral oil was used to seal the reaction, in order to avoid allelic drop-out for higher molecular weight alleles and increased primer dimer formation [5].

Alleles detection. From 0.5 to 3 μl of each reaction were combined with 6 fmol of commercial internal lane standard GS2500 (Applied Biosystem Division). After heat denaturation, samples were loaded onto a 6% polyacrylamide denaturing gel [2], electrophoresed for 5 hours and 30 minutes at constant power (36W) on an Applied Biosystems DNA Sequencer 373A Leon and analysed using Genescan 672 software (Applied Biosystems) employing the local Southern method. Amplified allelic ladders were run at the same conditions.

Statistical analysis. Observed frequencies were calculated both for alleles and genotypes. The Hardy-Weinberg equilibrium was tested by the chi-square method. Since some genotypes had expected frequencies smaller than 0.01 we also applied Smith's test [10]. For each marker expected homozygosity was computed.

Results and discussion

As expected all samples were successfully amplified and typed. Observed allele frequencies and allelic windows are shown in table 1. The use of a fluorescent-based technique allowed a better allele designation. Results confirmed databases worked out manually for single loci by silver staining. As expected, a better designation of alleles in HUMTH01 marker was reached; while by manual methods was possible to detect a single allele 10, analysis by flourescent labelled primers and Genescan 672 software showed 6 subjects presenting this allele. Frequencies for other markers were comparable to those obtained by manual techniques.

As referenced [5], allelic drop-out could occur for higher molecular weight markers (FES/FPS above all) when lower than 1 ng quantities of DNA are used.

For DNA quantities greater than 3 ng artefact peaks (stuttering) are very frequent because of polymerase slippage. In our experience, these bands range up to a maximum of 11 % of the allele.

The Hardy-Weinberg equilibrium was satisfied for all the analysed markers and even when Smith's test was employed a good agreement was found. Observed homozigosity was consistent with the expected for each marker:

HUMTH01	Observed= 0.1931	Expected= 0.2037
HUMvWA31/A	Observed= 0.1832	Expected= 0.1922
HUMF13A1	Observed= 0.2228	Expected= 0.2308
HUMFES/FPS	Observed= 0.2673	Expected= 0.2950

The use of these 4 markers determine an expected casual genotype sharing ranging from 0.6×10^{-9} to a maximum of 10^{-4} and a casual allelic sharing corresponding to a maximum of 10^{-3}.

In conclusion, fine allele designation is provided by comparing fluorescent labelled PCR products with an internal size standard and analysis with Genescan 672 software; obtained database shows, once more, usefulness of tetraplex amplification in forensic routine because of its high informativity and sensitivity.

References

1. Sullivan KM, Pope S, Gill P, Robertson JM (1992) Automated DNA profiling by fluorescent labelling of PCR products. PCR Methods Appl 2: 34-40
2. Kimpton CP, Gill P, Walton A, Urquhart A, Millican ES, Adams M (1993) Automated DNA profiling employing 'multiplex' amplification of short tandem repeat loci. PCR Methods Appl 3: 13-22
3. Kimpton CP, Fisher D, Watson S, Adams M, Urquhart A, Lygo JE, Gill P (1994) Evaluation of an automated DNA profiling system employing multiplex amplification of four tetrameric STR loci. Int J Leg Med 106:302-311
4. Urquhart A, Kimpton CP, Downs TJ, Gill P (1994) Variation in short tandem repeat sequences - a survey of twelve microstellite loci for the use as forensic identification markers. Int J Leg Med 107:13-20
5. Lygo JE, Johnson PE, Holdaway DJ, Woodroffe S, Whitaker JP, Clayton TM, Kimpton CP, Gill P (1994) The validation of short tandem repeat (STR) loci for use in forensic casework. Int J Leg Med 107: 77-89
6. Polymeropoulos MH, Xiao H, Rath DS, Merril CR (1991) Tetranucleotide repeat polymorphism at the human coagulation factor XIII A subunit gene (F13A1). Nucleic Acids Res 19: 4036
7. Polymeropoulos MH, Xiao H, Rath DS, Merril CR (1991) Tetranucleotide repeat polymorphism at the human tyrosine hydroxylase gene (TH). Nucleic Acids Res 19: 3753
8. Kimpton CP, Walton A, Gill P (1992) A further tetranucleotide repeat polymorphism in the vWF gene. Hum Mol Genet 1: 287
9. Polymeropoulos MH, Xiao H, Rath DS, Merril CR (1991) Tetranucleotide repeat polymorphism at the human c-fes/fps proto-oncogene (FES). Nucleic Acids Res 19: 4018
10. Smith CBA (1986) Chi-squared test with small numbers. Ann Hum Genet 50:163-167

Table 1. Allele frequencies for the coamplified HUMF13A1, HUMTH01, HUMVWA31/A and HUMFES/FPS loci in 202 Italian samples. Allelic windows were determined by analysis of ladders run 80 times across 20 gels.

STR Locus	Allele (repeat)	Frequency (n=404)	Windows-Minimum	Size range (bp) Maximum
HUMF13A1	3.2	0.1040	181.20	182.37
	4	0.0470	183.29	184.44
	5	0.2054	187.13	188.35
	6	0.2921	191.03	192.25
	7	0.2995	194.83	196.25
	8	0.0025	199.15	200.19
	9	0.0000	203.06	204.16
	10	0.0000	not present in the ladder	
	11	0.0074	211.05	212.35
	12	0.0025	215.03	216.40
	13	0.0074	219.06	220.57
	14	0.0050	223.24	225.18
	15	0.0074	227.73	230.01
	16	0.0198	231.88	234.20
	17	0.0025	235.53	237.58
HUMTH01	5	0.0025	152.43	153.87
	6	0.2574	156.65	157.95
	7	0.1510	161.11	162.19
	8	0.1559	165.22	166.21
	9	0.1634	169.54	170.42
	9.3	0.2574	172.88	173.56
	10	0.0173	174.06	174.86
	11	0.0000	177.60	179.56
HUMvWA31/A	13	0.0025	134.66	136.75
	14	0.0866	138.40	140.76
	15	0.1287	142.30	144.82
	16	0.2277	146.35	148.74
	17	0.2772	150.43	152.79
	18	0.1807	154.52	155.84
	19	0.0842	158.60	160.86
	20	0.0124	162.75	164.81
	21	0.0000	166.89	168.91
HUMFES/FPS	8	0.0049	212.19	214.05
	9	0.0025	216.24	218.12
	10	0.2673	220.39	222.41
	11	0.3663	224.79	226.72
	12	0.2921	229.21	231.68
	13	0.0594	233.36	235.74
	14	0.0074	236.86	239.29

n = number of studied chromosomes

MICROBIAL DNA CHALLENGE STUDIES OF PCR-BASED SYSTEMS USED IN FORENSIC GENETICS

Fernández-Rodríguez A., Alonso A., Albarrán C., Martín P., Iturralde M.J., Montesino M., Sancho M.

Sección de Biología, Instituto Nacional de Toxicología, Ministerio de Justicia e Interior, C) Luis Cabrera nº9, 28002 Madrid, España.

INTRODUCTION

The analysis of polymorphic DNA loci by PCR-based methods has extended DNA typing to a significant proportion of biological evidences that contain scarce and even highly degraded DNA. However, in many cases, biological samples presented for DNA analysis have also been subjected to contamination by microorganisms and, as a result of that, DNA isolated from such sources can potentially be a mixture of human and microbial DNA. To our knowledge only a few studies have been performed to address the specificity of the PCR-based systems against microbial DNA. (Budowle et al. 1995, Cosso et al. 1995).

The purpose of this study is to evaluate the influence of this source of foreign DNA on human PCR-based DNA typing by testing the specificity of 10 PCR-based systems widely used in forensic genetics (HLA-DQA1, LDLR, GYPA, HBGG, D7S8, GC, D1S80, HUMTH01, HUMTPOX and HUMCSF1PO) against microbial DNA templates obtained from 30 different microorganisms isolated from forensic casework or reference strains.

MATERIAL AND METHODS

A total of 30 microorganisms (10 Gram-negative bacterial strains, 16 Gram-positive bacterial strains and 4 yeasts) that can be usually found in forensic samples, as both environmental contaminants of biological samples and indigenous flora of skin and vagina was used in this study. The standard strains were: *Bacillus cereus* ATCC, *Escherichia coli* ATCC, *Klebsiella pneumoniae* ATCC, *Citrobacter freundii* ATCC, *Enterobacter aerogenes* ATCC, *Pseudomonas aeruginosa* ATCC, *Pseudomonas stutzeri* ATCC, *Salmonella enteritidis* ATCC, *Vibrio alginolyticus* ATCC, *Micrococcus luteus* ATCC, *Staphylococcus aureus* ATCC, *Staphylococcus epidermidis* ATCC, *Staphylococcus saprophyticus* ATCC, *Enterococcus faecalis* ATCC, *Streptococcus pyogenes* ATCC, *Streptococcus sanguis* ATCC, *Clostridium perfringens* ATCC, *Corynebacterium sp.* ATCC, *Saccharomyces cerevisiae* ATCC, *Candida albicans* ATCC, *Candida parasilopsis* ATCC, *Candida tropicalis* ATCC (kindly provided by the Spanish Collection of Culture Type) and *Listeria monocytogenes* L028 serotype 1,2 kindly provided by Dr. Pérez-Díaz (Ramón y Cajal Hospital, Madrid, Spain). The strains isolated from evidentiary items were: *P. stutzeri, V. alginolyticus, S. epidermidis, S. saprophyticus,* two strains of *Bacillus sp.* and one strain of *Staphylococcus sp.*

All the microorganisms were grown overnight in liquid Luria-Bertani (LB) culture medium at optima temperatures. High molecular weight DNA was isolated by the standard phenol/chloroform procedure after treatment with proteinase K and also by adding lysozime (10 mg/ml) (SIGMA) in the case of Gram-positive and yeasts strains. Genomic DNA was quantitated by fluorimetry. The absence of human DNA on the microbial DNA extracts was verified by slot-blot hybridization with the human-specific

D17Z1 probe (Walsh et al. 1992) using the QuantiBlot™ Kit (Perkin Elmer Corporation, Norwalk, CT).

The amplification and typing of the HLA-DQA1 and PM systems were performed according to the manufacturer's recommendations using the Amplitype PM and HLA-DQA1 forensic DNA amplification and typing kits (Perkin Elmer Corporation, Norwalk, CT). The amplification of HUMTH01, HUMTPOX and HUMCSF1PO was performed by a multiplex PCR reaction according to the manufacturer's recommendations using the GenePrint STR System (Promega Corporation, Madison, WI, USA). The amplification of D1S80 locus was performed using the AmpliFLP D1S80 PCR Amplification Kit (Perkin Elmer, Corporation, Norwalk, CT). In all the cases, PCR products were first analyzed by agarose (2-3% Nusieve, FMC) gel electrophoresis in the presence of ethidium-bromide. D1S80 PCR products were also analyzed by vertical polyacrylamide gel electrophoresis and silver stain (Budowle et al. 1991). All the extraction, amplification and detection procedures were performed twice by two different analyzers.

RESULTS AND DISCUSSION

Some nonspecific amplification products were observed in the post-amplification yield gel when some bacterial DNA templates were used for the amplification of the HLA-DQA1 and PM systems (Fig. 1). However, in no case false-positive results were found by the reverse dot-blot hybridization system used for the typing (data not shown). No PCR products were observed with the HUMTH01/ HUMTPOX/ HUMCSF1PO multiplex STR system for none of the microbial DNA templates tested (data not shown).

On the other hand, D1S80 amplifications from six of the bacterial DNAs analyzed showed some nonspecific amplification products of different sizes that were located within the range of length variability of the human D1S80 alleles, as analyzed by native polyacrylamide gel electrophoresis and silver stain (Fig. 2a). The amplification of bacterial DNA at different quantities (40 ng-100 pg) demonstrated that these nonspecific D1S80 PCR products were obtained even from trace amounts (100 pg) of bacterial DNA (Fig. 2b).

In conclusion, our results validate the specificity of the majority of PCR-based systems analyzed against microbial DNA templates, but also suggest that microbial DNA could be a potential source of extra bands when D1S80 typing is carried out from forensic biological samples subjected to contamination by microorganisms.

REFERENCES

Budowle B, Chakraborty R, Giusti AM, Eisenberg AJ and Allen RC.(1991). Analysis of the VNTR locus D1S80 by the PCR followed by high-resolution PAGE. Am J Hum Genet 48: 137-144.

Budowle B, Lindsey JA, DeCou JA, Koons BW, Giusti AM, Comey CT. (1995). Validation and population studies of the loci LDLR, GYPA, HBGG, D7S8, and Gc (PM loci), and HLA-DQA1 using a multiplex amplification and typing procedure. J Forensic Sci 40: 45-54.

Cosso S, Reynolds R. (1995). Validation of the ampliFLP D1S80 PCR amplification kit for forensic casework analysis according to TWGDAM guidelines. J Forensic Sci 40: 424-434.

Walsh PS, Varlaro J, Reynolds R (1992). A rapid chemiluminescent method for quantitation of human DNA, Nucleic Acids Res 20: 5061-5065.

HLA-DQA1

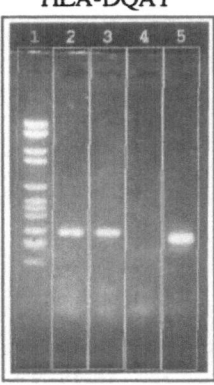

PM

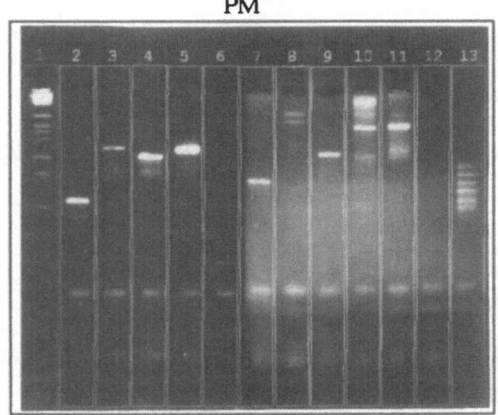

Figure 1: Nonspecific PCR products obtained with microbial DNA templates for HLA-DQA1 and PM loci. **HLA-DQA1:** Samples: (1) Molecular weight marker. (2) *V. alginolyticus* from an evidentiary item. (3) *V. alginolyticus* ATCC. (4) Negative control. (5) Human positive control. **PM:** Samples: (1) Molecular weight marker. (2) *C. perfringens* ATCC. (3) *K. pneumoniae* ATCC. (4) *S. saprophyticus* from an evidentiary item. (5) *P. stutzeri* from an evidentiary item. (6) *S. cerevisiae* ATCC. (7) *S. enteritidis* ATCC. (8) *C. parapsilosis* ATCC. (9) *C. tropicalis* ATCC. (10) *Corynebacterium sp.* ATCC. (11) *S. pyogenes* ATCC. (12) Negative control. (13) Human positive control.

D1S80

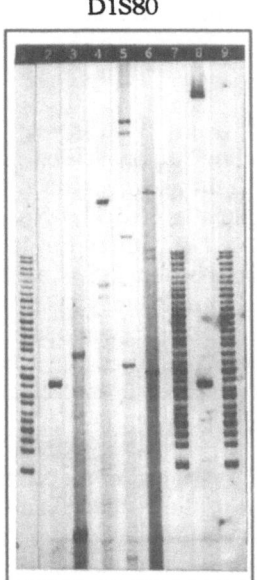

D1S80

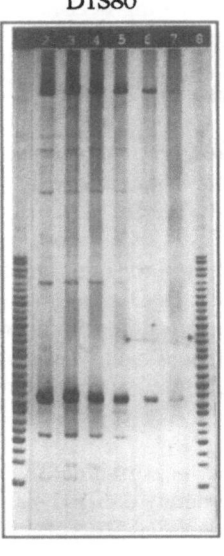

Figure 2a: Nonspecific PCR products obtained with bacterial DNA templates for D1S80 system as analyzed by polyacrylamide gel electrophoresis and silver stain. Samples: (1) Allelic ladder. (2) *Corynebacterium sp.* ATCC. (3) *S. sanguis* ATCC. (4) *M. luteus* ATCC. (5) *K. pneumoniae* ATCC. (6) *P. stutzeri* ATCC. (7) Allelic ladder. (8) *P. stutzeri* from an evidentiary item. (9) Allelic ladder.
2b: Nonspecific D1S80 PCR products obtained from different quantities of bacterial DNA template extracted from *P. stutzeri* . Samples: (1) Allelic ladder. (2) 40 ng of bacterial DNA template. (3) 20 ng. (4) 10 ng. (5) 5 ng. (6) 1 ng. (7) 0,1 ng. (8) Allelic ladder.

SOME CRITICAL COMMENTS AND EXPERIMENTAL CALCULATIONS USED AS VALIDATION STANDARDS IN THE IMPLEMENTATION OF RFLP ANALYSIS.

IC Flores, G Repetto and P Sanz.

National Institute of Toxicology, P.O. Box 863, 41080 - Sevilla, Spain.

INTRODUCTION

Analysis of restriction fragment length polymorphisms (RFLP's) has become one of the most powerful methods in forensic DNA analysis. In the last few years we have implemented in routine case work in our laboratory the use of 5 single locus probes. The forensic use of this technique is regarded as valid and reliable (NRC, 1992; Lander and Budowle, 1994). However, a critical interpretation of test results should be carried out according to the potency of the technique (i.e. reproducibility or sizing error and power of resolution) and the distribution of the allele of a locus in a given population.

The aim of this study was to assess the validity of RFLP analysis and to comment some interpretation difficulties in parentage testing. Moreover we present a conflicting paternity case with band sizing similarities between non-related mother and alleged father, in which matching decisions conducted either to father or to mother exclusion.

MATERIALS AND METHODS

DNA was extracted from blood samples according to the method of Gill et al (1987) using phenol/chloroform and was restricted with the enzyme Hinf I. Size separation of restricted DNA and K562 / Hinf I digest genomic control DNA was achieved by electrophoresis in a 0.7% agarose gel running in TBE buffer for 18 hours (Gill et al, 1992). Alkaline phosphatase conjugated single locus probes MS31, MS43a, G3, MS8 and MS43a from Cellmark Diagnostics and YNH24 from Promega Corporation were used sequentially. All autoradiographs were analysed using a computerized digital image analysis system (Bioimage, Millipore Corp.) which utilised the Elder and Southern method (1987) for band size calculation with reference to molecular weight markers (BRL/NICE).

The sizing error or measurement of reproducibility (sigma) of the electrophoretic system was estimated by determining the size variation of the genomic control (K562 / Hinf I digest) run on every gel. The ability of the system to resolve close bands (defined as delta, power of resolution) was estimated through a critical analysis of samples in which closely spaced bands occur in the same lane (heterozygous individuals or DNA mixtures from alleged father and child).

Percent homozygosity and heterozygosity for each VNTR-locus was calculated from the study of DNA from blood samples of 110 unrelated individuals of Southern Spain. The average power of exclusion ($A = h^2(1-hH^2)$) and the typical paternity index (TPI=1/2H) were estimated according to Brenner and Morris (1990).

RESULTS AND DISCUSSION

The sizing error (sigma) obtained for the system ranged from 0.54 to 2.7 % depending on the VNTR-locus and the size of the K562 / Hinf I digest fragment (Table 1). In this sense, sigma was higher for the low molecular weight fragment for all the loci studied, except for the D12S11. The power of resolution (delta) ranged from 2.6 to 3.6 %.

Table 1: Measurement reproducibility of the electrophoretic system calculated as allele sizing error (sigma) determining the size variation of the two fragments (high and low molecular weight fragments) of the genomic control (K562 / Hinf I digest) run on every gel (n=25). The power of resolution (delta) was calculated from closely spaced bands of the same lane (n > 10).

VNTR locus	D2S44		D12S11		D7S21		D7S22		D5S43	
DNA-probe	YNH24		MS43a		MS31		G3		MS8	
Fragment	HMW F	LMW F	HMWF	LMW F	HMW F	LMW F	HMW F	LMW F	HMW F	LM WF
Mean (bp)	4011	2909	13599	5253	7812	6963	7059	1964	5538	4774
SD (bp)	21.8	55.5	183.2	29.2	58.3	54.0	51.5	53.2	35.7	33.1
Sigma (%)	0.54	1.91	1.35	0.55	0.75	0.78	0.73	2.71	0.64	0.69
Maximum	4051	3079	13950	5309	7905	7079	7163	2027	5613	4836
Minimum	3986	2858	13270	5191	7694	6844	6963	1799	5481	4716
Resolution power (δ)	2.6		3.6		2.8		2.8		2.9	

Table 2: Percent homozygosity and heterozygosity for each VNTR-locus, average power of exclusion and typical paternity indexes were calculated for the andalusian population (S Spain), (N=110).

Genetic locus	D2S44	D12S11	D7S21	D7S22	D5S43
DNA-probe	YNH24	MS43a	MS31	G3	MS8
Heterozygosity (%)	95.75	95.10	95.05	83.33	85.06
Homozygosity (%)	4.25	4.90	4.95	16.67	14.94
Average power of exclusion (%)	88	86	86	61	76
Typical paternity index	0.118	0.102	0.101	0.030	0.033

The heterozigosity of the andalusian population was higher than 95 % for the D2S44, D12S11 and D7S21 loci, with an average power of exclusion higher than 86 % (Table 2). The tipical paternity index was particularly high for the D2S44 locus, and very low for the D7S22 and D5S43 loci. The average power of exclusion was very high for the

D2S44, D12S11 and D7S21 loci. This data confirms the validity of RFLP analysis, but also shows that some locus are more useful than others.

The results of a paternity case are presented in Table 3. Clear father exclusion was produced for the D12S11 locus. D7S22 locus showed also a clear exclusion of the father, however a possible mother exclusion was also present. The run of a mixture of the alleged father and the child DNA was very useful to detect exclusions when alleles from the mother and the father have similar molecular weights, as occurred with D7S21 and D2S44. In these case the mixture of child and mother DNA should be also included.

Table 3: RFLP analysis of a paternity case showing the allele size (bp) of the child, the mother, the alleged father and the mixture of the child and the father DNA. The conclusion of the study are expressed as excluded (E) or non-excluded (NE).

VNTR locus	D2S44		D12S11		D7S21		D7S22		D5S43	
DNA-probe	YNH24		MS43a		MS31		G3		MS8	
Fragment	HMW F	LMW F	HMWF	LMW F	HMW F	LMW F	HMW F	LMW F	HMW F	LM WF
Child	4059	2636	7895	5150	7882	5379	3216	3216	6349	6257
Mother	2652	2652	11919	7957	6364	5414	6674	6674	6257	4776
Putative father	4321	2684	9522	4867	7774	5685	6212	5790	6303	4688
Mixture (child + p. father)	4351	2701	9739	5182	8032	5722	6257	3216	6395	4688
	4089	2668	7957	4897	7882	5396	5825		6303	
Conclusion	F or M E		FE		FE		F or M E		F NE	

REFERENCES

Brenner C and Morris JW (1990) Paternity index calculations in single locus hypervariable DNA probes: validation and other studies. In: Proceedings for the International Symposium on Human Identification 1989. Data adquisition and statistical analysis for DNA laboratories. Promega Corporation. 21-53

Elder JK and Southern EM (1987) Computer aided analysis of one dimensional restriction fragment gels. In: Bishop MJ and Rawlings CJ (eds) Nucleic acid and protein sequence analysis. IRL Press, Oxford, pp 165-172.

Gill P, Lygo JE, Fowler SJ and Werrett DJ (1987) An evaluation of DNA fingerprinting for forensic purposes. Electrophoresis 8: 38-44.

Gill P, Woodroffe S, Bär W, Brinkman B, Carracedo A, Eriksen B, Jones S, Kloosterman AD, Ludes B, Mevag B, Pascali VL, Rudler M, Schmitter H, Scneider PM and Thompson JA (1992) A report of an international collaborative experiment to demonstrate the uniformity obtainable using DNA profiling techniques. Forensic Science International 53: 29-43.

Lander ES and Budowle B (1994) DNA fingerprinting dispute laid to rest. Nature 371: 735-738.

NRC (1992). DNA technology in forensic science. National Research Council. National Academy Press, Washington DC.

Analysis of somatic mutations at short tandem repeat loci in colorectal carcinomas

P. Hoff-Olsen, G.I.Meling, and B.Olaisen

Institute of Forensic Medicine, University of Oslo, Rikshospitalet, 0027 Oslo, Norway

INTRODUCTION

To further analyse the variability at tandem repetitive loci, we have studied somatic mutation events in a subset of four short tandem repeats (STRs or microsatellites). Pairs of human blood leukocyte and colorectal adenocarcinoma DNA were adopted as a somatic model system.

The existence of new tumour alleles in colorectal (Lothe et al. 1993; Thibodeau et al. 1993; Hoff-Olsen et al. 1995) and other tumours (Han et al. 1993; Risinger et al. 1993; Orth et al. 1994) have been extensively described. Most reports focus on dinucleotides and the mere registration of new tumour alleles. The somatic instability recorded is called replication error (Aaltonen et al. 1993), reflecting the mutation mechanism. With focus on the evolution, maintenance and variability of repetitive loci, the nature of mutational events becomes an important issue.

Several reports addressing the mutational mechanism responsible for the occurrence of new microsatellite alleles, conclude that the most likely definitive event is intra-chromosomal, i.e. strand slippage or sister chromatide exchange. These reports are based mainly on either studies of flanking sequences (Morrall et al. 1991; Mahtani et al. 1993) or evaluation of the fitness of the observed mutations to a certain mutation model (Pena et al. 1993; Shriver et al.1993).

Microsatellite mutations in CEPH pedigrees show an almost 2:1 ratio of gains over losses of alleles (Weber and Wong 1993). Rubinsztein et al. (1995) most recently pointed to the fact that microsatellite allele length distributions more often show positive than negative skews, consistent with a bias toward gains over losses. There is also evidence that *mini*satellites display a tendency toward allelic expansion vs. contraction at mutation (Jeffreys et al. 1988; Olaisen et al. 1993). The instability of trinucleotide repeats associated with several heritable diseases is also associated with a bias toward expansion at mutation (Kuhl and Caskey 1993).

We here report data on the nature and distribution of new tumour alleles at the four tetranucleotide STRs HUMTHO1, HUMFES/FPS, HUMVWA31/A and HUMF13A1.

MATERIALS AND METHODS

DNA was extracted from blood and carcinoma of 217 unselected patients. Meling et al. (1991) have presented the carcinoma material. Polymerase chain reaction (PCR) with fluorescent dye-labelled primers (Kimpton et al.1993), electrophoresis and analysis were performed using a 373A DNA Sequencer (Applied Biosystems,Inc.) as described (Hoff-Olsen et al. 1995).

RESULTS

Mutations are detected with all four markers . The somatic mutation frequencies range from 0.009 (HUMF13A1) to 0.122 (HUMVWA31/A). In the four STRs as a group, there is a significant excess of allelic expansion vs. contraction at mutation (43 vs. 24 tumours).

The mutant alleles are consistently composed of perfect integers of the four base pair repeats. Electrophoretogram reading confirmed this by locating the mutated alleles 4, 8, 12, or 16 base pairs to either side of the assigned constitutional allele (fig. 1). Furthermore, the new tumour bands could all be assigned to known alleles in the parent (Norwegian) population (Myhre Dupuy et al. 1993).

46 of the 61 tumours (75%) with mutant bands display only a single new band which differ with one (74%), two (15%) or three (11%) repeats from the constitutional band. The remaining 15 samples (25%) show either biallelic events (53%) or multiple consecutive mutant bands ("smears") (47%) (fig 1).

Figure 1

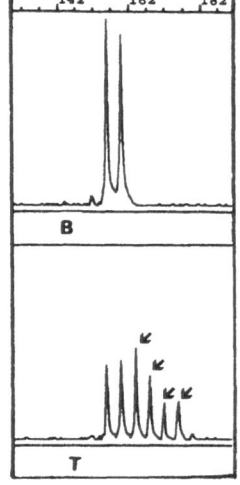

Electrophoretogram image.

Periferal blood (B) and colorectal carcinoma (T) DNA amplified with microsatellite marker HUMVWA31/A displaying "smear" of expanded new tumour alleles.

New alleles indicated (arrowheads).

Scale, X-axis: Basepairs (allele sizes).

DISCUSSION

Several reports conclude that human polymorphic tandem repeats tend to expand vs. contract at both somatic and germline mutation (Jeffreys et al. 1988; Olaisen et al. 1993; Weber and Wong 1993). The present study of somatic STR mutations strongly supports this observation.

Wooster et al (1994) found that alleles with greater number of repeats seem more likely to exhibit instability in tumours, supporting the suggestion that new mutants in triplet diseases originate from population subgroups with the longest "normal" repeats (Richards and Sutherland 1994). In contrast, in the four STR`s of this study we observe that the assigned constitutional alleles of the mutant tumour alleles are nearly evenly distributed over the allele frequency distributions of the parent population (data not shown).

185

Others have shown that colorectal adenomas display single mutant bands at mutation, while carcinomas tend to show smears (Lothe et al, 1993; Lothe RA, pers. comm.). Our present results also indicate that there are at least two such different types of somatic mutations. We will perform further analyses to clarify any eventual clinical significance of this observation.

REFERENCES

Aaltonen LA, Peltomäki P, Leach FS, Sistonen P, Pylkkänen L, Mecklin J-P, Järvinen H, Powell SM, Jen J, Hamilton SR, , Petersen GM, Kinzler KW, Vogelstein B, de la Chapelle A (1993) Clues to the pathogenesis of familial colorectal cancer. Science 260: 812-816

Han H-J, Yanagisawa A, Kato Y, Park J-G, Nakamura Y (1993) Genetic instability in pancreatic cancer and poorly differentiated type of gastric cancer. Cancer Res 53: 5087-5089

Hoff-Olsen P, Meling GI, Olaisen B (1995) Somatic mutations in VNTR-locus D1S7 in human colorectal carcinomas are associated with microsatellite instability. Hum mutat 5: 329-332

Jeffreys AJ, Royle NJ, Wilson V, Wong Z (1988) Spontaneous mutation rates to new length alleles at tandem-repetitive hypervariable loci in human DNA. Nature 332: 278-281

Kimpton CP, Gill P, Walton A, Urquhart A, Millican ES, Adams M (1993) Automated DNA profiling employing multiplex amplification of short tandem repeat loci. PCR methods appl 3: 13-22

Kuhl DPA,Caskey CT (1993)Trinucleotide repeats and genome variation.Curr Op Gen Dev 3: 404-407

Lothe RA, Peltomäki P, Meling GI, Aaltonen LA, Nyström-Lahti M, Pylkkänen L, Heimdal K, Andersen TI, Møller P, Rognum TO, Fosså SD , Haldorsen T, Langmark F, Brøgger A, de la Chapelle A, Børresen A-L (1993) Genomic instability in colorectal cancer: Relationship to clinicopathological variables and family history. Cancer Res 53: 5849-5852

Mahtani MM, Willard HF (1993) A polymorphic X-linked tetranucleotide repeat locus displaying a high rate of new mutation: implications for mechanisms of mutation at short tandem repeat loci. Hum Mol Genet 2: 431-437

Meling GI, Lothe RA, Børresen A-L, Hauge S, Clausen OPF, Rognum TO (1991) Genetic alterations within the retinoblastoma locus in colorectal carcinomas. Relation to DNA ploidy pattern studied by flow cytometric analysis. Br J Cancer 64: 475-480

Morral N, Nunes V, Casals T, Estivill X (1991) CA/GT microsatellite alleles within the cystic fibrosis transmembrane conductance regulator (CFTR) gene are not generated by unequal crossingover. Genomics 10: 692-698

Myhre Dupuy B, Berg ES, Olaisen B (1993) Four STRs in 300 Norwegians. In: Proc 15th Int Conf of the International society of forensic haematogenetics, Lido de Venezia 13-15 October 1993, p 157

Olaisen B, Bekkemoen M, Hoff-Olsen P, Gill P (1993) Human VNTR mutation and sex. In: Pena SDJ, Chakraborty R, Epplen JT, and Jeffreys AJ (eds) DNA fingerprinting: State of the science. Birkhäuser Verlag, Basel/Switzerland p 63

Orth K, Hung J, Gazdar A, Bowcock A, Mathis JM, Sambrook J (1994) Genetic instability in human ovarian cancer cell lines. Proc Natl Acad Sci USA 91: 9495-9499

Pena SDJ, de Souza KT, de Andrade M, Chakraborty R (1994) Allelic associations of two polymorphic microsatellites in intron 40 of the human von Willebrand factor gene. Proc Natl Acad Sci USA 91: 723-727

Richards RI, Sutherland GR (1994) Simple repeat DNA is not replicated simply. Nat Genet 6: 114-116

Risinger JI, Berchuck A, Kohler MF, Watson P, Lynch HT, Boyd J (1993) Genetic instability of microsatellites in endometrial carcinoma. Cancer Res 53: 5100-5103

Rubinsztein DC, Amos W, Leggo J, Goodburn S, Jain S, Li S-H, Margolis RL, Ross CA, Ferguson-Smith MA (1995) Microsatellite evolution - evidence for directionality and variation in rate between species. Nat Genet 10: 337-343

Shriver MD, Jin L, Chakraborty R, Boerwinkle E (1993) VNTR allele frequency distributions under the stepwise mutation model: A computer simulation approach. Genetics 134: 983-993

Thibodeau SN, Bren G, Schaid D (1993) Microsatellite instability in cancer of the proximal colon. Science 261: 816-819

Weber JL, Wong C (1993) Mutation of human short tandem repeats. Hum Mol Genet 8: 1123-1128

Wooster R, Cleton-Jansen A-M, Collins N, Mangion J, Cornelis RS, Cooper CS, Gusterson BA, Ponder BAJ, von Deimling A, Weistler OD, Cornelisse CJ, Devilee P, Stratton MR (1994) Instability of short tandem repeats (microsatellites) in human cancers. Nat Genet 6: 152-156

SIMPLE AND RAPID DUPLEX PCR FOR FORENSIC AND PATERNITY TESTING

K. LALU and M. LUKKA[*]

Department of Forensic Medicine, P.O.Box 40, 00014 University of Helsinki, Finland

[*]National Public Health Institute, Helsinki, Finland

INTRODUCTION

Short tandem repeat (STR) loci are a subclass of the highly polymorphic variable tandem repeat (VNTR) loci, which occur throughout the human genome. They are composed of repeated sequences of 1-7 bp in length. Their hypervariability and amenability to amplification by the polymerase chain reaction (PCR) make them ideal markers for use in the identification of individuals.

One tempting possibility of the PCR-technique is to amplify two or more loci simultaneously. In this study we describe a duplex PCR of two STR loci with non-overlapping allele size ranges: HumvWA (Kimpton 1992, Sajantila 1994) and HumFES/FPS (Polymeropoulos 1991) residing in chromosomes 12 and 15, respectively.

MATERIALS AND METHODS

DNA-samples

DNA was extracted from 3 ul EDTA-blood using Chelex^R method (Walsh 1991). Bone samples were pulverized, decalcified with 0.5 M EDTA and DNA was extracted using conventional organic extraction method (Sambrook 1989). From the shaver samples DNA was prepared by rapid lysis technique described by Higuchi et al.(1989).

Analysis of DNA-samples

The singleplex (both loci) or duplex PCR reactions were performed using primer sequences as follows:

HumFES/FPS	5' GGG ATT TCC CTA TGG ATT GG 3' 5' GGG AAA GAA TGA GAC TAC AT 3'
HumvWA	5' CCC TAG TGG ATG ATA AGA ATA ATC 3' 5' GGA CAG ATG ATA AAT ACA TAG GAT GGA TGG 3'

The PCR was carried out in 50 ul reaction volumes containing 0.2 mM of each dNTP and 1.25 U Taq polymerase (Promega) in PCR buffer (50 mM Tris-HCl, pH 8.8, 15 mM $(NH_4)_2SO_4$, 1.5 mM $MgCl_2$, 0.1% Triton X-100, 0.01% gelatin). The primer concentrations for the singleplex reactions were 1.0 uM and for duplex reaction 1.0 uM and 2.0 uM, for the HumFES/FPS and HumvWA loci, respectively. The amplification was performed with Gene AmpTM PCR System 9600 and each amplification was initiated with a hot start (Chou 1992). Denaturation for 30 sec. at 95°C, annealing for 30 sec at 58°C and extension for 60 sec. at 72°C was used for 30 cycles to amplify the locus HumvWA. In the amplification program for the HumFES/FPS locus and the duplex-PCR the annealing temperature was lowered to 54°C and 27 cycles were performed.

The amplified products were separated in 8.5% T, 4.8% C polyacrylamide gel (12cmx14cmx0.75mm) using 3.0% T, 4.8% C stacking gel (4cmx14cmx0.75mm) as described by Sajantila et al. (1993). The electrophoresis was runned for 1000 Vh and 100 mM Tris, 100mM boric acid, 2mM EDTA, pH 8.5 was used as a running buffer. The separated alleles were visualized by silver staining (Allen 1989).

RESULTS AND DISCUSSION

The size of the amplified fragments in the HumvWA and HumFES/FPS loci range between 134-170 and 211-231 base pairs, respectively. Because of the non-overlapping allele size ranges it is possible to amplify the loci simultaneously without labeling the primers and to separate and to visualize the amplified alleles using PAGE and silver staining (Fig.1.)

In 100 mother-child-putative father combinations from paternity testing material the HumvWA and HumFES/FPS loci were succesfully amplified with both duplex and single PCR. In this material no differences were obtained between the results of the single and the duplex PCR. Also no mother-child exclusion was found. In Finnish population the combined exclusion propability (Gurtler 1956) in paternity testing of the HumvWA (64.6)% and HumFES/FPS (41.3%) loci is 79.2%. In forensic analyses the duplex PCR has been used succesfully with semen and blood stains, hairs, epithelial cells as well as postmortem tissue samples (Fig. 2.)

Duplex PCR described is a simple method to increase the information obtained from one analysis. Co-amplification of the HumvWA and HumFES/FPS loci reduces the costs, labour and the time which is needed to perform the analyses.

REFERENCES

Allen RC, Graves G, Budowle B (1989) Polymerase chain reaction amplification products separated on rehydratable polyacrylamide gels and stained with silver. Biotechniques 12:736-744

Chou Q, Russell M, Raymond J, Bloch W (1992) Prevention of pre-PCR mispriming and primer dimerization improves low copy-number amplifications. Nucleic Acids Res 20:1717-1723

Gurtler H (1956) Principles of blood-group statistical evaluation of paternity cases at the University Institute of Forensic Medicine Copenhagen. Acta Med Leg Soc 9:83

Higuchi R (1989) Simple and rapid preparation of samples for PCR. In: Erlich HA (ed) PCR Technology-Principles and applications for DNA amplification. Stockton press New York pp. 34-39

Kimpton CP, Walton A, Gill P (1992) A further tetranucleotide repeat polymorphism in the vWF gene. Hum Mol Genet 1:287

Polymeropoulos MH, Rath DS, Xiao H, Merril CR (1991) Tetranucleotide repeat polymorphism at the human c-fes/fps proto-oncogene (FES). Nucleic Acids Res 19:4018

Sajantila A, Lukka M (1993) Improved separation of PCR amplified VNTR alleles by a vertical polyacrylamide gel electrophoresis. Int J Legal Med 105:355-359

Sajantila A, Pacek P, Lukka M, Syvänen A-C, Nokelainen P, Sistonen P, Peltonen L, Budowle B (1994) A microsatellite polymorphism in the von Willebrant Factor gene: comparison of allele frequencies in different population samples and evaluation for forensic medicine. Forensic Sci Int 69:161-170

Sambrook J, Fritsch EF, Maniatis T (1989) Analysis and cloning of eukaryotic genomic DNA. In: Molecular Cloning. Cold Spring Harbor Laboratory Press New York (A Laboratory Manual)

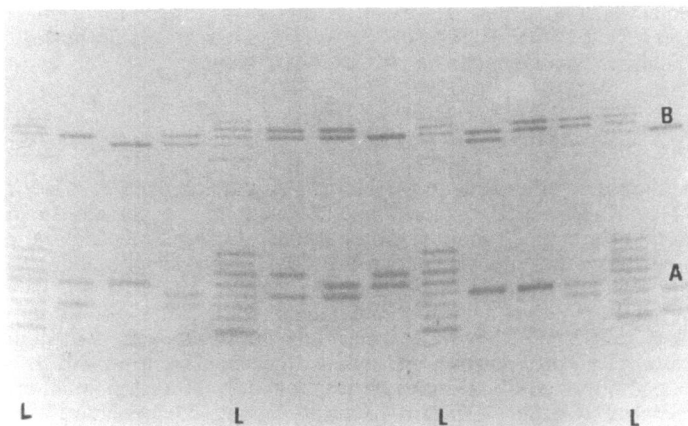

Figure 1. Analysis of the HumvWA (A) and HumFES/FPS (B) loci after duplex PCR and PAGE and silver staining. L= allelic ladder containing alleles 14-20 for the HumvWA locus and alleles 8,10,11,12 and 13 for the HumFES/FPS locus.

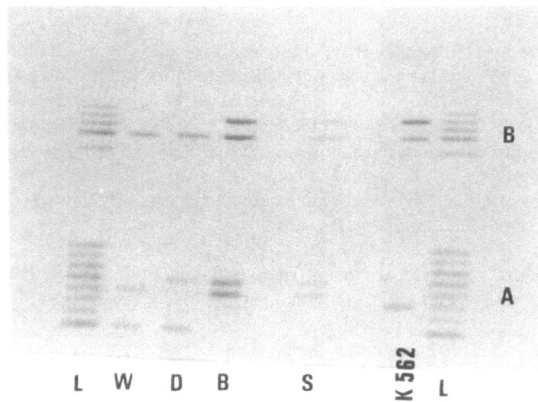

Figure 2. Identification of human skeletal remains which were found about one year after the death. The presumed identity was found by the police from the file of the lost persons. The silver staining pattern after duplex PCR of the HumvWA (A) and HumFES/FPS (B) loci and PAGE is shown. L= allelic ladders as in figure 1. Reference blood samples were obtained from the wife (W) and the daughter (D) of the presumed person. In addition the shaver (S) of this lost person was also available for DNA-analyses. B= bone sample obtained at the autopsy.

GENETIC STUDIES OF A STR AT THE UGB LOCUS

P. Leyenda and B. Caeiro

Section of Anthropology, Faculty of Biology
University of Santiago, 15706 Santiago de Compostela
Galicia (Spain)

The so called Short Tandem Repeats (STR) constitute nowadays one of the most interesting sources of information in human genetic studies. This paper deals with the analysis of a tetranucleotide repeat in the Uteroglobin Gene (UGB) (Stöhr & Weber 1994), localised in chromosome 11q (Wolf et al. 1992). Thus, an initial survey in a sample of the population of Galicia is carried out aimed at assessing the technical conditions for UGB phenotyping and evaluate its usefulness in the genetic profiling of human populations.

MATERIALS AND METHODS

Blood samples were obtained from 200 unrelated individuals from the population of Galicia (NW Spain). DNA was extracted by standard chelating resins method (Singer-Sam 1993) or phenol/chloroform (Maniatis et al. 1982).The primer sequences were as described (Stöhr & Weber 1994):
UGB-1: 5'-CAT CTT CCT TGC CCA TTT C-3'.
UGB-2: 5'-TGC ATC CCT CCC CTC TTA-3'.

PCR was carried out from a total volume of 12.5 μL, containing 0.8 μM each primer, 75 μM dNTPs, 0.5 Units of Taq DNA Polymerase (Boehringer Mannheim), in 10 mM Tris-HCl buffer, pH 8.3, containing 50 mM KCl and 1.5 mM $MgCl_2$. PCR was performed in a Perkin Elmer 2400 apparatus according to the following cycling conditions: 94 $^{\circ}$C (30 sec), 52 $^{\circ}$C (30 sec), 72 $^{\circ}$C (30 sec) for 30 cycles, and a final extension at 72 $^{\circ}$C for 5 min. Molecular separation took place in 12 cm wide x 19 cm long x 0.4 mm thick polyacrylamide gels (T=5, C=3, Glycerol 7.1%) in a discontinuous Tris-HCl-Glycine buffer, pH 8.8 according to Ornstein (1964) with modifications. Electrophoresis was conducted at 18 $^{\circ}$C, at a constant 200 V for 3 h, after which the gel was silver stained (Budowle et al. 1991) for UGB band detection.

RESULTS AND DISCUSSION

The abovementioned conditions achieve a good signal of amplification for UGB, $MgCl_2$ being, however, a critical factor; so, non-specific bands or low signal of amplified product were observed respectively at concentrations of 2-3 mM or lower than 1.5 mM (Fig. 1).

Given the size of alleles,(ranging between 387 to 411 bp), the most critical parameters for UGB phenotyping rely on the conditions for molecular separation of alleles. In our experience polyacrylamide matrixes using Tris-HCl-Glycine buffers, followed by silver staining for detection, constitute a reliable modality for UGB phenotyping (Fig. 2).

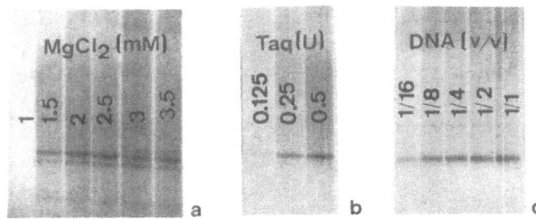

Fig. 1: Effects of MgCl₂ (a), Taq DNA Polymerase (b) and amount of DNA (c) in UGB amplification.

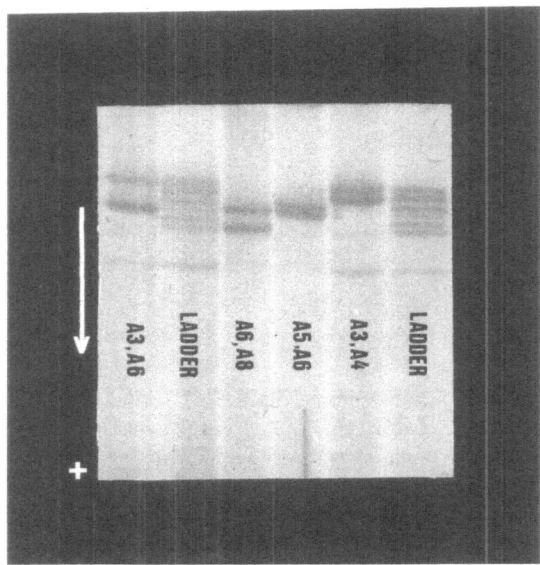

Fig. 2: Phenotype patterns of UGB after electrophoresis of polyacrylamide and Silver Staining. Alleles are denominated according to Stöhr & Weber 1994: A1 (415bp), A2 (411bp), A3 (407 bp), A4 (403 bp), A5 (399 bp), A6 (395 bp), A7 (391 bp) and A8 (387 bp).

Long distance electrophoretic runs and temperature of electrophoresis are crucial factors for an accurate discrimination of the alleles. Preliminary data in family groups (including 25 meioses from 10 informative families) are consistent with an autosomal codominant way of inheritance for this system. Notwithstanding, enlarging the number of cases is advisable in order to estimate its mutation rate.

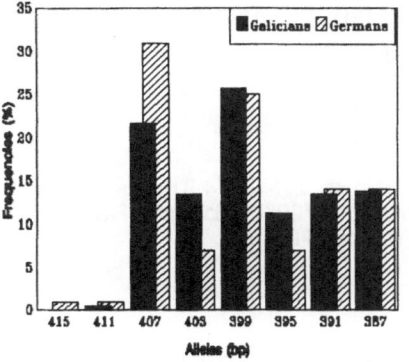

Fig. 3: Allele frequencies of UGB. Galicians (n=200), Germans (from general, n=57).

The distribution of allele frequencies obtained in this study (Fig. 3), configure unbiased values of $H = 0.790$ and $PIC = 0.818$, which indicates the degree of variability of this system. Statistical comparisons with the only data so far available, corresponding to unrelated Germans (Stöhr & Weber 1994), does not evidence significant differences after multinomial derived analyses ($G = 11.212$, $0.1 < p < 0.2$, 7 d.f.) (Sokal & Rohlf 1969).

As UGB demands long gels for molecular separation of the alleles, this makes it less suitable than other shorter systems for co-migration of multiplexed loci, unless very log gels (i.e. sequencing gels or similar) are employed. However, the well balanced degree of polymorphism of its alleles, denotes the potential interest of this STR in this type of studies.

REFERENCES

Budowle B, Chakraborty R, Giusti AM, Eisenberg AJ and Allen RC (1991). Analysis of the VNTR locus D1S80 by the PCR followed by high-resolution PAGE. *Am. J. Hum. Genet.* *48*, 137-144.

Maniatis T, Fristch EF and Sambrock J (1982). Molecular cloning: a laboratory manual. Cold Spring Harbor Laboratory, New York.

Ornstein L (1964). Disc electrophoresis I. Background and theory. *Ann. N. Y. Acad. Sci.* 121, 321-349.

Singer-Sam J, Tanguay EF and Riggs AD (1989). Use of chelex to improve the PCR signal from a small number of cells. *Amplifications 3*, 11.

Sokal RR, Rohlf FJ (1969). Biometry. Freeman and Company, San Francisco.

Stöhr H, Weber BFH (1994). (ATTT)$_n$-tetranucleotide repeat polimorphism in the 5'-flanking region of the UGB gene. *Hum. Mol. Genet. 3*, 2086.

Wolf M, Klug J, Hackenberg R, Gessler M, Grzeschik K-H, Beato M, Suske G (1992). Human CC10, the homologue of rabbit uteroglobin: genomic cloning, chromosomal localization and expression in endometrial cell lines. *Hum. Mol. Genet. 1*, 371-378.

ACKNOWLEDGMENTS

This work was partially supported by grants from the Ministerio de Educación y Ciencia (CICYT SAF92-0557) and Xunta de Galicia (XUGA 20001B94).

TUMOR INOCULATION BETWEEN TWO UNRELATED HUMAN INDIVIDUALS: STR ANALYSIS OF PARAFFIN-EMBEDDED TISSUE SECTION

C. Luckenbach*, V.H. Gärtner**, C. Seidl***, H. Ritter*

* Inst. f. Anthroplogie und Humangenetik, Wilhelmstr. 27, 72074 Tübingen, FRG
** Inst. f. Pathologie, Liebermeisterstr.8,Wilhelmstr. 27, 72074 Tübingen, FRG
***Blutspendedienst DRK,Sandhofstr.1, 60528 Frankfurt,FRG

1. Introduction

In this study we used the STR (short tandem repeat) technology to check the possibility of tumor inoculation between two unrelated individuals, first described by Gärtner et al. (1995).

Case report: A surgeon injured his hand with a sharp instrument during a resection of an intestinal soft tissue tumor (tumor I). After one year a tumor (tumor II) was detected in his hurt hand. Histological and morphological analysis revealed these two tumors (I and II) as identical.

Only paraffin-embedded tissue of these tumors was available to perform DNA-profiling. We succeeded in DNA extracting from these tissues, but the material was unsuitable for molecular techniques which require high-molecular-weight genomic DNA. Although significant DNA degradation was observed, three STR loci could be detected: CYP 19 (15q21.1), TH01 (11p15.5), SE 33 (ACTBP2).

We present the DNA extracting protocol for paraffin embedded tissue, the STR analysis method and the exeptional findings.

2. Materials and Methods

2.1. Samples

Tumor tissue
Paraffin embedded tumor tissue from autopsies or biopsies were obtained from the files of the Department of Pathology of the University of Tübingen, FRG.
Samples measuring approximately 5 x 5 x 3 mm were fixed by immersion in 10% buffered formalin, were processed into paraffin blocks and stored at ambient temperature.

EDTA-Blood
DNA was prepared from EDTA-blood of the surgeon according to the protocol of Miller et al. (1988)

2.2. Histological Examination
Gärtner et al. (1995)

2.3. DNA Extraction
- according to Goelz et al. (1985) with modifications
- paraffin was cut away before tinely mincing the tumor tissue
- suspension in TE-buffer (500mM Tris, 20mM EDTA, 10mM NaCL, pH 9.2)
- homogenization in a 50 ml falcon tube with 10 ml of TE-buffer containing 10% SDS and 0.5% Proteinase K, incubation for 30 hrs at 50 °C
- addition of 1.5 ml 0.5% Proteinase K and 1.5 ml 10% SDS
- vortex with high speed 4 min., incubation for 50 hrs at 50 °C
- DNA extraction once with 1 volume of phenol; three times with 1 volume of phenol-chloroform (3 parts phenol, 2 parts TE-buffer, 4 parts chloroform); once with 1 volume of chloroform
- addition of ammonium acetate (0.3 volumes of a 10M solution)
- DNA precipitation by 3 volumes of cold ethanol, incubation for 12-24 hrs at -70 °C, centrifugation 9500 xg for 30 min.
- resuspension of the pellet in TE-buffer (10 mM Tris, 1mM EDTA, pH 8)

2.4. PCR and STR-Characterisation

All oligonucleotides were commercially synthesized and 5'primers were labeled with fluorescence dye markers (Applied Biosystems (ABI), Weiterstadt, FRG) according to the allelic size distribution of the different STR-systems. PCR amplification was performed in a 9600 DNA thermal cycler system (Perkin Elmer, Weiterstadt, FRG) using 100 ng genomic DNA, 25 pmol of each primer 200 nmol dNTPs, 1x PCR buffer and 0.5 units Taq polymerase in a final volume of 50 ul.

HumCYP19:

- name: Human aromatose gene at the **CYP19** locus, Polymeropoulos et al. (1992)
- location: 15q21.1
- repeat: TTTA
- primer (5'-3'):   P5 GCAGGTACTTAGTTAGCTAC, P3 TTACAGTGAGCCAAGGTCGT
- cycle conditions: 95 °C 5 min., 95 °C 60 sec (35 cycles), 54 °C 30 sec., 72 °C 60 sec, final extension 72 °C, 5 min.

HumACTBP2:

- name: Human cytoplasmic beta actin related pseudogene **(SE 33)** Polymeropoulos et al. (1992)
- location: chromosome 6
- repeat: AAAG
- primer(5'-3'): P5 AATCTGGGCGACAAGAGTGA, P3 ACATCTCCCCTACCGTATA
- cycle conditions: 95 °C 5 min., 95 °C 45 sec (35 cycles), 54 °C 30 sec., 72 °C 60 sec, final extension 72 °C, 5 min.

HumTH01:

- name: Human tyrosine hydroxylase gene, intron 1 **(TC11)**, Polymeropoulos et al. (1991)
- location: 11p15.5
- repeat: TCAT
- primer (5'-3'): P5 GTGGGCTGAAAAGCTCCCGATTAT, P3 GTGATTCCCATTGGCCTGTTCCTC
- labeling: HEX (6-carboxy-2',4',7',4',7-Hexachlorofluorescin):
- cycle conditions: 95 °C 5 min., 95 °C 60 sec (35 cycles), 54 °C 30 sec., 72 °C 60 sec, final extension 72 °C, 5 min.

2.5. Allele Size Analysis:

Electrophoresis: automated DNA sequencer model 373A (ABI), 6% polyacrylamide sequencig gel, 30 W for 8 hrs
Internal standard: generated by amplification using various primer combinations from the vector pGL2-basic (Promega, Heidelberg, FRG), 6 ul
Samples: 2.5 ul of each amplification product, heat denatured
The relative position of fragments are determined by measuring the laserlight induced fluorescence emission. Fragment sizes are calculated automatically with the Genescan 672 software (ABI) using the local reciprocal method described by Southern (1979).

3. Results and Discussion

We have tried to determine wether DNA can be prepared from tissue which has been fixed and embedded for routine histopathological examination. Our findings confirm that it is possible to extract DNA from such specimens, but the revealed DNA is not completely intact. The isolated DNA was unsuitable for molecular techniques which require high molecular weight genomic DNA. Although significant DNA degradation was observed, three STR-loci could be detected: CYP19, SE33 and TC11. Because of their small sizes (< 300 bp) STRs are more likely to be successful on old or degraded material.
Figure 1 shows the electropherogram from a 6% denaturating polyacrylamide gel concerning the STR-locus TC11 of three different samples: tumor tissue of the surgeon (lane 13), blood sample of the surgeon (lane 14), tumor tissue of the patient (lane 15). Peaks represent fluorescent intensities of dye-labeled TC11-alleles.
Table 1 summarizes all results of Fig.1 indicating the peak height (measured against an arbitrary scale displayed on the y-axis) and the calculated sizes of the different alleles (shown along the x-axis) . Table 2 shows the detected alleles from the anlaysed samples at the STR-loci CYP19, SE33 and TC11.

Table 1: Summary of the calculated TC11 allele sizes and peak height

Peak	Lane	Allele size	Peak height
1	13	157.68	479
2	13	165.85	474
3	13	173.03	286
1	14	157.68	470
2	14	172.96	487
1	15	165.84	1507
2	15	173.03	344

Table 2: Alleles of the three samples at CYP19, SE33 and TC11

STR-locus	Surgeons tumor	Surgeons blood	Patients tumor
CYP19	168 bp	168 bp	168 bp
	187 bp		187 bp
SE33	252 bp	300 bp	252 bp
	277 bp		277 bp
	300 bp		
	158 bp	158 bp	166 bp
TC11	166 bp	173 bp	173 bp
	173 bp		

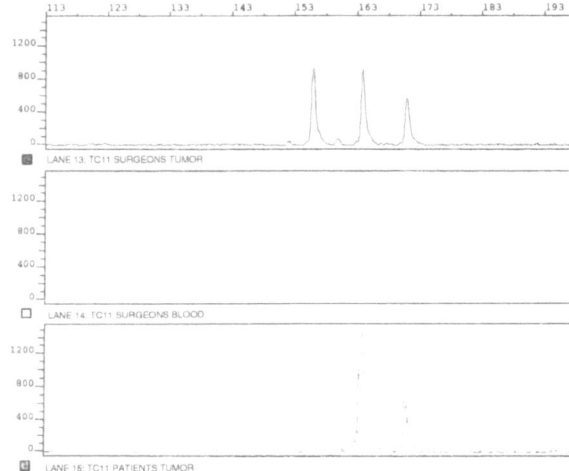

Fig. 1: Electropherogram from a 6% denaturating polyacrylamide gel at the TC11-locus; lane 13: tumor tissue (surgeon); lane 14: blood sample (surgeon); lane 15: tumor tissue (patient). Peaks represent fluorescent intensities of dye-labeled TC11-alleles.

The comparison of the surgeons blood sample with the tissue sections of his tumor (tumor II) and the tumor of the patient (tumor I) gave exceptional findings: tumor II showed at each STR locus all alleles from tumor I. These results point at the chance of tumor inoculation between humans, a new exciting finding in cancer research.

Thus we demonstrate the bridge between molecular genetics and classical histology meaning that the world-wide collection of archival paraffin-embedded tissues may be used to study rare cancers and genetic changes which occur in human tumors.

References
Gärtner HV, Seidl C, Luckenbach C et al. (1995) Accidental MFH-Transplantation from a patient to a surgeon: proof with molecular genetic methods. (in press)

Goelz SE, Hamilton SR, Vogelstein B (1985) Purification of DNA from foraldehyde fixed and paraffin embedde human tissue. Biochem. Biophys. Res. Comm.130: 118-126

Miller SA, Dykes DD, Polesky HF (1988) A simple salting out procedure for extracting DNA from human nucleated cells. Nucleic Acids Res 16:1215

Polymeropoulos MH, Xiao H, Rath DS , Merril CR.(1991) Tetranucleotide repeat polymorphism at the human tyrosine hydrolase gene (TH). Nucleic Acids Res.19:3753

Polymeropoulos MH, Xiao H, Rath DS , Merril CR.(1992) Tetranucleotide repeat polymorphism at the human aromatase cytochrome P-450 gene (Cyp19).Nucleic Acids Res.19(1):195

Polymeropoulos MH, Xiao H, Rath DS , Merril CR.(1992) Tetranucleotide repeat polymorphism at the human beta-actin related pseudogene H-beta-Ac-psi2 (ACTPB2). Nucleic Acids Res.20(6):14

Southern EM (1979) Measurement of DNA length by gel electrophoresis. Anal Biochem 100:319-323

MOLECULAR PHENOTYPING OF TWO TRINUCLEOTIDE REPEATS (XT00444 AND D5S373). EXPERIMENTAL CONDITIONS.

J.R. Luis and B. Caeiro.

Department of Anthropology, Faculty of Biology, University of Santiago de Compostela, Galicia, Spain.

In this work the genetic analysis of two trinucleotide repeats XT00444 (Yandava et al., 1994) and D5S373 (Dixon and Dixon, 1993) located in the chromosomes 13 and 5q32 respectively, is carried out. The main objectives consist not only in analysing their degree of variability in this initial approach, but mainly to study their molecular behaviour with a view towards developing robust phenotyping conditions for routine analyses.

MATERIAL AND METHODS

DNA samples were extracted from whole blood of 200 autochtonous Galician individuals (NW Spain) by standar chelating resins method (Singer-Sam et al., 1989) or phenol/chloroform (Maniatis et al., 1982).

The primer sequences for the D5S373 were as described by Dixon and Dixon (1993):
5' GGT AAC AAG AGA GAA ACT CC 3'
5' CAA TTT CTT AGT GCA CAC ATC 3'.
The temperature cycling conditions were 92°C/30 sec, 60°C/30 sec, 72°C/30 sec for 35 cycles and an additional extension step at 72°C for 10 min in the Linus Dualcicler. The DNA was amplified in a final volume of 12.5 μl containing 1μM of each primer, 200 μM dNTPs, 0.5 units of Taq DNA Polymerase (Boehringer Mannhein), 1.5 mM Mg Cl$_2$.

The XT00444 amplification was carried out according to the following primer sequences (Yandava et al., 1994):
5' GAA TAA AGT GCC CAG CTT GT 3'
5' GTT GTC CTT AAA GCC CCG T 3'.
The temperature profile consisted of an initial denaturation at 94°C for 6 min, followed by 35 cycles of 94°C/15 sec, 62°C/23sec, 72°C/30sec and an final extension step at 72°C for 5 min, in the Gene Amp PCR 2400 System (Perkin Elmer). The amplification mixture consisted of 20-50 ng of DNA, 0.4 μM of both primers, 200 μM dNTPs, 0.75 units of Taq DNA Polymerase (Boehringer Mannhein), 3 mM Mg Cl$_2$ in a total volume of 12.5 μl.

PCR amplified products were separated by semy-dry discontinuous polyacrylamide gel electrophoresis, in horizontal plates with 400 μm of thickness. The gel composition was 9% T, 4% C for XT00444 and 10% T, 5% C for D5S373 using piperazine diacrylamide as a crosslinker, Glycerol (7.1% v/v). A 0.375 M Tris-HCl pH 8.8 buffer was used for the gel and a 0.125 M Tris-Glycine pH 8.8 buffer for the bridge. Electrophoresis was carried out at constant 12.5 V/cm for 2 hours, and the bands were visualised by a specific DNA Silver Staining (Budowle et al., 1991).

RESULTS AND DISCUSSION

A non-specific constant band in the reading zone (Fig.1) of D5S373 was observed according to the conditions reported elsewhere (Dixon and Dixon, 1993). In our experience, the concentration primers and temperature of annealing are the critical factors. Thus, increasing the temperature up to 60°C leads to a progressive decrease of the non-specific bands which gives a remarkable improvement for the phenotype diagnosis (Fig. 1a). With regard to XT00444 a poor signal of amplification was obtained, despite diverse PCR parameters (reagents, cycling conditions) being assayed.

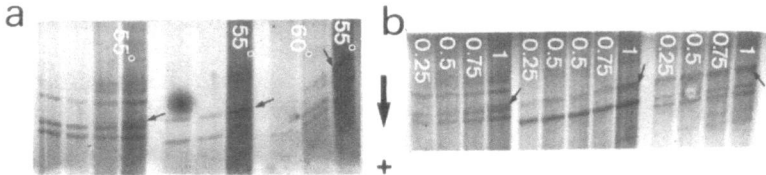

Figure. 1. Influence on the amplification of the D5S373 of the annealing temperature (a) and of the primer concentration (μM)(b). Arrows indicate the constant bands referred in the text.

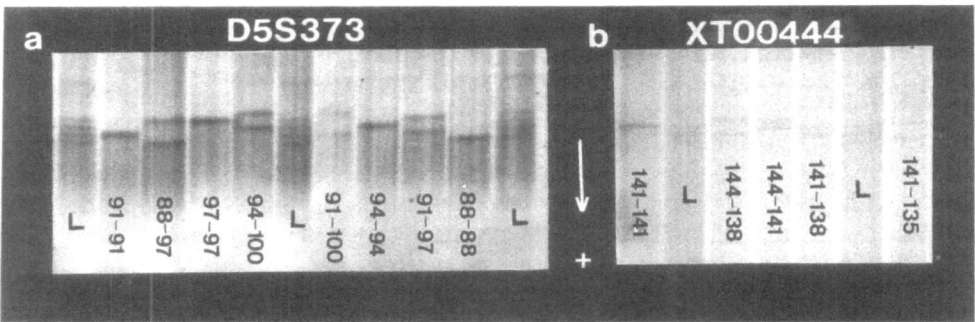

Figure. 2. Phenotype patterns after polyacrylamide gel electrophoresis : a) D5S373 and b) XT00444.

Polyacrylamide supports are revealed as a suitable modality for molecular separation of the alleles of both systems (Fig 2a/2b), regardless of the efficiency of the amplification as mentioned above.

The allele frequencies distributions in 200 individuals of the population of Galicia are summarised in Table I. No deviations from the Hardy-Weinberg proportions, were registered ($\chi^2 = 31.541$, $0.6 < p < 0.7$ for XT00444 and $\chi^2 = 4.035$, $0.9 < p < 0.95$ for D5S373). Finally, the weak bands frequently observed after PCR amplification of XT00444, leads us to not recommend this marker for routine analysis. Conversely, the robustness of D5S373 phenotyping and its degree of polymorphism deserves its potential inclusion as a suitable marker for these type of studies.

Table 1.- Allele frequencies distribution of the XT00444 and the D5S373.

XT0044		D5S373	
Alleles (bp)	Frequencies ± s.e.	Alleles(bp)	Frequencies ± s.e.
147bp	0.0100 ± 0.005	100bp	0.0125 ± 0.006
144bp	0.2125 ± 0.020	97bp	0.1800 ± 0.019
141bp	0.2275 ± 0.021	94bp	0.2825 ± 0.023
138bp	0.4225 ± 0.025	91bp	0.3700 ± 0.024
135bp	0.0950 ± 0.015	88bp	0.1550 ± 0.018
132bp	0.0050 ± 0.004	PIC = 0.678; H = 0.727	
129bp	0.0025 ± 0.002		
126bp	0.0050 ± 0.004		
123bp	0.0200 ± 0.007		
PIC = 0.672; H = 0.715			

REFERENCES

Budowle B., Chakraborty R., Giusti A.M., Eisenberg A.J. and Allen R.C. (1991) Analysis of the VNTR locus D1S80 by the PCR followed by high-resolution PAGE. *Am J Hum Genet 48*:137-144

Dixon J. and Dixon M.J. (1993). Trinucleotide repeat polymorphism at the D5S373 locus. *Hum Mol Genet 2*:829

Maniatis T, Fritsch E.F., Sambrook J. (1982) Molecular cloning: a laboratory manual. Cold Spring Harbor Laboratory, Cold Spring Harbor, New York, pp 438-454

Singer-Sam J., Tanguay R.L. and Riggs A.D. (1989) Use of Chelex to improve the PCR signal from a small number of cells. *Amplification 3*:11

Yandava C.N., Meyers V., Watkins H. and Duyk G. (1994) A trinucleotide repeat polymorphism in XT00444 (D13S635E). *Hum Mol Genet 3*:1209

ACKNOWLEDGMENTS

This work was partially supported by grants from the Ministerio de Educación y Ciencia (CICYT SAF92-0557) and Xunta de Galicia (XUGA 20001B94).

DEVELOPMENT AND OPTIMISATION OF A HIGHLY DISCRIMINATING MULTIPLEX PCR SYSTEM SUITABLE FOR FORENSIC IDENTIFICATION

N. J. OLDROYD, A. J. URQUHART, C. P. KIMPTON, E. S. MILLICAN, S. K. WATSON, R. R. E. FRAZIER & P. GILL.

THE FORENSIC SCIENCE SERVICE, PRIORY HOUSE, GOOCH STREET NORTH, BIRMINGHAM, B5 6QQ, UK.

INTRODUCTION

Forensic DNA profiling in the UK has in recent years targeted the analysis of short tandem repeat (STR) loci which consist of simple tandemly repeated sequences of 1-6 bp in length. Such loci can exhibit a high degree of length polymorphism due to variation in the number of repeat units displayed and as such can be highly informative in situations of human identification.

STRs are highly abundant in the genome, occurring approximately every 6-10 kb, and as such provide a considerable resource from which to select the most promising loci for use in forensic identification. In addition, the introduction of multiple dye technology enabling co-amplification of STR loci with overlapping size ranges combined with their hypervariable nature and PCR amplification efficiency has allowed the realisation of efficient and highly discriminating multiplex PCR systems. Such systems have several advantages over existing technology in that they are more sensitive, requiring as little as 0.5 ng of DNA (SLP analysis requires in excess of 50 ng), can be used on highly degraded DNA since the maximum length of DNA amplified is usually below 400 bp compared with 1-20 kb lengths probed by SLPs, and eliminate the need for radioactivity. The intrinsically rapid nature of the protocol afforded by single step PCR reactions and computer-controlled gel-running, analysis and allele designation means that the process is ideally suited for use in high throughput situations where the number of samples precludes the use of existing and time consuming methods of DNA analysis.

The system described here was developed as a result of the evaluation of several multiplexes including the quadruplex (Kimpton et al, 1993), heptaplex (Urquhart et al, 1995) and octoplex (Oldroyd et al, 1995) systems. Now known as the Second Generation Multiplex (SGM), the new system contains six tetranucleotide STR loci including three which exhibit alleles differing in size by 2 bp, and retains the X-Y homologous gene amelogenin (Sullivan et al, 1993) described in both the heptaplex and octoplex systems. It was intended that as a minimum requirement SGM would combine an integrated sex test with PCR integrity and a discriminating provide the Forensic Science Service with a system suitable for rapid, routine analysis of a large number of samples submitted to the UK National DNA Database.

MATERIALS AND METHODS

DNA Isolation

DNA was prepared from whole blood as described previously (Gill et al, 1990). Blood samples were collected from unrelated Caucasians, Afro-Caribbeans and Asians residing in the UK. Quantification of DNA was carried out using a primate-specific alpha satellite probe assay (Walsh et al, 1992).

Optimised Amplification Conditions

Primer sequences for the loci employed have been described previously (Oldroyd et al 1995). All oligonucleotide primers were synthesised commercially by Oswel DNA Services (Southampton, UK.) and selected primers labelled with one of the fluorescent dye markers 6-FAM 6-carboxyfluorescein (6-FAM), hexachloro-6-carboxyfluorescein (HEX) or tetrachloro-6-carboxyfluorescein (TET) all from ABD (Warrington, UK.), coupled with an aminohexyl linker.

PCR amplification was carried out using 1-5 ng genomic DNA in a 50 μl reaction volume containing 1 x PARR-Excellence buffer (Cambio Ltd, Cambridge UK.), 1.25 U Amplitaq™ DNA polymerase (Perkin-Elmer, Norwalk, CT, USA) and 200 μM each dNTP (Boehringer Mannheim GmbH, Mannheim, Germany). Samples were amplified for 30 cycles of 30 s at 93 °C, 75 s at 58 °C and 15 s at 72 °C followed by a 10 minute extension period at 72 °C on a Perkin-Elmer 9600 thermal cycler. Primer concentrations employed were 0.05 μM Amel 1/2; 0.32 μM VWA 1/2; 0.22 μM TH01 1/2; 0.28 μM D6S502 1/2; 0.08 μM FGA 1/2; 0.20 μM D21S11 and 0.08 μM D18S11 1/2.

Electrophoresis and Analysis

1.5μl of PCR product were combined with 2 μl formamide and 6 fmol of internal size standard GS350 (ABD) comprising *Pst 1*-digested plasmid DNA ligated to a TAMRA-labelled (N,N,N',N'-tetramethyl-6-carboxyfluorescein) 22-mer oligodeoxynecleotide at the cut ends. Subsequent digestion with BstU 1 results in DNA fragments containing a single TAMRA dye yielding a single peak for each fragment under denaturing and non-denaturing conditions. Samples were denatured for 2 min at 90 °C and loaded onto 6% denaturing 24 cm well-to-read polyacrylamide gels. National Diagnostics ultra-pure sequagel 6 and matched buffer batches were commercially supplied by Flowgen (Sittingbourne, UK.). Gels were electrophoresed for 8 h at 38 W constant power on an ABD 373A sequencer and fragment sizes determined automatically by GeneScan 672 software (ABD) using the Local Southern sizing algorithm. Allele designations determined by sequencing a selection of alleles from each locus were automatically assigned using the Genotyper DNA fragment analysis software (ABD).

Statistical Calculations

Discriminating power and matching probabilities were calculated by the method of Jones (1972).

RESULTS AND DISCUSSION

All of the loci contained within this system have previously been demonstrated to co-amplify effectively as part of a multiplex containing 7 STR loci previously described by this laboratory (the octoplex, Oldroyd *et al*, 1995). The system described here evolved as a result of forensic difficulties encountered with one of the loci (D20S85) in the octoplex. When multiplexing several loci together in this fashion, interaction between the primers can result not only in the production of desired allele peaks but also in the formation of artefactual bands caused by the interaction of mismatched primer pairs with the genomic DNA. In a forensic context, the presence of additional bands unrelated to the genotype of an individual could lead to confusion during interpretation of the profile. The locus D20S85 was found to be particularly problematic in this area and it was decided to remove it from the multiplex and optimise the conditions for the remaining loci in the system.

The loci in the revised system were found to co-amplify effectively and employed identical buffer, dNTP and enzyme concentrations as the heptaplex and octoplex systems previously described. Comparable band intensities for all the loci contained within the system were obtained by the adjustment of individual primer concentrations within the reaction. Optimum amplification was achieved through manipulation of PCR cycle parameters. Genescan 672 analysis (ABD) generated electropherograms in which DNA fragments were depicted as coloured peaks. Examples shown in Fig. 1 indicate the consistency in peak areas generated both between alleles and across loci. Co-amplification of loci whose size ranges overlap was afforded by the combination of 3 dye labels.

Preliminary statistical calculations for each STR locus were carried out on a minimum of 50 unrelated individuals from each of the three British populations: Caucasians, Afro-Caribbeans and Asians (amelogenin was not included in these calculations). The individual and combined matching probabilities (pM) for each locus in each of the stated race codes are given in table 1 and correspond with previously published values. SGM produces a matching probability of between 1.2×10^{-8} and 1×10^{-9}, a value equivalent to that produced by 4 RFLP probes and when used in conjunction with the quadruplex system (Kimpton *et al*, 1993), the value approaches 1×10^{-10}.

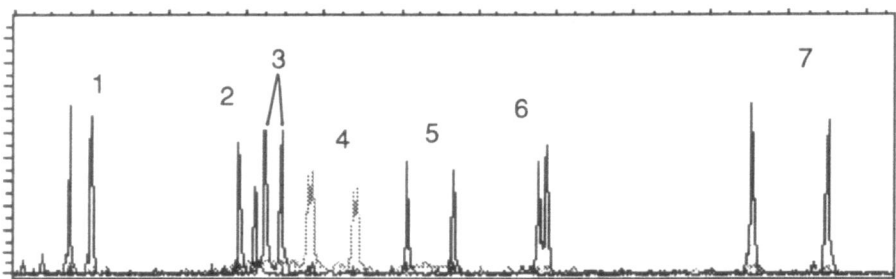

Figure 1: Example of an electropherogram generated by Genescan 672 software. Key to locus numbers: 1: Amelogenin, 2:HUMVWFA31/A, 3: HUMTH01, 4: D6S502, 5: HUMFIBRA, 6: D21S11, 7: D18S51. (Loci 1, 3, 6 & 7 labelled with 6-FAM; 2 & 5 labelled with HEX; 4 labelled with TET).

Table 1: The individual and combined matching probabilities of each locus for each of the three stated race codes. * indicates loci displaying alleles differing in size by 2bp.

Locus	Location	Probability of a Match		
		White Caucasians	Afro-Caribbeans	Indo-Pakistani
HUMVWFA31/A	12p12-pter	0.064	0.057	0.075
HUMTH01	11p15-15.5	0.086	0.100	0.084
HUMFIBRA*	4q28	0.044	0.027	0.031
D21S11*	21	0.051	0.042	0.046
D18S51*	18q21.3	0.029	0.024	0.042
D6S502	6	0.047	0.061	0.054
COMBINED (SGM)		1.7×10^{-8}	9.5×10^{-9}	2.0×10^{-8}

SGM has been demonstrated to be robust and reproducible with profiles demonstrated to be consistent across a range of sample types (results in prep.). The system is currently used for the analysis of hair root and buccal scrape samples submitted to the UK National DNA Database.

REFERENCES
- Clarke, J. M. (1988) Nucleic Acids Res: 16, 9677-9686.
- Gill, P., Woodroffe, S., Lygo, J. E., Millican, E. S., Int. J. Leg. Med. 1991, 104, 221-227.
- Hauge, X. Y., Litt, M. Hum. Mol. Genet. 1993, 2, 411-415.
- Jones, A. D. J. (1972) Forensic Sci. Soc: 12, 355-359.
- Kimpton, C. P., Gill, P., Walton, A., Urquhart, A., Millican, E. S., Adams, M. (1990). PCR Methods Applic: 3, 13-22.
- Kimpton C. P., Walton, A., Gill, P. (1992) Hum. Molec. Genet: 1, 287.
- Mells, R., Beadley, P., Elsner, T., Robertson, M., Lawrence, N., Gerken, S., Alvertson, N., White, R. (1993) Genomics: 16, 56-62.
- Mills, K. A., Even, D., Murray, J. C. (1992) Hum. Molec. Genet: 1, 779.
- Oldroyd, N. J., Urquhart, A. J., Kimpton, C. P., Millican E. S., Watson, S. K., Downes, T. J., Gill, P. (1995) Electrophoresis: 16, 334-337.
- Polymeropoulos, M. H., Xiao, H., Rath, D. S., Merril, C. R. (1991) Nucleic Acids Res: 19, 3753
- Sharma, V., Litt, M. (1992) Nucleic Acids Res: 1, 67.
- Straub, R. E., Speer, M. C., Luo, Y., Rojas, K., Overhauser, J., Otto, L., Gilliam, T. C. (1993) Genomics: 15, 48-56.
- Sullivan, K. M., Mannucci, A., Kimpton, C. P., Gill, P. (1993) BioTechniques: 15, 636-641.
- Urquhart, A. J., Kimpton, C. P., Downes, T. J., Gill, P. (1994) Int. J. Leg. Med: 107, 13-20.
- Urquhart, A., Oldroyd, N. J., Kimpton, C. P., Gill, P. (1995) Biotechniques: 18, 116-121
- Walsh, P. S., Varario, J., Reynolds, R. (1992) Nucleic Acids Res: 20, 5061-5065.

MANUAL DNA TYPING VIA THE SHORT TANDEM REPEATS (STRs): KW 426, TH AND hTPO

R. Pöttl, C. Luckenbach, H. Ritter

Inst. f. Anthropologie und Humangenetik, Wilhelmstr. 27, 72074 Tübingen, Germany

SUMMARY
Short tandem repeats (STRs) represent a rich class of highly polymorphic markers in the human genome. Usually they are composed of tandemly repeated sequences, 2 to 5 bp in length. Alleles range from 100 to 350 bp.
STRs have gained increasing popularity for genetic mapping and linkage analysis, trimeric and tetrameric loci are especially suited for identity testing.
We present a new combination of three unlinked tetrameric STR - loci (hTPO: 2p23 - 2pter, TH: 11p15.5, KW 426: 8q) performing the same polymerase chain reaction (PCR) - recipe for all three loci.
The amplification products of the three STR loci are separated together in one lane using a polyacrylamide-gradient-gel- electrophoresis (PAGGE) - system.
Thus we can type STRs with increased throughput and discrimination power by use of manual techniques which can easily be carried out by most laboratories.

1. INTRODUCTION
Short tandem repeats (STRs), also referred to as microsatellites or simple sequence length polymorphisms, occur approximately every 6 to 10 kb in the human genome (Olroyd 1995; Litt 1989; Tautz 1989).
Due to their abundance and high polymorphism they have become useful markers for physical and genetic mapping, personal identification and in some cases for disease diagnosis.
PCR fragment sizes are more and more often automatically determined by so-called "gene-scanners". Using these machines even octoplex STR typing is possible (Olroyd 1995).
Nevertheless many laboratories do manual DNA profiling because of the high costs of automatic systems. We have developed a procedure for:
1) the simultaneous PCR amplification and
2) the separation of three STR loci in one lane of a denaturing polyacrylamide-gradient-gel-electrophoresis (PAGGE) - system.

2. MATERIALS AND METHODS

2.1. DNA - PREPARATION:
Genomic DNA was isolated from leucocytes according to Miller et al. (1988).

2.2. OLIGONUCLEOTIDES
Oligonucleotides were synthesized with the DNA synthesizer "Gene Assembler Plus" (Pharmacia, Freiburg, Germany) and cleaned with NAP - 10 columns (Pharmacia).

2.3. POLYMERASE CHAIN REACTION
Reaction conditions:
PCR-reaction conditions were: 1cycle 94°C/5min; 30 cycles 94°C/30 sec, 60°C/45 sec, 72°C/30 sec; 1 cycle 72°C/5 min.
Cycling conditions:
PCR was carried out in a 25 μl reaction mixture containing 200mM dNTPs, 0.5 U Taq DNA polymerase, 1 mM $MgCl_2$, 2.5 pmol of each primer for hTPO and 12.5 pmol of each primer for TH and KW 426 and 10 ng DNA.

Primers:
KW 426 (Lu 1993):
Primer 1: 5´- GTA GCC TCC CTG CCA TTT CCT AA -3´
Primer 2: 5´- TAT TGT GGT CCA GAG CTC CTT GG -3´
TH (Polymeropoulos 1991):
Primer 1: 5´- CAG CTG CCC TAG TCA GCA C -3´
Primer 2: 5´- GCT TCC GAG TGC AGG TCA CA -3´
hTPO (Anker 1992):
Primer 1: 5´- CAC TAG CAC CCA GAA CCG TC -3´
Primer 2: 5´- CCT TGT CAG CGT TTA TTT GCC -3´

2.4. Polyacrylamidegel electrophoresis and detection
PCR - fragments were separated in 6 - 10% denaturing polyacrylamide-gradient-gels at 600 V, 30 mA, 30 W for three hours.
Analysis was possible after silver staining.
Photographs were taken with the "Easy - Plus" - System (Herolab, Wiesloch, Germany).

2.5. Sample application
Samples were diluted 1 : 5 with water. 7.5 µl were then applied to the gel 2 cm from the cathode using paper sample sheets (0.5 x 0.5 cm; Pharmacia).

3. Results and Discussion
We describe a PCR procedure which enables simultaneous amplification of the three STR loci KW 426 (length: 322 - 382 bp), TH (244 - 260 bp) and hTPO (106 - 134 bp).
Table 1 summarizes characteristics of these loci.
Furthermore we demonstrate a new method of STR - PCR fragment analysis by using 6 - 10% denaturing polyacrylamide-gradient- gels (see figure 1).
Thus we present an easy reproduceable and cheap manual method to do STR DNA - profiling.
   Exact allele typing demands an allelic ladder which is still in preparation. Large formal and population genetic studies will show whether this STR loci combination represents a highly informative genetic marker system.

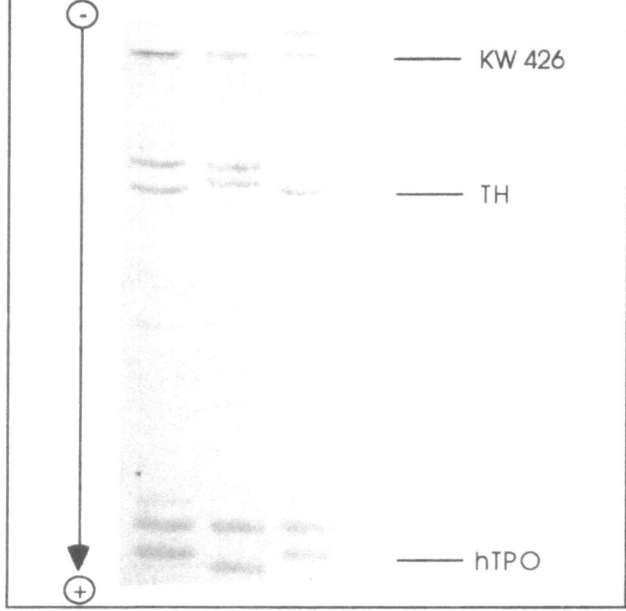

Fig.1: 6 - 10% PAGG showing STR separation; 600 V, 30 mA, 30 W for 3 hours

Table 1: Characteristics of the three STR - loci under investigation

STR:	description:	locus:	Genbank No:	alleles (bp):	repeat unit:	author:
KW 426	D8S347	8q	L12268	322-382	AGAT	Lu
TH	human tyrosine hydroxylase gene	11p15.5	D00269	244-260	TCAT	Polymer-opoulos
hTPO	human thyroid peroxidase gene	2p23-2pter	M68651	106-134	AATG	Anker

References
Anker R, Steinbrueck T, Donis - Keller H, (1992) Tetranucleotide repeat polymorphism at the human thyroid peroxidase (hTPO) locus. Hum. Mol. Gen. 1: 137.
Litt M, Luty JA, (1989) A hypervariable microsatellite revealed by in vitro amplification of a dinucleotide repeat within the cardiac muscle actin gene. Am. J. Hum. Gen 44: 397 - 401.
Lu J, Riley R, Robertson M, Nelson L, Ward K, (1993) Tetranucleotide repeat polymorphisms at the D8S342, D8S323, D8S345, D8S315 and D8S347 loci on 8q. Hum. Mol. Gen. 2: 1743.
Miller SA, Dykes DD, Polesky HF, (1988) A simple salting out procedure for extracting DNA from human nucleated cells. Nuc. Acid. Res. 16: 1215.
Olroyd NJ, Urquhart AJ, Kimpton CP, Millican ES, Watson SK, Downes T, Gill PD, (1995) A highly discriminating octoplex short tandem repeat polymerase chain reaction system suitable for human individual identification. Electrophoresis. 16: 334 - 337.
Polymeropoulos MH, Xiao H, Rath DS, Merril CR, (1991) Tetranucleotide repeat polymorphism at the human tyrosine hydroxylase gene (TH). Nuc. Acid. Res. 19: 3753.
Tautz D, (1989) hypervariability of simple sequences as a general source for polymorphic DNA markers. Nuc. Acid. Res. 17: 6463 - 6471.

A MULTIPLEX AMPLIFICATION APPROACH FOR SIMULTANEOUS TYPING OF FIVE LOCI IN DNA OF ANCIENT BASQUE POPULATIONS

Prieto[*], E. Arroyo[*], A. Pérez-Pérez[**], C. Asperilla[*], I. Arenal[***], J. M. Ruiz de la Cuesta[*], D. Turbón[**]

[*]   Escuela de Medicina Legal. Fac. Medicina. U. Complutense. Madrid-28040. Spain.
[**] Sec. Antropología. Dep. Biol. Animal. Fac. Biol. U.de Barcelona. Spain.
[***] Dep. Genética y Biol. Animal. Fac. Ciencias. U. Lejona. Bilbao. Spain.

INTRODUCTION

We tried to test the commercial forensic kit worldwide known as "Polymarker" in cases of samples of very old DNA. We will try to type ancient DNA samples for five genetic systems (LDLR, GYPA, HBGG, D7S8 and GC) all of them comprised in this multiplex PCR commercial kit. Our hypothesis is that given that the amount of target ancient DNA is very small, only standardized systems already tested for succesful amplification of a few nanograms can be suitable for very scarce and damaged DNA. This kit, in the routine forensic casework, produces good results with a template DNA amount of 2-40 ngr in a final reaction volume of 100 µl.

Ancient DNA samples (teeth) from the Basque Country (Spain) were chosen for this study due to the special demographical and anthropological characteristics of this human population (Calderón, 1994).

MATERIAL

Samples were selected to cover a wide range of time periods, but only specially well preserved tooth samples were studied. The Basque sites studied included Atxuri (Vizcaya, Neolithic and Calcolithic period, 5000-3600 B.P.), Urbiola (Navarra, Early Bronze Age, 3700 B.P.) and Garai (Vizcaya, XI-XIII centuries A. D.). Samples from Atxuri are quoted AT-; Urbiola, UR-; and Garai, GA-.

DNA EXTRACTION

Teeth have been immersed in 15% chlorhydric acid (10') to remove dirt and carbonate deposits, 70% ethanol (30') to remove acid residues, distilled water (30') and posteriorly irradiated 10-15 minutes under UV light (254 nm). The methodology proposed for the treatment of the teeth is a modification of that of Ginther et al. (1992). The cleaning of the external surface of the ancient material is essential in order to eliminate possible exogenous DNA from the archaeologist and the curators and also to reduce the presence of soil inhibitors. The DNA extraction procedure mainly follows that described by Hagelberg (1994) with slight modifications. The samples were ground in a freezer mill (Spex Industries Inc.) refrigerated with liquid nitrogen, and the teeth powder was stored in sterile plastic tubes (Corning 50 mL) at -20ºC. The tubes and impactors of the Freezer mill were cleaned with ethanol and distilled water, and placed 10 minutes under UV for sterilization, between each grinding. Samples were washed by adding 0.5 M EDTA pH 8.0, and centrifugating them. The aquaeus fase was discarded and the washing repeated 2 or 3 times, for removing some of the brown coloration from the sample. Ten mL lysis buffer, containing 8.5 mL 0.5 M EDTA pH 8.0 - 8.5, 1 mL 5% SDS, 0.5 mL 1M Tris and 100 μl. Proteinase K (1 mg/mL), was added to the tubes,and incubated overnight at 37°C with agitation. After the incubation, the tubes were centrifugated 5' at 2000 rpm, and the supernatant stored in sterile tubes for the extraction with phenol/chloroform. Phenol was previously saturated with 0.02 M Tris (pH 8). After the addition of phenol to the sample, the tube is agitated and centrifugated for 5 minutes at 2000 rpm, until the phenol and the aqueous fases become separated. The aqueous fase is recuperated and extracted once more with phenol/chloroform (1:1), and finally only with chloroform. The 10 mL of the resultant sample were concentrated and purified with Centricon-30 microconcentrators (Amicon Inc.), by adding 6 mL of sterile water in 3 consecutive centrifugations during 30' at 4000 rpm. The final volume obtained was 100-300 μl. depending of the coloration of the sample. Dark brown samples were more diluted, to try to dilute the soil inhibitors, otherwise discarded.

AMPLIFICATION AND TYPING PROTOCOLS

The whole protocol was carried out in a sterile environment. Nine μl. of ancient DNA solution were added to a volume of 20 μl. of reaction mix, 20μl.of primers dilution and 1μl. of Bovine Serum Albumine (BSA) at a final concentration of 160 mgr/mL. The 50 μl. final volume was amplified in a first round of 94 1'/ 60 1'/ 72 1' 32 cycles. After checking the results in a 4% agarose gel electrophoresis (NuSieve 3: Seakem 1), a second round of amplification was started with 4 μl. of the last reaction product plus 5 μl. of distilled water, 20 μl. of mix, 20 μl. of primers dilution and 1 μl. of the former BSA dilution. Amplification conditions were 94 1'/ 60 1'/ 72 1' but this time for just 30 cycles. Definitive reaction products were checked in a 4% agarose gel electrophoresis before reverse dot blot typing, according to the manufacturer's protocol. DNA-1 Polymarker kit control (Perkin Elmer. USA) was used as a positive control for every amplification turn and subsequently sterile double distilled water was used as negative control. As recommended by the manufacturer, the control spot of the strips was considered as a reference of the quality of the amplification.

RESULTS AND DISCUSSION

Highly amplified bands were observed after the second PCR round in the case of the fresh DNA positive control . No signal was observed in the case of the negative control and DQA1 showed almost always a clear band, though this marker was not included in the typing strips. Damaged or not amplified systems produced always a lack of a band in the gel and subsequently no signal (hybridization) was observed in the corresponding site at typing strip. Reverse dot blot produced several kinds of results *(See table 1)*.

According to manufacturer's protocol, only the strips with hybridization in its control spot were considered for the study. A sample (AT-95) was correctly amplified and typed in the first PCR round and showed an invariant dot-blot pattern in three further repetitions. Other samples showed variation in some markers when repetition was performed, probably due to jumping PCR effect or inespecific hybridization.

All the samples were repeated (twice minimum) and at least one marker out of the five tested was persistently typed the same, the average being 1.8 markers per sample. This value scores below our previous results (Prieto et al., 1995). However, given that the intensity of the signal of the hybridization spots varies - and sometimes the typing remains unclear -, perhaps it would be better to try a sequencing approach given the high amount of DNA contained in the amplification band.

Table 1.

Sample	Amplified bands	Typed loci
UR-71	All but DQA1, GYPA	GC
UR-85	All but LDLR	GC
UR-95	All	All
UR-98	All but DQA1, LDLR	HBGG
AT-117	All but LDLR	GYPA
AT-118	All	GYPA, HBGG
AT-119	All	D7S8
AT-120	All but DQA1	GYPA
AT-121	All	LDLR, HBGG, D7S8
AT-122	All but HBGG	D7S8, GYPA
AT-123	All	LDLR, GYPA, GC
AT-124	All but LDLR	HBGG, D7S8
AT-125	All but DQA1, LDLR, GYPA	HBGG
AT-126	All	LDLR
GA-132	All	GYPA, D7S8
GA-133	All	HBGG
GA-136	All	All but GYPA
GA-138	All but GYPA	D7S8

REFERENCES

Calderón R (1994) Allelic frequency patterns in basques: Evolutionary deductions. Journal of Human Ecology 4: 37-54.

Ginther C, Issel-Tarver L., King MC (1992) Identifying individuals by sequencing mitochondrial DNA from teeth. Nature genetics 2: 135-138.

Hagelberg E (1994) Mithocondrial DNA from Ancient Bones. In: Herrmann and Hummel (Eds.) Ancient DNA. Springer-Verlag. Berlin-Heidelberg-New York, pp. 195-204.

Prieto L et al. (1995) Simultaneous typing of five loci in ancient DNA of three basque populations. Ancient DNA III meeting. 20-22 July. Oxford. UK. (in press).

TRIPLEX PCR OF THREE STR LOCI WITH NON-OVERLAPPING ALLELE SIZES

I. Rostedt and M. Lukka

National Public Health Institute, Helsinki, Finland

INTRODUCTION

One of the advantages in the PCR methodology is the possibility
to amplify simultaneously several loci (multiplex PCR) which
improves remarkably the information obtained from one analysis.
Here we describe a triplex PCR of three STR loci: HumTPO (Anker
1992) in chromosome 2, HumTHO1 (Edwards 1991) in chromosome 11
and D3S1359 (Li 1993) in chromosome 3.

With suitable primers the allele size ranges in the HumTPO
(106-130 base pairs; bp), HumTHO1 (155-179 bp) and D3S1359
(197-265 bp) loci do not overlap which made it possible to
amplify the loci simultaneously using unlabeled primers and perform the size separation and allele detection using electrophoresis and silver staining without expensive automation.

MATERIALS AND METHODS

Sample preparation: DNA was extracted from 3 μl blood samples
with the Chelex (R) resin-extraction approach (Walsh 1991).
One μl from the 200 μl extract was used for triplex PCR amplification.

PCR-amplifications:

Locus	Primer sequences	Concentrations
HumTPO	5' CAC TAG CAC CCA GAA CCG TC 3'	0.40 μM
	5' CCT TGT CAG CGT TTA TTT GCC 3'	0.40 μM
HumTHO1	5' GTG ATT CCC ATT GGC CTG TTC CTC 3'	0.45 μM
	5' GTG GGC TGA AAA GCT CCC GAT TAT 3'	0.45 μM
D3S1359	5' ATG CTA AGT GCT AAG TCA ACT 3'	1.40 μM
	5' GTT GCC TCT GAC ATG GCT TT 3'	1.40 μM

In PCR-amplifications the nucleotide (dNTPs) concentration was
0.2 mM in a PCR buffer consisting of 10 mM Tris-HCl, pH 8.8,
50 mM KCl, 1.5 mM $MgCl_2$, 0.1% Triton x-100. The PCR was performed
in 100 μl volume under a layer of mineral oil using MJ-Research
PTC-100 thermal cycler.

Each amplification was initiated with a hot start (Chou 1992) and
2.5 U Dynazyme-polymerase (Finnzymes, Finland) were used as DNA-
polymerase.

Amplification program was as follows:
$94^{\circ}C$ 1', $55^{\circ}C$ 45'', $72^{\circ}C$ 45''; 32 cycles.

Electrophoresis: A 10 μl aliquot of PCR-product containing 2 μl
of sample buffer was applicated for electrophoresis in vertical
PAGE (Sajantila 1993).

The separation gel 12 x 14 x 0.075 cm (10% T, 4.8% C) and the
stacking gel 4 x 14 x 0.075 cm (3.0% T, 4.8% C)were made from
acrylamide stock solution 30% T, 4.8 % C containing 21% glycerol
in the gel buffer (33mM Tris-sulfate, pH 4.5).

The electrophoresis was carried out for 17 hours at 200 V in $+4^{\circ}C$
using 100 mM Tris, 100 mM boric acid, 2 mM EDTA; pH 8.5 as the
running buffer.

The amplified fragments were visualised by silver staining (Allen
1989) and the gels were dryed for documentation.

RESULTS AND DISCUSSION

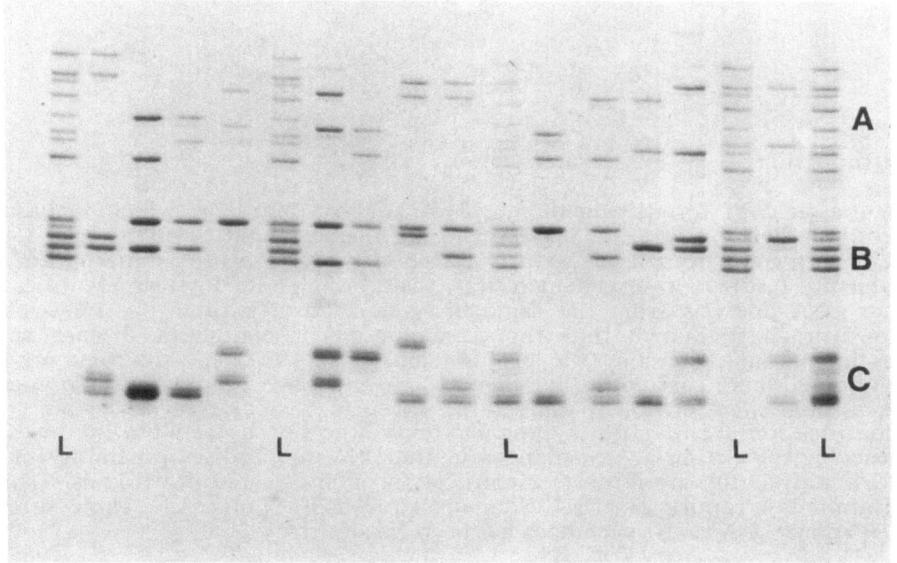

Silver stained patterns at the HumTPO (C), HumTH01 (B) and
D3S1359 (A) loci after triplex PCR and PAGE. L = allelic ladder
containing alleles 8 - 11 for the HumTPO locus, alleles 6 - 10
(9.3) for the HumTH01 locus and alleles 2, 4, 5, 7, 10, 12, 13
and 16 for the D3S1359 locus. The allele nomenclature for D3S1359
is tentative.

The HumTPO, HumTH01 and D3S1359 loci can be safely genotyped
simultaneously utilizing the triplex PCR method. No discrepancies
has been found between the results after single or triplex PCR.

In the Finnish population the mean exclusion probabilities (Gürtler
1956) of HumTPO, HumTH01 and D3S1359 loci in paternity testing are
33.4%, 58.5%, 76.6% respectively. The combined exclusion probability of these three loci is 93.5%.

References:
Allen RC et al (1989) Biotechniques 7:736-744
Anker R et al (1992) Hum Mol Genet 1:137
Chou Q et al (1992) Nucl Acids Res 20:1717-1723
Edwards A et al (1991) Am J Hum Genet 49:746-756
Gürtler H (1956) Acta Med Leg Soc 9:83-93
Li H et al (1993) Hum Mol Genet 2:1327
Sajantila A and Lukka M (1993) Int J Leg Med 105:355-359
Walsh PS et al (1991) Biotechniques 10:506-513

Visualization of Epigenetic Toxicological DNA Changes

T. Sawaguchi, S. Nakamura, X. Wang and A. Sawaguchi

Department of Legal Medicine, Tokyo Women's Medical College, Tokyo Japan

Introduction

In the field of forensic medicine, DNA analysis methods, which include DNA profiling (Jeffreys et al. 1985) and the polymerase chain reaction (PCR) (Saiki et al. 1985), have been used extensively for identification in criminal cases and in paternity testing with excellent results. One principle of forensic identification is that DNA analysis from the same body must always show the same pattern. However, it is known that the development of malignant disease such as carcinoma, may alter the DNA profile (Saito et al. 1991) and the same possibility may exist where carcinogen or other toxic agents have been active. No study has been published on DNA analysis of forensic toxicological cases as regards identification. Thus DNA typing methods may not be reliable in the case of toxicological victims. Any changes in the DNA, jeopardises possibility of using DNA analysis for the forensic identification of intoxicated individuals. This is a preliminary report on DNA changes caused by poisons. Their effect on well-known DNA analysis methods has been examined.

Materials and methods

In this experiment, we evaluated epigenetic toxicological DNA changes using five methods indicated in Table 1. Southern hybridization with multi-locus probes and with single-locus probe, AmpFLP for minisatellite loci and for microsatellite and HLADQα were carried out according to the manufacturer's instructions.

Table 1 Experimental procedures

Chronic methamphetamine toxication: rabbit experimental case

Materials: 5 - 10 mg/kg methamphetamine intravenous toxication each two days

Methods: 1. southern blotting with MLP (33.15, 33.6)
with SLP (MS31, MS43a, MS1, g3)

2. PCR (AmpFLP by minisatellite): D1S80 (MCT118)

3. PCR (AmpFLP by microsatellite): TH01, TPOX, CSF1PO

4. PCR: HLADQα

Results and discussion

DNA changes caused by methamphetamine could be evaluated by southern hybridization with a multi-locus probe, but not with a single-locus probe. DNA profiles produced bands with probe 33.15 in the high molecular area where no bands exist in humans. In this area the DNA changes were clearly observed. Two pre-intoxication bands disappeared and one pre-intoxication band was discolored. With HLADQα DNA typing, pre-intoxication positive spots became negative after intoxication and pre-intoxication negative spots became positive after intoxication. With AmpFLP on D1S80 locus, a band appeared in an area where no bands exist in humans. This band appeared clearly before intoxication but disappeared after intoxication. Besides, the pre-intoxication negative band changed to post-intoxication positive band. This also happened at the TH01, TOPX and CSF1PO. Sensitivity to detect the changeability of DNA was highest in AmpFLP of microsatellite loci. There were any changes in 7 cases among total 8 cases in AmpFLP of microsatellite loci.

From the above results, epigenetic DNA changes caused by methamphetamine intoxication were detected in the same individuals, the results of well-established forensic DNA analysis methods showing changes which could confuse identification procedures.

Acknowledgment

The authors are grateful to Prof. Bernard Knight for editing the manuscript. This work was prepared under Yamakawa awards from Tokyo Women's Medical College.

References

Jeffreys AJ, Wilson VW and Thein SL (1985) Hypervariable 'minisatellite' regions in human DNA. Nature 314: 67-73.
Saiki RK, Scharf S, Faloona F, Kary B, Mullis G, Horn T, Erlich HA and Arnheim N (1985) Enzymatic amplification of β-Globin genomic sequences and restriction site analysis for diagnosis of sickle cell anemia. Science 230: 1350-1354.
Saito J, Inoue M, Azuma C, Saji F and Tanizawa O (1991) Histogenetic analysis of ovarian teratoma by DNA fingerprinting. Eur J Cancer 27: 813.

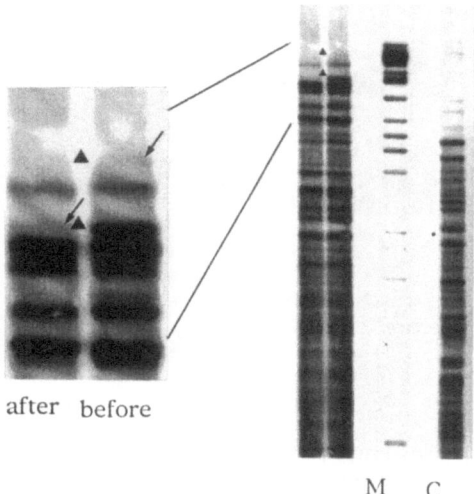

Fig. 1 DNA fingerprint with MLP33.15 before and after methamphetamine toxication.

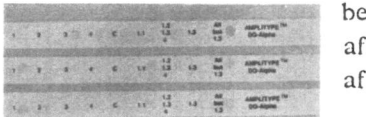

before
after (2w)
after (death)

Fig. 2 HLADQα type before and after
methamphetamine toxication.

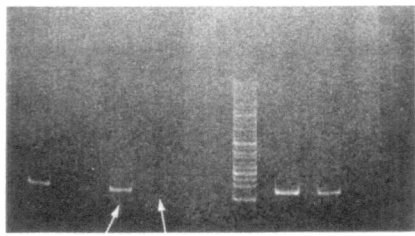

before   after   M

Fig. 3 D1S80 DNA fragments before
and after methamphetamine toxication.

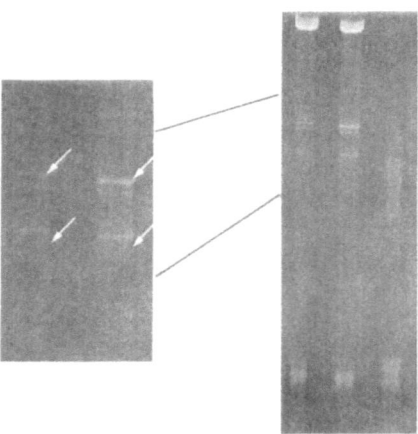

before   after

M

Fig. 4 TH01 DNA fragments before and
after methamphetamine toxication.

THE 3' HYPERVARIABLE VNTR-LOCUS APO B:
THREE DIFFERENT ANALYSING METHODS REVEALING DIFFERENT ALLELES AND LARGE FAMILY STUDIES.

S. Sedlmayr, R. Pöltl, C. Luckenbach, H. Ritter

Institut für Anthropologie und Humangenetik, Wilhelmstr. 27, 72074 Tübingen, Germany

SUMMARY
Separation of polymerase chain reaction (PCR) amplification of the Apo B 3'- VNTR was carried out on horizontal, 4%, denaturing polyacrylamide(PAA)/piperazindiacrylamide(PDA)-gels crosslinked with 3% C using a discontinuous buffer system, providing an efficient typing system. Furthermore we compared three different electrophoretic systems and proved that in several samples, alleles showed a completely different migration velocity in agarose- and PAA-gels.
Fifteen different alleles containing 14-53 repeats of the basic 15-bp unit were distinguished in a population study of 220 individuals from 38 northwest-portuguese families. For population studies the Hardy-Weinberg-equilibrium was checked by forming groups of phenotypes and no significant deviation could be found. Family studies confirmed the formal conception of an autosomal codominant type of inheritance. Two children of one family showed a new mutation to allele 49 on the condition of their legitimacy.

1. INTRODUCTION
Genotyping hypervariable regions (HVR) is a widely used method for gene mapping as well as for forensic applications and it has become even more important with the implication of HVRs as a cause of genetic and somatic diseases including e.g. the fragile X syndrome, myotonic dystrophy, Huntington's disease and coronary heart disease.
One of these well-known tandemly repeated sequences is the apolipoprotein 3'- hypervariable region, located 73 bp downstream from the second putative polyadenylation signal at the 3'- end of the human Apo B-gene which maps to chromosome 2p24. It consists of a dimeric AT-rich core repeat sequence of 30bp, respectively of two structurally related sequences "x" and "y" with an average length of 15bp (Knott et al. 1986).
Using PCR and agarose gel electrophoresis Boerwinkle et al. (1989) found 12 different alleles, while Ludwig (1989) used the more rapid and high-resolution denaturing polyacrylamide gel electrophoresis (PAGE) to detect 14 different alleles. To date, 24 alleles have been identified, containing between 14 and 55 repeats.
In fact, VNTR-alleles differing in length may not represent the total allelic polymorphism of the Apo B 3'- Minisatellite due to sequence microheterogeneity of the hypervariable elements (HVE) (Heliö 1991; März et al. 1993; Ellsworth et al. 1995).

2. MATERIALS AND METHODS
DNA-Isolation: genomic DNA samples were extracted from peripheral blood leucocytes according to Miller et al. (1988).
PCR: Amplification was carried out for 31 cycles under the following conditions: 3 cycles 94°C-2', 62°C-3' and 28 cycles 95°C-90", 61°C-3'.
The amplification mix contained 2.5 U Taq Polymerase, 200mM of each dNTP, 1.5mM $MgCl_2$ and 100µl reaction buffer (all Perkin Elmer-Appl. Biosyst. Weiterstadt, Germany), 10 pmol each primer and 25ng genomic DNA up to a total volume of 100µl, layered with 60µl mineral oil.
Molecular weight markers: 100bp-ladder (Gibco BRL) 100-1500bp, Amplisize standard (BioRad) 50-2000bp.
Allelic ladder: a home made, reamplified allelic ladder was used for classifying phenotypes.
Electrophoresis:
a) 2% agarose gel (NuSieve 3:1 Agarose, Biozym, Oldendorf, Germany) in 1xTBE-buffer at 70V for 16h.
b) horizontal denaturing PAA-gel (4%T, 3%C) with PDA as crosslinker, using a discontinuous buffer system (Tris-Formiat/Tris-Borat), at constant 1000V and 5W for 1h, 10W for 1h and 15W for 1.5h (190x250x0.5 mm).
c) horizontal native PAA-gel (4%T, 3%C), on same conditions as b).

Detection:
- agarose gels were stained with ethidiumbromide and the separated products visualized by means of UV-light.
- PAGE was followed by silver staining.

The alleles were typed by comparing the products with an allelic ladder which was constructed from alleles observed during this study and previous studies by R.Pöltl in the same lab.

Family-studies: The phenotypes of the children were pooled into eight groups in order to obtain a suitable number for X^2 calculation under Hardy-Weinberg law.

Population genetics: Alleles, respectively phenotypes of all unrelated individuals of the population sample were pooled into six groups. Heterozygosity rate and allelic diversity were calculated.

3. RESULTS AND DISCUSSION

3.1 Denaturing PAGE

Fig.1 shows the fragment pattern of family 22. The allelic ladders run in lanes 1 and 7, the 100bp ladder runs in lane 8. We obtained very good resolution with the described gel formulation which yields sharp bands for almost error-free interpretation. Using this method, we were able to easily distinguish 15bp differences in VNTR allele length.

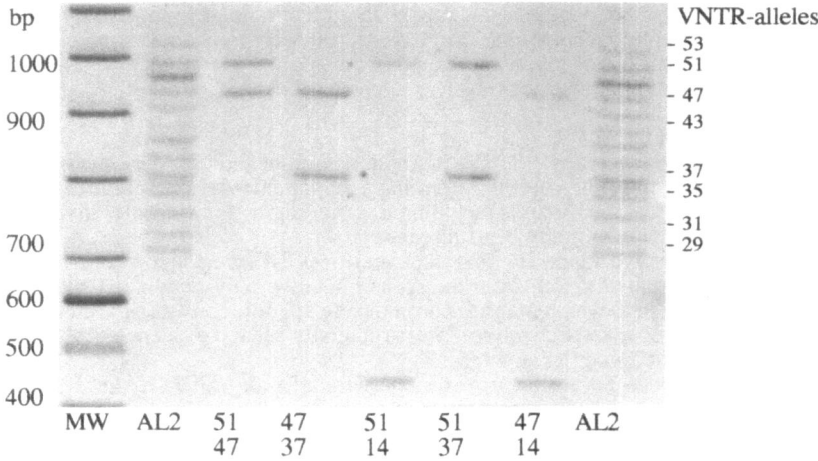

Fig.1 3´- Apo B alleles after denaturing PAGE and silver staining. From left to right, lane: 1= 100bp ladder, 2= allelic ladder 2, 3-5=three children of the family, 6= mother, 7=father, 8=allelic ladder2.

3.2 Comparison of three different analysing methods

It is evident that alleles in certain samples show a completely different migration whether they are seperated in agarose or in PAA. An example is given in fig.2. It shows two different allelic ladders separated in agarose and PAA. Both of them seem to be identical in the agarose gel. PAGE reveals a completely different allele composition of both ladders. Exact characterization of the alterations could be obtained by single separation of each sample that contributes to the allelic ladder in both gel types.

One reason for this effect could be the impact of varying secondary structures due to sequence differences within the repeat units. So far unknown correlations between these secondary structures and the both gel types might influence the migration velocity. Moreover, computer analysis of tertiary structures of minisatellites showed varying curvation of repeat sequences, depending on their base composition. This effect may lead to the same observed consequences (Trifonov 1985; Bachmann 1990). In any case it is evident that sequence differences interfere with the base pair number in determining the migration velocity. As this can lead to most profound forensic consequences, agarose gel electrophoreses has to be used with extreme caution in analysing repetitive DNA.

Native and denaturing PAGE produced identical results, except for a more rectilinear migration front and sharper bands in the denaturing system.

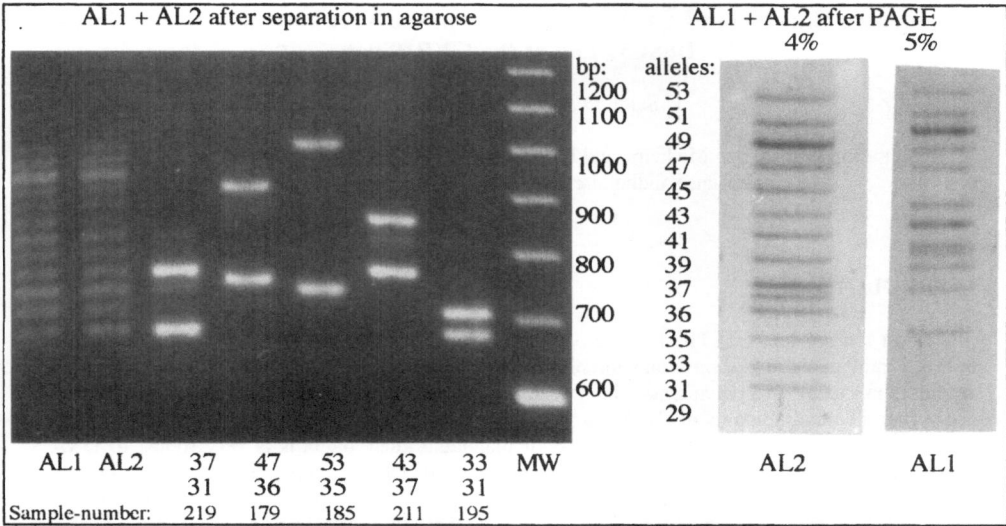

Fig.2 Two different allelic ladders after separation in agarose and PAA. MW=100bp ladder

Tab.1 Altered migration of alleles in agarose- and PAA-gels.

sample	agarose	PAA
195	33	33
	31	29
185	53	53
	35	36
211	43	39
	37	37

It is obvious that there are blank spaces in AL1(PAA), because alleles 31 and 43 show up as alleles 29 respectively 39 after PAGE. In AL2 the alleles 29 and 36 are not detectable in agarose, but they can be clearly identified in PAA.

3.3 Family studies

For this report 38 families (140 meioses) were analysed. Segragation analysis confirmed the formal conception of an autosomal codominant type of inheritance for the Apo B VNTR. In one family we found two children with a putative new mutation to allele 49. This indicates a relatively high mutation rate of 0,011, on the condition of legitimacy of both children. The validity of this mutationrate needs further investigation. In all, no significant deviation of the Hardy-Weinberg equilibrium could be found (X^2=18.6; d.f.=24; 0.2<P>0.3).

3.4 Population genetics

The analysis demonstrated 44 phenotypes, representing products of 15 alleles containing 14-53 repeats. The distribution of the phenotypes is in Hardy-Weinberg equilibrium (X^2=17.557, d.f.=22, 0.2<P>0.3). The observed heterozygosity was 72%. The most frequent alleles were 37 (38%), 35 (26.1%), 47 (9.9%) and 49 (4.9%). Two new alleles were found with 14 and 27 repeat units. Allele 14 is the smallest allele yet described, but sequencing has to reveal the exact number of repeats.

4.REFERENCES

Bachmann L (1990) Dissertation, University Tübingen.
Boerwinkle E, Xiong W,Fourest E, Chan L **(1989)** Proc. Natl. Acad. Sci. 86: 212 - 216.
Ellsworth DL, Shriver M.D, Boerwinkle E **(1995)** Hum. Mol. Gen. 4 (5): 937-944
Heliö T (1991) Biochem. a. Biophys. Res. Comm. 181 (2): 846-851.
Knott TJ, Wallis SC, Pease RJ, Powell ML, Scott J **(1986)**Nucl. Acids Res. 14 (22): 9215 - 9216.
Ludwig EH, Friedl W, McCarthy BJ **(1989)** Am.J.Hum.Gen. 45: 458 - 464.
März W, Ruzicka V, Fisher E, Russ AP, Schneider W, Groß W **(1993)** Electrophoresis 14: 169 - 173
Miller SA, Dykes DD, Polesky HF **(1988)** Nucleic Acid Res. 16 (3): 1215.
Trifonov EN (1985) C.R.C. Crit. Rev. Biochem.19: 89-106.

Automated fluorescent PCR based analysis of the STR polymorphism at locus D8S639 and at the CYP19 gene

C.Seidl, O.Jäger, M.Kilp, E.Seifried

Institute for Transfusion Medicine and Immunohematology, Red Cross Blood Donor Service Hessen, Sandhofstrasse 1, 60528 Frankfurt, Germany

INTRODUCTION

Short tandem repeat (STR) loci are polymorphic markers that can be used for discrimination between individuals in paternity and forensic testing. The feasability to analyse these markers by amplification using the polymerase chain reaction (PCR) has improved the sensitivity of DNA analysis from small amounts of DNA. Furthermore, due to the allele distribution of most of these markers between 100 - 500 bp, the analysis of individual allele patterns is very robust to DNA degradation. Unfortunately, the analysis of the common dinucleotide repeat polymorphism can be problematic due to the occurence of 'shadow bands'. The less common tri-, tetra- and pentanucleotide repeats in contrast are less sensible for these PCR artefacts and are more preferable for PCR analysis in paternity or forensic casework. We have studied the allele distribution and sequence structure of two tetranucleotide repeat polymorphism, one at locus D8S639 (Nelson 1994) and the second starting at base pair 682 of the human aromatase cytochrome P-450 gene (CYP19) (Polymeropoulos 1992).

Systems and locus:	HUMD8S639 (8p21-p11)
	HUMCYP19 (15q21.1)
Population and sample size:	Hesse (Germany)
	N: 110 (HUMD8S639)
	N: 132 (HUMCYP19)

METHODS

Locus D8S639: Primersequences were choosen according to Nelson (1994). The 5' primer was labelled with HEX (6-carboxy-2',4',7',4,7-Hexachlorofluorescein, Perkin Elmer - ABD)
PCR amplification conditions: 95 C - 5 min; 28 cyles 95 C - 30 sec , 54 C 40 sec, 72 C 30 sec; 72 C 5 min. (Perkin Elmer 9600).
PCR reaction conditions: 10-100ng DNA, 5pmol 5'and 3' primer, 200 µmol dNTP's, 0,5 Units Taq DNA polymerase (Appligene) and the corresponding buffer (Appligene) in a final volume of 50 µl.

Locus CYP19: Primersequences were choosen according to Polymeropoulos (1992). The 5' primer was labelled with FAM (5-carboxylfluorescein, Perkin Elmer - ABD).
PCR amplification conditions: 95 C - 5 min; 28 cyles 95 C - 30 sec , 54 C 40 sec, 72 C 30 sec; 72 C 5 min. (Perkin Elmer 9600).
PCR reaction conditions: 10-100ng DNA, 10pmol 5'and 3' primer, 200 µmol dNTP's, 0,5 Units Taq DNA polymerase (Appligene) and the corresponding buffer (Appligene) in a final volume of 50 µl.

Electrophoretic methods: 6% polyacrylamide denaturing gel electrophoresis. The gels were run for 8h at constant power (30W) 1600V and 28mA on an ABD automated DNA seqencer 373A. Typing was performed by comparison with an ROX (6-carboxy-X-rhodamine) labelled internal standard generated from the vector pGL-2-Basic (Promega) using the Southern local method for fragment size assignement (Genescan software, Perkin Elmer - ABD).

Sequence analysis: Individual alleles were sequenced using the solid-phase sequence strategy. Biotin labelled PCR primers were included in the amplification reaction and PCR fragments were subsequently separated by streptavidin coated magnetic beads (Dynal). Sequence reaction were performed using the T7 DNA polymerase and Dye terminators (Prism T7 sequence kit, Perkin Elmer - ABD). Analysis of sequence reaction was conducted on an ABD 373A automated DNA sequences using the Sequence Navigator software. Allele assignement was conducted according to the number of repeat units of the individual alleles.

Statistical analysis: The polymorphic information content (PIC) was calculated using the formula of Botstein (1980). The discrimination index (DI) and the matching probability (pM) were calculated by the method of Jones (1972). The sample gene diversity (geneD) (frequency of heterozygotes expected under Hardy Weinberg equilibrium was calculated as described by Kimpton (1993).

RESULTS

HUMCYP19 - Observed genotypes

Gen.	Obs. (N)	Gen.	Obs.(N)	Gen.	Obs.(N)	Gen.	Obs.(N)
7-3 - 7-3	16	7-3 - 12	9	7 - 12	1	9 - 11	1
7-3 - 8	13	7 - 7	1	8 - 8	1	10 - 11	2
7-3 - 9	7	7 - 8	4	8 - 9	1	11 - 11	18
7-3 - 10	1	7 - 10	2	8 - 10	1		
7-3 - 11	28	7 - 11	18	8 - 11	9		

HUMCYP19 - Allele frequencies

Allele (bp*)	Frequency	Allele (bp*)	Frequency	Allele (bp*)	Frequency
7-3** (168)	0,341	9 (179)	0,004	12 (191)	0,038
7 (171)	0,152	10 (183)	0,023		
8 (175)	0,087	11 (187)	0,356		

* lenght as detected by Genescan software
** allele 7-3 has a 3bp deletion in the 5'flanking region

HUMD8S639 - Observed genotypes

Gen.	Obs. (N)	Gen.	Obs. (N)	Gen.	Obs. (N)	Gen.	Obs. (N)
22 - 26	2	25 - 30-1	2	27 - 28	9	28 - 32-1	2
23 - 27	2	25 - 31-1	1	27 - 29	5	28 - 34-1	2
24 - 25	2	25 - 33-1	1	27 - 30	2	28 - 36-1	1
24 - 27	1	26 - 26	2	27 - 31-3	1	29 - 29	1
24 - 28	3	26 - 27	12	27 - 31	1	29 - 30	2
25 - 25	1	26 - 28	5	27 - 33-1	1	29 - 31-1	1
25 - 26	2	26 - 29	5	28 - 28	3	29 - 34-1	1
25 - 27	7	26 - 30	1	28 - 29	4	30-1 - 31	2
25 - 28	8	26 - 33-1	1	28 - 30	4		
25 - 29	2	27 - 27	8	28 - 31	1		

HUMD8S639 - Allele frequencies

Allele (bp*)	Frequency	Allele (bp*)	Frequency	Allele (bp*)	Frequency
22 (317)	0,009	28 (341)	0,200	32-1 (356)	0,009
23 (321)	0,009	29 (345)	0,100	33-1 (360)	0,014
24 (325)	0,027	30-1 (348)	0,018	34-2 (363)	0,005
25 (329)	0,123	30 (349)	0,041	34-1 (364)	0,005
26 (333)	0,145	31-1 (352)	0,014	36-1 (372)	0,005
27 (337)	0,259	31 (353)	0,018		

* lenght in base pairs as detected by Genescan software
** number of trinucleotide repeats are indicated by (-n).

COMMENTS

STR locus	HR	gene D	PIC	DI	pM	mean exclusion change
HUMCYP19	0,727	0,724	0,719	0,88	0,12	48,9
HUMD8S639	0,857	0,838	0,819	0,95	0,05	67,5

Hardy Weinberg equilibrium was observed for both STR loci.

The sequence analysis of alleles at the HUMCYP19 locus revealed a regular tetranucleotide repeat structure. Alleles 7-3 (168bp) and allele 7 (171bp) exhibit the same repeat unit structure containing 7 tetranucleotide repeat units, but allele 7-3 has a 3bp deletion in the 5' flanking region.

Alleles at locus D8S639 contain tri- and tetranucleotide repeat units leading to allele sizes that differ only by one base pair. In addition, several alleles at this locus contain structural differences in their repeat order but have the same number of repeat units leading to PCR fragments of identical sizes.

REFERENCES

Botstein D, White RL, Skolnick M, Davis RW (1980) Construction of a genetic linkage map in man using restriction fragment lenght polymorphisms. Am.J.Hum.Genetics 32: 182-190

Jones DA (1972) Blood samples: Probability of discrimination. J.Forens.Sci.Soc.12: 355-359

Kimpton CP, Gill P, Walton A, Urquhart A, Millican ES, Adams M (1993) Automated DNA profiling employing multiplex amplification of short tandem repeat loci. PCR methods and applications 3: 13-22

Nelson L, Lu J, Petterson M, Riley R, Ward K (1994) Tetranucleotide repeat polymorphism at the D8S639 locus. Human Molecular Genetics Vol. 3 (7): 1209

Polymeropoulos MH, Xiao H, Rath DS, Merril CR (1992) Tetranucleotide repeat polymorphism at the human aromatase cytochrome P-450 gene (CYP19). Nucleic Acids Research Vol.19(1): 195

MUTATIONS OF D2S44 AND D4S139 ALLELES AND PRESENCE OF TWO-FRAGMENT ALLELES FOR D4S139

A. Vandenberghe, N. Mommers, I. Peeters, M. Vandenbroeck and L. Muylle.

Department of Biochemistry, University of Antwerp, B-2610 Wilrijk, Belgium, Blood Transfusion Center, B-2650 Edegem, Belgium, and Faculty of Pharmacy, University Claude Bernard, F-69373 Lyon CEDEX 08.

INTRODUCTION

Short DNA sequences with a variable number of tandem repeats (VNTR) are highly polymorphic and informative and are frequently applied to solve a number of genetic problems. A major condition for using these probes in paternity testing is the absence of mutations upon transmission which could be interpreted as false negatives. We studied the transmission of alleles from three VNTR probes frequently applied in paternity testing: YNH24 (D2S44), pH30 (D4S139) and MS43A (D12S11). Mutations, albeit at low frequency, were found with the first two. In some cases, interpretation of the D4S139 locus becomes more complex due to the presence of an additional RFLP and of methylation events.

MATERIALS AND METHODS

DNA was digested with the restriction enzyme *Hinf*I following the instructions and using the solutions of the manufacturer (Boehringer, Mannheim, Germany). Separation, transfer onto nylon membranes and hybridization with radiolabelled DNA probes was done according to routinely applied laboratory procedures. Manually measured migration distances were plotted on a standard curve obtained with Analytical Marker DNA Wide Range (Promega corp., Madison, WI). Values were rounded off to the closest 100pb, 50pb was rounded up to the higher value.

RESULTS AND DISCUSSION

Mutations

No mutations for MS43A were found. Smith et al.(1990) described 2 mutations during the transmission of 298 alleles while others did not find mutations for this probe when analyzing 688 gametes (Jeffreys et al., 1988). We observed 2 mutations for YNH24 and 4 for pH30 (Figures 1a, 1b and Table 1). No allelic association of the mutation was observed (Table 2) and the sex of the receiving offspring seems not to be involved (3 boys and 3 girls). The age of the parent does not seem to play any role: the mean age of the fathers of the mutated children at birth was 29.6 year, while for 100 controls this was 31.3 years. Only expansions were observed. Expansions are also seen in a growing number of pathologies (reviewed by Wieringa, 1994). These mutations involve the expansion of the number of repeats of a triplet sequence. Although VNTR core sequences are longer (31 for YNH24, 32 for pH30, 45 for MS43A), an analogous mutation mechanism cannot be excluded. Recently the involvement of a certain genetic environment predisposing to the instability of triplet repeats (Neville et al.1994) or VNTRs (Jeffreys et al. 1994) was suggested. Weber and Wong (1993) reported mutations of short tandem repeats (STRs) and observed a preference for increasing over decreasing (31:9). Similar results were reported by Vergnaud et al. (1991) (30:12) for a new VNTR locus. Although STRs have shorter repeat sequences than VNTRs, the majority of studies conclude to absence of unequal recombination between homologous chromosomes but favours rather polymerase or strand slippage (Jeffreys et al. 1990;) or even more complex reactions (Jeffreys et al. 1994) as the mechanism of choice.

One of the mutations is from maternal origin while the others all are from paternal origin. The parental origin of the mutation was derived considering the parental allele most similar in size to the mutant allele. Another maternal mutation for YNH24 was reported by Endean (1989) but a superior mutation rate for paternal VNTR alleles was reported by Jeffreys et al. (1990) (15:5), Vergnaud et al. (1991) (51:1) and Nürnberg et al.(1989) (7:1) and for STR alleles by Weber and Wong (1993) (15:4). It remains to be proven wether the higher male bias in the generation of new alleles is simply the reflection of a larger number of cell divisions during spermatogenesis.

The pH30 complex polymorphism

In 10 unrelated persons from the 782 examined, a third fragment was observed with probe pH30 (Figure 1c) including one case with 4 fragments (see use of *Hinf*I). The other VNTR probes did not detect such complex patterns. From 8 persons this third fragment was transmitted to their offspring. The occurrence of an additional fragment for pH30 has been described by Waye and Fourney (1990) for genomic DNA digested with the restriction enzyme *Hae*III in about 1% of 547 individuals. They conclude to the occurrence of a VNTR polymorphism on both chromosomes with, in addition, a bi-allelic RFLP on one of the two chromosomes. We here conclude to the presence of an internal additional *Hinf*I site. This site should be situated in the repeat sequence since no unique fragment length was observed for persons with three fragments (see Table 3).

By observing the transmission, the chromosome carrying the VNTR in combination with the biallelic polymorphism could be identified. Since all fragments show distinct fragment sizes, we can reasonably assume the presence of linkage equilibrium between the VNTR and the RFLP. However the RFLP is clearly associated with longer VNTR fragment lengths (allele frequencies of D4S139 show a maximal value around 6 kb for DNA hydrolyzed with *Hinf*I).

Use of the restriction enzyme *Hinf*I

An unusual observation was made with a 2 fragment allele of D4S139 (pH30) (Fig. 1d), where a weak fourth fragment is present in the mother and in the child profile. The *Hinf*I recognition site contains a cytosine residue in the 3′position that can be followed by a guanine residue. Methylation can reduce the activity of the enzyme (Nelson and McClelland, 1987) and produce partial digestion patterns. An almost identical observation was made earlier by Budowle et al. (1990). Since the additional fragment is also transmitted to the child, we suppose that one of the *Hinf*I sites present in this family contains a methylable CpG sequence and that partial digestion occurred. Since the length of the third fragment (12.5 kb) is not the sum of the two other fragments (11.3 and 6.6 kb), the methylable CpG should not be part of the additional internal restriction site but should belong to one of the sites at the extremities of the detected region. Although not really bothering the interpretation for paternity testing, the phenomenon of methylation and partial digestion is disavantageous for the comparison of forensic samples.

REFERENCES

Budowle B, Waye JS, Shutler GG, Baechtel FS (1990) *Hae*III -a suitable restriction endonuclease for restriction fragment length polymorphism analysis of biological evidence samples. J Forens Sci 35:530-536.

Endean DJ (1989) RFLP analysis for paternity testing: observations and caveats. In: Proceedings of the International Symposium on Human Identification, Promega Corp., Madison, pp. 55-69.

Jeffreys AJ, Royle NJ, Wilson V, Wong Z (1988) Spontaneous mutation rates to new length alleles at tandem-repetitive hypervariable loci in human DNA. Nature 332:278-281.

Jeffreys AJ, Neumann R, Wilson V (1990) Repeat unit sequence variation in minisatellites: a novel source of DNA polymorphism for studying variation and mutation by single molecule analysis. Cell 60:473-485.

Jeffreys AJ, Tamaki K, MacLeod A, Monckton DG, Neil DL, Armour JAL (1994) Complex gene conversions events in germline mutation at human minisatellites. Nature Genet 6:136-145.

Nelson M, McClelland M (1987) The effect of site-specific methylation on restriction modification enzymes. Nucl Acids Res 15:r219-r230.

Neville CE, Mahadevan MS, Barceló MS, Korneluk RG (1994) High resolution genetic analysis suggests one ancestral predisposing haplotype for the origin of the myotonic dystrophy mutation. Hum Mol Genet 3:45-51.

Nürnberg P, Roewer L, Neitzel H, Pöpperl A, Hundrieser J, Pöche H, Epplen C, Zischler H, Epplen JT (1989) DNA fingerprinting with oligonucleotide probe $(CAC)_5/(CTG)_5$: somatic stability and germline mutations. Hum Genet 84:75-78.

Smith JC, Anwar R, Riley J, Jenner D, Markham AF, Jeffreys AJ (1990) Highly polymorphic minisatellite sequences: allele frequencies and mutation rates for five locus-specific probes in a Caucasian population. J Forens Sci Soc 30:3-18.

Vergnaud G, Mariat D, Apiou F, Aurias A, Lathrop M, Lauthier V (1991) The use of synthetic tandem repeats to isolate new VNTR loci: cloning of a human hypermutable sequence. Genomics 11:135-144.

Waye JS, Fourney RM (1990) Identification of complex DNA polymorphisms based on variable number of tandem repeats (VNTR) and restriction site polymorphism. Hum Genet 84:223-227.

Weber J, Wong C (1993) Mutation of human short tandem repeats. Hum Mol Genet 2:1123-1128.

Wieringa B (1994) Myotonic dystrophy reviewed: back to the future. Hum Mol Genet 3:1-7.

Table 1. Observed mutation frequencies.

probe	# meioses	# mutations	frequency
YNH24	536	2	0.37 %
pH30	536	4	0.75 %
MS43A	517	0	-

Table 3. Length of the D4S139 fragments transmitted as a fragment-pair to the offspring.

lengths of the transmitted fragments (kb)		sum (kb)
14.3	2.8	17.1
8.5	1.8	10.3
10.1	5.1	15.2
12.7	4.6	17.3
10.7	4.2	14.9
11.3	6.6	17.9
4.9	3.5	8.4
4.0	3.3	7.3

Table 2. Origin (p:paternal; m:maternal) and lengths (kb) of mutant alleles.

probe	origin	transmitted alleles	mutant allele
YNH24	p	2.6 & 3.7	2.7
YNH24	m	5.9 & 3.5	3.7
pH30	p	9.7 & 4.8	5.0
pH30	p	10.0 & 5.4	10.1
pH30	p	11.5 & 4.7	11.9
pH30	p	7.1 & 5.1	5.2

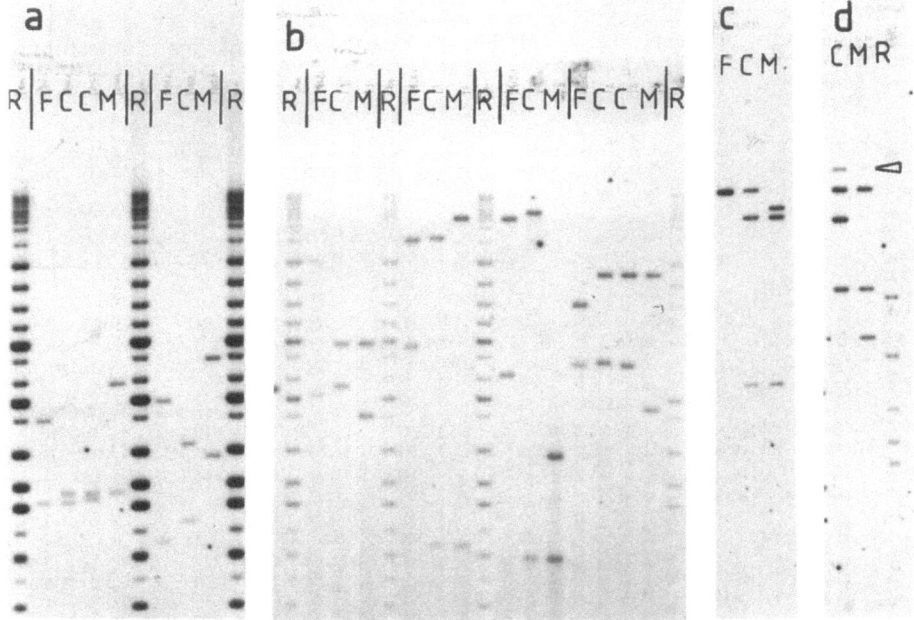

Figure 1.

Mutations found with probe YNH24 are shown in (a) and with pH30 in (b). With probe pH30, sometimes a third fragment is revealed (c) and is transmitted to the offspring. In one case a weak fourth fragment was observed (d, arrowhead) believed to result from methylation of a restriction site sequence. R, reference ladder; F, (alledged) father; C, child; M, mother.

NON-AUTOMATIC MULTIPLEX ANALYSIS AND DETECTION OF SIX STR-LOCI:
HPRT, FABP2, CD4, F13A1, CYP19 AND LPL

R. Weispfenning, C. Luckenbach, H. Ritter

Institut für Anthropologie und Humangenetik, Wilhelmstr. 27, 72074 Tübingen, GER

SUMMARY

We present a DNA-typing method using six unlinked STR loci (HPRT, FABP2 CD4, F13A1, CYP19, LPL). All loci are separated in one gel, using one lane for three different loci .
Electrophoretic analysis was non-automatically performed, followed by silverstaining in a native, vertical gel system.

INTRODUCTION

Personal identification by use of DNA typing methodologies has been an issue in the popular and scientific press. Many years of experience have demonstrated that DNA typing methodologies, using a battery of highly polymorphic RFLP-VNTR probes (Jeffreys et al. 1985; Nakamura et al. 1987) offer reliable, feasible and rapid DNA analysis and are consequently efficient for resolving personal identification in many cases. But there are limiting factors for these VNTR analysis, for example in circumstances, where only small DNA amounts or partially degraded DNA are available. Because of the small sizes of STRs (≤ 350 bp), they can be informative in cases where VNTR analysis would fail.

STRs are a subset of microsatellite loci, containing a repeated motif of 2 to 7 nucleotids in length (Edwards, A. et al. 1991; Hammond et al. 1994; Weber et al. 1989; Alford et al. 1994). STRs differ in their number of nucleotids within their repeated sequence. The vast majority of STRs reported to date have been dinucleotide STRs, but increasing numbers of tri- and tetranucleotide STRs are being detected. The polymorphisms are due to the variable number of repeats of three, four and five nucleotide sequences. Three-, four-, and five-base repeats amplify more authentically and provide more easily interpretable results, than dinucleotide repeat loci do (Hammond et al. 1994; Edwards, M.C. et al. 1991; Huang et al. 1991). The tri- and tetranucleotide STRs have another significant advantage over dinucleotide STRs in that strand slippage artifacts (also called shadow or stutter bands), are greatly reduced (Dubovsky et al. 1995).

We have developed a PCR-based DNA typing method that uses 6 unlinked STR loci to provide a rapid and reliable typing system for personal identification with a highly discriminating power.

MATERIAL AND METHODS

Preparation of DNA
DNA was isolated from leucocytes, according to Miller et al. (1988).

Oligonucleotides
Oligonucleotides were synthesized with the DNA synthesizer „Gene Assembler Plus"(Pharmacia, Freiburg, GER) and cleaned with NAP-10 columns (Pharmacia).

STR Loci

The STR loci used in this study are one trinucleotide STR locus (FABP2), four tetranucleotide STR loci (HPRT, F13A1, CYP19 and LPL) and one pentanucleotide STR loci (CD4).

Table 1 summarizes the STR locus names, Genome Database (GDB) designations, chromosomal locations, PCR primers and allele weight ranges of the six STR loci used in this study (Hammond et al. 1994).

Table 1: Characteristics of six unlinked STR-loci

Genbank Locus [STR]ₙGDB Designation	Gene (chromosome location)	PCR Primers	Product Length (bp)
HUMHPRTB[AGAT]ₙ/HPRT	Hypoxanthine phosphoribosyltransferase (Xq26)	A:ATGCCACAGATAATACACATCCCC B:CTCTCCAGAATAGTTAGATGTAGG	259-299
HUMFABP[AAT]ₙ/FABP2	Intestinal fatty acid-binding protein (4q28-q31)	A:GTAGTATCAGTTTCATAGGGTCACC B:CAGTTCGTTTCCATTGTCTGTCCG	199-220
HUMCD4[AAAAG]ₙ/CD4	Recognition/ surface antigen (cd4) (12p12-pter)	A:TTGGAGTCGCAAGCTGAACTAGCG B:CCAGGAAGTTGAGGCTGCAGTGAA	125-175
HUMF13A01[AAAG]ₙ/F13A1	Coagulation factor XIII (6p24-p25)	A:GAGGTTGCACTCGAGCCTTTGCAA B:TTCCTGAATCATCCCAGAGCCACA	281-331
HUMCYAR04]AAAT]ₙ/CYP19	Aromatase cytochrome P-450 (15q21.1)	A:GGTAAGCAGGTACTTAGTTAGCTAC B:GTTACAGTGAGCCAAGGTCGTGAG	173-201
HUMLIPOL[AAAT]ₙ/LPL	Lipoprotein lipase (8p22)	A:CTGACCAAGGATAGTGGGATATAG B:GGTAACTGAGCGAGACTGTGTCT	125-175

PCR Conditions

DNA amount:
10-15 ng of genomic DNA.
Cycling conditions: (Gene Amp PCR System, 2400; Perkin Elmer thermocycler)
94°C, 5 min, 1 cycle; 94 °C, 30 s, then 60 °C, 45 s, then 72 °C, 30 s, 30 cycles; and 72 °C, 5 min, 1 cycle.

Reaction conditions:

Reagent:	Final concentration:
Buffer (100mM Tris-HCl, pH 8,3; 500mM KCl)	1 x
dNTPs	200 µM (of each)
Primers	0,25 µM (of each)
MgCl₂	1,5 mM
Taq	1 unit/PCR

Electrophoresis and silverstaining

Amplified fragments were separated in a native polyacrylamide gel (7,5% T, 2% C), using a vertical electrophoresis system (17,1 x 32,5 x 0,08 cm, Model SA 32, GIBCO BRL). The amplified products of three different STR loci (HPRT-FABP2-CD4; F13A1-CYP19-LPL) were applicated into one lane using a time distance of 15 minutes of intervening electrophoresis.
Settings: 500 V, 40 mA, 40 W, 2,5-3 hrs, detection by silverstaining (Bassam et al. 1991).

Allele designation

Exact allelic designation needs sequenced allelic ladders, which are still in preparation, according to the recommendations of Puers et al. (1994).

RESULTS AND DISCUSSION

Fig. 1 shows several DNA-profiles analyzed by PCR and vertical polyacrylamide gel electrophoresis, followed by silverstaining. All fragments are well separated and can be distinguished without any doubt. If the allelic ladders are finally developed, is it possible (i) to differentiate clearly alleles differing by only one repeat unit and (ii) to achieve a high output of efficient results. Together these findings suggest that these 6 STR loci are well suited for separation in one gel system.

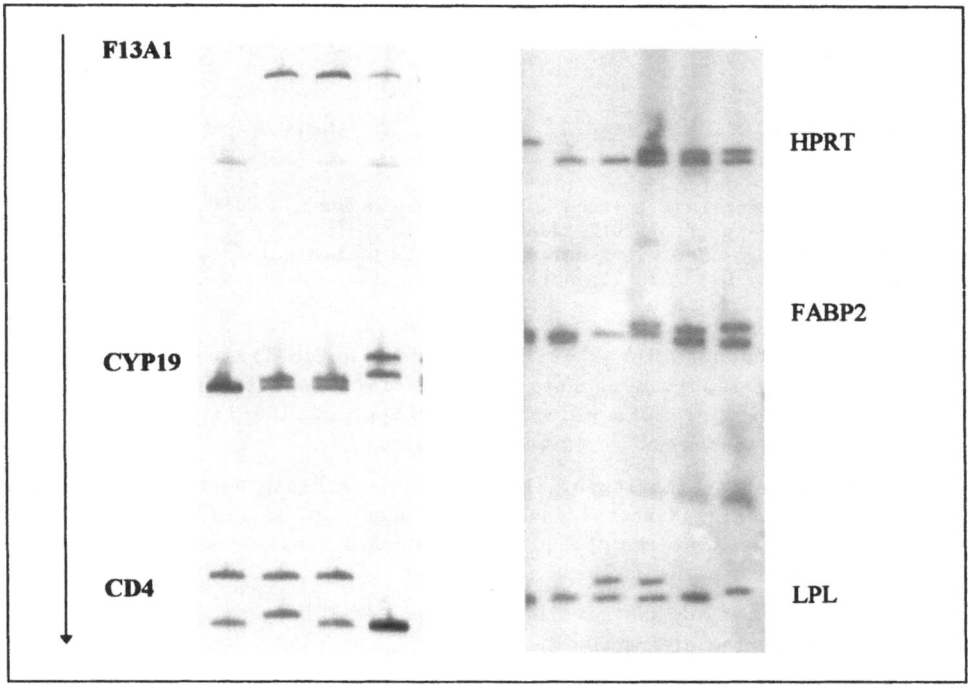

Figure1: Separation of six unlinked PCR-loci

REFERENCES
Alford, R.L., Hammond, H.A., Coto, I. and Caskey C.T. (1994). Rapid and efficient resolution of parentage by amplification of short tandem repeats. Am. J. Hum Genet. 55: 190-195.

Bassam, B.J., Caetano-Annollés, G. and Gresshoff, P.M. (1991). Fast and sensitive silver staining of DNA in polyacrylamide gels. Anal-Biochem. 196 (1): 80-83.

Dubovsky, J., Sheffield, V.C., Duyk, G.M. and Weber J.L. (1995). Sets of short tandem repeat polymorphisms for efficient linkage screening of the human genome. Hum. Mol. Genet. Vol.4, No. 3: 449-452.

Edwards, A., Civitello, A., Hammond, H.A. and Caskey, C.T. (1991). DNA typing and genetic mapping with trimeric and tetrameric tandem repeats. Am. J. Hum. Genet. 49: 746-756.

Edwards, M.C:, Clemens, P.R., Tristan, M., Pizzuti, A.and Gibbs, R.A. (1991). Pentanucleotide repeat length polymorphism at the human CD4 locus. Nucleic Acids Res 19: 4791.

Jeffreys, A:J:, Wilson, V. and Thein, S.L. (1985). Hypervariable 'minisatellite` regions in human DNA. Nature 314: 67-73.

Hammond, H.A., Jin, L., Zhong, Y., Caskey, C.T. and Chakraborty, R.C. (1994). Evaluation of 13 STR loci for use in personal identification applications. Am. J. Hum. Genet. 55: 175-189.

Huang, TH.-M., Hejtmancik J.F., Edwards, A., Pettigrew, A.L., Herrera, C.A.,Hammond, H.A.,Caskey, C.T., et al.(1991). Linkage of the gene for an X-linked mental retardation disorder to a hypervariable (AGAT)n repeat motif within the human hypoxanthine phosphoribosyltransferase (HPRT) locus (Xq26). Am. J. Hum. Genet. 49: 1312-1319.

Miller, S.A., Dykes, D.D. and Polesky, H.F. (1988). A simple salting out procedure for extracting DNA from human nucleated cells. Nucleic Acids Res. 16: 1215.

Nakamura, Y., Leppert, M., O'Connell, P., Wolff, R., Holm, T., Culver, M. and Martin, C., et al. (1987). Variable number of tandem repeat (VNTR) markers for human gene mapping. Science 235: 1616-1622.

Puers, C., Hammond, H.A., Caskey, C.T., Lins, A.M., Sprecher, C.J., Brinkmann, B. and Schumm, J.W. (1994). Allelic ladder characterization of the STR polymorphism located in the 5`flanking region to the human coalgulation factor XIII A subunit gene. Genomics 23: 260-264.

Weber, J.L. and May, P.E. (1989). Abundant class of human DNA polymorphisms which can be typed using polymerase chain reaction. Am. J. Hum. Genet. 44: 388-396.

DNA Analysis of Polymorphism in Drug or Xenobiotics Metabolism.

Yamada M[1], Sato M[2], Ushiyama I[2], Yamada Y[1], Nishimura A[2] and Nishi K[2]

[1] Department of Human Life Science, Seibo Jogakuin Women's College,
Fukakusa, Fushimi-ku, Kyoto 612, Japan
[2] Department of Legal Medicine, Shiga University of Medical Science,
Seta-Tsukinowacho, Otsu 520-21, Japan

Hereditary differences in activities of drug metabolizing enzymes among individuals have led to a phenotypic classification of humans as poor or extensive metabolizer. The metabolic genotype may be important in drug overdose with substances subjected to detoxication.

Here we present determination of the GSTM1 (glutathione S-transferase) gene deletion and the NAT2 (N-acetyltransferase) genotype, and also the influence of allelic difference at the ALDH2 (aldehyde dehydrogenase) gene locus on the ethanol loading in healthy Japanese individuals' DNAs.

Genotyping assays using DNA sample can be of great help at drug therapy and clinical or postmortem diagnosis.

GSTM1 POLYMORPHISM

GSTM1, one of the genetic loci encoding human GST isoenzymes, is associated to the GSTμ isoenzyme. In three alleles at the GSTM1 locus, GSTM1*0 (null) corresponds to a gene deletion. Almost 50% of people show the μ isoenzyme deficiency, which is caused by GSTM1*0/*0. Absence of the detoxifying role of GST against xenobiotics is considered to increase the risk of lung cancer (Comstock 1990; Groppi 1991).

We have examined the distribution of the GSTM1*0/*0 genotype in a Japanese population. According to Comstock (1990) and Groppi (1991), the regions from exon 4 to exon 5 and from intron 4 to exon 5, respectively, in the GSTM1 gene were amplified by PCR. Among 65 subjects, 32 lacked the PCR product and were determined as null homozygote.

NAT2 GENOTYPE

Polymorphic NAT2, which catalyzes the N-acetylation of various arylamines and hydrazines, divides into slow or rapid acetylator. The acetylation polymorphism is considered to be susceptible to bladder cancer and colorectal cancer. Four NAT2 alleles differ at single base substitutions which modify the restriction enzyme cleavage sites. About 40% of Caucasians are slow acetylators, who do not possess NAT2*1 allele (Hickman 1991).

We have amplified the sequence containing the polymorphic sites in the NAT2

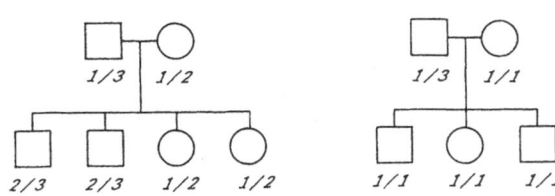

Figure 1. Determination of the NAT2 Genotype in Two Families.

Table 1. NAT2 Genotype Distribution in Healthy Japanese Examined.

Genotype	No. subjects	%	Genotype	No. subjects	%
1/1	30	46	2/4	0	0
1/2	10	15	3/3	1	2
1/3	19	29	3/4	0	0
1/4	0	0	4/4	0	0
2/2	1	2	Total	65	100
2/3	4	6			

Table 2. ALDH2 Genotype Distribution in Healthy Japanese Examined.

ALDH2 Genotype	No. subjects	%
ALDH2*1/ALDH2*1	35	48
ALDH2*1/ALDH2*2	32	44
ALDH2*2/ALDH2*2	6	8
Total	73	100

Table 3. Relationship between ALDH2 Genotype and the Ethanol Sensitivity.

	n	ALDH2 Phenotype	Mean Max. Acetaldehyde Level (μM)	Mean β_{60} Value (mg/mℓ/hr)
ALDH2*1/ALDH2*1	11	active	3.9± 1.9	0.16±0.03
ALDH2*1/ALDH2*2	15	inactive	20.6± 7.5	0.14±0.02
ALDH2*2/ALDH2*2	4	inactive	84.8±29.4	0.11±0.03

gene by PCR (Abe 1993) and the allele was determined as NAT2*2, *3 or *4 when the fragment was not cleaved by BamHI, TaqI or KpnI, respectively. The NAT2*1 allele was detected by cleavage of three enzymes (Fig. 1). The allele NAT2*4 was not detected and 6 Japanese among 65 were slow acetylators (Table 1).

ALDH2 GENOTYPE AND ALCOHOL LOADING TEST

In an individual ethanol sensitivity, allelic differences at the ADH2 and ALDH2 loci (Hsu 1985; Xu 1988) have an important role.

We distinguished the polymorphism at the ALDH2 locus in Japanese individuals' DNAs using the technique of PCR and allele-specific oligonucleotide probes. The activity of the ALDH2 isozyme in their hair roots was also detected. The subjects were orally administered 0.4 g/kg of ethanol to investigate the sensitivity (Yamada 1992; Yamamoto 1993). In people possessing the ALDH2*2 allele a consequent elevation of blood acetaldehyde after alcohol intake due to less or no enzyme activity causes strong sensitivity to ethanol (Tables 2 and 3).

ACKNOWLEDGEMENTS

The study was partially supported by Grants-in-Aid for Scientific Research (#02670257 and #07670489) from the Ministry of Education, Science and Culture of Japan.

REFERENCES

Abe M, Suzuki T, Deguchi T (1993) An improved method for genotyping of N-acetyltransferase polymorphism by polymerase chain reaction. Jpn J Hum Genet 38:163-168

Comstock KE, Sanderson JS, Claflin G, et al (1990) GST1 gene deletion determined by polymerase chain reaction. Nucl Acids Res 18:3670

Groppi A, Coutelle C, Fleury B, et al (1991) Glutathione S-transferase class μ in French alcoholic cirrhotic patients. Hum Genet 87:628-630

Hickman D, Sim E (1991) N-Acetyltransferase polymorphism. Biochem Pharmacol 42:1007-1014

Hsu LC, Tani K, Fujiyoshi T, et al (1985) Cloning of cDNAs for human aldehyde dehydrogenases 1 and 2. Proc Natl Acad Sci USA 82:3771-3775

Xu Y, Carr LG, Bosron WF, et al (1988) Genotyping of human alcohol dehydrogenase at the ADH2 and ADH3 loci following DNA sequence amplification. Genomics 2:209-214

Yamada M, Yamamoto K, Ueno Y, et al (1992) Genotypes of alcohol-metabolizing enzymes and ethanol sensitivity. In: Kaempe B (ed) Forensic Toxicology. Mackeenzie Press, Copenhagen, pp.497-504

Yamamoto K, Ueno Y, Mizoi Y, et al (1993) Genetic polymorphism of alcohol and aldehyde dehydrogenase and the effects on alcohol metabolism. Jpn J Alcohol Drug Depend 28:13-25

FORENSIC EFFICIENCY AND GERMAN POPULATION DATA FOR THE TETRAMERIC STR POLYMORPHISM DHFRP2 (HUMFOLP23)

Mark Benecke, Cornelia Schmitt, Mechthild Prinz

Institute for Forensic Medicine, University of Cologne, DNA Research Dept., D-50923 Koeln

Introduction

Hypervariability in short tandem repeated sequences of genomic DNA (STRs) is one of the most reliable ways of personal identification from biological samples. We examined the allelic distribution of the human dihydrofolate reductase psi-2 pseudogene (Polymeropoulos et al. 1991) in a Western German population (Rhine area). These were compared to population data first described by Polymeropoulos et al. and by Kimpton et al.. To reach highest possible detection sensitivity, separation and detection of PCR products were performed using an Automatic Laser Fluorescence Detection Unit (A.L.F. sequencer, Pharmacia) (Schmitt & Prinz, in press).

Material and Methods

Whole blood DNA of unrelated West Germans was amplified using fluorescent primers (FPLCpure, Pharmacia) as given in Polymeropoulos et al. 1991 (20-/21-mer, resp.) on the Perkin Elmer GeneAmp PCR System 2400 (29 cycles, 58°C annealing) and on the Biometra Thermoblock (28 cycles, 60°C annealing). Mastermix: Primer 0,5 µM each in 25 µl, 2 U Taq Polymerase (Promega), 150 µM dNTPs, 10 mM Tris-HCl pH 9,0, 0,1% Triton X-100 (Promega buffer).
1-5 µL of PCR product each were loaded on a Pharmacia A.L.F. Sequencer (green laser); data processing was performed by internal software exclusively. Quantitation of DNA was done with the ACES Human DNA Quantification System (Gibco Life Technologies).

Results

Analysing the allelic distribution of 102 unrelated Germans we detected six alleles; minor differences to the allelic distribution given in the original paper were found (Fig. 1). Heterozygosity was 72 %. Using the exact test (Guo & Thompson 1992; formula implemented in the „DNA View" software package (Charles Brenner, Berkeley)) and assuming 15 degrees of freedom, alleles were in Hardy-Weinberg equilibrium. No slippage bands were observed.

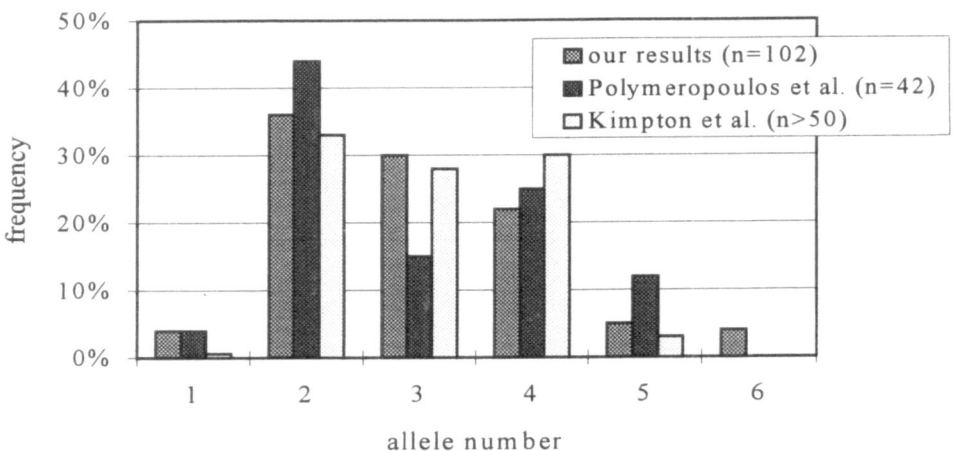

Figure 1: Allele frequencies of DHFRP2 (HUMFOLP23) in Caucasians. Alleles 1-5 are alleles A5-A1 at Polymeropoulos et al.. Accordingly, #1 is the shortest allele.

Amplification of samples containing less then 50 pg of DNA led to clear signals on the A.L.F. sequencer (Fig. 2) in homozygous genotypes. No DNA-dependent band shifts occurred but baseline sometimes got triflingly fuzzy at lowest DNA level.

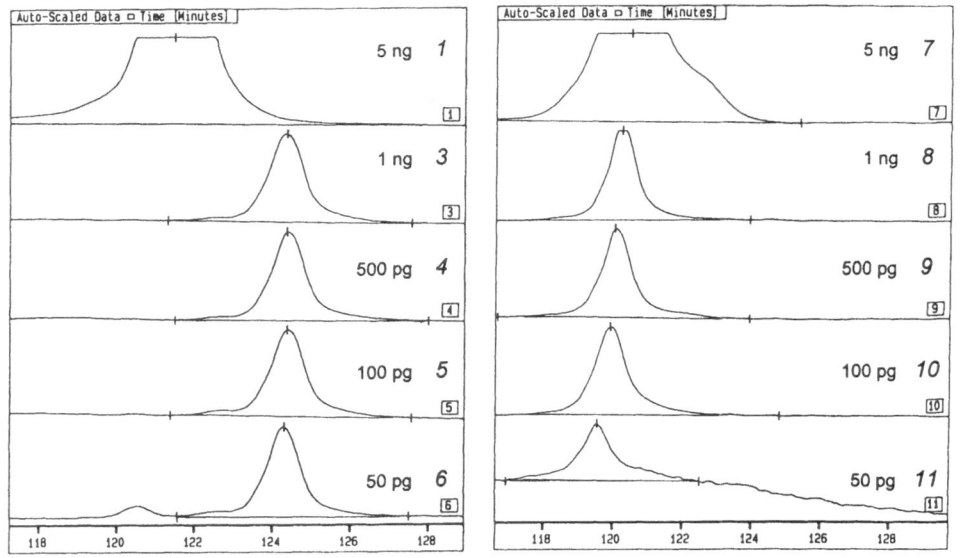

Figure 2: Sensitivity of DHFRP2/HUMFOLP23. 1-6: Decreasing amounts of homozygous DNA of person A. Band/allele shift of the 5 ng signal is due to the use of the first slot of the A.L.F.-PAG. 7-11: Decreasing amounts of DNA of person B.

Discussion

Due to
- the simple repeat structure (Urquhart at al. 1994),
- the short fragment length,
- the low detection limit and
- the non-occurrence of slippage bands

this locus should be a valuable forensic marker.
Another primer sequence for the same locus which we did not try out was suggested by Urquhart et al. 1994.

References

GUO SW, THOMPSON EA (1992) Performing the exact test of Hardy-Weinberg proportion for multiple alleles. Biometrics 48, 361-372

KIMPTON CP, GILL P, WALTON A, URQUHART A, MILLICAN ES, ADAMS M (1993) Automated DNA profiling multiplex amplification of short tandem repeat loci. PCR Methods and Application, 13-22

POLYMEROPOULOS MH, XIAO H, RATH DS, MERRIL CR (1991) Tetranucleotide repeat polymorphism at the human dihydrofolate reductase psi-2 pseudogene (DHFRP2). Nucleic Acids Research 19, 4792

SCHMITT C, PRINZ M (1995) Anwendbarkeit eines DNA-Sequenzierautomaten für die PCR-Typisierung von forensischen Spuren. (Applicability of a DNA sequencer for forensic PCR typing.) Rechtsmedizin, in press

URQUHART A, KIMPTON CP, DOWNES TJ, GILL P (1994) Variation in short tandem repeat sequences-a survey of twelve microsatellite loci for use as forensic identification markers. International Journal of Legal Medicine 107, 13-20

5 Forensic Applications

Criminal intelligence databases and interpretation of STRs

P. Gill, A. Urquhart, E. Millican, N. Oldroyd, S. Watson, R. Sparkes and C.P. Kimpton

Forensic Science Service, Priory House, Gooch Street North, Birmingham B65QQ, UK

INTRODUCTION

DNA profiling in forensic science in the UK is focussed on the analysis of short tandem repeat (STR) loci using PCR. It is the technique of choice for the national strategy to create criminal intelligence databases. Apart from the increased sensitivity inherent with any PCR technique, with STRs there is also the advantage of definitive allelic identification. This is a consequence of lower measurement errors associated with the use of polyacrylamide gel electrophoresis to detect DNA fragments ranging between 200-400bp in size (Ziegle et al. 1992).Because of their small sizes STRs are more likely to be successful on old or badly degraded material (Gill et al. 1994; Hagelberg et al. 1991; Jeffreys et al. 1992; Weigand et al. 1993) an important aspect of forensic casework.

The National DNA database Unit

Recently, a change in the UK legislation allowed the formation of a national DNA database. The purpose is to store DNA profiles derived from individuals either suspected or convicted of crimes. DNA is sampled from either buccal scrapes or from hair-roots. The aim is to store 135,000 DNA profiles per year and it is envisaged that the database may eventually contain 5 million profiles. This is a significant proportion of the UK population of 60 million people. As the custodian of the DNA database, the Forensic Science Service (FSS) has constructed a unit at the FSS headquarters, Birmingham, UK, consisting of c.125 scientists, eight 373A ABD automated sequencers and six 377 ABD automated sequencers.

METHOD

To decide the method of choice, the following requirements must be fulfilled:
- It must be reliable (the quality of results must be high).
- Throughput must be high.
- The process must be cost-effective.

Automation is the key to achieving all three requirements.

Choice of loci

Several factors are considered when choosing candidate loci:
- Discriminating power (Jones 1972) of >0.9 (Observed heterozygosity >70%).
- The predicted length of alleles must be approximately between 90-500bp (the higher the molecular weight the lower the precision of measurement).

Also the lower the size of the STR locus, the less chance of locus or allelic drop-out because of degradation of the sample.

- Chromosomal location (to ensure that closely linked loci are not chosen).
- Robustness and reproducibility of results, low stuttering characteristics.

Dimeric loci cannot be used because slippage during amplification results in spurious bands that are difficult to interpret whereas trimeric and tetrameric loci are less prone to this problem. Complex hypervariable loci such as HUMACTBP2 have more than 30 alleles. Although originally described (Polymeropoulos et al. 1992; Warne et al. 1991) as a tetrameric repeat, sequencing by Urquhart et al. (1993) and Weigand et al. (1993) has revealed that repeats differ by 1,2, or 3 bps; in addition, different alleles the same size, may have different sequences. To designate alleles to these types of STRs is difficult, although there is no reason why interpretation cannot be carried out based using size estimates (bp), but the system is not discrete

To achieve higher discriminating powers required for large criminal intelligence DNA databases, we have chosen to utilise the advantages of complex tetrameric repeat loci described by Urquhart et al. (1993). Because these have alleles that differ in size by 2bp, the DPs are greater compared to those previously utilised by Kimpton et al. (1994) (Table 1). The loci used in the National DNA database are listed; there are 3 complex STRs included - D18S51 (15 common alleles); D21S11 (21 common alleles); HUMFIBRA/FGA (21 common alleles).

Table 1. List of loci used in the National DNA database; chromosomal locations and Pms for 3 different ethnic groups.

Locus	Chromosomal	Probability of Match (Pm)		
	location	Caucasian	Afro-Caribbeans	Indo-Pakistani
AMELOGENIN	Xp22, Yp11.2	X,Y	X,Y	X,Y
HUMVWFA31/A	12p12-pter	0.064	0.057	0.075
HUMTH01	11p15-15.5	0.086	0.100	0.084
HUMFIBRA*	4q28	0.044	0.027	0.031
D21S11*	21	0.051	0.042	0.046
D18S51*	18q21.3	0.029	0.024	0.042
D6S502	6	0.047	0.061	0.054
	Total Pm	1.7×10^{-8}	1×10^{-9}	1.2×10^{-8}

* Display alleles differing by 2bps

MULTIPLEXING

The availability of 4 distinguishable fluorescent dyes facilitates the development of STR multiplexes (i.e. single tube reactions) enables loci that have overlapping allele size ranges to be labelled with different colours.

To build a multiplex system, primers must be chosen so that annealing temperatures are similar and have low affinity either to each other or to regions of the DNA outside the specific target template; this is achieved with the help of computer programs such as Oligo^{TM}. Once a system has been designed, primer concentrations must be optimised so that even signals are obtained after PCR .

237

Accordingly, we have developed a quadruplex consisting of the loci HUMTH01, HUMVWFA31, HUMFES/FPS and HUMF13A1 for use in routine casework throughout the UK (Kimpton et al. 1994; Lygo et al. 1994). All four loci have discrete classes (Kimpton et al. 1993). An allelic class may comprise 2 or more alleles, for example we do not distinguish between the HUMTH01 9.3 allele and the rarer 10 allele which differs in size by 1bp. The combined frequency of the two alleles is therefore used for interpretation purposes.

The main purpose of using multiplexes, is to speed the process of analysis. Inevitably, there may be some loss of efficiency of amplification since the conditions used are a compromise. This has no significant implications for the database, since the operator has large quantities of undegraded DNA available for analysis. Furthermore, the DNA is never a mixture. In casework, where the sample is less predictable, singleplexes may sometimes be used to identify difficult (e.g. degraded) samples (i.e. singleplexing and multiplexing are not mutually exclusive techniques).

DETERMINING THE SIZE OF STR ALLELES

To determine the sizes of DNA fragments, standard marker ladders consisting of all the common alleles of a given locus can be used for comparison on an electrophoretic gel (Puers et al. 1993; Puers et al. 1994). They are made by mixing together DNA from different individuals displaying the entire range of alleles for comparison and carrying out PCR on the mixture. Ladder markers are widely utilised and available throughout the forensic community.

Fig. 1. Multiplexed allelic ladders for 3 STR loci.

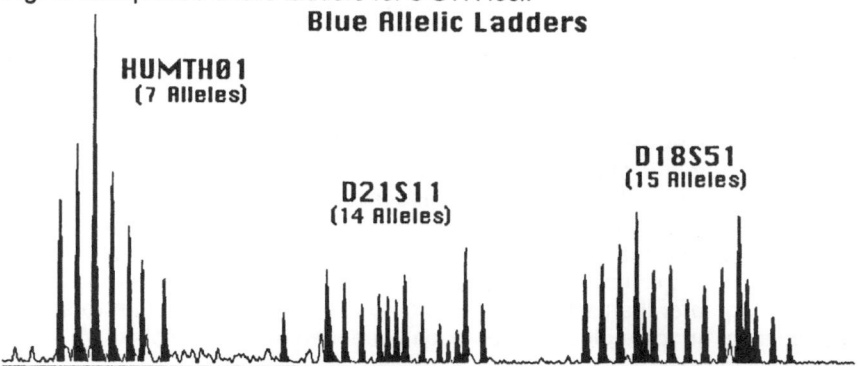

However, the major advantage of fluorescence is that internal size markers can be incorporated and this improves sizing accuracy both within and between gels (Mayrand et al. 1992; Ziegle et al. 1992; Kimpton et al. 1993). Whereas the use of allelic ladders is indispensable with non-automated systems, fluorescently tagging STR loci enables inclusion of size standards as an internal size marker within each lane. This reduces measurement errors and allows automatic sizing of STR-PCR products with GENESCAN™ 672 analysis software. For the majority of loci, reliable sizing can be achieved by direct comparison with a lambda *Pst I* restriction digests (ABD GS2500 or GS350). For calibration purposes allelic ladders are used in our laboratory (if new software is installed, for example).

The consistency of automatic size calling against the GS2500 or GS350 ladder markers was evaluated for each locus studied by examination of the distribution of computer-generated band sizes of allelic ladders for a large number of samples (72 allelic ladders run across 6 different gels). These experiments are used to set windows based on the range of observed sizes of any given allele. Accuracy has been demonstrated to be within a range of approximately 1.2 bp (Table 2 of Kimpton et al. 1993 ; Fig. 2). Ranges based on observations are programmed into the ABD GENOTYPER™ software, enabling automatic allele designations to be made.

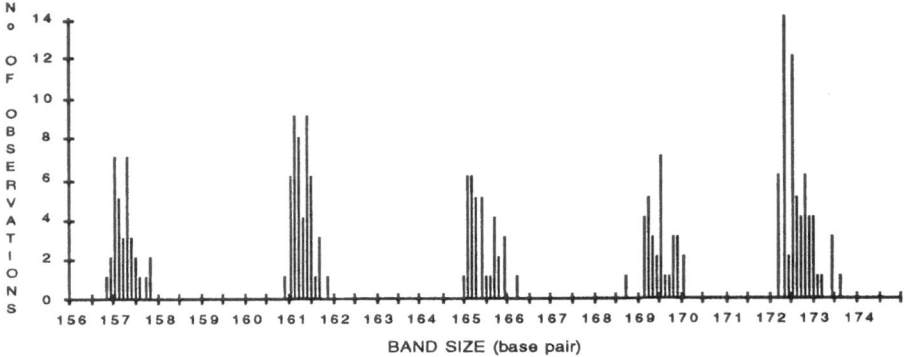

Fig. 3: Distribution of HUMTH01 alleles sized against the GS2500 standard (the allele at the far right comprises 9.3 and 10 alleles, hence the range is relatively large).

A NEW METHOD OF RULE-BASED INTERPRETATION USING ALLELIC LADDER CONTROLS

HUMFIBRA/FGA (Mills et al. 1992) is a complex repeat locus with 21 common alleles differing by increments of just 2bp. If complex loci were perfect 2bp repeats, then the window established to encompass measurement error for any given allele would be just ±1bp of its mean. However, intermediate alleles differing by 1bp may also occur. For example, we have recently discovered a 22.3 allele in HUMFIBRA/FGA. This means that to identify these very rare (p<0.001) alleles, windows must be no greater than ±0.5bp. The difficulty is that measurement errors may exceed this value, hence a different approach is needed to use complex STRs as discrete systems.

An alternative approach to that described above is to calculate the relative difference in size between a questioned sample and an allelic ladder marker control on the same gel. All sizes, in base pairs, are calculated by reference to the internal GS350 standard. If the distance is within a predetermined range, then the allele can be designated. This is a fundamentally different approach to that previously described. Whereas the former method calculates 'absolute' windows based upon repeated running of allelic standard markers, the new method calculates windows relative to ladder markers on the same gel - windows are therefore set for each individual gel.

Examination of the population distribution of HUMFIBRA/FGA (Fig. 3) reveals that the most common alleles such as 19,20,21 are complete tetramers, whereas intermediates (19.2,20.2,21.2) are much rarer (p<0.02). If α.0 represents a complete no. of repeats, we can generalise that α.0 repeats are common; α.1 and α.3 alleles are always very rare (p<0.001) and α.2 repeats are intermediate. In some systems we have examined e.g. (D21S11), some α.2 variants are relatively common, yet the extreme rarity of α.1 and α.3 alleles holds true for complex loci listed in Table 1.

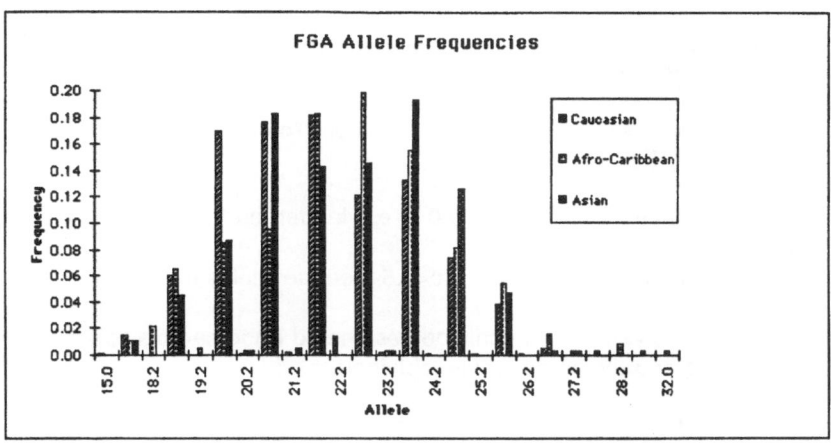

Fig. 3: HUMFIBRA/FGA population survey of 3 different ethnic groups

For HUMFIBRA/FGA, the following conditional logic applies:

- If an α.1 or α.3 allele is observed then this is an extremely rare occurrence.
- Given that the size distribution of individual STR alleles may be in the region of ±0.6bp, an explanation may be that an α.0 or α.2 variant is in a tail of its measurement error distribution such that it now resides in an adjacent window, normally occupied by an α.1 or α.3 variant.
- To test this possibility, re-run the sample to determine if the result is reproducible.
- If the allele is a true α.1 or α.3 variant then the locus would normally be heterozygous (unless, the population from which the sample is derived is atypical, or inbred). It follows that the partner allele must also normally be a common α.0 or α.2 variant.
- If a heterozygous sample is observed where both alleles are apparently α.1 or α.3 variants then that result suggests the strong possibility that 2 common variants are shifted into the tails of their error distributions. In fact band shifts are strongly correlated (Gill, unpublished observations).

240

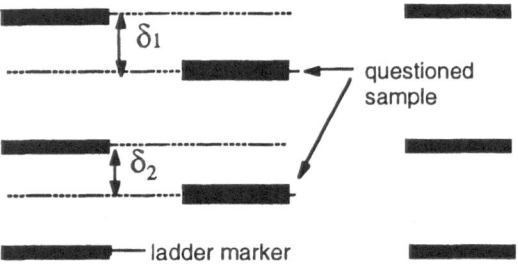

questioned
sample

ladder marker

Fig. 4: Exaggerated diagrammatic representation of band shift showing
correlation. The questioned sample is compared to ladder markers on the gel.

Measuring the correlation effect is a useful diagnostic tool. To do this the
following procedure is used (fig 4):

- **If** both alleles are <0.5bp from the closest $\alpha.0$ or $\alpha.2$ ladder marker then
continue to the next test.
- Measure the correlation effect $(c= \delta1-\delta2)$. **If** c<0.5 then the alleles may be
designated.
- Extremely rare $\alpha.1$ or $\alpha.3$ variants can only be designated **if** the sample has
been separately analysed and the same results obtained.

The utility of this procedure is best illustrated by reference to an actual example

Identification of a rare HUMFIBRA/FGA 22.3 allele

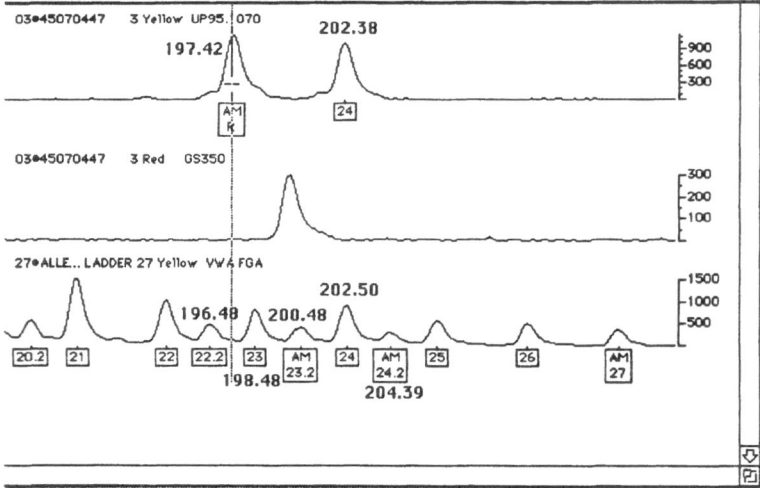

Fig 5: Interpretation of an extremely rare variant allele in HUMFIBRA/FGA -
showing designations made by GENOTYPER. The top lane is the questioned
sample; the bottom lane is the allelic ladder.

Table 2: Compilation of allele sizes illustrated in Fig 5.

Allele Designation	Size in questioned sample (bp)	Size in allelic ladder (bp)	Difference (δ)
22.3	197.42	197.48 '	-0.06 (δ1)
22.2		196.48	+0.98*
23		198.48	-0.98*
24	202.38	202.50	-0.12 (δ 2)

* If the questioned allele (designated 22.3) is truly a common allele it must be either 22.2 or 23. The test fails this condition since δ >0.5 (ignore sign).
' The 22.3 allele is not in the allelic ladder, but its size can be estimated as the mean of alleles 22.2 and 23. The difference passes the condition d <0.5 (ignore sign), if the allele is 22.3.

Correlation measurements

• If the questioned allele is 22.3 then the observed correlation with allele 24 (c=δ1-δ2) is +0.06bp, passing the condition since c<0.5

• If the questioned allele is 22, then the observed correlation with allele 24 is +1.1bp, failing the condition since c>0.5.

• If the questioned allele is 22.2, then the observed correlation with allele 24 is -0.86bp, failing the condition since c>0.5 (ignore sign) .

• Because the putative allele is an α.3 variant, the sample was separately reanalysed, confirming the above interpretation.

Modification of the above procedure may be needed for different loci but the same principles can be applied, given knowledge of rare and common variants; for example in HUMTH01, both 9.3 and 10 alleles are common, whereas 9.2 and 10.1 alleles are not observed (or extremely rare). Otherwise all remaining common alleles are α.0 variants.

Universal application of the relative measurement method

These principles, incorporating use of the 0.5bp rule, can be universally applied to interpretation of STRs, regardless of the platform or method used, provided that allele sizes are always cross-referenced to allelic ladders. The number of inconclusive results (apparent extremely rare alleles observed) is dependent upon the resolving power of the system used, but it is not a pre-requisite that the true measurement error <0.5bp.

In our hands the 'absolute' method of window estimation suffers from the drawback that windows must be reset when new acrylamide batches are prepared - other factors may necessitate the use of different windows in different laboratories. On the other hand, the relative measurement approach has a universal applicability because the windows are constant for each locus and independent of the method used. The principle of rule-based interpretation packages built upon experimental observations can be extended to enable construction of algorithms or computer based expert systems. This will automate the interpretation procedure, guiding the scientist to interpret results in the presence of artefacts, such as stutters, and to distinguish components of mixtures.

REFERENCES

DNA recommendations (1994) Int. J. Leg. Med. 107 159-160

Gill P, Ivanov PL, Kimpton C, Piercy R, Benson N, Tully G, Evett I, Hagelberg E, Sullivan K, (1994) Identification of the remains of the Romanov family by DNA analysis. Nature Genetics 6: 130-135.

Hagelburg E. Gray IC. Jeffreys AJ (1991) Identification of the skeletal remains of a murder victim. Nature 352: 427-429.

Jeffreys AJ, Allen MJ, Hagelburg E, Sonnberg A (1992) Identification of the skeletal remains of Josef Mengele by DNA analysis. For. Sci Int. 56: 65-76.

Jones D.A. (1972) Blood samples: Probability of discrimination. J. Forens. Sci. Soc. 12: 335-359.

Kimpton CP. Gill P. Walton A. Urquhart A. Millican ES. and Adams M (1993) Automated PCR profiling employing 'multiplex' amplification of short tandem repeat loci. PCR Methods and Applications 3: 13-22

Kimpton C. Fisher D. Watson S. Adams M. Urquhart A. Lygo. J.E. & Gill P (1994) Evaluation of an automated DNA profiling system employing multiplex amplification of four tetrameric STR loci. Int. J. Leg. Med. 106: 302-311.

Lygo JE, Johnson PE, Holdaway DJ, Woodroffe S, Whitaker JP, Clayton TM, Kimpton CP, Gill P (1994) validation of of short tandem repeat (STR) loci for use in forensic casework. Int. J. Leg. Med. 107: 77-89

Mills KA, Even D, Murray JC (1992) Tetranucleotide repeat polymorphism at the human alpha fibrinogen locus (FGA) Hum Molec. Genet. 1992 1 779

Polymeropoulos MH, Rath DS, Xiao H, Merril CR (1992) Tetranucleotide repeat polymorphism at the human beta-actin related pseudogene H-beta-Ac-psi-2 (ACTBP2). Nucleic Acids Res. 20 1432.

Puers C, Hammond H,A, Jin L, Caskey C,T, and Schumm J.W. (1993) Identification of repeat sequence   heterogeneity at the polymorphic short tandem repeat locus HUMTH01 [AATG]$_n$ and reassignment of alleles in population analysis by using a locus-specific allelic ladder. Am J Hum Genet. 53: 953-958.

Puers C, Hammond HA, Caskey CT, Lins AM, Sprecher CJ, Brinkmann B, Schumm JW (1994) Allelic ladder characterization of the Short Tandem Repeat polymorphism located in the 5' flanking region to the human coagulation factor XIII A subunit gene. Genomics 23: 260-264.

Urquhart A, Kimpton CP, Gill P (1993) Hypervariability of the tetranucleotide repeat of the human beta-actin related pseudogene H-beta-Ac-psi-2 (ACTBP2) locus. Hum Genet 96: 637-638

Urquhart A, Kimpton CP, Downes TJ, Gill P (1994) Variation in short tandem repeat sequences - a survey of twelve microsatellite loci for the use as forensic identification markers. Int J Leg Med. 107 13-20.

Warne D, Warkins C, Bodfish P, Nyberg K, Spurr NK (1991) Tetranucleotide repeat polymorphism   at the human beta-actin related pseudogene 2 (ACTBP2) detected using the polymerase chain reaction. Nucleic Acids Res. 1991 20 1432.

Weigand P, Budowle B, Rand S, Brinkmann B (1993) Forensic validation of the STR systems SE33 and TC11. Int J Leg Med. 105: 315-320.

Ziegle JS, Su Y, Corcoran KP, Nie L, Mayrand PE, Hoff LB, McBride LJ, Kronick MN, Diehl SR, (1992) Application of automated DNA sizing technology for genotyping microsatellite loci. Genomics 14: 1026-1031.

Identification through Genetic Typing of the victims of the Sect of the Solar Temple (Cheiry/Salvan, Switzerland)

C. Brandt-Casadevall, N. Dimo-Simonin, T. Krompecher

Institut universitaire de Médecine légale, Bugnon 21, 1005 Lausanne Switzerland

On october 5 1994, at approximately 1:00 a.m., a fire alarm was given in the village of Cheiry (Canton of Fribourg, Switzerland), at a farm lying just outside the village. The lifeless body of the owner was found in the living quarters. The fire had reached the upper parts of both the inhabited and the unhabited part. While searching for a vehicle in a space thought to be a garage, the police discovered a room that had been fitted for reunions. A concealed door led to other premises transformed into a chapel. Twenty two corpses were found scattered among the different rooms.

On the same fifth day of October 1994, at around 3:00 a.m., an alarm was raised in response to fires of chalets in the heights of Salvan (Canton of Valais, Switzerland). Inside one of the chalets, that was only slightly damaged by fire, fifteen corpses were discovered. Inside a second chalet, severely damaged by the flames, ten bodies were found. In a third chalet, that was completely destroyed by fire, no victims were present.

Our institute was commissioned to remove the corpses, to identify the victims, to determine the cause of the death and to help establish the surrounding circumstances of the tragedy.

It was later determined that the farm in Cheiry and the chalets in Salvan were owned or rented by members of the Sect of the Order of the Solar Temple.

In Cheiry, the 23 bodies had not been directly exposed to fire and could hence be identified visually by relatives, or through dactiloscopic or odontological examinations.

In Salvan, however, some of the corpses had been significantly damaged by fire, making their identification very difficult. In some cases, visual identification or identification through finger-prints was not possible; in other cases, odontological methods were useless (indeed, these were cases of either complete destruction by fire or complete lack of dentition). In these cases and as a last resort, it became necessary to search for available medical or radiological records or perform genetic typing. Importantly, four children were found among these victims. For these children, there were no odontological or radiological records of any nature prior to death.

We thus proceeded to determine the VNTR polymorphism on thirteen corpses, for which it was the only method that could lead to identification. The VNTR polymorphism was also determined in the case of several leading members of the Sect in addition to others means of identification.

This forensic investigation was carried out in close collaboration with the police which even occupied some office space in our institute for the occasion. Throughout the course of our work, we were able to request any and all material that was needed. This approach turned out to be quite advantageous : indeed, thanks to the collaboration between the police, family members and the institute, all medical records and samples were obtained on a very short notice, even in the case of foreign nationals (French people, Belgians and Canadians). It was equally simple to establish the family ties of the presumed victims.

With the exception of the removal of corpses on October fifth, the actual forensic investigation of the corpses from Salvan started only in October tenth. This delay made it possible for the police team to investigate the cases of the missing persons and establish the ties that existed between them. This, in turn, allowed to asign a presumed identity to most corpses in relation to their localization at the time of discovery. This presumed identity was eventually confirmed for each corpse from Salvan, thus greatly facilitating laboratory analyses, none of which having to be repeated.

The material taken from the victims and made available to us consisted of either a blood sample in EDTA or muscle tissue. The genetic profile was determined on the basis of VNTR polymorphism at the following loci : D12S11, D7S21, D16S309, D2S44 and in some cases D1S7 and D5S43. The probes consisted of MS43a, MS31, MS205, YNH24, MS1 and MS8.

For each victim, the polymorphism was compared with that of one or several other persons with an established identity, either victims or individuals without any connection to the tragedy.

The following method [1] was used :

- A saline extraction of fresh blood samples was performed. In the case of the victims, a phenol-chloroform extraction of the material was done. Controls carried out with our first extractions were troubling, since part of the DNA appeared degraded (Fig. 1).

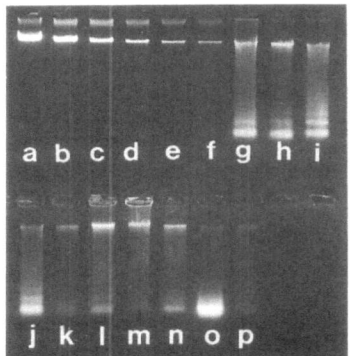

Fig. 1. Agarose gel electrophoresis with ethidium bromide :
- **a** to **f** : quantitation standard (from left : 500, 250, 125, 63, 31 and 15 ng)
- **g** to **p** : phenol-chloroform extracts from muscle tissues from victims of Salvan.

Our fears turned out to be injustified. The quantity of high molecular weight DNA samples was sufficient to allow Southern technique. Indeed, as you can see in some of our analyses (Fig. 2 and 3), the bands were well-defined and sharp, in spite of occasional background.

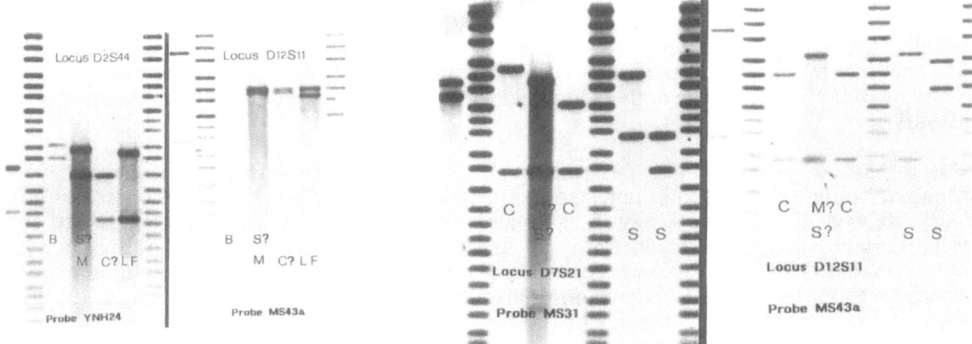

Fig. 2. VNTR polymorphisms determined with the probes YNH24 and MS43a

Fig. 3. VNTR polymorphims determined with the probes MS31 and MS43a

- The probes used were labeled with alkaline phosphatase and revealed by chemiluminescence.
- The results were analyzed visually and with the help of computerized equipment.

Every scenario of relatedness was encountered in the course of this work :

- Children identified relative to their mother and father
- Children identified relative to their mother
- Children identified relative to their mother and sibling(s)
- Individuals identified relative to their children and siblings
- Individual identified relative to her child
- Individual identified relative to his brother
- Individual identified relative her children and their father

Probabilities were calculated according to the method of Essen-Möller [2], using band frequencies found in the Swiss population.

All calculated probabilities were above 99.8%, the threshold accepted by the Swiss Federal Court above which a paternity is considered pratically proven.

An exemple is given by the case of a woman whose fraternity tie with her legal brother was estimated to be 99.98%. The corpse of the child was identified thanks to the determined maternity tie with the corpse of the legal mother (99.996%) and the paternity tie with the corpse of the legal father (99.993%).

In cases of multiple relatives, the calculation was performed solely for the main family tie, and the others were ignored. While we did considerer that the presence of the other common bands increased the probability of relatedness, we did not calculate any specific value.

An exemple is given by the case of a woman whose maternity tie with two legal children were respectively : 99.84 and 99.83%. She presented also some bands in common with two legal sisters.

Whenever a child was identified relative to one or both parents, the probability was calculated as in the other cases, but we always specified that the child was the offspring of a particular individual or couple, without excluding the possibility that the corpse actually was that of another child of similar age whose parents were the same individuals.

The same issue was important when a victim was identified relative to a brother only. While the corpse may indeed be that of the person presumed dead, it may also belong to another brother in the same group of siblings. This is especially true since it is more difficult to precisely evaluate the age of an adult.

The identification process through genetic typing of the victims of Salvan was completed in a period of three weeks. On Friday, November 4 1994 all the victims of the tragedy Cheiry/Salvan were formally identified.

Acknowledgements

The authors would like to thank Mrs C. Besançon and A. Grini for technical assistance.

References

1. Dimo-Simonin N, Brandt-Casadevall C, Gujer H.-R. Chemiluminescent DNA probes : Evaluation and usefulness in forensic cases. Forensic Sci. Intern. 57 (1992) 119-127.

2. Hummel K, Fukshansky N, Bär W, Zang K. Biostatistical approaches using minisatellite DNA patterns in paternity cases (mother-child-putative father trios). Advances in Forensic Haemogenetics 3. Ed by HF Polesky and W Mayr, Dpringer-Verlag, Berlin, Heidelberg (1990) 17-19.

Design of novel oligonucleotide probes for sex determination and its forensic application

R. Kobayashi, N. Iizuka*, and Y. Itoh

Department of Forensic Medicine, Juntendo University School of Medicine, Tokyo, Japan
*Medico-Legal Section, Criminal Investigation Laboratory, Metropolitan Police Department, Tokyo, Japan

INTRODUCTION

Sex determination of forensic samples is a very important element in the analysis of biological evidence submitted to forensic science laboratories. Although sex determination has been performed by Southern blotting (Gill 1987; Kobayashi 1988) or PCR (Kogan 1987; Witt 1989), we sometimes observed that the results obtained by PCR were different from those obtained by Southern blotting. Since the contamination of the samples found in criminal spots is usually unknown, PCR may sometimes give false results because of its high sensitivity. By contrast, although Southern blotting for sex determination is less sensitive and takes a long time, the findings obtained are reliable. The aim of our study was the design of the novel oligonucleotide probes for Southern blotting to lower the detection limit and to shorten the working time.

MATERIALS AND METHODS

Design of oligonucleotides

Two oligonucleotide probes (YJ1: TTC CAT TCC ATT CCA TT, Y1.3: TTC TAT TCC CTT CTA CTG CAT AC) were designed and synthesized. The region with 88.2% and higher homology with YJ1 is found in 45.8% of DYZ1 (Nakahori 1986). By contrast, the region with 80% and higher homology with Y1.3 is located in only 0.65% of DYZ1. These oligonucleotides were labeled with alkaline phosphatase by LIGHTSMITH II Luminescence Engineering System (Promega, WI).

Southern blotting

DNA was isolated from 123 bloodstains picked up in criminal spots as described elsewhere (Kobayashi 1988) and was digested with HaeIII or EcoRI. After electrophoresis of digested DNA on 0.8% agarose gel and transferring the fractionated DNA fragments onto a nylon membrane, the membrane was hybridized with each probe for 1 hour at 42°C. After hybridization, the membrane was washed three times with 6 x SSC for 5 min at 42°C. The probe-target hybrids was detected by development with NBT/BCIP. The DNA specimens were concluded to be male, when the 3.4-kb band was apparently observed.

PCR for sex determination

For comparison with Southern blotting, PCR was performed as described by Witt, M. et al. (1989). About 50 ng of DNA isolated from bloodstains was amplified using Y chromosome specific primers (Y1: ATG ATA GAA CGG AAA TAT G, Y2: AGT AGA ATG CAA AGG GCT CC) or X chromosome specific primers (X1: AAT CAT CAA ATG GAG ATT TG, X2: GTT CAG CTC TGT GAG TGA AA). PCR was run for 30 cycles of 94°C for 1 min, 65°C for 1 min, and 72°C for 2 min. After amplification, the PCR products were analyzed by electrophoresis on 2% agarose gels. The DNA specimens were concluded to be male, when the 170-bp band was apparently observed.

RESULTS AND DISCUSSION

1. In Southern blotting, the Y1.3 probe could determine the sex of specimens using 400 ng of DNA. By contrast, the YJ1 probe could also determine the sex using 25 ng of the DNA (Fig. 1).
2. The working time could be shortened from 23 hours to 3.5 hours by the use of the YJ1 or Y1.3 oligonucleotide probe.
3. Sexes were determined in 106/123 (86.2%) of bloodstains by Southern blotting with both probes (Table 1). Of the remaining 17 specimens, we could not determine the sex, because the yield of DNA isolated from these bloodstains was very low. However, no mistake in sex determination results occurred.
4. PCR was used to determine the sexes in 32/36 (88.9%) of bloodstains. The sex determined by PCR was different from that determined by Southern blotting in one case. In this case, the bloodstain spattered on men's underwear was used. Although the result of PCR demonstrated that the sex of specimen was male, the true sex of specimen was female. This indicates that PCR could detect not only a female's DNA isolated from bloodstains but also a man's slight DNA isolated from the man's underwear because of the high sensitivity of this method.
5. Although the sensitivity of Southern blotting is not higher than that of PCR, we did not obtained any false results by Southern blotting.
6. In conclusion, despite the lower sensitivity compared to PCR, Southern blotting using YJ1 or Y1.3 oligonucleotide as a probe is a suitable method for sex determination in forensic practical cases.

REFERENCES

Gill P (1987) A new method for sex determination of the donor of forensic samples using a recombinant DNA probe. Electrophoresis 8:35-38

Kobayashi R, Nakauchi H, Nakahori Y, Nakagome Y, Matsuzawa S (1988) Sex identification in fresh blood and dried bloodstains by a nonisotopic deoxyribonucleic acid (DNA) analyzing technique. J Forensic Sci 33:613-620

Kogan SC, Doherty M, Gitschier J (1987) An improved method for prenatal diagnosis of genetic diseases by analysis of amplified DNA sequences. Application to hemophilia A. N Engl J Med 317:985-990

Nakahori Y, Mitani K, Yamada M, Nakagome Y (1986) A human Y-chromosome specific repeated DNA family (DYZ1) consists of a tandem array of pentanucleotides. Nucl Acids Res 14:7569-7580

Witt M, Erickson P (1989) A rapid method for detection of Y-chromosomal DNA from dried blood specimens by the polymerase chain reacton. Hum Genet 82:271-274

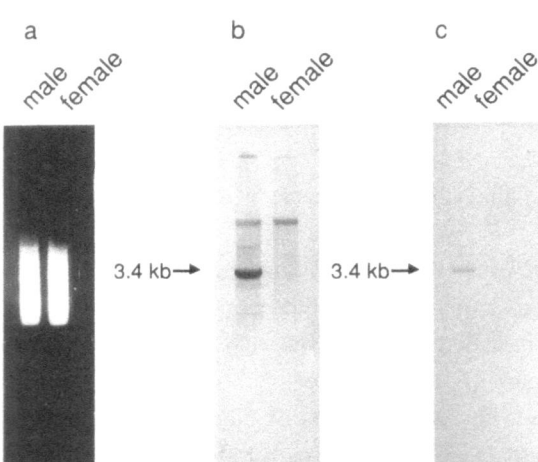

Fig. 1 Hybridization patterns of HaeIII-digested DNA. Four hundred nanograms of DNA was digested with HaeIII and fractionated on 0.8% agarose gel. After transferring DNA fragments onto a membrane, the membrane was hybridized with YJ1 or Y1.3 probe. a; ethidium bromide staining, b; hybridization with YJ1, c; hybridization with Y1.3

Table 1. The results of sex determination of bloodstains by Southern blotting with YJ1

Sex estimated prior to the test	Sex determined by Southern blotting: Case (%)			
	Male	Female	Undetermined	Total
Male	60 (89.6)	0 (0.0)	7 (10.4)	67 (100.0)
Female	0 (0.0)	40 (87.0)	6 (13.0)	46 (100.0)
Unknown	5 (50.0)	1 (10.0)	4 (40.0)	10 (100.0)
Total	65 (52.9)	41 (33.3)	17 (13.8)	123 (100.0)

CASEWORK EXPERIENCES WITH A MULTIPLEX STR SYSTEM.

M.J.Greenhalgh

Metropolitan Police Forensic Science Laboratory,
109 Lambeth Rd. London SE1 7LP
United Kingdom.

INTRODUCTION

DNA profiling using Short Tandem Repeat (STR) Loci has been used in casework at the Metropolitan Police Laboratory since August 1994. The system used is that devised by Kimpton et al.(1994). This uses multiplex amplification of four loci, (HUMVWA31, HUMTHO1, HUMF13A1 & HUMFES). Casework data have been collected over the first nine months of operation and a summary of the results is given in this paper.

METHOD

1) DNA extraction of stains by boiling with "Chelex" resin. (Walsh et al. 1991)
2) Quantification of the DNA using a slot blot which is hybridised to the Human specific probe D17Z1.
3) Multiplex PCR amplification using fluorescently labelled primers. 1-3 ng of target DNA where possible.
4) The PCR products are analysed using denaturing acrylamide gel electrophoresis on an ABI 373 Sequencer.
5) Sample details, processing details (gel number etc.) and final results are stored in a computer database and a report form is automatically generated for the Reporting Officer.

RESULTS

During a period of nine months from August 1994, 885 cases were analysed. This represents more than 5000 individual samples as each case often contains several crimestains. Reference blood samples are duplicated for QA purposes. In all 1497 blood reference samples were completely duplicated and no discrepancies were observed. A second sequencer is now in operation and additional staff are being trained for a planned increase in work. Estimates have been made that one sequencer and five staff could produce STR profiles from approximately 10,000 samples per year. It would be possible for fewer individuals to achieve this work rate for short periods of time but it has been found at the MPFSL that a considerable reserve of staff is required to cope with holiday absences, training and quality assurance activities.

Types of Reference samples:

SAMPLE TYPE	NUMBER	SUCCESS RATE (FULL PROFILES)
BLOOD	1497	> 95%
SALIVA	121	79%
HAIR	30	66%

Blood samples were the most numerous and the most successful samples in giving results at all four loci. (a full profile). Liquid saliva, mouth swabs and hairs were more variable samples and much depended on the manner in which the sample was taken. eg. some hair samples had no discernable roots and there was very little cellular material present on some of the mouthswabs.

Types of Cases Analysed:

CASE TYPE	STR CASES(%)	SLP CASES(%)
ASSAULT	26	4
SEXUAL ASSAULT	24	76
MURDER	21	16
ROBBERY	19	*
MISCELLANEOUS	10	4

* Results for SLP robbery cases were recorded under miscellaneous.

The sensitivity of the STR method has enabled it to be used in a much wider range of cases than Single Locus probe (SLP) analysis. The normal amount of target DNA for this STR system is between 1 and 3 ng however full profiles have been obtained with as little as 150 pg of DNA. Care has to be taken in interpreting results from such small amounts of DNA because of the increased dangers of contamination with extraneous DNA and possible loss of some of the loci. No instances of allelic "dropout" have been observed with these low amounts of target DNA. No attempts are made to amplify samples which have given a negative DNA assay.

At the Metropolitan Police Laboratory the relatively rapid turn round time of STR analysis and its sensitivity has meant that conventional blood grouping systems have been discontinued. STR analysis is used as an initial screening technique in complex cases prior to SLP analysis and it is often the only technique used where very small or degraded stains are encountered. Although SLP remains the system of choice if sufficient DNA is present, there has been a reduction in the number of samples submitted. This is probably because it is more important to get rapid results in some cases rather than powerful statistics. (The average frequency of occurrence of a Caucasian Quad STR profile is approx 1 in 10,000)

Types of Bodyfluid Analysed

BODY FLUID	% of ITEMS
BLOOD	77
SEMEN	8
VAGINAL EPITHELIA	7
SALIVA	3
OTHER	5 (hair, skin, bone etc)

Many of the assault cases involve the analysis of very small bloodstains which would be unsuitable for SLP. These were formally analysed using conventional markers such as EAP and PGM. STR profiles can also be obtained from the small amounts of saliva staining on items such as stamps,envelope flaps, cigarette butts and face masks with a reasonable chance of success. Items such as these, which are unlikely to work using SLP analysis could cause a considerable increase in the STR caseload as forensic scientists and police officers become more aware of the capability of the system.

Relative Success Rates of Different Types of Stain.

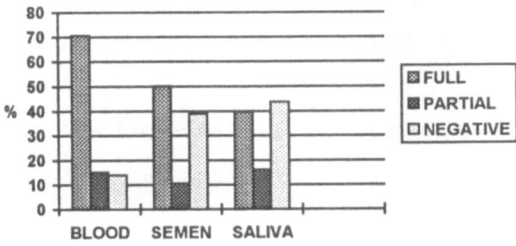

The overall success rate for STR profiling is high, especially for bloodstaining. There are indications that the lower success rates obtained with semen and saliva are due to contaminants which are not removed by the simple "Chelex" extraction method. From the survey data it can be seen that the higher the concentration of DNA in the stain extract, the greater the chance of obtaining a full profile, even when the same final amount of target DNA is analysed. Presumably this is because only a small volume of concentrated extract is required to give 3ng. in the reaction mix. This will cause any contaminant present to be diluted. If the DNA extract is dilute, a much greater volume of the extract and any contaminants present, will be required to give 3ng of DNA.

Mixture Profiles

Mixtures of bodyfluid have been detected in a wide range of STR profiling results. Approximately 7% of all STR profiling results showed the presence of a mixture of bodyfluids. When only cases with semen and saliva staining are considered this figure rises to 14% even though a method to preferentially separate semen from epithelial cells is used routinely. The relatively low number of alleles in the STR loci can be a problem as components from the different individuals are much more likely to overlap. Mixtures are relatively easy to detect if the components parts are present in approximately equal amounts. Where one profile is present as a minor component there can be difficulties in distinguishing the alleles from background noise and care needs to be taken.

CONCLUSION

The Quad STR multiplex is robust and reliable in casework operation giving results from a wide range of bodyfuids.
Its greater sensitivity than SLP anaysis will mean that more case types are suitable for DNA analysis.

References

Kimpton et al. Evaluation of an automated DNA profiling sustem employing multiplex amplification of four tetrameric STR loci. Int J. Leg Med (1994) 106: 302-311

Walsh et al. Chelex 100 as a medium for the simple extraction of DNA for PCR typing from forensic material. Biotechniques (1991) 1:91-98.

MULTIPLEXED DNA MARKERS FROM CIGARETTE BUTTS IN A FORENSIC CASEWORK

F. DE STEFANO, G. BRUNI, L. CASARINO, M.G. COSTA, A. MANNUCCI

Istituto di Medicina Legale dell'Università degli Studi di Genova, via De Toni 12, 16132 Genova, Italy

Introduction

As described by Hochmeister et al. [1], suitable amounts of DNA for Polymerase Chain Reaction (PCR) may be recovered from saliva cells present on cigarette butts. In such cases, detection of DNA markers may be limited both by degradation and poor amount of extracted DNA. The analysis of STR loci by fluorescent-based technology [2-3] may reduce these limitations. Moreover, coamplification of different markers in the same reaction [2-3] allows to reach more informativity in defining identity of samples.

A case where 53 cigarette butts found in 3 different cars were analysed by a fluorescent-base technology after a multiplex reaction and compared to 10 suspects is here described.

Case report

A truck-driver was compelled to drive his truck to a suburban place by 2 masked people got off a car (Car 1) in a parking area. Other 2 masked people reached the truck and they all transferred goods from the truck to a pick-up driven by another person. The 2 first assailants were transported by the truck-driver to an area where got into a second car (Car 2).

The truck-driver quickly informed the police and a man (suspect 1) in his car (Car 3) was arrested. A gun was found in this car. The day after, other 9 persons were checked because found into possession of the stolen goods. 2 among them (suspects 3 and 4) were seen to get off the car of suspect 1 the day before. Cars 1 and 2 resulted stolen a few days before the action. A total amount of 53 cigarette butts were found in the 3 cars and in the truck, according to the scheme in Table 1.

Our laboratory was charged to employ DNA techniques with the aim to reach a positive identification comparing DNA from cigarette butts to the suspects.

A multiplex amplification of 4 STR markers (HUMvWA31/A, HUMTH01, HUMF13A1 and HUMFES/FPS) was performed. Gendering of cigarette butts was done as previously described [4].

Materials and methods

DNA extraction. A rapid Chelex extraction followed by Centricon 100 concentration was performed for cigarette butts. Phenol/chlorophorm protocols were used for fresh samples from suspects.

PCR conditions. Up to 10 ng from fresh samples and 10 μl of Chelex extracted material was amplified by a multiplex reaction as suggested by literature [2-3]. Amelogenin amplification was done according to Mannucci et al. [4].

Products analysis. From 1 to 5 μl of amplification mixtures were combined with an internal lane standard (GS2500), heat denatured and loaded onto a 6 % polyacrylamide denaturing gel. Electrophoresis was carried out for 5 hours and 30 minutes at constant power (36W) on an Applied Biosystems automated DNA sequencer 373A. Genescan 672 software (Applied Biosystems) was used to determine fragment sizes.

Results and discussion

In 50 samples out of 53 results were obtained both by multiplex reaction and gendering. The most of the samples (38) were referred to 4 suspects and 12 to 7 unknown men and 5 women (Table 1). In 3 cases no amplification products were obtained from cigarette butt extractions.

Referring to the 4 suspects, PCR products analyses allowed calculation of casual phenotype sharing respectively of 0.8×10^{-4} for suspect 1, 10^{-4} for suspect 2, 0.4×10^{-4} for suspect 3 and 0.3×10^{-5} for suspect 4.

As expected, the use of a multiplex reaction by a fluorescent-based technology gave useful indications for individual identification of suspects (Table 1).

Identity values by manual methods and silver staining would surely be lower than that reached by fluorescent-based techniques, because of the poor amounts of DNA recovered from cigarette butts. The use of a multiplex reaction allows detection of different markers using the same amount of extracted DNA that is commonly used for a single reaction. Moreover fluorescent-based technologies assure higher sensitivity and may disclose results unidentifiable by manual methods.

Conclusively, it can be stressed that such a technique is a powerful tool for forensic casework both for sensitivity and liability, when it is used as suggested by validated protocols.

Table 1. Number of cigarette butts per car referred to the identified suspects and unkown people. In 3 samples out of 53 no amplification products were observed.

	Car 1	Car 2	Car 3	Truck	Total
Suspect 1	2	2	18	1	23
Suspect 2	=	6	=	=	6
Suspect 3	=	=	2	=	2
Suspect 4	=	=	7	=	7
Unknown	=	1	11	=	12
No results	=	=	3	=	3
Total	2	9	41	1	53

References

1. Hochmeister MN, Budowle B, Jung J, Börer UV, Comey CT, Dimhofer R (1991) PCR-based typing of DNA extracted from cigarette butts. Int J Leg Med 104:229-233

2. Kimpton CP, Fisher D, Watson S, Adams M, Urquhart A, Lygo JE, Gill P (1994) Evaluation of an automated DNA profiling system employing multiplex amplification of four tetrameric STR loci. Int J Leg Med 106:302-311

3. Lygo JE, Johnson PE, Holdaway DJ, Woodroffe DJ, Whitaker JP, Clayton CP, Kimpton CP, Gill P (1994) The validation of short tandem repeat (STR) loci for use in forensic casework. Int J Leg Med 107:77-89

4. Mannucci A, Sullivan KM, Ivanov PL, Gill P (1994) Forensic application of a rapid and quantitative DNA sex test by amplification of the X-Y homologous gene amelogenin. Int J Leg Med 106:190-193

DNA POLYMORPHISMS IN DENTAL PULP: EFFECT OF ENVIRONMENTAL FACTORS.

A. Alvarez García, I. Muñoz, C. Pestoni, M.V. Lareu, M.S. Rodríguez-Calvo, F. Barros and A. Carracedo.
Institute of Legal Medicine. Faculty of Medicine. 15705 Santiago de Compostela. Galicia. Spain.

This study was designed to observe the results of DNA typing on teeth subjected to aging, different temperatures and various environmental factors. The study includes the analysis of some DNA polymorphisms amplified by PCR, such as the HLA DQA1, D1S80, two STRs (HUMTH01 and HUMFES/FPS) and sex typing (XY homologous gene amelogenin).

Material and methods

Samples
Teeth were obtained from patients of oral surgeons (n=559), rinsed with distilled water, air dried and inmediately frozen at -20°C after the extraction until teeth were exposed to the experimental conditions.

Conditions of exposure (series)

1. Temperature
198 teeth were removed from the freezer and mantained at 4°C, 20°C and 40°C for periods of time ranging from 15 days (2weeks) to 36 months.
2. Water
96 teeth were submerged in the sea and in a river for periods of time ranging from 15 days to 6 months.
3. Burial
72 teeth were buried outdoors in a garden and in the sand of a beach (Pontevedra). They were placed approximately 20 cms into the ground for periods of time ranging from 15 days (2 weeks) to 6 months.
4. Outdoors air exposure
36 teeth were exposed to open air for periods of time ranging from 15 days (2 weeks) to 6 months.
5. Incineration
We incinerated 144 teeth by introducing them in a dental ceramic furnace (Programat P95, Ivoclar) for 1 and 2 min at 75°C, 100°C, 200°C, 300°C, 400°C and 500°C.
6. Aging (old samples)
Six teeth of 10 to 30 years old were mantained at indoor conditions.
7. Forensic casework
Three teeth from cremated bodies (corpses) and one from an exhumated body (of more than 50 years buried) from our forensic casework were included in our study.

Samples preparation and DNA extraction

After removing teeth from experimental conditions of exposure, they were rinsed with distilled water and air dried. The access to dental pulp was performed using three different methods (Smith et al 1993): mostly of the teeth were enterely crushed and the others were either opened by a conventional endodontic access or cut with a transversal section. Dental pulp was retrieved by a fine forceps and resuspended in water for DNA extraction with chelating resine (Singer-Sam 1989).
DNA was quantified using the DNA DipStick kit (Invitrogen Corp.)

Detection methods

System	Method
HLA DQA1	Dot-Blot with ASO probes
D1S80	PAGE+ Silver Staining
HUMTH01	PAGE+ Silver Staining
HUMFES/FPS	PAGE+ Silver Staining
XY Homologous gene amelogenin	ALF DNA Sequencer

Results

Table1. Results of HLA DQA1 system under different conditions of exposure and time periods.

Time	Conditions of exposure							
	4°C	20°C	40°C	fresh water	seawater	outdoors	sand buried	soil buried
15 days	6/6	6/6	6/6	3/6	6/6	6/6	6/6	5/6
1 month	5/6	6/6	6/6	1/6	1/6	6/6	4//6	5/6
3 months	5/6	6/6	6/6	1/6	0/6	4/6	3/6	4/6
6 months	4/6	5/6	5/6	1/6	1/6	4/6	2/6	2/6
12 months	6/6	5/6	5/6					
24 months	6/6	6/6	6/6					
36 months	5/6	6/6	6/6					

positive results/sample number

Table 2. Results of D1S80 system under different conditions of exposure and time periods.

Time	Conditions of exposure							
	4°C	20°C	40°C	fresh water	seawater	outdoors	sand buried	soil buried
3 months	6/6	6/6	6/6	2/6	2/6			
6 months				1/6	1/6	3/6	2/6	3/6
12 months	6/6	5/6	4/6					
36 months	5/6	4/6	3/6					

positive results/sample number

Table 3. Results of HUMTH01 locus under different conditions of exposure and time periods.

Time	Conditions of exposure							
	4°C	20°C	40°C	fresh water	seawater	outdoors	sand buried	soil buried
3 months				4/6	4/6			
6 months				2/6	2/6	5/6	4/6	3/6
36 months	6/6	6/6	6/6					

positive results/sample number

Table 4. Results of HUMFES/FPS locus under different conditions of exposure and time periods.

Time	Conditions of exposure							
	4°C	20°C	40°C	fresh water	seawater	outdoors	sand buried	soil buried
3 months				4/6	6/6			
6 months				3/6	2/6	5/6	5/6	3/6
36 months	6/6	6/6	6/6					

positive results/sample number

Table 5. Results of XY homologous gene amelogenin under different conditions of exposure and time periods.

Time	Conditions of exposure							
	4°C	20°C	40°C	fresh water	seawater	outdoors	sand buried	soil buried
3 months				6/6	6/6			
6 months				6/6	6/6	6/6	6/6	6/6
36 months	6/6	6/6	6/6					

positive results/sample number

Table 6. Results of the PCR markers analized after the teeth cremation with the temperatures and time used.

	HLA DQA1		D1S80	HUMTH01	HUMFES/FPS	XY Amelogenin
	1 min	2 min	2 min	2 min	2 min	2 min
75°C	6/6	6/6	6/6	6/6	6/6	6/6
100°C	6/6	5/6	6/6	6/6	6/6	6/6
200°C	6/6	6/6	5/6	6/6	6/6	6/6
300°C	6/6	5/6	1/6	6/6	5/6	6/6
400°C	6/6	2/6	0/6	4/6	4/6	6/6
500°C	2/6	0/6	0/6	0/6	0/6	5/6

positive results/sample number

Discussion

1. Temperature and aging

During the testing period of 36 months using temperatures of 4, 20 and 40°C positive results were obtained in most of the cases.

100% positive results were obtained for the two STRs studied and the amelogenin gene. Good results were also obtained for HLA DQA1 and D1S80 (more than 50% in the oldest samples).

There were no significant differences between the three temperatures studied (4, 20,40°C) and the results were similar for all three.

2. Water

Near 50% positive results were obtained typing STRs in samples submerged in water. Worst results (1/6) were obtained for HLA DQA1 and D1S80 and the best ones (6/6) for the XY homologous gene amelogenin. No significant differences were obtained between seawater and fresh water.

In general teeth submerged in water offer the poorest results. It is neccesary to keep in mind that the average temperatures of seawater and fresh water in Galicia range from 10-20°C and both are extremely rich in zooplankton. This explains the bad results obtained for this serie.

3. Outdoors/buried

Teeth exposed outdoors offer better results than burial teeth, but even in this case an average of 50% positive results were obtained in the 6 month old samples. Slightly better results were obtained when using STRs.

No significant differences were seen between teeth buried in sand or soil.

4. Incinerated teeth

With the exception of the amelogenin gene, complete negative results were obtained after exposure of 500°C during 2 min. The STRs offer clearly better results than HLA DQA1. The latter offers better results than D1S80 (only 1/6 at 300°C).

If the exposure time to high temperatures is reduced (1min), clearly better results are obtained.

5. Old samples

Teeth ranging from 10 to 30 years old were studied. 100% positive results were obtained for all the systems with the exception of D1S80 where only 50% positive results were observed.

6. Markers and aging

In general the best results were obtained with the amelogenin gene followed by the two STRs studied (HUMTH01 and HUMFES/FPS). The small sizes and the method of detection used after PCR amplification are the main factors in explaining this fact.

References

Singer-Sam, J., Tanguay, R.L., Riggs, A.D. (1989). "Use of chelex to improve the PCR signal from a small number of cells". *Amplications: A forum for PCR Users.*

Smith, B.C., Fisher, D.L., Weedn V.W., Warnock, G. R., Holland M.M. (1993) "A systematic approach to the samplingof dental DNA" *Journal of Forensic Sciences*, 38:1194-1209.

IDENTIFICATION OF HUMAN REMAINS USING DNA AMPLIFICATION (PCR).

J. Andradas, E. García, T. Cámara, L. Prieto, J. López.

Comisaría General de Policía Científica. Servicio de Analítica. C/ Gran Vía de Hortaleza s/n. 28043 Madrid. Spain.

INTRODUCTION

Positive identification of human remains has always been one of the main goals of Forensic Science. Fingerprints, dental or skeletal data were considered useful tools for this purpose until now (Farinelli 1993; Sopher 1993). However, the application of molecular biology methods in forensic laboratories has achieved new perspectives in the direct identification by resolving cases with critical amount of sample for analysis (Hagelberg 1991; Sullivan 1992). This can be made through the study of inherited characters in parents or relatives and direct matching with human remains samples. In this comunication we show the results in two cases received in the Servicio de Analitica de la Comisaría General de Policía Científica, Madrid (Spain). In one of them, human remains were buried over four years, in the other they suffered the effect of high temperatures because of a fire. These two cases were selected because they express critical factors in the necroidentification.

CASE REPORT

Case 1: on 11th August 1994, Police sent to our laboratory a purse containing several bones and a photograph of a possible person. These remains were found buried in lime soil in 1992 and they were studied in others laboratories but no clear results were obtained. After morphologycal studies (craneal and dental measurement, cephalic indexes, apical radiographies in the maxillaries and image superpositions) we asked for 5 mL. of fresh blood from the putative parents to compare with DNA extracted the from human remains.

Case 2: Police of Almería (Spain) sent us both maxillaries of a person who comitted suicide by setting fire to his home. As the former case, after mophologycal studies, fresh blood was obtained from the putative parents.

MATERIALS AND METHODS

DNA extraction and quantification

Extraction from fresh blood samples was made by standard methods (Phenol/Chloroform) (Sambrook 1989). In the first case, a femur bone and several teeth were selected. A layer of approximately 1 mm. was removed from the surface of the bone sample in order to reduce contamination from previous handling. The sample was ground to a fine powder and washed by adding 0.5 M EDTA pH 8.0 to remove salts (Manfred 1991). A lysis buffer was added to the tubes, and the extraction was made with the adition of phenol/chloroform. After this organic extraction, the aqueous layers were dialyzed and concentrated to approximately 40 µL. by using Centricon-100 microconcentrators (Amicon, USA). In case of teeth samples, after mechanical opening and recovery of pulp tissue, they were trated the same than the bone, except decalcification. In case N. 2 we only had upper and lower maxillaries. Subsequently, just dental pulps could be used for DNA extraction like in the former case. DNA quantification was made through agarose gel electrophoresis and "Quantiblot" (Perkin-Elmer, USA). RFLP's polymorphism was not tried because of the scarce amount DNA extracted from the human remains.

Amplification and typing

A total of 11 loci were amplified by PCR, using 10 ng. of DNA for each amplification. Bovine serum albumine (BSA, 160 mgr./mL.) was added to the samples extracted to facilitate amplification (Hochmeister 1991). Comercial Kits were used for D1S80, HLA DQA1, Polymarker (Perkin-Elmer, USA), HUMTH01, HUMFES/FPS, HUMvWFA31 and HUMF13A01 (Promega, USA) under conditions recommended by the manufacturer. Amplification products were analysed by reverse dot-blot for HLA DQA1 and Polymarker, Gene Amp detection gel (Perkin-Elmer, USA) for D1S80 and 6% denaturing polyacrilamide gel electrophoresis (PAGE) for the others markers. PAGE separations and D1S80 were silver stained.

RESULTS

In the first case, a positive identification resulted from morphologycal and molecular methods. The shape of upper central incisors of the skull overlaps with those in the photograph of the alleged person. In Table 1 genetic profiles of the human remains together with those of his alleged parents are shown. No exclusion can be seen in the markers and no result for HUMF13A01 locus could be obtained for sure. In the second case, a positive identification did not results through morphologycal methods. The possible race and sex, and the approximate age of the individual were made. In Table 2, genetic profiles of human remains and alleged parents can be seen. As in the former case, no exclusion was observed. These results were analyzed by calculation of Likelyhood Ratio (LR) or "Correspondence index" between the putative parents and doubtful remains: LR = X/Y, where X is the probability of the human remains if the couple is the progenitors and where Y is the probability of the human remains if the couple isn't the progenitors. In the first case, the LR was 68.721 and 3.146.873 in the second. If we assume an "a priori" probability of 0.5, the alleles obtaines from the human remains showed a match with the putative parents with a probability of 99.998545% in the first case and 99.99996% in the second one.

DISCUSSION

In our first case, human remains were found in 1992. Our laboratory analyzed this remains in 1994, and this demonstrates that in spite of delayed time and the conditions of the burial, the positive identification by PCR is possible.

Table 1. Genetic profiles in case 1.

L O C I	HUMAN REMAINS	PROGENITOR 1	PROGENITOR 2
DQA1	2-4	3-4	2-2
D1S80	18-31	18-31	18-24
LDLR	A-A	A-A	A-B
GYPA	B-B	A-B	B-B
HBGG	A-A	A-A	A-A
D7S8	A-A	A-B	A-A
GC	A-C	A-B	C-C
TH01	9-9.3	9-9.3	8-9.3
FES	11-13	11-13	11-12
vWF	17-18	17-18	16-17

In second case, the remains suffered the effect of high temperatures and equally positive results were obtained. In general, the traditional identification methods via fingerprint, dental records, clinical or personal reports are commonly considered as sufficient for identification of bodies when all available characters match to confirm an assumption (Farinelli 1993; Sopher 1993). But this comparison is not always possible because of the absence of antemortem data. In such cases, only DNA polymorphism test can provide a useful mean of identification (Hagelberg 1993; Gill 1994). PCR has the advantage of needing little amounts of sample and the results are positive even when degraded DNA is extracted from samples.

Table 2. Genetic profiles in case 2.

L O C I	HUMAN REMAINS	PROGENITOR 1	PROGENITOR 2
DQA1	1.2-4	1.2-4	4-4
D1S80	30-31	18-31	20-30
LDLR	B-B	B-B	B-B
GYPA	A-B	A-A	A-B
HBGG	A-B	A-A	A-B
D7S8	A-A	A-B	A-A
GC	C-C	C-C	B-C
TH01	9-9.3	8-9.3	9-9.3
FES	10-11	11-11	10-10
vWF	14-18	14-18	16-18
F13	5-7	7-7	5-6

REFERENCES

Farinelli M, (1993) In: Spitz W.V. (ed.) Medicolegal investigation of death, 3rd edn. Charles C. Thomas, Springfield, Ill, pp. 71-117.

Gill P, Ivanov P L, Kimphon C, Piercy R, Benson N, Tully G, Evett I, Hagelberg E, Sullivan K, (1994) Identification of the remains of Romanov family by DNA analysis. Nature Genetics 6: 130-135.

Hagelberg E, Gray I C, Jeffreys A J, (1991) Identification of the skeletal remains of a murder victim by DNA analysis. Nature 352: 427-429.

Hochmeister M N, Budowle B, Jung J, Boer U V, Comey C T, Dimhofer R, (1991) PCR-based typing of DNA extracted from cigarette butts. Int. J. Leg. Med., 104: 229-233.

Hochmeister M N, Budowle B, Borer U V, Eggmann U, Comey C T, Dimhofer R,(1991) Typing of Deoxyribonucleic acid (DNA)extracted from compact bone from human remains. J. For. Sci. 36, 6: 1649-1661.

Sambrook J., Fritsch E.F., Maniatis T. (1989) Molecular clonning: a laboratory manual. Cold Spring Harbor Laboratory Press, Cold Spring Harbor N.Y.

Sopher I.M. (1993). In: Spitz W.V. (ed.) Medicolegal investigation of death, 3rd edn. Charles C. Thomas, Springfield, Ill, pp. 118-136.

Sullivan K.M., Hopgood R., Gill P. (1992) Identification of human remains by amplification and automated sequencing of mitochondrial DNA. Int. J. Leg. Med. 105: 83-86.

THE SO-CALLED ALCOHOL-BLOOD-SAMPLE IDENTITY EXPERTISE

Huckenbeck W and Bonte W

Institute of Forensic Medicine, Heinrich-Heine-University Düsseldorf, Germany

Summary

From August 1986 to August 1994 the Institute of Forensic Medicine in Düsseldorf was engaged by courts to prove the identity of blood-ethanol samples in 157 cases. Non-identity was found in 11 cases. In the last years the total number of expertises has been declining but the number of expertises concerning non-identity has remained relatively constant. So in 1994 we found non-identity in every fifth case. This paper reports on the population data of the collective and especially on the efficiency of 'traditional' serological markers used in serological identity examinations.

Results and Discussion

In Germany - in cases of suspected dwi-driving - a blood sample can be taken by order of the police (Huckenbeck et al 1989; Huckenbeck and Schweitzer 1985; Huckenbeck et al 1987). In some cases the defendant asserts that blood samples have been interchanged (Haurich 1981; Henke and Hummelsheim 1985; Henke et al 1990; Huckenbeck and Bonte 1988; Kleiber 1987; Oepen 1986; Oepen and Trautner 1968; Püschel et al 1994). From 1986 - 1994 we were ordered by the court to check 157 identities by reexamination of the 'alcohol blood sample' and comparison to a freshly taken blood sample. Figure 1 shows the chronological development of expertises. There has been a significant decrease from year to year. In contrast the share of female defendants has remained relatively constant. The same phenomenon was observed in the cases of real non-identity (Figure 2). In our total sample (157) 11 cases of non-identity were found (7%) but in 1994 the share was nearly 20% (Figure 3). We found no interchanging of blood samples in the laboratories. In all the cases the non-identity was caused by third persons giving false particulars at the police station. Figure 4 shows the meaningfulness of the markers used in such examinations. Sometimes difficulties occurred because of the age of the 'alcohol blood samples', which are stored up to 2 years.

Figures 5 and 6 presents a comparison between the age distributions among dwi-drivers and defendants claiming non-identity with their blood samples. We found a significant deviation to the elder age groups (identity expertises). The reason is unclarified.

But back to serology: comparing the 11 cases of real non-identity the number of exclusions varies from 2 to 7 (Figure 7). Figure 8 shows the effectiveness of the serological markers used. The most exclusions were found in the Gm, MNSs, PGM_1 and GLO system.

In summary the presented data proves that the so-called conventional serological markers have been a sufficient powerful tool for identity expertises. Nevertheless in 1995 we started to use DNA systems in addition to some established conventional markers (Bär and Kratzer 1989; Henke et al 1990; Roewer et al 1989).

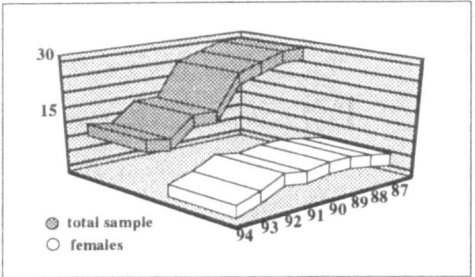

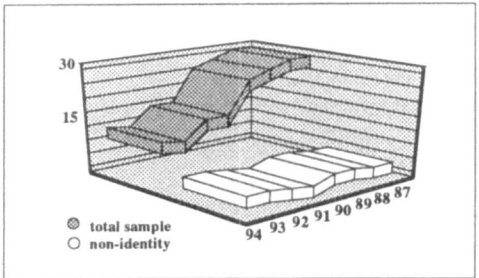

Figure1 Chronological development of expertises per anno.

Figure 2 Chronological development of expertises per anno

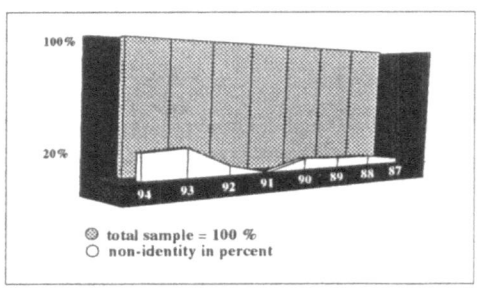

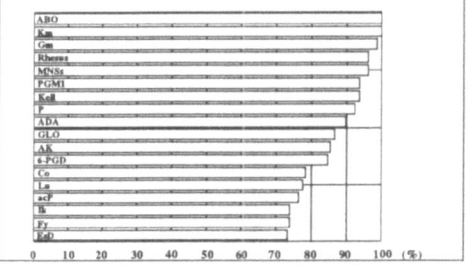

Figure 3 Relative share of non-identity

Figure 4 Successful typing of phenotypes in percent (n=157)

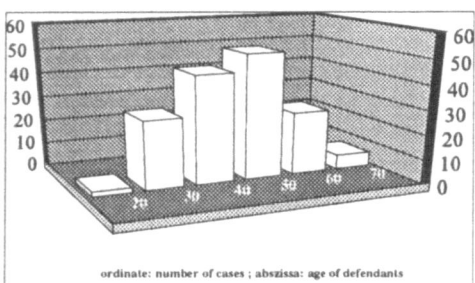

Figure 5 Age distribution (identity expertises)

Figure 6 Age distribution (dwi-drivers)

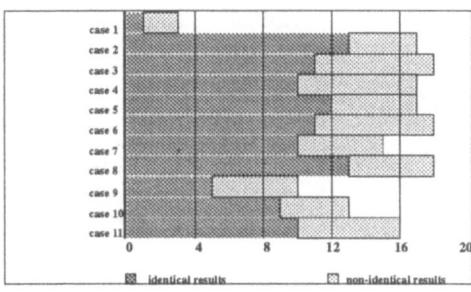

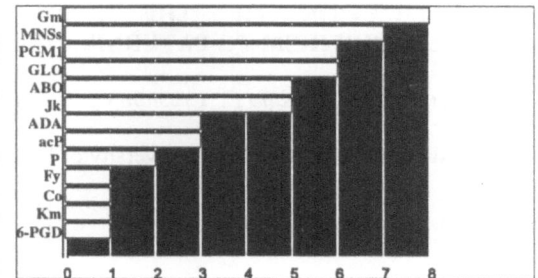

Figure 7 Number of exclusions in 11 cases of non-identity

Figure 8 Number of exclusions found per system

References

Bär W, Kratzer A (1989) Abklärung strittiger Identität von Blutalkoholproben mit DNA-Fingerprinting. Z Rechtsmed 102: 263-270; **Freudenstein P, Schmidt P, Bonte W** (1989) Female dwi offenders: the situation in Düsseldorf. In: Valverius M. (Hrsg.) Women, Alcohol, Drugs and Traffic. Stockholm, Dalctraf, S 63-64; **Haubrich T** (1981) „Vergleichende Blutprobe" als Prozeßverschleppung. NJW 34: 2507-2508; **Henke J, Hummelsheim G** (1985) Zwei serogenetische Blutalkohol-Identitätsüberprüfungen mit ungewöhnlichen Resultaten. Blutalkohol 22: 261-263; **Henke L, Hummelsheim G, Springer E, Henke J** (1990) Zur Bedeutung und Aussagekraft des hämogenetischen Identitätsgutachtens unter besonderer Berücksichtigung der DNA-Analyse. Arch Kriminol 186: 107-115; **Huckenbeck W, Daldrup T, Bonte W** (1989) Female drivers under influence of drugs. In: Valverius M. (Hrsg.): Women, Alcohol, Drugs and Traffic. Stockholm, Dalctraf, S 111-117; **Huckenbeck W, Schweitzer H** (1985) Atemalkoholbestimmungen mit den Blutalkoholkonzentrationen in den Grenzbereichen um BAK 0,8 und 1,3 Promille - Erfahrungen mit dem Gerät „Alcotest 7310" in Düsseldorf 1984 -. Blutalkohol 22: 417-431; **Huckenbeck W, Bonte W** (1988) Zur Möglichkeit der Falschetikettierung von Alkoholblutproben. Blutalkohol 25: 14-17; **Huckenbeck W, Barz J, Huch R** (1987) Abschließende Untersuchung des Gerätes „Alcotest 7310" im polizeilichen Einsatz in Düsseldorf. Blutalkohol 24: 1-10; **Kleiber M** (1987) Häufigkeit und Bedeutung von Identitätsuntersuchungen an gelagerten Alkoholblutproben. Blutalkohol 24: 253-261; **Oepen I, Trautner R** (1968) Zum Ausschluß einer Blutprobenverwechslung durch vergleichende Blutgruppenuntersuchung. Blutalkohol 5: 270-276; **Oepen I** (1986) Untersuchung gealterter Blutproben. In: Forster, B. (Hrsg.) Praxis der Rechtsmedizin. Thieme, Stuttgart - New York; **Püschel K, Krüger A, Wischhusen F** (1994) Identitätsprüfungen an gelagerten Blutproben. Blutalkohol 31: 315-322; **Roewer L, Rose M, Semm K, Correns A, Epplen JT** (1989) Typisierung gelagerter, haemolysierter Blutproben durch „DNA-Fingerprinting". Arch Kriminol: 103-107

APPLICATION OF THE STR ANDROGEN RECEPTOR (HUMARA) POLYMORPHISM TO PATERNITY CASES

Caenazzo L., Ponzano E., Crestani C., Bonan G., Cortivo P.

Istitute of Legal Medicine, University of Padova, V. Falloppio 50, 35121 Padova, Italy

INTRODUCTION

The human Androgen Receptor gene located on chromosome X (Xcen-q13) contains an high polymorphic trinucleotide repeat (acg)n in the coding region of the first exon (1). The polymorphism, was first described by Sleddens (2) for its usefulness in the diagnosis of Androgen Intensitivity Syndromes. The Androgen Receptor polymorphism was studied by Edwards et al. (3,4) for personal identification pourposes.

In order to valuate the possibility of application of this system to forensic casework of our laboratory we have studied a population sample and a group of paternity with femeale son.

MATERIALS AND METHODS

The sample consists in 123 unrelated individuals living in Veneto (Italy): 56 female and 67 male.

DNA was extracted in according to a non-organic procedure. Each sample containing: 10 ng of template DNA, 1 U Taq polymerase (Pharmacia), 1 μM each primer, 200 μM each nucleotide, 1X PCR Buffer (Pharmacia), diluted with distilled water to a final volume of 25 μl, were amplified in GeneAmp 2400 PCR System.

Primer sequences and amplification parameters are in according to Hammond et al. (5) with minor modification:

5' TCCAGAATCTGTTCCAGAGCGTGC
5' GCTGTGAAGGTTGCTGTTCCTCAT

95°C 45 sec, 64°C 45 sec, 72°C 45sec 28 cycles.

PCR amplified DNA samples were separated in a non denaturanting vertical polyacrylamide gels 12% 25 cm long. Running time: 12 hours 20 mA.

The bands were visualised by silver staining and classified by comparation with an homemade allelic ladder.

This system was succesfully co-amplified, with HumTH01 with the same conditions.

RESULTS AND DISCUSSION

Allele frequencies for the HUMARA were first determined. Among the Veneto sample 8 different alleles in the range 250-310 bp were detected as reported in table 1. The alleles number is less to that found by Edwards (4) this could be due to the sample dimension, and there are little discrepances in the number of repeats of the alleles in comparison to the study of Hammond (5), for this reason we don't called our alleles with the number of repeats but from A1 to A8.

To evaluate the usefulness of this marker in paternity testing we studied 52 family trios with female son previously studied with convetional and VNTR systems. In all 26 attribution cases there was allelic concordance as expected. For the others 26 exclusion cases, 18/26 were confirmed, this correspond to a 70% informativity rate.

In conclusion these preliminary results, suggest that HUMARA can be valuable, additional marker for paternity disputes relatively to the parental origin of the X chromosome.

Table 1. Allele frequency of HUMARA system

allele	frequency ± S.E.	allele	frequency ± S.E.
A1	0.0218 ± 0.009	A5	0.2363 ± 0.027
A2	0.0953 ± 0.060	A6	0.1172 ± 0.020
A3	0.1281 ± 0.021	A7	0.0535 ± 0.031
A4	0.3418 ± 0.030	A8	0.0059 ± 0.004

REFERENCES

1. Kuiper GGJM, Faber PW, van Rooij HCJ, van der Korput JAGM, Ris-Stalpers C, et al (1989) Structural organization of the human androgen receptor gene. J Mol Endocrinol 2: R1-R4

2. Sleddens HFBM, Oostra BA, Brinkmann AO, Trapman J (1991) trinucleotide repeat polymorphism in the androgen receptor gene (AR). Nucleic Acid Res 20: 1427

3. Edwards A, Civitello A, Hammond HA, Caskey CT (1991) DNA typing and genetic mapping with trimeric and tetrameric tandem repeats. Am J Hum Genet 49: 746 -756

4. Edwards A, Holly HA, Jin L, Caskey T, Chakraborty R (1992) Genetic variation at five trimeric and tetrameric tandem repeat loci in four human population groups. Genomics 12: 241-253

5. Hammond HA, Jin L, Zhong Y, Caskey CT, Chakraborty R (1994) Evaluation of 13 short tandem repeat loci for use in personal identification applications. Am J Hum Genet 55: 175 - 189

MULTIPLEX GENETIC TYPING OF CSF1PO, TPOX AND HUMTH01 LOCI IN FORENSIC SAMPLES

Castro A[1], Fernández-Fernández I[1], Alonso S[1], García-Orad A[1], Tamayo G[2], Martínez de Pancorbo M[1,2].

[1]Servicio de Diagnóstico de la Paternidad Biológica e Identificación Genética. Fac. Medicina. [2]Instituto Vasco de Criminología. Universidad del País Vasco. 48940. Leioa. Bizkaia. SPAIN.

INTRODUCTION

Due to their abundance, polymorphic nature and simplicity of amplification by PCR, microsatellite DNA loci (Small Tandem Repeats), represent a rich source of markers for genetic identification. Edwards et al. (1992) introduced the analysis of 3-4 bp repeat unit STRs which enabled the analysis of even 0.1 ng DNA samples. Moreover, these STR systems are suitable for the analysis of ancient or badly preserved specimens, which only contain very degraded DNA (Hagelberg et al. 1991; Gill et al. 1992; Jeffreys et al. 1992).

The 3 loci chosen for this work, CSF1PO, TPOX and TH01, have the advantage that can be analyzed in approximately 24 h, as they can be amplified and typed simultaneously. To evaluate the applicability of these systems to forensic casework, we have examined several samples such as hair-roots, semen stains, vaginal swabs and blood stains, each of these of varying ages. We could type unambiguously 30 day old hair-roots, up to 6 months old phenol-chloroform or Chelex 30%-extracted semen-stains and up to 13 year old blood-stains, showing the high applicability of this Multiplex system.

MATERIALS AND METHODS

Extraction of DNA from whole blood: DNA extraction from 700µl of whole blood was performed using the phenol-chloroform method and the concentration adjusted to 30 ng/µl.

Extraction of DNA from hair-roots: the DNA from hair roots was extracted by rapid lysis. The hair root was washed with sterile milli-Q H_2O and incubated in 200 µl of the lysis buffer (0.01M Tris-HCl pH 8, 0.09% Triton X-100, 35 mM DTT, 0.35 mM NaAc pH 5.2) for 30 min at 56°C. After boiling for 10 min and mixing for 10 s, it was spun at 12000 rpm and the supernatant recovered.

Extraction of DNA from semen stains: the DNAs from semen stains were extracted using phenol-chloroform or Chelex resin (Jung et al. 1991). With the aim of increasing the concentration of the DNA extracted, the following modifications were made: a 30% stock solution of Chelex resin was prepared and 30 µl of this were added to the sample.

Extraction of DNA from vaginal swabs: a differential lysis was performed followed by a phenol-cloroform extraction.

Extraction of DNA from blood stains: the extraction procedure was as Chelex resin above described.

Quantification of the human DNA: the quantities of DNA extracted were measured by slot-blot using the probe D17Z1 (Gibco-BRL) following the manufacturer´s protocol.

Mulitplex amplification: amplification were performed in a Perkin-Elmer 2400 thermocycler, using the multiplex system GenePrint™ (CSF1PO, TPOX y TH01) (Promega, USA) with minor modifications: increase to 0,75 U of Taq polymerase per sample and adition of 1 µl of BSA (10 mg/ml). Amplifications were checked by electrophgoresis in 2% agarose gels stained with ethidium bromide.

Typing of the amplification product: electrophoresis was performed in acrylamide denaturing gels (4%, 7 M urea) in a Cambrige Electrophoresis sequentiation chamber; bands were visualized by silver staining as Budowle et al. (1991), except that the ethanol step was omitted.

RESULTS

The analysis of CSF1PO, TPOX and TH01 loci in 161 individuals from the resident population of the Basque Country showed heterozygosities of 0.78, 0.64 and 0.72. The probability of two individuals sharing the same genotype with each of these loci is 0.08, 0.21 and 0.13 respectively, being their combined value 0.002.

The hair roots from 5 different individuals showed identical results when analized 7 and 30 days after pulled out.

The semen stains from 4 individuals were extracted by the methods of phenol-chloroform and Chelex at the end of 1 day and 6 months. Good results were obtained with these samples; only one of the 6 month old samples extracted with Chelex showed faint bands.

Three 1 h post-coital and three 10 h post-coital semen samples obtained through vaginal swabs were also analyzed. It was possible to obtain the male genetic profile in all the samples taken in the first hour, while, of the samples taken after 10 h or more, one of them could be typed for the three loci, another one only showed faint bands in loci TH01 and TPOX, and the last one did not show spermatic bands at all.

Twenty blood stains of 13 years old stored at enviromental conditions were estudied. The human DNA concentrations ranged between 0.2 to 1 ng/µl. A 72.5 % of the blood stains whose human DNA concentration was greater than 0.4 ng/µl could be directly typed. The remaining percentage could not be amplified in a first assay, despite showing a DNA content higher than the detection limit of the applied technique. To eliminate any possible inhibitor, every sample was microfiltrated by Microcon 30, removing simultaneously small DNA fragments that can interfere in the amplification reaction. Following this procedure, it was possible to type 95% of the analyzed samples.

DISCUSSION

One of the characteristics that an identification protocol should include is rapidity. Multiplex analysis considerably reduces the time required to obtain the genetic typing. Moreover, a protocol of extraction based on Chelex-100 can be used as PCR amplification does not require higly purified DNA, though it has to be taken into account that DNAs from whole blood or blood stains extracted by Chelex resin must be amplified as soon as possible because the continuous release of Fe^{++} from the hemo group interferes with the amplification process as was also described by Prinz and Schmitt (1994).

Another characteristic is that the analized loci must show enough power of discrimination. The probability of genotype matching with the 3 loci CSF1PO, TPOX and TH01 that we have calculated for the population residing in the Basque Country is $2x10^{-3}$. Therefore a multiplex genetic identification protocol of STR loci with high probability of discrimination can be proposed that should allow, in a first step, to straightforwardly reduce the number of cases of no exclusion that must be analyzed further employing a high number of loci.

ACKNOWLEDGEMENTS

This work was supported by a grant from the following institutions: University of the Basque Country (1994 Research Project) and Gobierno Vasco (Aquitania-Euskadi, 1994).

LITERATURE

Edwards A,Hammond H. A, Jin L, Caskey C. T, Chakraborty R. (1992). Genetic variation at five trimeric and tetrameric tandem repeat loci in four human population groups. Genomics. 12:241-253.

Gill P, Kimpton C. P, Sullivan K. M. (1992). A rapid polymerase chain reaction method for identifying fixed specimens. Electrophoresis 13:173-175.

Hagelberg E, Gray I. C, Jeffreys A. J. (1991). Identification of the skeletal remains of a murder victim by ADN analysis. Nature 352:427-429.

Jeffreys A. J, Allen M. J, Hagelberg E, Sonnberg A. (1992). Identification of the skeletal remains of Josef Mengele by ADN analysis. Forensic Sci. Int. 56:65-76.

Jung JM, Comey CT, Bair DB, Budowle B (1991) Extraction strategy for obtaining DNA from blood stains for PCR amplification and typing of the HLA DQα gene. Int J Leg Med 104:145-148.

Prinz and Schmitt (1994). Effect of degradation on PCR based DNA typing. Advances in Forensic Haemogenetics, 5: 375-378

A FIVE MINUTE PROCEDURE FOR EXTRACTION OF GENOMIC DNA FROM WHOLE BLOOD, SEMEN AND FORENSIC STAINS FOR PCR

J. Dissing, L. Rudbeck and H. Marcher

Department of Forensic Genetics, Institute of Forensic Medicine, University of Copenhagen, Frederik V's Vej 11, DK-2100 Copenhagen, Denmark.

INTRODUCTION

PCR does not require highly purified DNA and various methods have been devised to simplify the extraction of DNA for PCR. However, most methods consist of several steps and include harsh treatments to liberate the DNA; for example the widely used "Chelex 100®️ method" includes a boiling step and takes an hour or more to perform (Ohhara et al. 1994; McCusker et al. 1992; Nordvåg et al. 1992; Walsh et al. 1991).

It has been shown that incubation of isolated single cells with KOH and DTT at 65°C renders genomic DNA accessible to PCR (Li et al. 1991); also an alkaline extraction procedure for plant tissues was recently reported (Wang et al. 1993). Strong alkaline solutions exert a high denaturing and solubilizing effect on proteins due to ionization of aspartic, glutamic, cysteic and tyrosine residues (Ghélis and Yon, 1982). Incubation at alkaline pH may therefore disrupt and solubilize cell and nucleus membranes and denature nucleases whereas the primary structure of DNA is relatively stable to such treatment (Feliciello and Chinali, 1993). Furthermore, strong alkaline solutions may also dissolve denatured biological stains. For these reasons we have studied the applicability of alkaline extraction for the preparation of human genomic DNA from blood, semen and stains for PCR.

MATERIALS AND METHODS

Pooled blood drawn in sodium citrate from 5 individuals and pooled semen from 3 men with normal cell counts were used for the extraction experiments.

Extraction of DNA was performed by incubation of $5\mu l$ of blood or $1\mu l$ of semen or the equivalents of stain material with $20\mu l$ 0.1M NaOH in a 1.5ml centrifuge tube for various amounts of time and at different temperatures. The incubations were terminated by the addition of 180 μl 0.02M Tris, pH 7.5, bringing the pH of the solution from 13 to 8.5. The extracts ($5\mu l$ of supernatant) were tested for the presence of liberated DNA by PCR amplification (30 cycles) of a 404 bp segment at the ACP1 locus using primers 10 and 16 as previously described (Lazaruk et al. 1993). For extracts of whole blood the quantity of liberated DNA in the supernatant was also estimated by slot-blotting and hybridisation[1]. Removal of plasma proteins and hemoglobin from whole blood was performed by mixing the blood ($5\mu l$) with 1ml of distilled water, incubation for 5 min at room temperature, centrifugation at 12,000xg for 5 min and removal of the supernatant. The pellet was extracted with $20\mu l$ NaOH as described above. This removed about 85% of the protein content as determined by elementary analysis of crude and washed extracts[2].

---

[1] Kindly performed by Dr. B. Eriksen and G. Masumba using the ACES 2.0 Human DNA Quantization System (Life Technologies).

[2] Elementary analysis of Nitrogen, Carbon and Hydrogen was kindly performed by Karin Lindtog, Department of Organic Chemistry, H.C. Ørsted Instituttet, University of Copenhagen.

Blood and semen stains were prepared by spotting $5\mu l$ of blood or $1\mu l$ of semen onto clean cotton cloth. The stains were dried and stored in the dark at room temperature for 2 weeks.

RESULTS AND DISCUSSION

Initially the solubilizing power of NaOH was tested on heat denatured dry (90°C for 5 min) pellets of whole blood. It was found that incubation with 0.1 M NaOH at 70°C (or higher) for 5 min. completely dissolved the pellet whereas water or 0.02M NaOH had no effect. PCR on the neutralized extract showed that genomic DNA was rendered accessible as template. Extraction with 0.1M NaOH was hereafter attempted on whole blood and semen as well as on stains of these.

Whole blood:
Incubation of whole blood with 0.1M NaOH for 1 min or more at room temperature liberated high amounts of genomic DNA. Longer incubation time or higher temperature did not increase the yield (approx. 60%). For comparison $5\mu l$ of blood were also extracted by the "Chelex method" (Walsh et al. 1991). The yield of DNA extracted was significantly lower being about 50% of the yield of the NaOH procedure as estimated by the slot blot method (Fig. 1).

To test whether the extracted genomic DNA was generally usable for PCR, DNA segments at 3 structural loci (ACP1, GC and ABO) and two tandem repeat loci (D1S80, 16bp repeat and HUMTH01, 4bp repeat) were amplified (Lazaruk et al. 1993; Witke et al. 1993; Yamamoto and Hakomori, 1990; Thymann et al. 1993; Nellemann et al. 1994; Dissing, unpubl. results). Five μl of extract were used as template throughout. In all cases specific PCR product were obtained and the yields were consistently greater than when the same quantity of Chelex extract was used as source of DNA (Fig. 1). Silver staining of D1S80 bands as separated by polyacrylamide gel electrophoresis gave rise to some background staining. This was probably caused by the high protein content of the crude NaOH extract, and did not occur when a brief "washing step" of the blood sample was introduced prior to the NaOH extraction step.

Semen:
Incubation of fresh semen with 0.1M NaOH (with or without added DTT) did not give consistently high yields of DNA at any of the temperatures tested (ambient to 90°C) as indicated by the results of PCR with the extracts. However, the yields were greatly increased if the semen was dried briefly (75°C for 5 min) prior to extraction. Incubation with NaOH was far more effective at 75°C or 90°C than at room temperature. DTT had no positive effect at elevated temperatures. The time was not critical and similar results were obtained after incubation for 5 to 60 min.

Blood and semen stains:
Incubation of the stains with NaOH at 75°C for 5 min was effective with both types of stains, whereas incubation at room temperature or prolonged incubation (> 30 min for blood stains) at 75°C or 90°C yielded less DNA or less intact DNA as indicated by a decrease in the amount of PCR product (Fig. 2).

CONCLUSION

A simple short alkaline extraction step is sufficient for extraction of genomic DNA for PCR. Incubation of 5 μl of whole blood or 1 μl of semen (or the equivalents of stain material) with 0.1 M NaOH for 5 min at either room temperature (with whole blood) or 75°C (with semen and stains) results in the release of high amounts of DNA. After the addition of $180\mu l$

0.02M Tris pH 7.5 the extract is ready for PCR; no washing, treatment with proteases, boiling or centrifugation are required. Five µl of the 205µl extract are usually adequate as template in a 50µl PCR reaction. The extract is stable at 4°C for months indicating that endogenous nucleases are effectively denatured by the extraction process.

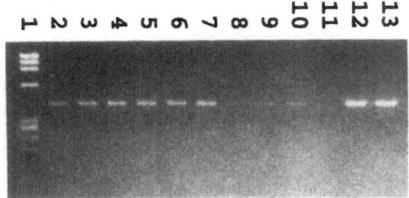 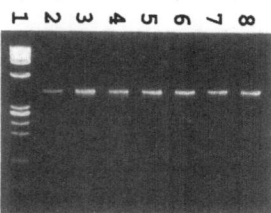

Fig. 1 (left). Comparison of DNA extracts prepared from 5µl of whole blood using different extraction conditions. Agarose gel electrophoresis of a 404bp fragment (ethidium bromide stained) PCR amplified with the human ACP1 locus as template (PCR using 5µl of DNA extract, 50µl reaction volume, 30 cycles of 94°C, 30 sec., 62°C, 30 sec., 72°C, 30 sec. DNA was extracted with 0.1M NaOH for 1 min (lanes 2,3), 5 min (lanes 4,5), 20 min (lanes 6,7) at room temperature or by the "Chelex method" (lanes 8-11). A control extract was prepared from 5µl of phenol/chloroform purified DNA (50ng/µl) by treatment with NaOH for 5 min as described above (lanes 12,13). Lane 1, φX 174 RF DNA HaeII digested 72-1353bp size markers (Stratagene).

Fig. 2 (right). Extracts of DNA prepared from blood and semen stains. PCR and agarose gel electrophoresis of PCR product as described in Fig. 1. Blood stains were incubated with 0.1M NaOH for 5 min. at room temperature, 75°C and 90°C (lanes 2-4, respectively). Semen stains were incubated with 0.1M NaOH at 75°C for 5, 20, 30 and 60 min. (lanes 5-8, respectively). Lane 1, size markers (see Fig. 1).

REFERENCES

Feliciello I, Chinali G (1993)   A modified alkaline lysis method for the preparation of highly purified plasmid DNA from Escherichia coli. Anal Biochem 212:394–401

Ghélis C, Yon J (1982)   Protein Folding. Academic Press, New York: 223-296

Lazaruk KDA, Dissing J, Sensabaugh GF (1993)   Exon Structure at the Human Acp1 Locus Supports Alternative Splicing Model for f-Isozyme and s-Isozyme Generation. Biochem Biophys Res Commun 196:440-446

Li H, Cui X, Arnheim N (1991)   Analysis of DNA sequence variation in single cells. Methods 2:49-59

McCusker J, Dawson MT, Noone D, Gannon F, Smith T (1992)   Improved method for direct PCR amplification from whole blood. Nucleic Acids Res 20:6747

Nellemann LJ, Møller A, Morling N (1994)   PCR typing of DNA fragments of the short tandem repeat (STR) system HUMTH01 in Danes and Greenland Eskimos. Forens Sci Int 68:45-51

Nordvåg B-Y, Husby G, El-Gewely MR (1992)   Direct PCR of Washed Blood Cells. Biotechniques 12:490-492

Ohhara M, Kurosu Y, Esumi M (1994)   Direct PCR of whole blood and hair shafts by microwave treatment. Biotechniques 17:726-728

Thymann M, Nellemann LJ, Masumba G, Irgens-Møller L, Morling N (1993)   Analysis of the locus D1S80 by amplified fragment length polymorphism technique (AMP-FLP). Frequency distribution in Danes. Intra and inter laboratory reproducibility of the technique. Forens Sci Int 60:47-56

Walsh PS, Metzger DA, Higuchi R (1991)   Chelex 100 as a Medium for Simple Extraction of DNA for PCR-based Typing from Forensic Material. Biotechniques 10:506-513

Wang H, Qi M, Cutler AJ (1993)   A simple method of preparing plant samples for PCR. Nucleic Acids Res 21:4153-4154

Witke WF, Gibbs PE, Zielinski R, Yang F, Bowman BH, Dugaiczyk A (1993)   Complete structure of the human Gc gene: differences and similarities between members of the albumin gene family. Genomics 16:751-754

Yamamoto F-I, Hakomori S-I (1990)   Sugar-nucleotide donor specificity of histo-blood group A and B transferases is based on amino acid substitutions. J Biol Chem 265:19259-19262

FALSE RESULTS IN THE HLA-DQα TYPING: TWO CASES REPORTED

P. Fattorini*, N. Malusa'*, A. Junge &, F. Cossutta*, F. Florian §, BM. Altamura*, G. Furlan* and G. Graziosi §

*) Istituto di Medicina Legale e delle Assicurazioni dell' Universita' di Trieste, Trieste (Italy)
&) Institut für Rechtsmedizin, Westfälische-Wilhelms Universität, Münster (Germany)
§) Dipartimento di Biologia dell'Universita' di Trieste, via Giorgieri 5, 34100, Trieste (Italy)

INTRODUCTION

DNA analysis by PCR-based polymorphisms is routinely carried out in the forensic laboratory. The most relevant advantage of the *in vitro* amplification is the high sensitivity of this technique that permits successful characterisations from nanograms of (also degraded) DNA samples (Bloch, 1991; Reynolds and Sensabaugh, 1991).

The HLA-DQA1 locus (DQα according to the old nomenclature) is one of the systems most used and the genetic polymorphisms of this locus can be shown by several methods: sequence analysis (Gyllensten and Herlich, 1988), revers dot blot hybridisation with Allele Specific Oligonucleotides (ASO) (Saiki, 1989) and digestion with restriction enzymes.

We present here two cases where the characterisation of the HLA-DQA1 locus by ASO gave unreliable results.

MATERIALS AND METHODS

Case 1

A 55-year-old woman was murdered, 13 years previously, by multiple head injures (laceration of the scalp and fissured fractures of the skull); her clothes, however, showed 2 large bloodstains (ref. n. 418 and 419) and 4 other bloodstains (ref. n. 414-417) that were used, at the time of DNA analysis, as reference samples of the victim. The reference sample of the suspect (who is the child of the victim) was the Na2EDTA blood collected at the time of the DNA analysis (ref. n. 423).

Case 2

A paternity test was carried out on Na2EDTA blood samples of a mother-son couple (ref. n. 487 and 486) and on tissue samples collected at autopsy from the body of the alleged father who has died 6 years before. The tissue samples were the following: cartilage of the sternum (497/5), cartilage of the ear (497/1) and ligamentus of the acetabulum (497/17).

DNA extraction

The DNA was extracted from all the samples by SDS/Proteinase K buffer, phenol purification and ethanol precipitation. Chelex procedure was also employed for DNA purification from the bloodstains for PCR amplification. The presence of human DNA was demonstrated in all the samples by slot blot hybridisation with a P^{32} alphoid sequence.

PCR-based polymorphisms analysis

The following systems were amplified: Coll2AI, D1S80, HumTH01, HumVWA, MBP-B and SE33. The PCR products of STR systems were separated by electrophoresis in polyacrylamide gels (5-8%) in 1xTBE buffer. TBE-agarose gel electrophoresis (3.3 %) was carried out to type D1S80 and Coll2AI loci. The HLA-DQA1 system was amplified and typed by the Amplitype Kit (Perkin-Elmer) according to the manufacturer's instruction.

The DQA1 locus was furthermore amplified by published protocols (Saiki, 1989) in 25 μl reaction tubes and the amplification products direct sequenced by PCR (Gyllensten, 1989). A

373A Sequencer (Applied Biosystem) was employed to analyse the sequence reactions. Negative and positive amplification controls were always included.

<u>HPLC (High Performance Liquid Chromatography) analysis</u>
About 10 μg of the DNA extracted from bloodstains 418 and 419 and from 2 postmortem tissue samples (ref. n. 497/5 and 497/17) were hydrolysed in 90 % formic acid at 170 C for 30' (Pääbo, 1989). After lyophilization, the samples were redissolved in 1 % HCl and analysed by reverse-phase HPLC using a Res Elut C18 5 μ column (Varian) in acetonitrile/Na-acetate buffer. Hydrolysed human DNA was used as reference standard; the base-specific peaks were identified by comparison wiht hydrolysed dNTPs (Boëhringer).

RESULTS
<u>Case 1</u>
The first characterisations at the HLA-DQA1 locus showed a 1.1/4 genotype in the samples 416T and 418 (Fig. 1). As these results excluded the parental relationship between the victim and her child (sample 423; genotype: 2/3), further characterisations were carried out: new amplification solutions were used and others bloodstains typed. The results are shown in Fig. 1. New extractions were then carried out from the bloodstains and all typed at locus HumTH01 as genotypes 6/9; the son of the victim was typed as 9/9.3. The bloodstains 418 and 419 were further typed in 3 other STR systems and they have been shown to share the same genotypes (7/11 at locus MBP-B; 14/18 at locus HumVWA, 14/21 at locus SE33); however there was always a "match" with the sample of the suspect.
Moreover, sequence analysis of the amplification products of the samples 418 and 419 demonstrated the presence of 239 bp fragments that show a 0201 genotype.
HPLC analysis shows the presence of anomalous peaks.

<u>Case 2</u>
The results of the characterisations at VNTR and STR systems are reported in Table 1.
By ASO, the HLA-DQA1 results were 1.1/4 in the mother and 4/4 in the son while the samples 497/5 and 497/17 were typed as 1.1/1.3 and 1.2/4 respectively. Samples 486 and 487 were sequenced and the results confirmed. However, sequence analysis of amplification products of the samples 497/5 and 497/17 shows the presence in both of 239 bp fragments corresponding to 0501 genotype. These two DNA templates were also analysed by HPLC: this shows the presence of an anomalous chromatogram.

DISCUSSION
Two cases are reported where ambiguous results by HLA-DQA1 typing by ASO were obtained. The case 1 refers to the DNA typing of 13-year-old bloodstains. The reasons of these results are unknown and several mechanism could be involved: contamination by exogenous DNA, inhibitors, etc. Nevertheless, in samples 418 and 419 only the presence of 239 bp long PCR products was identified; these fragments, however, have been sequenced as 0201 genotypes (a 2/2 genotype was also clearly typed by AS0 in sample 414T) (Fig. 1).
More reliable was the PCR analysis of STR loci. Four of them (MBP-B, HumTH01, HumVWA and SE33) were successfully typed and the results obtained were in agreement with those expected: same genotype in the samples 418 and 419 and one allele shared with the sample of the child.
As regards the paternity here presented (Case 2), it has been practically proven by six PCR-based polymorphisms. Moreover, the sequence analysis at HLA-DQA1 locus shows the presence in the alleged father of 239 bp fragments, corresponding to allele 0501 (allele 4 in the

old denomination). These data further confirm the paternity (genotype of the son: 4/4). The reasons of these ambiguous results obtained by ASO typing are being investigated.

As the HPLC analysis shows the presence, in both cases, of anomalous peaks, also the role of highly damaged templates is being considered (Golenberg, 1994).

REFERENCES

Bloch W (1991) A biochemical perspective of the Polymerase Chain Reaction. Biochemistry 30 (11):2735-2747

Golenberg EM (1994) DNA from plant compression fossils. In: Hermann B and Hummel S (eds) Ancient DNA. Springer-Verlag, New York, pp. 237-256

Gyllensten UB and Erlich HA (1988) Generation of single-stranded DNA by the Polymerase Chain Reaction and its application to direct sequencing of the HLA-DQα locus. Proc.Natl.Acad.Sci.USA 85:7652-7656

Gyllensten UB (1989) PCR and DNA sequencing. BioTechniques 7:700-708

Pääbo S (1989) Ancient DNA: extraction, characterisation, molecular cloning and enzymatic amplification. Proc.Natl.Acad.Sci.USA 86:1939-1943

Reynolds R and Sensabaugh G (1991) Analysis of genetic markers in forensic DNA samples using the Polymerase Chain Reaction. Analytical Chemistry 63:2-15

Saiki RK, Walsh PS, Levenson CH, Erlich HA (1989) Genetic analysis of amplified DNA with immobilised sequence-specific oligonucleotides probes. Proc.Natl.Acad.Sci.USA 86:6230-6234

ACKNOWLEDGEMENTS

We thank Prof. B. Brinkmann and Dr. S. Rand (University of Münster, Germany) for their helpful suggestions in proceeding of this work.

Table 1. The alleles shared between the son and alleged father are underlined. *: not performed; **: the sequence analysis of others PCR products are being carried out.

System	mother	son	497/1	497/5	497/1
Coll2AI	13/13	13/13	13/13	13/13	13/13
D1S80	18/24	17/18	*	17/18	17/18
WVA-A	17/19	15/19	15/18	15/18	15/18
MBP-B	10/12	7/10	7/7	7/7	7/7
THO1	6/9.3	6/9.3	6/6	6/6	6/6
SE33	20/26	16/20	*	16/19	16/19
HLA-A1	0101/0501	0501/0501	*	01../0501**	01../0501**

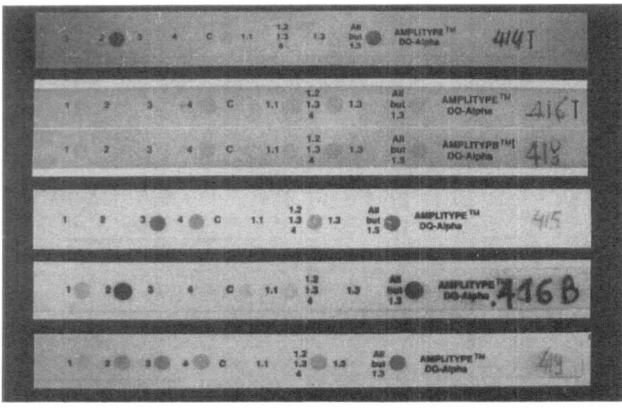

Fig. 1. HLA-DQA1 system. Revers dot blot hybridisations of the PCR products of 13-year-old bloodstains.

FORENSIC USE OF PCR DNA ANALYSIS IN HAIRS, ENVELOPES AND CIGARETTE ENDS

R. Fernández, E. Ramírez, M. Crespillo, J.A. Luque, P. García and J.L. Valverde

Sec. BiologÍa, Instituto Nacional de Toxicología, .Mº Justicia e Interior. Mercè, 1
08002 Barcelona. Spain

INTRODUCTION

The advances in the polymerase chain reaction (PCR) development enables a great discrimination in analysis of forensic traces. Samples such as bloodstains and semen stains can be identified, but it also allows to have a great information about forensic samples that contain a limited amount of DNA, such as single hair, salival cells in cigarette ends, stamps or envelopes and skin residues found in nails although they were old samples with degraded DNA.

This work is a revision of forensic traces analysed in our laboratory, the majority resulting from forensic cases, in the last three years.

MATERIALS AND METHODS

Samples preparation
Hairs: They are washed with distilled water and are examined by microscopy to ensure that root is present. They are cut 0.5cm from the root and put in an eppendorff tube.

Salival cells in envelopes, stamps and cigarettes ends: the sample is cut and put into an eppendorff tube with distilled water.

Extraction

Chelex 100 extraction (Walsh 1991)

Phenol-Chloroform extraction procedure is based on the related by Higuchi (1988) with minor modifications according to the samples.

Amplification

Amplification of specific regions of the following genetic loci HLA-DQA1, LDLR, GYPA, HBGG, D7S8 and GC is performed using the Amplytipe® HLA-DQα Forensic DNA Amplification and Typing Kit and Amplitype® PM PCR Amplification and Typing Kit supplied by Perkin-Elmer. Typing of these six loci is performed according to the kits protocols.

D1S80 Forensic DNA Amplification Reagent Set (Perkin-Elmer) is used to amplify the alleles at the D1S80 locus according to the protocol. The amplified products are analysed by vertical electrophoresis using 0.75 mm thick native polyacrylamide gel (GeneAmp Detection Gel, Perkin-Elmer). The electrophoresis runs for one hour at a constant voltage or 500 Volts. To size de PCR products, a 27-allelic ladder, supplied by the manufacturer, is used. After electrophoresis the DNA fragments are silver stained (Bassam 1991).

HUMTHO1 locus is amplified in 25 ml of PCR mix (Gene Print STR systems Promega) according to the manufacturers instructions. The amplified products are analysed by vertical electrophoresis on 0.75 mm thick 4% denaturing polyacrylamide gel (19:1 acrylamide: bisacrylamide, 7 M urea, 24 cm length) and silver stained. The electrophoresis runs for one hour at constant voltage of 1000 Volts with a fixed temperature of 51°C. Alleles were assigned by a ladder supplied by Promega.

All the DNA amplifications are carried on a Linus DualCycler Thermocycler.

RESULTS AND DISCUSSION

DNA extraction method differs according to the samples. At first, chelating resin was used for minute samples because is a simple and fast procedure. At present, this is the used method in cigarette butts, stamps, envelopes and salival cells in fabrics, often combined with Microcon 100 in order to concentrate and purify. In analysis of single hairs, the DNA is obtained by phenol-chloroform extraction because it provides better results in VNTR analysis.

The found hairs in crime scenes are not, in most of cases, freshly plucked hairs samples but shed hair and contain too little DNA amounts to analyse all the markers and often only HLA-DQA1 and PM can be analysed.

SAMPLES	N. SAMPL.	DNA EXTRACTION		POSITIV. EXTRAC.	DQA1	PM	D1S80	TH01
		CHELEX	PHE/ CHLOR					
HAIRS	88	36	52	64	44	6	1	1
CIGARETTE BUTTS	28	28	0	25	16	6	1	1
SALIVA	8	8	0	8	8	8	1	1
ENVELOPES	4	4	0	4	4	4	1	0
STAMPS	4	4	0	4	4	4	1	1
TISSUES REMAINS	3	1	2	3	3	3	0	0
TOTAL	135	81	54	108	79	31	5	4

Table 1 shows the different kind of samples, extraction methods and loci studied in this sort of evidences, in the last years.

The progressive use of VNTR loci at the same time as DQA1 and PM loci can be seen on Fig. 1. In 1994 we began to analyse D1S80 and HUMTH01 in hairs, salival cells and cigarette butts.

Figure 2 shows the rate of successful DNA extraction. In 1994, DNA extraction seems to give worst results because we began to receive some older and older samples so as re-examined cases.

In Fig. 3, the different sort of samples are related.

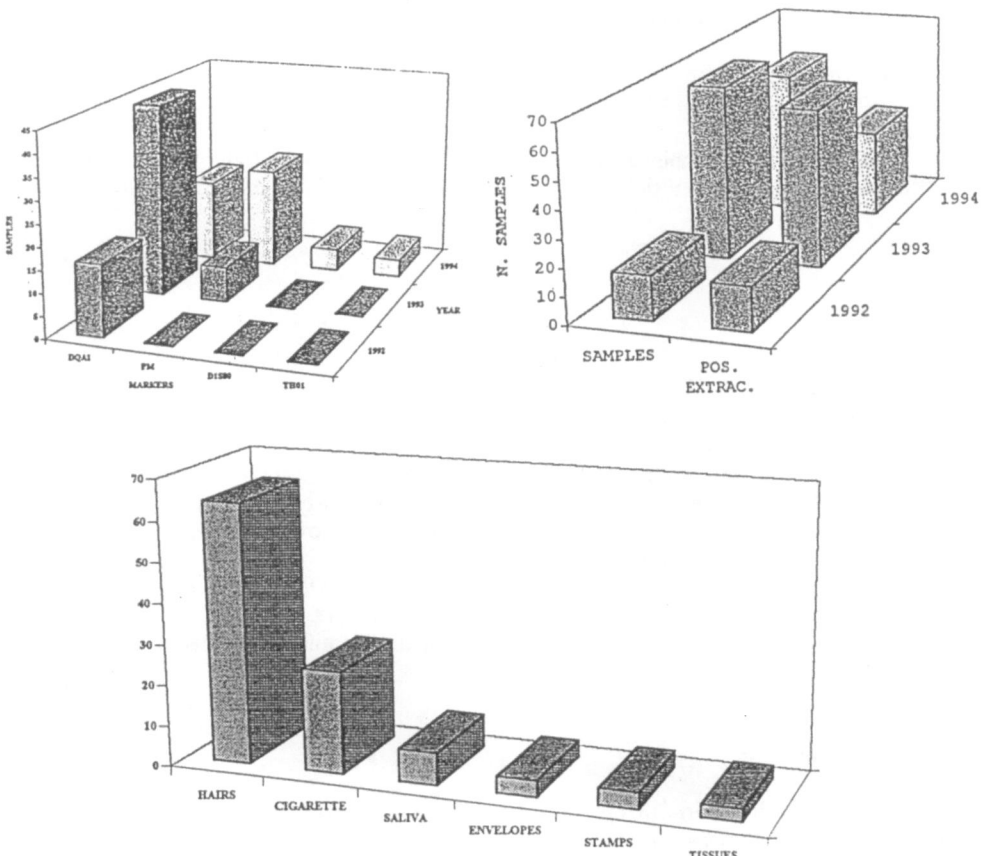

REFERENCES

Bassam B, Caetano-Anolles G , Gresshof PM (1991) Fast and sensitive silver staining of DNA in polyacrylamide gels. Anal. Biochem. 196: 80-83
Higuchi R, von Beroldingen CH, Sensabaugh GF, Erlich HA (1988) DNA typing from single hairs. Nature 332:543-546
Walsh PS, Metzger DA, Higuchi R (1991) Chelex® 100 as a Medium for Simple Extraction of DNA for PCR Based Typing from Forensic Material. Biotechniques 10:506-513.

PCR-DNA typing from beard samples

*Garofano L., *Lago G., *Zanon C., *Bruno M., *Carresi P., *Zignale G.,
**Gino S. and **Torre C.

*Servizio Carabinieri Investigazioni Scientifiche, Roma, Italy.
**Istituto di Anatomia e Fisiologia Umana, Università degli Studi di Torino, Italy.

Introduction

The analysis of DNA polymorphisms by means of PCR (Erlich H.A., 1989; Innis M.A. et al., 1990) has drastically increased the possibility of using some evidence that was not suitable until a short while ago.

Moreover, the introduction of STRs (Edwards A. et al.; 1991), HLA-DQα (Saiki R.K. et al., 1986) and Polymarker system (Amplitype[R] PM user guide, 1994) kits in forensic applications has greatly improved the discriminating power of these tecniques also in the case of a small amount of target DNA.

In this study we tried to extract, amplify and type DNA from the material remained after shaving, on blades and inside the electric razors. We think this kind of samples could be considered an interesting specimen about identification aims in forensic biology.

Materials and methods

We used both electric razors and blades specimens, sampling, at the end of a single shaving, the material remained inside the electric razor or between the blades of 10 individuals. Besides we took their blood as control.

Samples of material obtained from electric razors (Braun and Philips) were examined with the light microscope and the Scanning Electon Microscopy (Cambridge 110) to seek for the presence of cells, expecially nucleated ones. We collected the material with bi-adhesive tape stuck on a slide for the observation with the light microscope and on stub for the SEM. The former samples were stained with toluidine blue at 60°C, while the latter were gold-coated. As to the samples obtained from blades, to avoid possible inhibition by chemicals in shave soaps, this material underwent successive washings and centrifugations to pellet the skin evidence. The hair fractions were separated from the cells at low centrifugal force (2-3 g) to eliminate the hair constituents that could interfere with PCR (Yoshii T. Et al., 1993). The pellets were resuspended adding 300 µl of lysis buffer (Tris 0.01 M, pH 8.0, EDTA 0.01 M, NaCl 0.1 M, DTT 0.06g/ml, SDS 2%).

After a 3-hour incubation at 56°C, the evidence was digested with 10 µl of proteinase K (20 mg/ml) at 37°C overnight. According to our previous experience on the same kind of evidence the extraction was performed following the "salting-out" protocol (Miller S. et al., 1988), that proved to be more efficient than phenol-chloroform (Sambrook J. et al., 1989) and Chelex[R] ones (Walsh P.S. et al., 1991). DNA extracts were finally purified with Centricon-100.

The DNA was then quantified by means of both agarose gel electrophoresis (0.8%) stained with ethidium bromide and UV Spectrophotometry (Beckman DU 650).

We amplified 3 STR systems: HUMTH01 (Polymeropoulos M.H. et al., 1991), HUMVWFA31 (Kimpton C. et al., 1992), HUMBFXIII (Nishimura D.Y. et al., 1992); one AMP-FLP: D1S80 (Budowle B.J. et al., 1991); the HLA-DQα sequences and the 5 different loci of the Amplitype^R PM system (LDLR, GYPA, HBGG, D7S8, GC).

PCR protocols were carried out on a Perkin-Elmer 9600 Thermal Cycler according to the literature for D1S80 and as suggested by Promega (Geneprint^{TM} STR System) for HUMVWFA31, HUMTH01 and HUMBFXIII and by Perkin-Elmer (AmpliType^R HLA-DQα and AmpliType^R PM) for HLA-DQα and Polymarker loci. The typing of PCR products was achieved by horizontal polyacrylamide gel electrophoresis with silver staining for D1S80 and STRs and by means of reverse dot blot procedure as concern HLA-DQα and Polymarker.

Results and discussion

The observation with light microscope and SEM showed the presence of hair debris and epidermal cells. The aspect of the debris changes according to the different electric razors used. Rare nucleated cells are always present. These cells could explain the outcome that we obtained in extraction, amplification and typing of DNA. The successful typing percentage changes from 60% to 73% according to the different loci. We didn't note a significatively different rate about positive results from blades and electric razors (respectively 65% and 69%).

The results we obtained are summerized in the table, that shows the relatively successful typing rate, according to the systems used and the kind of specimens (razor or blade). We think this method could be used for forensic purposes in identification casework.

Table 1

Successful typing rate

Locus	electric razors (samples typed: **61**)	blades (samples typed: **66**)
HUMVWFA31	70 %	70 %
HUMBFXIII	60 %	60 %
HUMTH01	73 %	70 %
D1S80	67 %	70 %
HLA-DQα	70 %	60 %
Polymarker system	70 %	60 %

References

Amplitype[R] PM user guide, (1994). Roche Molecular System Inc., Branchburg, New Jersey.

Budowle B.J. et al., (1991). Analysis of the VNTR locus D1S80 by the PCR followed by high-resolution PAGE. Am. J. Hum. Genet. 48, 137-144.

Bugawan T.L., Saiki R.K., Levenson C.H., Watson R.W. and Erlich H.A., (1988). The use of non-radioactive oligonucleotide probes to analyse enzymatically amplified DNA for prenatal diagnosis and forensic HLA typing. Bio-Technology 6, 943-947.

Edwards A. et al., (1991). DNA typing and genetic mapping with trimeric and tetrameric tandem repeats; Am. J. Hum. Genet. 49, 746-751.

Erlich H.A. (1989) PCR technology: principles and applications for DNA amplification. Stockton Press, New York.

Innis M.A. et al., (1990). PCR protocols: a guide to methods and applications; Academic Press, San Diego.

Kimpton C., Walton A. and Gill P., (1992). A further tetranucleotide repeat polymorphism in the vWF gene. Hum. Mol. Genet. 1, 287.

Miller S.A., Dykes D.D. and Polesky H.F., (1988). A simple salting out procedure for extracting DNA from human nucleated cells. Nucl. Acids Res. 16, 1215.

Nishimura D.Y. and Murray J.C., (1992). A tetranucleotide repeat for the F13B locus. Nucl. Acids Res. 20, 1167.

Polymeropoulos M.H., Rath D.S., Xiao H. and Merril C.R., (1991). Tetranucleotide repeat polymorphism at the human tyrosine hydroxylase gene (TH). Nucl. Acids Res. 19, 3753.

Saiki R.K., Bugawan T.L., Horn G.T., Mullis K.B.and Erlich A.A., (1986). Analysis of enzimatically amplified β-globin and HLA-DQα DNA with allele specific oligonucleotide probes. Nature 324, 163-166.

Sambrook J., Fritsch E.F. and Maniatis T., (1989). Molecular Cloning: a laboratory manual. Second edition, Cold Spring Harbor, New York.

Walsh P.S., Metzer D.A. and Higuchi R., (1991). Chelex [R] 100 as a medium for simple extraction of DNA for PCR- based typing from forensic material. Biotechniques 10, 506-513.

Yoshii T., Akiyama K., Tamura K. and Ishiyama I., (1993). PCR inhibitor: water soluble melanin, which inhibits DNA polimerases and DNases. Jpn. J. Legal Med. 47, 393-396.

PCR based analyses of epidermal cells found on adhesive tape

*Garofano L., *Lago G., *Zanon C., *Virgili A., *D'Errico G., *Vespi G.,
**Gino S. and **Torre C.

*Servizio Carabinieri Investigazioni Scientifiche,
**Istituto di Anatomia e Fisiologia Umana, Università degli Studi di Torino, Italy.

Introduction

Adhesive tapes are commonly used by Police Forces to collect Gun Shot Residues (GSR). In a previous experiment (Torre C. and Gino S., submitted to J. Forensic Sci.) it was observed that enough DNA can be extracted, amplified and typed for the HLA-DQα locus (Saiki et al., 1986), in order to attribute with certainty a GSR stub and/or to obtain samples for DNA analyses.

Adhesive tapes are often used in kidnapping cases or to wrap packages, and can represent important evidence related to crimes. For this reason, we investigated whether the cellular material stuck on different adhesive tapes could be employed for genetic analyses.

Materials and methods

We used common available tapes (plastic packing tape, Comet[TM]; strapping tape, Asirom90[TM]; transparent tape, Syrom[TM]; stub). The samples (54) from 6 individuals were collected from various skin areas as perioral region, wrist, back of hand and fingers.

All samples were obtained pressing many times the adhesive tapes on the collecting surface until the adhesive power was lost. From the same individuals blood samples were also taken for a comparative study.

For each specimen, a fragment of about 1.5 cm^2 was cut and then placed into 1.5 ml Eppendorf tube adding 300 μl of lysis buffer (Tris 0.01 M pH 8.0, EDTA 0.01 M, NaCl 0.1 M, DTT 0.06 g/ml, SDS 2%). After 1-hour incubation at 37°C, the evidence was digested with 10 μl of proteinase K (20 mg/ml) at 37°C overnight. Then we carried out three different extraction procedures: phenol-chloroform (Sambrook et al., 1989); Chelex[R] method (Walsh et al., 1991) and the "salting-out" protocol (Miller et al., 1988). All extracts were purified using Centricon[R]-100.

The extracted DNA was then quantified by means of both agarose gel electrophoresis (0.8%) stained with ethidium bromide and UV Spectrophotometry (Beckman DU 650).

DNA was amplified (Erlich H.A., 1989; Innis M.A. et al.,1990) to investigate some STRs (Edwards et al., 1991) and a AMP-FLP commonly used in our laboratory: HUMTH01 (Polymeropoulos M.H. et al., 1991), HUMVWFA31 (Kimpton C. et al., 1992), HUMBFXIII (Nishimura D.Y. et al., 1992), D1S80 (Budowle B.J. et al., 1991); as well as HLA-DQα and Polymarker loci (Amplitype[R] PM user guide, 1994).

Amplifications were carried out in a Perkin-Elmer 9600 Thermal Cycler according to: literature for D1S80, Promega Technical guide (Geneprint™ STR System) for STRs, and Perkin-Elmer AmpliType^R HLA-DQα and AmpliType^R PM.

Typing of PCR products was achieved by horizontal polyacrylamide gel electrophoresis followed by silver staining (D1S80 and STRs) and by means of reverse dot blot procedure (HLA-DQα and Polymarker system loci).

From the same anatomic regions some samples were prepared in order to be studied, to check for presence of cells, by light microscope and Scanning Electron Microscope (SEM, Cambridge 110). The SEM specimens were gold coated, while the light microscope ones were stained with toluidine blue at 60°C .

Results and discussion

Microscopical study of adhesive tapes showed the presence of cells coming from the stratum corneum in all the examined regions. There were few cells in the palm of hand, while in the other regions there was an almost continous layer of cells. All samples showed some nucleated cells.

The DNA results (see tables) were quite homogeneous in the different collecting areas. The perioral surface proved to be the best source of sampling (31% successful typings); this is probably related to the contribution provided by the epithelial tissue cells coming from the oral cavity and a thinner stratum corneum layer in this region. Negative results came only from the fingers skin area, probably because this area is more exposed than others to mechanical and chemical stresses. We would like enphasize the effectiveness of the method on the perioral and the wrist regions for investigative purposes.

Till now we achieved the best results with the "salting-out" method.

As regards the plastic packing tape, the strapping one, and the stub, they showed good possibilities of success (20%, 14% and 33%, respectively). The reason could be the more powerful tackiness of these tapes compared to the conventional transparent one.

In conclusion, even tough, as a matter of fact, the present study had a generally low parcentage of positive results (16% in 248 typings), we think the material stuck on the adhesive tapes can be considered an interesting source of DNA for investigation purposes.

Successful typing rates

Table 1

Locus	samples typed: 248
HUMVWFA31	25 %
HUMBFXIII	5 %
HUMTH01	24 %
D1S80	14 %
HLA-DQα	19 %
Polymarker system	25 %

Table 2

Sample source	samples typed: **248**
Mouth	**31 %**
Wrist	**20 %**
Back of Hand	**15 %**
Fingers	**2 %**

Table 3

Type of tape	samples typed: **248**
Plastic Packing Tape	**20 %**
Strapping Tape	**14 %**
Transparent Tape	**4 %**
Stub	**33 %**

References

Amplitype[R] PM User Guide, (1994). Roche Molecular System Inc., Branchburg, New Jersey.

Budowle B.J. et al., (1991). Analysis of the VNTR locus D1S80 by the PCR followed by high-resolution PAGE. Am. J. Hum. Genet. 48, 137-144.

Edwards A. et al., (1991). DNA typing and genetic mapping with trimeric and tetrameric tandem repeats; Am. J. Hum. Genet. 49, 746-751.

Erlich H.A. (1989). PCR technology: principles and applications for DNA amplification. Stockton Press, New York.

Innis M.A. et al., (1990). PCR protocols: a guide to methods and applications. Academic Press, San Diego.

Kimpton C., Walton A. and Gill P., (1992). A further tetranucleotide repeat polymorphism in the vWF gene. Hum. Mol. Genet. 1, 287.

Miller S.A., Dykes D.D. and Polesky H.F., (1988). A simple salting out procedure for extracting DNA from human nucleated cells. Nucl. Acids Res. 16, 1215.

Nishimura D.Y. and Murray J.C., (1992). A tetranucleotide repeat for the F13B locus. Nucl. Acids Res. 20, 1167.

Polymeropoulos M.H., Rath D.S., Xiao H. and Merril C.R., (1991). Tetranucleotide repeat polymorphism at the human tyrosine hydroxylase gene (TH). Nucl. Acids Res. 19, 3753.

Saiki R.K., Bugawan T.L., Horn G.T., Mullis K.B.and Erlich A.A., (1986). Analysis of enzimatically amplified β-globin and HLA-DQα DNA with allele specific oligonucleotide probes. Nature 324, 163-166.

Sambrook J., Fritsch E.F. and Maniatis T., (1989). Molecular Cloning: a laboratory manual. Second edition, Cold Spring Harbor, New York.

Walsh P.S., Metzer D.A. and Higuchi R., (1991). Chelex[R] 100 as a medium for simple extraction of DNA for PCR-based typing from forensic material. Biotechniques 10, 506-513.

DETERMINATION OF SEX IN DENTAL PULP USING PCR

Gremo A, Martínez MA, Sanchez J, Landete C

Toxicología y Legislación Sanitaria. UCM. 28040 Madrid. Spain.

INTRODUCTION

Dental pulp has proven to be a very good source of biological evidence for forensic casework. It location in a especially protected cavity makes dental pulp very valuable. The diagnosis of the sex has been elected like parameter of study by being a binary variable of easy confirmation and included the only variable that could be contrasted in samples of human bones remains. This simple parameter allows to study the behavior of the DNA obtained of dental pulp subjected to different external agents and as well as the antiquity.

MATERIALS AND METHODS

532 pieces has been analized to teeth (the half of the masculine sex and the half of the femenine).

The extraction of DNA of the pulps was carried out for the method of the phenol/chloroform (Maniatis 1989). The amplifications were performed in a final volume of 25 µl in a Perkin-Elmer thermocycler. Each reaction contained 20-500 ng of DNA relying of the characteristics of the samples, 1 U taq polymerase (Boehringer), 10 mM tris-HCl pH 8.3, 50 mM KCl, 1.5 mM Mg Cl_2, 200 µM of each dNTP and 0.4 µM of each primer X_{145} and X_{146} for the amplification of the fragment of the X chromosome and 0.1 µM of each primer Y_{1-3} and Y_{1-4} for the amplification of Y-specific fragment. The cycles temperatures were as follows: 95 ºC (1 min), 54 ºC (1min), 72 ºC (1 min), 28 cycles with an increment in the phase of extension of 6 seconds. Prior to the first cycle the DNA was denatured at 95 ºC for 10 min and after the last cycle an additional extension at 72 ºC for 10 min was performed. This protocol was based in Pfitzinger et al. (1993) but carrying out the amplification for separating of the fragment of the X chromosome and the Y chromosome.

The fragments was visualized on submarines agarose gels with tris/acetic/edta (pH 8.0) 1x as buffer.

RESULTS AND DISCUSSION

A) Results in relationship to the state of the dental piece:
Number of studied pieces:198, conserved at room temperature, maximal antiquity one week.
The healthful pieces and with cavities, but without pulp damage they allow to get excellent results (100% of success), however the pieces with cavities and pulp damage they offer results but less satisfactory (94,73% of success).

B) Results in relationship to the class of piece in function of the concentration of obtained DNA:
Number of studied pieces: 160, conserved at room temperature, maximal antiquity one week.
A direct relationship between the volume of pulp is observed and the concentration of DNA extracted in each class of piece, returning the maximal efficiency at first molar.

C) Results in pieces subjected to incineration :
Number of studied pieces : 80, all were subjected to 8 levels of temperatures (100-800 ºC) during 5 min.
In pieces subjected 100-200 ºC during 5 min, the results have been satisfactory (100% of success).The pieces subjected to 300ºC during 5 min. they offer difficulties in approximately the 50% of the cases (56% of success). To 400 ºC during 5 min. the pieces could rarely have been studied (12,5 % of success). It through 500 ºC has not been possible to us study the DNA of dental pulp.

D) Results in connection with the antiquity:
- pieces with an antiquity 0-2 years and subjected to different

conditions of conservation:

Number of studied pieces 378.

For an antiquity until 2 years, the frozen (-20 ºC) is the method that offers the best result (100% of success), although the room temperature and the interment doesn't disable the study of the DNA. (98,98% of success and 98,33% respectively). The conservation in saline serum seems to affect the posterior study of DNA of more notable form (91,66% of success).

- pieces with an antiquity 2-20 years:

Number of studied pieces 68.

For their study we formed a group in intervals of years: from 2 to 5, of 5 to 10, of 10 to 15 and of 15 to 20; the results were as follows: 90,0%, 100%, 85,71% and 92,85% of success.

The results are not very uniform, probably due the conditions of coservation; this condition could not have been standarized, being in many cases unknown for us. All the pieces treated with oxygenous water must be discarded, since the DNA is destroyed completely.

We believe that in this type of samples should take special caution: increase the quantity of sample (2 pulps); use more efficient methods of extraction (e.g.: Centricon Perkin-Elmer); an accurately control of the method.

REFERENCES

Pfitzinger H, Ludes B, Mangin P (1993) Sex determination of forensic samples: co-amplification and simultaneous detection of a Y-specific and X-specific DNA secuence. Int J Legal Med 105: 213-216

Sambrook I, Fritsch EF, Maniatis T (1989) In: Molecular Cloning. Cold Spring Harbor Laboratory Press.

Schwartz TD, Schwartz EA, Mieszersky BS, Mc Nally L, Kobilinski L (1991) Characterization of deoxyribonucleic acid (DNA) obtained from teeth subjected to various enviromental conditions. J Forensic Sciences 4:979-990

USE OF PCR IN FORENSIC CASEWORK
IN THE AREA BERLIN - BRANDENBURG:
ALLELE FREQUENCY DISTRIBUTION OF SIX MICROSATELLITES

G.Bläß[*], B.Jauert[*], W.Oesterreich, E.Ackermann, A.Pieper, S.Herrmann[*]

LKA Berlin, 12099 Berlin, Germany [*]
LKA Brandenburg, 16352 Basdorf, Germany

Introduction:

During the last few years a great variety of polymorphic DNA loci was introduced into forensic science.
In the forensic police laboratories of Berlin and Brandenburg (Germany) we routinely amplify the polymorphic loci D1S80, VWA31A, F13A1, THO1 (TC11), FESFPS and ACTBP22 (SE33). At these six DNA loci we analysed the allele distributions in the region of Berlin - Brandenburg (population size ca. 500 individuals) according to the recommendations of the ISFH.

Material and Methods:

DNA was isolated according to standard methods (Gill et al 1987).
Amplification of D1S80 was carried out with the commercial kit from Perkin Elmer Kasai et al. (1990); the analysis of the four STR systems VWA31A, F13A1, THO1 and FES was performed as described by Edwards et al. (1991) and Kimpton et al. (1993), amplification of SE33 as described by Polymeropoulos et al. (1992) with modifications according to an optimized protocol developed by the LKA Hessen, Germany.
The AMFLP system D1S80 can easily be separated by vertical or horizontal native PAGE (6%), whereas the STR systems (especially SE33) require an improved and standardized separation on denaturing PAGE (6%). In our hands we found that analysis of the above mentioned STRs were easiest and most reliable by working on the DNA sequencer (ABI 373A) in connection with the Genescan 350-ROX or 500-ROX fragment size standard. The evaluation was done with the Genescan and Genotyper software from Applied Biosystems on a Macintosh computer.

Results:

The distribution of the observed allele frequencies at six DNA loci in a population sample of about 500 unrelated individuals is shown in the following table. The results were compared with the data of other european studies (see references). In spite of the heterogeneity of the population in the Berlin - Brandenburg region which is composed of several national groups the allele frequency distribution does not differ significantly from these data.

The most useful system is SE33, but the non-standardized nomenclature presents a problem still to be solved.

D1S80   (n=635)

Allel	%	Allel	%	Allel	%	Allel	%	Allel	%
14	0	20	2,7	26	1,5	32	0,3	38	0
15	0,1	21	2,3	27	0,9	33	0,3	39	0,1
16	0,4	22	4,4	28	6,9	34	0,2	40	0,2
17	0,3	23	0,9	29	3,8	35	0,3	41	0,1
18	22,3	24	35,6	30	1,4	36	0,6	>41	0,2
19	0,7	25	5,3	31	8	37	0,3		

SE33   (n=568)

Allel	%	Allel	%	Allel	%	Allel	%	Allel	%
227	0,1	246	4,2	264	1,5	284	3,9	314	0,2
231	0,1	250	6,6	266	2,9	288	4,4	316	0,5
235	1,3	253	0,2	268	1,9	292	6,7	320	0,1
237	0,1	254	8,2	270	0,9	296	8,2	323	0,1
238	3,9	256	0,1	272	4,6	300	6,5	326	0,1
240	0,1	258	7	276	3	304	6,3		
242	4,1	260	0,4	280	3	308	2,4		
244	0,1	262	4,6	282	0,3	312	1,5		

F13   (n=552)

Allel	%	Allel	%	Allel	%	Allel	%
3.2	9,4	7	32,2	11	0,1	15	1,4
4	3,4	8	0,4	12	0,5	16	1,6
5	19,2	9	0	13	0,5	17	0
6	29,8	10	0	14	1,4	18	0,1

VWA   (n=597)

Allel	%	Allel	%	Allel	%	Allel	%
11	0	14	10	17	27,4	20	1,3
12	0,1	15	10,7	18	21,6	21	0,1
13	0,6	16	20,8	19	7,5		

FES   (n=460)

Allel	%	Allel	%
7	0,2	12	23,7
8	1,9	13	5,4
9	0,2	14	0,1
10	25,9	15	0,1
11	42,4		

TC11   (n=589)

Allel	%	Allel	%
5	0,1	9.3	30,1
6	22,4	10	2,5
7	16,2	11	0,0
8	11,2		
9	17,5		

References:

Budowle B, Chakraborty R, Giusti AM, Eisenberg AJ, Allen RC (1991) Analysis of the VNTR locus D1S80 by the PCR followed by high resolution PAGE. Am J Hum Genet 48:137-144

Cabrero C, Diez A, Valverde E, Carracedo A, Alemany J (1995) Allele frequency distribution of four PCR amplified loci in the Spanish population. Forensic Sci Int 71:153-164

Dupuy BM, Berg ES, Olaisen B (1995) Four STRs in 300 Norwegians. In: Baer W, Fiori A, Rossi U (eds) Advances in Forensic Haemogenetics 5.Springer, Berlin Heidelberg New York, p 539-541

Edwards A, Civitello A, Hammond HA, Caskey CT (1991) DNA typing and genetic mapping with trimeric and tetrameric tandem repeats. Am J Hum Genet 49:746-756

Gill P, Lygo JE, Fowler SJ, Werrett DJ (1987) An evaluation of DNA fingerprinting for forensic purposes. Electrophoresis 8:38-44

Hochmeister MN, Jung JM, Budowle B, Borer UV, Dirnhofer R (1994) Swiss population data on three tetrameric short tandem repeat loci--VWA, HUMTHO1, and F13A1--derived using multiplex PCR and laser fluorescence detection. Int J Legal Med 107:34-36

Holgersson S, Karlsson JA, Kihlgren A, Rosen B, Savolainen P, Gyllensten U (1994) Fluorescent-based typing of the two short tandem repeat loci HUMTHO1 and HUMACTBP2: reproducibility of size measurements and genetic variation in the Swedish population. Electrophoresis 15:890-895

Kasai K, Nakamura Y, White R (1990) Amplification of a variable number of tandem repeats (VNTR) locus (pMCT118) by the polymerase chain reaction (PCR) and its application to forensic science. J Forensic Sci 35:1196-1200

Kimpton CP, Gill P, Walton A, Urquhart A, Millican ES, Adams M (1993) Automated DNA profiling employing multiplex amplification of short tandem repeat loci. PCR Methods Appl 3:13-22

Meyer E, Wiegand P, Brinkmann B (1995) Phenotype differences of STRs in 7 human populations. Int J Legal Med 107:314-322

Polymeropoulos MH, Rath DS, Xiao H, Merril CR (1992) Tetranucleotide repeat polymorphism at the human beta-actin related pseudogene H-beta-Ac-psi-2 (ACTBP2). Nucl Acids Res 20:1432

Schnee-Griese J, Blaess G, Herrmann S, Schneider HR, Foerster R, Baessler G, Pflug W (1993) Frequency distribution of D1S80 alleles in the German population. Forensic Sci Int 59:131-136

Wiegand P, Budowle B, Rand S, Brinkmann B (1993) Forensic validation of the STR systems SE33 and TC11. Int J Legal Med 105:315-320

THE NEVERENDING STORY: A NEW TSAREVITCH ?

W. Huckenbeck[a], W. Bonte[a], V. Hees[b], S. West[b], K.W. Alt[a]

[a] Institute of Forensic Medicine, Heinrich-Heine-University, Düsseldorf
[b] Landeskriminalamt of Northrhine-Westphalia, Düsseldorf

Summary

A case of assumed lineal descent from the family of the Russian Tsars was investigated. Using 4 STR-system two exclusion constellations were found. These results emphasize the importance of STR systems for the assessment of such cases.

Introduction

In 1944 we were privately charged to examine a case of possible lineal descent from the family of the Russian Tsars. In the course of the last decades individuals have been claiming such a descent time and again, but since the publication of a British-Russian team of scientists in 1994 (1) there is an opportunity of testing such claims by molecular-biological means. The investigation of the skeletons from a mass grave in Ekaterinburg made their identification as the last Tsar and his family highly probable, although two skeletons (one male and one female descendant) were missing. In our case the individuals concerned are 4 brothers and sisters and their mother. Except for one daughter the family lives in St. Petersburg. Various circumstances suggested that the deceased father of the siblings could have been the Tsarevitch. The siblings came in person to Düsseldorf to have blood samples taken, the mother's blood was transported via aeroplane from St. Petersburg. It also seems worth mentioning that the results of a preliminary anthropological investigation in St. Petersburg seemed promising by the written report we received. The assumed family tree is shown in Tab. 1. Photographs of the missed Tsarevitch Alexeij and of Oleg F. are presented in Fig. 1.

Materials and Methods

DNA extraction and typing were realized by routine methods.

Results and Discussion

To test the genetic relations between siblings and mother, a total of 33 systems were investigated (Tab. 2). There were no contradictions to the laws of heredity. The investigations of the British-Russian research team on the skeletons referred to the STR-systems HumTC11, HumVWA, HumFES, HumF13A and SE 33, so these systems were decisive in the evaluation of the paternal hereditary traits. Because of differences in nomenclatures, we refrained from including the SE33 system in our analysis. The genetic traits of the deceased father corresponded in the HumVWA3 1 and HumF13A systems. There was one classical exclusion constellation in each the HumTHO1 and HumFES systems.

The results of the present case emphasize the importance of STR systems for the assessment of deficiency cases in paternity testing.

(1) P Gill, PL Ivanov, C Kimpton, R Piercy, N Benson, G Tully, I Evett, E Hagelberg, K Sullivan (1994) Identification of the remains of the Romanov family by DNA analysis. Nat Genet 6, 130-135

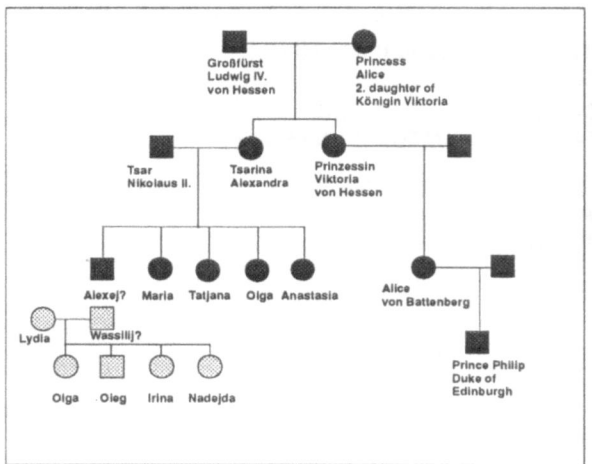

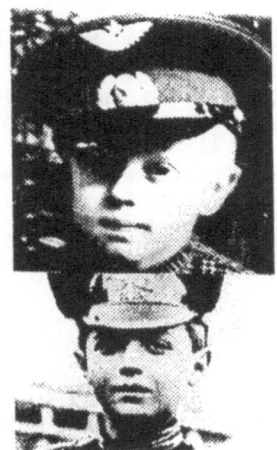

Table 1   The pedigree: Wassilij = Alexej ?

Fig. 1   Oleg and Alexej

	Oleg Child	Irina Child	Nadeja Child	Olga Child	Lydia Mother	Wassilij Father	Tsar*	Tsarina*
ABO	A1	A1	O	A1	A1	O		
MNSs	Nss	MNSs	MNSs	Nss	Nss	MS		
Rhesus	R2r	R1R2	R2r	R2r	R₁r	R₂		
Kell	K·k+	K·k+	K·k+	K·k+	K·k+	k+		
Duffy	a+b+	a·b+	a·b+	a+b+	a·b+	a+		
P	P+	P+	P·	P+	P+			
Kidd	a·b+	a·b+	a·b+	a·b+	a·b+	b+		
Lutheran	a·	a·	a·	a·	a·			
Colton	b·	b·	b·	b·	b·			

	Oleg	Irina	Nadeja	Olga	Lydia	Wassilij		
Hp	2	·	2	2	2	2		
Gc	2-1F	2	2	2	2	1F		
Gm	1-2 3 10	-1-2 3 10	-1-2 3 10	-1-2 3 10	-1-2 3 10	1		
Km	-1 3	-1 3	-1 3	-1 3	-1 3	3		
C 3	S	FS	S	FS	FS	S		
Tf	C1	C1	C1	C1	C1	C1		
Bf	S	S	S	S	S	S		
Pi	M1	M1	M1	M1	M1	M1		
acP	BC	AB	B	AC	BC	AB		
PGM₁	a3a1	a1	a1	a3a1	a1	a3		
ADA	1	1	1	1	1	1		
GPT	2	2	2-1	2	2-1	2		
EsD	1	1	1	1	1	1		
GLO	2	2	2	2	2	2		
PGP	1	1	1	1	1	1		

	Oleg	Irina	Nadeja	Olga	Lydia	Wassilij	Tsar*	Tsarina*
HumTH01	7-9.3	7-9	9-9.3	9-9.3	7-9.3	9	7-10	8-8
HumVWA	16-16	16-16	16-16	16-16	16-16	16	15-16	15-16
HumFES	11-13	11-11	11-13	11-13	11-13	11	12-12	12-13
HumF13A	3.2-7	6-7	6-7	3.2-6	3.2-6	7	7-7	3-5
HLA-DQα	1.2-3	1.2-3	3-3	3-3	1.2-3	3		
D1S80	24-30	24-28	24-30	24-28	24-24	28-30		
LDRL	BB	BB	AB	AB	BB	AB		
GYPA	BB	AB	AB	BB	BB	AB		
HBGG	BB	BB	BB	AB	BB	AB		
D7S8	AB	AA	AB	AA	AB	AA		
GC	AB	AA	AA	AA	AA	AB		

Table 2 Serological findings (* according to Gill et al., 1994)

INFLUENCE OF MEDIAEVAL CLOTHES COLOUR PIGMENTS ON DNA EXTRACTION AND AMPLIFICATION

C. KEYSER [1], D. MONTAGNON [2], B. LUDES [1], E. CRUBEZY [3], D. CARDON [4], P. WALTON ROGERS, J. WOUTERS [5], P. MANGIN [1]

(1) Institut de Médecine Légale et (2) Laboratoire d'Embryologie, 11rue Humann 67085 Strasbourg, France. (3) Laboratoire d'Anthropologie, Université de Bordeaux I, URA 376 du CNRS et (4) UMR 99 67 du CNRS, France. (5) Instituut voor Kunstpatrimonium, Belgique.

INTRODUCTION

Different factors affect DNA preservation and recovery such as depth of burial, soil pH, presence of humic acids or pigments of ancient clothes.

We examined bone fragments (vertebra, talus and heel bones) from a mediaeval skeleton burial (810-900 AD) excavated from a burial vault. This skeleton belonged to a duke dressed with mediaeval clothes stained with kermes vermilio binded to the wool by elagic acid and alun [$Al_2(SO_4)_3$]. The vertebra was slightly brown coloured and we showed in a previous (Crubézy, 1995) study that cytochrome b mtDNA had been successfully amplified.

The talus and the heel bone showed red-brown color due either to the kermes vermilio or to the putrefaction processes and the extracts were also brown coloured from the previous contaminants. These extracts could not be amplified.

To investigate the inhibition power of these four contaminants (alun, kermes vermilio, kermes coloured wool and elagic acid), modern DNA was extracted with those pigments.

MATERIALS AND METHODS

DNA extraction : modern genomic DNA (20 μg) was isolated and purified from 1 ml of human blood sample by the organic extraction protocol (Maniatis *et al.* 1982) in absence or presence of 10 mg of different types of coloured clothes contaminant (kermes, kermes coloured wool, alun, elagic acid).

Polymerase Chain Reaction : PCR amplification was performed in 50-μl volume of 20 mM Tris-buffer (pH 8,4) containing 50 mM KCl, 1.5 mM $MgCl_2$, 200 μM of each dNTPs, 0.05 % Tween, 10 μg of bovine serum albumin, 5 pmole of each primer, 10μl of the extracted DNA and 2.5 units of Taq DNA Polymerase (Gibco BRL). Primers used for amplification and sequencing were L14841 and H15149 (Kocher *et al.*, 1989). Each cycle of the polymerase chain reaction, carried out in a Perkin Elmer-Cetus Thermal Cycler, consisted of denaturation for 1 mn at 94°C, hybridization for 1 mn at 50°C, and extension for 2-5 mn at 72°C. This cycle was repeated 35 times.

The PCR products were separated on 3 % NuSieve agarose gels and stained with ethidium bromide.

RESULTS

The DNA extraction was not affected by the component added except when carried out in the presence of 10 mg of alun, which interfered with the DNA recovering by the formation of a precipitate.

Following agarose electrophoresis and ethidium bromide staining, PCR products of expected size were detected with the DNA extracted without contaminant and with kermes coloured wool and kermes. Faintly PCR product was observed for the DNA extracted in the presence of alun. A band of smaller size than the region of the cytochrome b gene flanking by the two primers used was also observed and was probably due to a DNA degradation. No amplification product occurred with the DNA extracted in the presence of 10 mg of elagic acid.

In order to test the influence of the elagic acid concentration and to determine a possible inhibitory threshold value, DNA extraction was carried out with seven different concentrations of elagic acid (0,5; 1; 3; 6; 8; 10; 16 mg) in the experimental conditions primary used.

As shown in the figure, fewer products appeared with increasing elagic acid concentration in the extraction solution. No visible bands were detected beyond 10 mg of elagic acid.

DISCUSSION

After death, the conservation of DNA depends mostly on either environmental factors or artificial treatment of the body. Humidity combined with anaerobic conditions and a high concentration of humic acids may lead to complete conservation of the body (Hauswirth et al., 1994).

If the soft tissues are decomposed, the organic structures in bones may persist even under normal burial conditions. This observation can be explained by the situation in little caves of the osteocytes or osteoblastes which are surrounded by protective hard tissues protecting the DNA against physical and biochemical aggressions.

In previous studies, it was shown that this mediaeval crypt burial belonged to a count of Toulouse (France). In fact, one of the skeletons was dressed with rich mediaeval clothes and the lord was wearing red socks. We showed that the extracted DNA from the vertebra was suitable for PCR and a part of the cytochrome b gene could be amplified. On the opposite, the DNA yielded from talus and heel bones could not be amplified. Macroscopically these bones showed a brown-red colour coming either from the degradation processus or from the coloured clothes contaminants. In the present study, we tried to highlight the effects of these tannins on the DNA molecule by adding 10 mg of the four contaminants (kermes, kermes coloured wool, alun and elagic acid) to the extracted modern genomic DNA.

Kermes seems to have no visible effects, neither on the DNA extraction, neither on the amplification reaction. In contrast, our results suggest that alun alters the DNA extraction and the efficiency of the amplification reaction whereas elagic acid might have inhibitory effects on the amplification reaction.

CONCLUSION

This study allowed us to conclude that the lack of amplification results on talus and heel bones might be attributed to the coloured mediaeval clothes tannins which contamine the bone DNA and inhibit the amplification reaction.

REFERENCES

Crubézy E., Dieulafait C. Etudes historiques, archéologiques, anthropologiques et des textiles du sarcophage dit de Guillaume Taillefer à Saint Sernin. Aquitania, in press.

Hauswirth WW., Dickel CD., Lawlor DA. (1994) DNA Analysis of the Windover population. In Ancient DNA , B. Herrmann, S. Hummel eds, Springer-Verlag , 1994, pp 104-121.

Kocher TD, Thomas WK, Meyer A, Edwards SV, Pääbo S, Villablanca FX, Wilson AC (1989) Dynamics of mitochondrial DNA evolution in animals : amplification and sequencing with conserved primers. Proc. Natl. Acad. Sci. USA 86:6196-6200.

Maniatis T, Fritsch EF, Sambrook J (1982) Molecular cloning. A laboratory manual. Second Edition C. Nolan (ed.) Cold Spring Harbor Laboratory Press. Printed in USA.

Figure legend :
Conventional 3 % NuSieve agarose-gel electrophoresis of the amplified products after staining with ethidium bromide. Part of the cytochrome b gene was amplified from human genomic DNA extracted without any contaminant (lane 1) or with 10 mg of vermilio kermes (lane 2), 10 mg of kermes coloured wool (lane 3), 10 mg of alun (lane 4), 0.5 mg of elagic acid (lane 5), 1 mg of elagic acid (lane 6), 3 mg of elagic acid (lane 7), 6 mg of elagic acid (lane 8), 8 mg of elagic acid (lane 9), 10 mg of elagic acid (lane 10), 16 mg of elagic acid (lane 11). Lane 12 denote a DNA mass ladder marker (Gibco BRL).

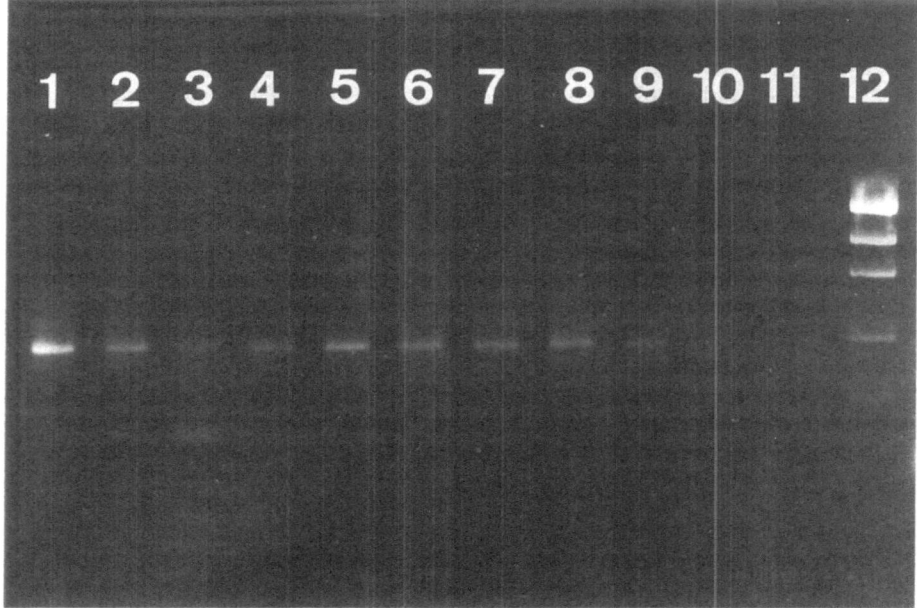

Forensic investigations after sexual abuse of several infants: a criminal case report.

J. Kreike[*], A. Lehner[*], E. Friedrich[*] and O. Tauscher[**]

[*])Institute of Forensic Medicine, Sensengasse 2, A-1090 Vienna, Austria;
[**])Security Bureau of the Viennese Police Department, Roßauer Lände 5, A-1090 Vienna, Austria.

INTRODUCTION

Sexual violence against women and sexual abuse of male and female infants are crimes of major social importance and form a large part of the forensic stain analysis work. The development of sensitive forensic DNA analysis techniques based on the polymerase chain reaction (PCR), e.g. HLA-DQα (Saiki et al. 1989; Schneider and Rittner 1993), D1S80 (Budowle et al. 1991) and Amplitype PM (Budowle et al. 1995), as well as the selective lysis procedure to enrich sperm cells (Giusti et al. 1986) highly facilitated stain analysis with these crimes. Here we report on a successful collaborate search for a sexual offender of young girls based on concommitant criminal investigations and forensic DNA analyses.

CASE REPORT

Materials and Methods

DNA was isolated from vaginal swabs and underwear after selective lysis and from blood samples using standard forensic methods with small modifications (Kreike and Lehner, 1995). PCR (HLA-DQα, D1S80 and PM) and the analysis of the amplified products were performed as described by the supplier (Perkin-Elmer/Cetus), except that the number of cycles during D1S80 amplification was increased to 32. D1S80 allele frequencies and distribution of HLA-DQα and PM genotypes were taken from Hochmeister et al. (1994).

Results

In the first week of June 1994 four girls, between 9 and 12 years of age, were sexually abused. Medical examination did not show major injuries of the abdomen, nor indications of defloration. Serological examination revealed sperm in vaginal secretions and underwear from two of the victims. Since all four cases showed prominent similarities in the course of events presumably a single offender was involved. This assumption was confirmed by HLA-DQα analysis of sperm enriched fractions from the stains. In the vaginal swab from victim #1 HLA-DQα alleles 2 and 3 were present in addition to the female alleles 1,3 and 4. Also in the slip from victim #2 HLA-DQα allele 3 was present in combination with alleles 2 and 4 from the girl itself (Fig. 1). From the other two victims no sperm containing material could be identified.

Several months later, between September and November 1994, three more girls were abused in a similar way. From one of them (victim #3) sperm was detected in vaginal and anal swabs and the underwear. In DNA isolated from the sperm stain in the slip again HLA-DQα alleles 2 and 3 could be determined in addition to the alleles 1.1 and 4 from the victim (Fig. 1). A still unsolved earlier case of infant sexual abuse was compared with these three current cases. A sperm stain on

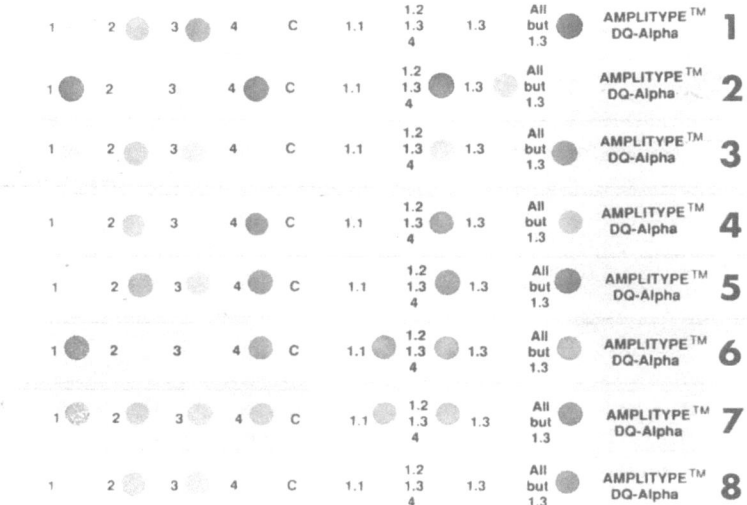

Fig. 1: Results of HLA-DQα analysis of blood samples and stains. *Strip 1:* blood, suspect; *strip 2:* blood victim #1; *strip 3:* stain, victim #1; *strip 4:* blood, victim #2; *strip 5:* stain, victim #2; *strip 6:* blood, victim #3; *strip 7:* stain, victim #3; *strip 8:* stain, victim #4.

a girl´s jacket from January 1994 was analysed and it showed HLA-DQα alleles 2 and 3 (Fig. 1). These results were confirmed by D1S80 analysis of the stains, which all showed D1S80 alleles T24 and T25, and by PM analysis (data not shown). The frequencies of HLA-DQα alleles 2 and 3 and D1S80 alleles T24 and T25 were calculated to be 0.04 % (Hochmeister et al. 1994). The similarities in the crimes and the forensic DNA results prompted us to perform a computer search of known sexual offenders in Austria. From over 3000 possible candidates 6 were selected out using several criteria: offenders known in Vienna, personal description, no additional crimes (drugs or brutal violence), place of crime or living appartment in three viennese districts, not in prison at the time of the crime. On photographs of these six men, two closely resembled the personal description of the offender and one of them was unequivocally identified by one of the victims.

The putative offender, who had been convicted of four similar crimes in 1986, was arrested at his place of work and, after he had been told that DNA analysis from the stains may prove his guilt, he made a partial confession. Later he admitted sexual abuse on nine girls between 6 and 12 years old, one of which is still unidentified. He was sentenced to 12 years imprisonment in May, 1995.

Discussion

After HLA-DQα, D1S80 and PM analysis the probability of this man to be the offender lies between 99.7% (victim #2)and 99.9998% (victim #4). However, due to his confession to the authorities and in court, in this particular case these probabilities should not be interpreted primarily as strong evidence for sexual abuse by this accused man. The primary result from the forensic analyses is the presence in the swabs and underwear of sperm cells, which highly likely originate from the suspect. This indicates clear evidence for executed sexual intercourse with three of the victims.

	victim #1 (12 years)		victim #2 (9 years)		victim #3 (8 years)		victim #4 (7 years)		accused man
	blood	stain	blood	stain	blood	stain	blood	stain	blood
HLA-DQα	1,3 4	1,3 2 3 4	2 4	2 3 4	1,1 4	1,1 2 3 4	n.d.	2 3	2 3
D1S80	T18 T26	T18 T24 T25 T26	T18	T18 T24 T25	T18 T24	T18 T24 T25	n.d.	T24 T25	T24 T25
LDLR	AB	AB	n.d.	n.d.	AB	AB	n.d.	AB	AB
GYPA	AA	aB	n.d.	n.d.	AA	AB	n.d.	BB	BB
HBGG	BB	AB	n.d.	n.d.	BB	aB	n.d.	AB	AB
D7S8	BB	Ab	n.d.	n.d.	AA	AA	n.d.	AA	AA
GC	BC	BC	n.d.	n.d.	AC	abC	n.d.	BC	BC
genotype frequency (%)		0.002		0.3		0.1		0.0002	

Fig. 2: Schematic presentation of the results of HLA-DQα, D1S80 and PM analysis of DNA from stain material (sperm enriched fractions) from four sexually abused female infants. Weak PM alleles are indicated by small letters; n.d., not done

REFERENCES

Budowle B, Chakraborty R., Giusti AM, Eisenberg AJ, Allen RC (1991) Analysis of VNTR locus D1S80 by the PCR followed by high resolution PAGE. Am J Hum Genet 48: 137-144

Budowle B, Lindsay JA, DeColl JA, Koons BW, Giusti AM, Comey CT (1995) Validation and population studies of the loci LDLR, GYPA, HBGG, D7S8 and GC (PM loci) and HLA-DQα using a multiplex amplification and typing procedure. J Forensic Sci 40: 45-50

Giusti A, Baird M, Pasquale S, Balasz I, Glassberg J (1987) Application of deoxyribonucleic acid (DNA) polymorphisms to the analysis of DNA recovered from sperm. J Forensic Sci 31: 409-417

Hochmeister M, Budowle B, Borer U, Dirnhofer, R (1994). Swiss population data on the loci HLA-DQα, LDLR, GYPA, HBGG, D7S8, GC and D1S80. For Sci Int 67: 175-184

Kreike J, Lehner A (1995) Sex determination and DNA competition in the analysis of forensic mixed stains by PCR. Int J Leg Med 107: 235-238

Saiki RK, Walsh PS, Levenson CH, Erlich HA (1989) Genetic analysis of amplified DNA with immobilized sequence-specific oliogonucleotide probes. Proc Natl Acad Sci USA 86: 6230-6234

Schneider PM, Rittner, (1993) Experience with PCR-based HLA-DQα DNA typing system in routine forensic casework. Int. J Leg Med 105: 295-299.

SEX DETERMINATION IN ANCIENT BONES

Kuntze K, Huckenbeck W, Bonte W, Alt KW
Institute of Forensic Medicine, Heinrich-Heine-University Düsseldorf

Summary

Using the PCR based amelogenin system anthropological results could be proved and be completed: the 'Velké Pavlovice grave' contains the skeletons of two adults (female and male) and six children (one female, five males). The anthropological theory of a family grave could not be refuted.

Introduction

The remains of eight individuals of the Early Bronze Age Veterov culture found at Velké Pavlovice (distr. Breclav, Moravia, CR) were subjected to a PCR-based sex determination. The skeletal material represents two adult individuals and six children from two to ten years of age (Fig.1). To verify the hypothesis that this group of individuals represent a proper family, at first the sex of the individuals was determined.

Material and Methods

Sample Pretreatment: Since samples probably have been touched during excavation or previous investigations it is necessary to decontaminate the sample properly. Irradiation with shortwave UV light (254 nm) induces covalent bindings of opposite thymine bases and prevents therefore double-stranded DNA from melting during PCR.

DNA-Extraction: A small piece of bone is ground to a fine powder in a bone-mill. About 500 mg of the bone meal is transferred into an microtube and mixed with 1 ml extraction buffer (0.3M Sodium-acetate, 10 mM Tris-HCl, 1 mM EDTA, 1% SDS, ph 7.8) and 0,5 mg proteinase K. This mixture is incubated overnight at 55°C in a shaking water bath or in an incubator. Periodical vortexing should be performed to achieve an optimal intermix.

DNA-Isolation: After incubation two 340 µl aliquots of the supernatant are transferred into sterile microtubes. After addition of 100 µl 5 M sodium perchlorate the DNA-isolation was carried out according to the protocol of the Nucleon DNA Extraktion Kit (Nucleon, Scotlab).

DNA-Amplification: Amplification is performed using the GenePrint STR System DC4080 (Amelogenin) (Promega) according to the technical manual. To obtain the recommended concentration of DNA, it was diluted in the ratio of one to four with 10mM Tris-HCl, pH 8,7. *Electrophoresis*: The electrophoresis is carried out as a semidry, ultrathin horizontal polyacrylamide-gel electrophoresis. The following protocol is for the preparation of a polyacrylamide gel with the dimensions of 26 cm x 20 cm x 800 µm (w x h x thickness): 30% Acryl-PDA, 8,7 ml; Aqua bidest., 21,0 ml; CHES, 4,0 ml; 500 mM Tris-Formiat, 6,6 ml; 10 % APS, 300µl; TEMED, 15,5 µl. 2% Agaroseplugs in 2 x Tris-Borat-Buffer, pH 9,0 stored in 2 x Tris-Borat-Buffer/0,01% Bromphenolblue serve as reservoir for the buffer. 4 µl of the DNA samples were applied on small pieces of filter paper. Electrophoresis was carried out on a cooling plate (15°C) for 1,5 h at 5 W, 40 mA, 1000V, 1 h at 10 W, 40 mA, 1000 V and ca. 1 h (until bromphenolblue reaches the anode) at 15 W, 40 mA , 1000 V. Silver staining was performed according to Budowle et al. (1991).

Results and Discussion

The traditional prehistoric kinship analysis represents an attempt to establish the similarity or dissimilarity of individuals on the basis of external skeletal variants. In principle it is a polysymptomatic estimation of similarity based on morphognostic characteristics like anthropological (non-genetic) paternity testing (Knussmann, 1988). For morphognostic traits the exact processes of transmission are more or less unknown. although there is agreement on the facts that genetic factors play a role in their development and that environmental factors modify their expression. Morphognostic characteristics can therefore not be used for genetic analysis s.s. but for establishing phenotypical similarities beetween individuals. In the case of „Velké Pavlovice" the skeletons partly are in too bad a state to get definite results from the anthropometric sex analysis, especially the hypothetical mother. Nevertheless, a family (father, mother and six children) is suggested. Typing the sex of the children - by anthropological methods - was impossible (Alt et al., in press).

The results of the genetic sex determination (amelogenin) proved the results of the anthropological investigation: the skeleton of the hypothetical "mother" is female. In addition the children's skeletons were typed: five male and one female remains. These results represent the importance of DNA-PCR analyis for the investigation of prehistoric bones. Further investigations on the Velké Pavlovice material - kinship analysis using STR systems - are planed.

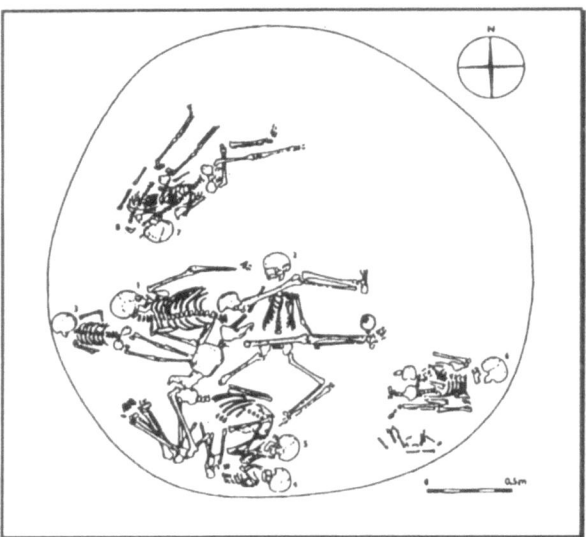

Fig.1 The 'family burial' from Velké Pavlovice.

References

Alt KW, Pichler S, Vach W, Huckenbeck W, Stoukal M; Early Bronze Age family burial from Velké Pavlovice. Homo, in press

Budowle B, Chakraborty R, Giusti AM, Eisenberg AJ, Allen RC (1991) Analysis of the variable number of tandem repeat locus D1S80 by the polymerase chain reaction followed by high resolution polyacrylamide gel electrophoresis. Am J HumGenet 48, 137-144

Knussmann R (1988) Methoden des morpholgischenVergleichs in der forensischen Anthropologie. In: Knussmann R (ed) Anthropolgie Vol. 1, Fischer, Stuttgart, 368-407

IDENTIFICATION OF THE SKELETAL REMAINS OF TWO 12-YEARS OLD BODIES BY NUCLEAR DNA POLYMORPHISMS ANALYSIS.

P. Martín, A. Alonso, C. Albarrán and M. Sancho.

Sección de Biología. Instituto de Toxicología. Mº de Justicia e Interior. Madrid. SPAIN.

INTRODUCTION

The ability to analyse by PCR-based methods trace amounts of human DNA isolated from old bone material (Hagelberg et al. 1989; Hochmeister et al. 1991) offers the opportunity to identify unknown skeletal remains by a comparative genetic analysis with their presumptive relatives (Hagelberg et al. 1991; Gill et al. 1994).

We here report the successful identification of two 12-years-old bodies by comparative typing of nuclear DNA polymorphisms in the remains and in their presumptive parents. We also describe the main methodological challenges that we have found during this investigation.

CASE BACKGROUND

Two skeletons buried with quicklime were found in a grave near Alicante (Eastern Spain) in 1985. Autopsy findings revealed that both skulls had bullet wounds as well as other signs of violence and mistreatment before death, but the cadavers were kept unidentified. On 1995, the police obtained some kind of evidence which indicated that the two bodies would corresponded with those of two individuals, disappeared in 1983, that presumably collaborated with a terrorist group from the Basque Country. The anthropological analysis carried out by forensic experts allowed to perform stature and age estimation as well as sexing of the remains, but no clinical or odontology records were available for comparison. To confirm the identification, DNA analysis was requested.

MATERIALS AND METHODS

Laboratory Organization

The following conditions were fullfilled to minimize the risk of contamination: Bone extractions were set up in a laminar flow cabinet with dedicated equipment (treated with 5% Sodium hypochlorite and UV light). Amplifications were set up in a laminar flow cabinet with a strict physical separation from the laboratory area where bone DNA was extracted. Negative controls were used in all experiments. At least two extractions per sample on different occasions and from different parts were performed. The DNA profile of the investigators involved in the case was available.

DNA Extraction and Quality Control

The outer surfaces of a femur and a tibia from each cadaver were removed by sanding and three cleaned bone fragments from each body were independently pulverized to obtain three portions of aproximately five grams of bone powder. DNA was extracted from one of the bone powder portions using the protocol described by Hochmeister et al. (1991) that included a decalcification step for three days in 0.5 M EDTA at pH 7.5. DNA was extracted from the two remainning bone powder portions following the protocol described by Gill et al. (1994) without previous decalcification. In all cases the mixture that resulted from the Proteinase K treatment was extracted three times with equal volumes of phenol/chloroform/isoamyl alcohol (25:24:1). DNA extracts were washed and concentrated with TE buffer. using Centricon-100 microconcentrator devices. Total DNA was determined by agarose gel electrophoresis and ethidium bromide staining and by fluorimetry. Human DNA was quantitated by slot-blot hybridization with the human-specific D17Z1 probe using the Quantiblot system (Perkin-Elmer). About 1-3 µg/µl of total DNA were recovered in each extract, but only a small proportion (20-60 pg/µl) was of human origin. DNA was extracted from the blood of the presumptive parents by the standard phenol/chloroform extraction procedure.

PCR Amplification and Typing

The amplification of STR loci was performed by single-locus PCR reactions in the case of HUMFES/FPS, HUMVWA, HUMF13B and HUMF13A1 or by a multiplex PCR reaction in the case of HUMTH01, HUMTPOX and HUMCSF1PO according to the manufacturer's recommendations using the GenePrint STR System (Promega Corporation, Madison, WI, USA). PCR products were typed by denaturing polyacrylamide gel electrophoresis followed by silver stain (Budowle et al. 1991; Martín et al. 1995). The amplification and typing of HLA-DQA1 and PM systems were performed according to the manufacturer's recommendations using the Amplitype PM and HLA-DQalpha forensic DNA Amplification and Typing kits (Perkin-Elmer Corporation, Norwak, CT).

Statistical Analysis

The statistical weight of the evidence linking the skeletal remains to the presumptive parents was evaluated using Spanish allele frequencies. The likelihood ratio (LR) of the probabilities of obtaining the precise combination of alleles seen in the presumptive parents and in the skeletal samples, under the alternative assumptions that the skeletal remains are either derived, or not derived, from an offspring of their presumptive parents, was determined for each locus.

RESULTS AND DISCUSSION

Given the low quantity (20-60 pg/µl) and the extent of degradation of the nuclear human DNA recovered from the bone samples we opted for a PCR-based typing of polymorphic markers with very short alleles (STRs, HLA-DQA1 and PM systems) as the unique suitable typing approach of nuclear DNA in this case.

All 13 loci were reproducibly amplified and typed from at least two independent bone DNA extracts (Fig.1 illustrates the STR profiling) and the typing results were fully consistent with the bone DNA from each body being derived from an offspring of their respective presumptive parents. It should be noted, however, that in one of the three DNA extracts obtained from one of the bodies, in addition to the bone-alleles, other PCR-products which could not be attributed to none of the presumptive parents were also detected (Fig. 2). A comparison of the typing results obtained from this DNA extract with the DNA profile of the researchers involved in this investigation allowed to demonstrate in this sample a contamination with modern human DNA originating from the investigator who performed DNA extraction. Apart from contamination, another methodological challenge found in this investigation during STR typing was the difficulty to detect some alleles (specially larger alleles which showed lower amplification efficiency) due to the presence in the bone DNA extracts and consistently in the PCR-reaction mix of vast amounts of irrelevant microbial DNA that often produced a high background when silver stain detection was attempted. In these cases, typing was confirmed by reamplification of a dilution (10^{-3}-10^{-6}) of the original PCR-product (Fig. 3).

The statistical weight of the evidence linking the skeletal remains to their respective presumptive parents was evaluated using Spanish allele frequencies. The cumulative likelihood ratio for all 13 loci was very high in both cases (LR/cadaver 1 = 35973; LR/cadaver 2 = 657117) establishing with a high degree of confidence the identification of the cadavers.

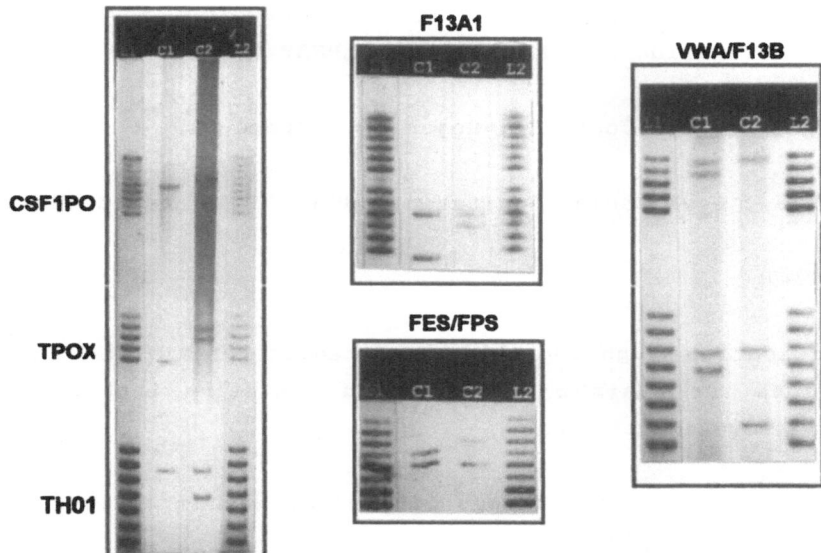

Figure 1. Representative STR profiles obtained from the bone DNA extracts.
(C1): cadaver 1; (C2): cadaver 2, (L): allelic ladder.

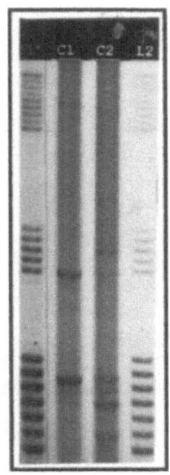

Figure 2. Example of STR typing (TH01, TPOX and CSF1PO loci) showing a DNA contamination in the bone extract recovered from cadaver 2.
(C1): cadaver 1
(C2): cadaver 2
(L): allelic ladder

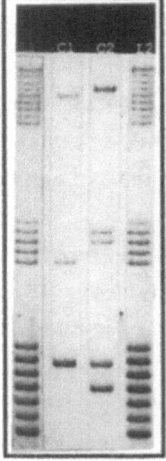

Figure 3. STR profiles (TH01, TPOX and CSF1PO loci) obtained by reamplification of a 10^{-4} dilution of the original PCR-products.
(C1): cadaver 1
(C2): cadaver 2
(L): allelic ladder.

REFERENCES

Budowle B, Chakraborty R, Giusti AM, Eisenberg AJ, Allen RC (1991) Am J Hum Genet 48: 137-144

Gill P, Ivanov PL, Kimpton C, Piercy R, Benson N, Tully G, Evett I, Hagelberg E, Sullivan K (1994) Nature Genet 6: 130-135

Hagelberg E, Gray IC, Jeffreys AJ (1991) Nature 352: 427-429

Hagelberg E, Sykes B, Hedges R (1989) Nature 342: 485

Hochmeister MN, Budowle B, Borer UV, Eggmann U, Coney CT, Dimhofer R (1991) J Forensic Sci 36: 1649-1661

Martín P, Alonso A, Budowle B, Albarrán C, García O, Sancho M (1995) Int J Leg Med (in press)

IDENTIFICATION IN VESTIGES FROM DIVERSE BIOLOGICAL SOURCES USING DUPLEX AMPLIFICATION OF SHORT TANDEM REPEAT LOCI

Martínez, M.A.; San José, S.; Rojas, A.; Gremo, A.

Toxicología y Legislación Sanitaria. UCM. 28040 Madrid. Spain.

INTRODUCTION

The amplification of polymorphic short tandem repeat (STR) loci by PCR provides the basis of a rapid and sensitive technique for individual identification.

We have studied DNA of vestiges biological humans employing the amplification by duplex PCR with STRs.

The two loci analyzed there HUMTHO1 and HUMFES/FPS. The samples were: hair roots, saliva, sperm, bloodstain and dental pulp.

MATERIALS AND METHOD

The extraction of DNA of the samples from hair roots, sperm, bloodstain and dental pulp was carried out for the method of the phenol/chloroform. DNA from saliva was extracted using the chelex method (Chelex 100 chelating resin, Bio-Rad labs).

The amplifications were performed in a final volume of 25 μl in a Perkin-Elmer thermocycler. Each reaction contained 2-50 ng of genomic DNA, 10 mM Tris-HCl, pH 8.3, 50 mM KCl, 1.5 mM Mg Cl$_2$, Triton X-100, 0.5 μl of each dNTP (10 mM stoks), 0.5 μl U Amplitaq polymerase and 0.25 μM of each primer. The cycle temperatures were as follows: 95 °C (1 min), 54 °C (1min), 72 °C (1 min), 29 cycles. Prior to the first cycle the DNA was denatured at 95 °C for 10 minutes and after the last cycle an additional extension at 72 °C for 7 minutes was performed. Both amplifications were run as a multiplex-PCR in a single reaction. The primers were:
HUMTHO1: $^{5'}$ GTGGGCTGAAAAGCTCCCGATTAT$^{3'}$
$^{5'}$ GTGATTCCCATTGGCCTGTTCCTC$^{3'}$

HUMFES/FPS: 5' GGGATTTCCCTATGGATTGG 3'
            5' GCGAAAGAATGAGACTACAT 3'

After PCR the amplified alleles were separated in a vertical
polyacylamide gel (T6,C5), under denaturing conditions. The time
for assay was 45 minutes.

The alleles were visualized using a silver staining procedure,
according to Budowle et al (1991). Genotype assignment was done by
side-by-side comparison with an allelic ladder. Allele ladders
were constructed by mixing, amplified samples of validated
genotype in appropiate ratios.

RESULTS AND DISCUSSION

The results were satisfactory included in the cases in those that
there was little quantity of DNA or that the sample was
degradated.

The amplification of polymorphics STRs by PCR is specially useful
when we have a very small amount of biological material.

The present work indicates that multiplex-PCR should be applicable
to forensic specimens that yield limiting amounts of DNA.

REFERENCES

Budowle B, Chakraborty R, Giusti A, Eisenberg A, Allen R (1991)
Analysis of the VNTR locus D1S80 by the PCR followed by high
resolution PAGE. American Journal of Human Genetics 48:137-144

Hopkins B, Williams N, Webb M, Debenham P, Jeffreys A (1994) The
use of minisatellite variant repeat-polymerase chain reaction
(MVR-PCR) to determine the source of saliva on a used postage
stamp. Journal of Forensic Sciences 39:526-531

Lorente J, Lorente M, Budowle B, Wilson M, Villanueva E (1994)

Analysis of the HUMTHO1 allele frecuencies in the spanish population. Journal of Forensic Sciences 39:1270-1274

Valverde E, Cabrero C, Cao R, Rodriguez M, Díez A, Barros F, Alemany J, Carracedo A (1993) Population genetics of three VNTR polymorphisms in two differents spanish population. Int J Leg Med 105:251-256

A rare paternity case with PP 99,99% and exclusion at three loci derived from the 33.15 sequence

E.Seifried, C.Seidl, R.Grigorean**, E.Brude*, O.Jäger, U.Langenbeck*, K.D. Zang**

Institute for Transfusionsmedicine and Immunohematology,
Red Cross Blood Donor Service Hessen, Sandhofstrasse 1, 60528 Frankfurt / Main
* Inst. for Human Genetic, J-W Goethe University, Theodor-Stern Kai 7, 60528 Frankfurt / Main
** Inst. for Human Genetic,University of Saarlandes, Universitätskliniken Bau 68, 66421 Homburg
Germany

INTRODUCTION

In general in cases of proven paterbnity (p > 99.99%) by analysis of conventional blood groups and the HLA system paternity exclusion by analysis of VNTR or STR-Loci is very rare. We present a case report with PP > 99.99% after analysis of 21 conventional systems, HLA, 5 SLP and 5 STR but 3 exclusions with SLP G3, MS1 and MS205 all derived from MLP 33.15.

CASE: Paternity quartet: Mother , child I, child II and putative father

METHODS AND MATERIALS

Blood group antigens (ABO-, MNSs-, Rh-, Kell-, Duffy- and Kidd-system), plasma protein polymorphisms (PLG-, Gm-, Km-, C3-, Tf-, Pi-, Hp- and Gc-system) and erythrocyte enzyme polymorphisms (PGM-, GPT-, ACP-, AK-, ADA-, EsD- and PGD-system) were determined for each case following standard procedures. HLA-A, HLA-B and HLA-C antigens were typed by the microlymphocytotoxicity test (LCT).
VNTR (SLP/MLP) polymorphism analysis: Genomic DNA was extracted from 8ml of peripheral blood following the salting-out method. Electrophoresis conditions, hybridisation, southern blot transfer to nylon membranes (Quiabrane from Diagen Inc, Hilden, Germany) and detection of probes were performed as recommended by the manufacturers (NICE™ ICI/CELLMARK, GenePrint Light™ Promega, (GTG)5 Fresenius, 33.15 ICI/CELLMARK). The results were analysed by an semiautomatic computerised system (DNA-Auswertungssystem Version 2.40 from M.Muche Immucor Medizinische Diagnostik GmbH, Rödermark, Germany) and the biostatistical calculation of paternity was performed with the Essen Möller probability (W).
STR polymorphism analysis: Fluorescence based PCR based analysis of STR loci was conducted on an 373A automated DNA sequencer (Perkin-Elmer) as described (Seidl 1995).The single/multi locus probes and STR polymorphism used in this study are summarized in table1. Chromosome staining: Staining of metaphase chromosomes in situ was performed according to standard protocols.

Table.1: SLP/MLP and STR polymorphism

SLP	SLP	MLP	STR
yNH24 (D2S44)	MS1 (D1S7)	33.15	TH01 (11p15.5-p15)
MS31 (D7S21)	MS205 (D16S309)	(GTG)5	D8S639 (8p21-p11)
MS43A (D12S11)	G3 (D7S22)		CYP19 (15q21.1)
LH1 (D5S110)			ACPP (3q21)
PH30 (D4S139)			SE33 (ACTPB2)

RESULTS AND DISCUSSION

DNA analysis using three VNTR loci, G3, MS205 and YNH24 did give conclusive results for child I but revealed paternal fragments for child II regarding the loci G3 and MS205 that could not be observed in the putative father (Fig. 1). Extended VNTR analysis using 5 additional single locus probe (SLP's) (Table 1) exhibited a third mutation with probe MS1 affecting the paternal fragment of child II (Fig.1). Table 2 summarizes the results of the VNTR analysis. All potential mutations were affecting paternal fragments of child II resulting in size differences of 110 (MS205), 110 (MS1) and 460 (G3) bp's between the observed and expected fragments and were reproducible with new DNA samples. Child II exhibited in all cases larger fragments sizes as we expected from the fragment sizes observed in the father.

Table 2: Results obtained by the VNTR analysis of child I and II. Shifted fragments are printed in bold

SLP	Mother	Child I	Child II	Put.Father
MS205	2,38 / 3,10	1,75 / 3,08	**1,86** / 3,09	1,75 / 2,92
yNH24	2,83 / 3,24	2,89 / 3,22	2,82 / 4,04	2,89 / 4,05
LH1	3,67 / 4,58	2,37 / 4,59	3,87 / 4,57	2,37 / 3,88
pH30	2,90 / 4,59	2,90 / 17,09	4,58 / 16,86	3,60 / 16,98
MS1	2,20 / 2,68	2,67 / 3,35	2,67 / **5,12**	3,33 / 5,01
MS43A	9,81 / 10,76	10,47 / 10,77	9,14 / 10,66	9,14 / 10,58
G3	1,67 / 9,43	1,67 / 6,16	9,45 / **10,39**	6,15 / 9,93
MS31	6,50 / 9,26	6,43 / 9,24	6,44 / 9,21	6,42 / 6,42

In contrast to the analysis of VNTR loci, the analysis of five STR-PCR loci (HUMTH01, D8S639, CYP19, ACPP and ACTBP2), 22 conventional serum protein and erythrocyte membrane systems including HLA-Class I (ABC) analysis did not reveal any exclusion patterns. Biostatistical calculation using the results obtained by the conventional, HLA and STR analysis resulted in an PP value of 99,99%. In addition, calculation of the results obtained from all analysed polymorphisms including the analysis of VNTR loci resulted in an PP value of 99,97% giving clear evidence for paternity.

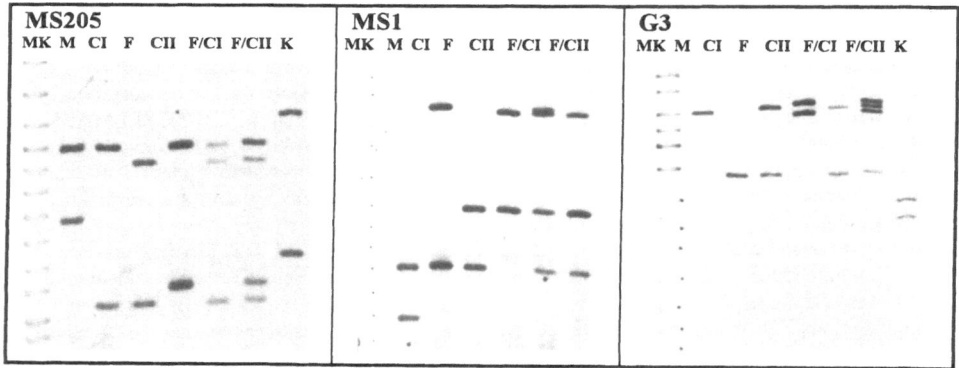

Figure 1. Mutations observed with SLP's MS205, MS1 and G3. Marker (MK) Gibco-BRL bp ladder, mother (M), child I (CI), child II (CII), father (F), mixed samples father and child (F/CI F/CII), control cell line K562 (K)

In order to verify the observed mutations in the VNTR systems, we performed DNA analysis using the multilocus probes 33.15 and (GTG)$_5$. The three SLP's MS1, MS205 and G3 have been originally cloned out from probe 33.15. In this respect, we were interested to study if the observed discrepancies in paternal fragment size of child II could be explained by a general shift of all bands generated with 33.15 or if there are single shifted bands that indicate a mutation event. Interestingly, with probe 33.15 we observed a single band difference between child II and the putative father that corresponds to the G3 mutation (Fig. 2). Unfortunately, the MLP 33.15 showed a very homogeneous pattern in the short fragment region, therefore we could not identify similar band shifts corresponding to SLP MS1 and MS205. In contrast, the results obtained from (GTG)$_5$ were in accordance with the expected paternity of the putative father for both children.

MK CII M CI F F/CII F/CI

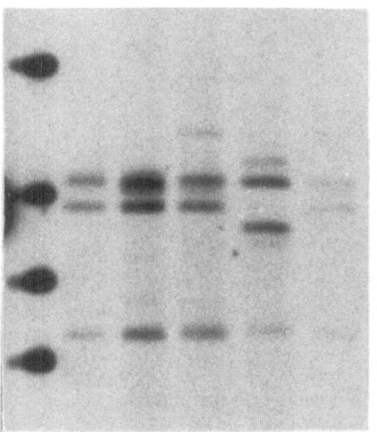

Figure 2. Multilocus probe 33.15 reveals band shift corresponding to the G3 mutation in child II.

Complex chromosome translocations may cause such phenomenon. Metaphase chromosome in situ staining results, however, did show regular caryotypes with no structural variations. In this respect, we interpretate the observed band shifts of child II as the result of at least three individual events leading to an increased fragment size of the paternal alleles. The mutation rate for SLP MS1 has been reported to be 4,16%, while the mutation rates of SLP's MS205 and G3 are 0,4% and 0,69%, respectively (Henke 1993, Jeffreys 1988, Royle 1992). Thus the possibility that these paternal mutations occur in one case is $1,15 \times 10^{-6}$ or 0,0001%. If 6 VNTR loci (including MS31, MS43A, LH1) are analysed the possibility of such an event is $0,96 \times 10^{-5}$ or 0,001%. Since the individual band shifts are relatively small (between 110 - 460 bp) the possibility that the enlarged fragments are due to the loss of a restriction enzyme site in the flanking region of the VNTR loci may not be very likely. Restriction enzyme sites in the human genome have in genral a distance between several thousand to 50 kb (Linn 1968, Smith 1970). Instead, we would propose two alternative explanations: a multiple unequal crossing over affecting the chromosomes 1 (MS1), 7 (G3) and 12 (MS205) occurred during paternal meiosis. An unequal crossing can result in a changed number of repeats in the core-sequence itself and thus explains the increased fragment sizes that we observed in child II. Alternatively a systematic slippage effect occurred during the last premeiotic paternal S phase. Both possibilities may represent rare event but emphasize the importance to combine the analysis of several VNTR loci and/or other genetic marker, i.e. STR or conventional marker, in the evaluation of paternity or human identification cases.

References

Henke J, Fimmers R, Baur MP, Henke L (1993) DNA minisatellite mutations: recent investigations concerning distribution and impact on parentage testing. Int.J.Leg.med. 105: 217-222

Jeffreys AJ, Royle NL, Wilson V, Wong Z (1988) Spontaneous mutation rates to new lenght alleles at tandem-repetitive hypervariable loci in human DNA. Letter to Nature Vol.332(17): 278-281

Linn S, and Arber W (1968) Host specificity of DNA produced by E.coli X. In vitro restriction of phage fd replicative form. Proc.Natl.Sci. 59: 1300-1306

Royle NJ, Armour JA, Webb M, Thomas A, Jeffreys AJ (1992) A hypervariable locus D16S309 at the distal end of 16p. Nucleic Acids Res. 20 (5): 1164

Seidl C, Löliger C, Jäger O, Kühnl P, Seifried E (1995) Analysis of chimerism after bone marrow transplantation by multiplex PCR of the STR-Loci TC11, CYP19, D8S639 and ACPP. Eur.J.Immunogenetics, Vol 22 (1): 35

Smith HO, Wilcox KW (1970) A restriction enzyme from Hemophilus Influenza I. Purification and general properties. J.Mol.Biol. 51: 379-391

Three intriguing identification cases.

B. Mevåg, S. Jacobsen, B. Olaisen.

Institute of Forensic Medicine, University of Oslo, Norway.

Introduction:
The use of DNA analysis has proved to be a powerful tool in cases where identification by ordinary means is impossible. The three cases presented here, involved highly decomposed bodies.
I. A decapitated body was found in the sea March-94 in northern Norway. The police related the finding to a missing person - a man born in 1916 who was last seen December-93. The only relative was a nephew.
II. A young Norwegian sailor disappeared at Crete in November-93. A headless body was found at the seaside of Crete in January-94 and remains of the clothing indicated that this might be the missing man. Relatives: parents.
III. A body with a high degree of adipocere was found in a lake in september-94. The only missing person in the area was a man born in 1896 who disappeared in 1972. His only relatives were two sons living in the USA.

Materials:
Different kinds of samples were taken from all three bodies, including soft tissue, organs and cartilage.

Methods:
Preparation and quantitation of DNA:
DNA was extracted from all the samples, using the common procedure with proteinase K, phenol extraction and ethanol precipitation.Then the DNA was purified by dialysis.
The DNA was quantified by the slot-blot system detailed by Walsh et al.(Nucleic Acids Research 20: 5061-5065), using the QuantiBlot™ Human DNA Quantitation Kit(Perkin Elmer).

HLA DQ A1:
HLA DQ A1- typing was performed using the Amplitype™- kit from Perkin Elmer.

STR-primers:
HUMTHO1 (Polymeropoulos et al. 1991a), HUMF13A1 (Polymeropoulos et al. 1991b), HUMFES(Polymeropoulos et al. 1991c), HUMVWA (Kimpton et al. 1992), D8S347 (Lu et al. 1993), D8S306 (Nelson et al. 1993), D3S1349 (Li et al. 1993).

STR amplification conditions and fragment analysis:
Amplification was performed in a Perkin Elmer 9600 thermo cycler. The fragments were analysed in an ABI model 373 Seqencing System using Genescan 672 software.

Statistics:
Odds calculations were performed using the PATER computer program (Mostad et al. 1995).

Results:

Case I:

	The body	Nephew
HLA DQ A1	1.2/2	1.2/2
HUMTHO1	9,3 (173)	6/9,3 (158/173)
HUMVWA	16/18 (147/155)	16 (147)
HUMF13A1	5/7 (187/195)	7 (195)
D3S1349	129/134	129/134
D8S306	255/270	256/264
APOA1	285/287	280/286

Case II:

	The body	Mother	Father
HLA DQ A1	3/4	1.2/3	4
X/Y	107/113	107	107/113
HUMTHO1	7/9,3 (162/173)	7/9,3 (162/173)	7/9 (162/170)
HUMFES	10/11 (221/225)	10/12 (221/229)	10/11 (221/225)
HUMVWA	14/17 (139/151)	15/17 (143/151)	14/18 (139/155)
HUMF13A	6 (191)	6 (191)	6 (191)
D3S1349	134	134/138	134
D8S347	352/356	352/372	356/380
D8S306	256/264	256/280	264

Case III:

	The body	son no. 1	son no. 2
HLA DQ A1	1.1/4	1.1/4	1.1/4
HUMFES	10/12 (221/229)	10 (221)	10/12 (221/229)
HUMACTBP2	249/263	249/298	263/298

The odds in favour of the missing persons were 22 (case I), 46454 (case II) and 5339 (case III).

Discussion:

In these three cases, the bodies were heavily decomposed and the DNA yield in the samples was low/degraded. Positive results were therefore not expected.

In case I and II the presence of inhibitors made amplification difficult. This was most likely related to the seawater. To avoid the inhibitors, the samples were diluted and reamplified. The results of reamplification have to be interpreted with care regarding contamination. When such results match with the patterns of the relatives, this may be regarded as a positive identification. However, a non-match cannot be used as a proof of nonidentity.

Comparing the different kinds of samples, cartilage proved to be the best source of DNA for PCR.

Even though the bodies were heavily decomposed, HLA DQ A1 and the STR's gave sufficient information for the identification purpose.

References:

Dupuy BM, Olaisen B (1994) Type distribution and allele frequencies of ten STR loci in a Norwegian population. *XII Scandinavian Conference in Forensic Medicine*

Kimpton CP, Walton A, Gill P (1992) A further tetranucleotide repeat polymorphism in the vWF gene. *Hum Mol Genet 1:287*

Kimpton CP, Fisher D, Watson S, Adams M, Urquhart A, Lygo J, Gill P (1993) Evaluation of an automated DNA profiling system employing multiplex amplification of four tetrametric STR loci. *Int J Leg Med 106 : 302-311*

Kimpton CP, Gill P, Walton A, Urquhart A, Millican ES, Adams M (1993) Automated DNA profiling employing multiplex amplification of short tandem repeat loci. *PCR Methods Appl., 3: 13-22*

Li H, Schmidt L, Wei M-H, Hustad T, Lerman MI, Zbar B, Tory K (1993) Three tetrametric repeat polymorphisms on human chromosome 3: D3S1349, D3S1350, D3S1351. *Hum Mol Genet 2 :819*

Lu J, Riley R, Robertson M, Nelson L, Ward K (1993) Tetranucleotide repeat polymorphisms at the D8S342, D8S323, D8S345, D8S315 and D8S347 loci on 8q. *Hum Mol Genet 2 : 1743*

Lygo JE, Johnson PE Holdaway DJ, Woodroffe S, Whitaker JP, Clayton TM, Kimpton CP, Gill P (1994) The validation of short tandem repeat (STR) loci for use in forensic casework. *Int J Leg Med*

Mostad PF, Egeland T (1995) Probability assessments of family relations using the program 'pater'. *Norwegian Computing Center, P.O. Box 114, Blindern, N-0314 Oslo, Norway*

Nelson L, Riley R, Lu J, Robertson M, Ward K (1993) Tetranucleotide repeat polymorphism at the D8S306 locus. *Hum Mol Genet 2 :1984*

Polymeropoulos MH, Xiao H, Rath DS, Merril CR (1991a) Tetranucleotide repeat polymorphism at the human tyrosine hydrolase gene (TH). *Nucleic Acids Res 19:3753*

Polymeropoulos MH, Rath DS, Xiao H, Merril CR (1991b) Tetranucleotide repeat polymorphism at the human coagulation factor XIII A subunit gene (F13A1). *Nucleic Acids Res 19: 4036*

Polymeropoulos MH, Rath DS, Xiao H, Merril CR (1991c) Tetranucleotide repeat polymorphism at the human c-fes/fps proto-oncogene (FES). *Nucleic Acids Res 19: 4018*

Polymeropoulos MH, Rath DS, Xiao H, Merril CR (1992) Tetranucleotide repeat polymorphism at the human beta-actin related pseudogene H-beta-Ac-psi-2 (ACTBP2). *Nucleic acids Res.20 :1432*

Sullivan KM, Manucci A, Kimpton CP, Gill P (1993) A rapid and quantitative DNA sex test : fluorescence-based PCR analysis of X-Y.

FORENSIC DNA-TYPING IN THE SPANISH POLICE USING VNTRs SINGLE PROBES

E. Rivas, T. Vicente, C. Gamella, J. González, J. Andradas

Comisaría General de Policía Científica. Servicio de Analítica. Gran Vía de Hortaleza S/N 28043 Madrid. Spain.

Introduction.

In the last years, our Laboratory has included DNA profiling in forensic case work as a substitutive technique of traditional analysis of proteins. This technique has been employed primarily in case of sexual assault; more than 230 stains and other biological specimens deriving from 125 Spanish crime cases were subjected to this technique, during 1994.

Variable number of tandem repeats (VNTRs) base secuences are one of the most informative genetic DNA Polymorphism for indentification purposes. We have implemented the analysis of VNTRs loci at the Spanish Police using the single locus probe hybridization technique; this analysis includes four independent DNA VNTRs systems: D1S7 (Probe MS1); D2S44 (Probe YNH24); D12S11 (Probe MS43a) and D7S21 (Probe MS31).

This paper describes the case types in which DNA profiling was carried out and shows the rate of obtained profiles from evidence samples in reference to suspect's profile.

DNA extraction.

The extraction of DNA in samples containing semen is done in a differential way. Vaginal cells found in washings and swabs are lysed in presence of Proteinase K and SDS. A second lysis of the spermatozoa is done later in presence of DTT and Proteinase K. Purification is carried out by standard Phenol-Chlorophorm methods, or by ultrafiltering by Centricon 100 (Amicon, USA). The presence of high molecular weight DNA was determined electrophoretically.

Electrophoretic system and DNA Probes.

DNA aliquots were partially digested with Hinf I and quantificated using fluorometric methods. Afterwards, DNA was completly digested and fragments were separated by gel electrophoresis, according to the EDNAP protocol. Gels contained: Lambda DNA/Hind III, to see the movility of the fragments; DNA control Ladders (BRL), as marker and DNA from cell line K562/Hinf I, as allelic control. After electrophoresis, the DNA was transfered to a nylon membrane, by Southern blotting. Hybridization was done using oligonucleotide probes, which were already labelled with alkaline phosphatase. The membrane was sprayed with Lumi-Phos 530 (Lumigen, Inc.) and the light emission was detected with X-ray film by exposing overnight. (Fig. 1).

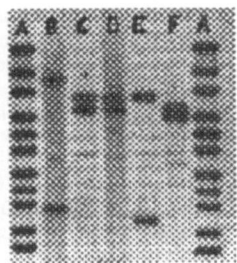

Fig. 1. Hinf 1 / MS43a profile. A)Ladder. B) Allelic control. C) Suspect blood. D) Semen Evidence. E) Victim blood. F) Anonymous Evidence.

Analysis of band position.

The length of DNA-fragments was calculated (Elder 1983) by reference to the DNA control ladder (BRL) using a computerized scanner system (EQUIDNA Pharmagen/Filosoft). This system allows many profile comparison possibilities. Generally, the suspect's profile (if it is available) is compared with the profile obtained in the evidence. This comparison is made band to band using a previously defined coincidence margin (criterion of defined coincidence margin (criterion of matching). If the band sizes are coincident, the identification is established and using the sliding window method, the possibility of finding the identified profile among the Spanish population is calculated. If the suspect's sample is not available, then the profile obtained from the evidence is stored as anonymous in a special data-base which allows the relationship between different offences. (Fig. 2).

Results and discussion.

The types of semen stained exhibits examined at the DNA Laboratory of the Spanish Police are recorded in table N. 1.

Table 1. Exhibit types examined

EXHIBIT TYPE	NUMBER	SUCCESS RATE (%)
Vaginal swabs or washings	89	73
Knickers	30	96
Fabric clothing	30	96
Bed linen	12	83
Other semen remains	1	100
Condoms	2	100
Papers	12	75

Vaginal swabs or washings are the most common items submitted for DNA profiling in rape cases. The DNA is generally of good quality because swabs are taken in controlled conditions so that there is little opportunity for the DNA to degrade, but however the samples are sometimes contaminated, for instance with blood, which does not suppose any problem or with microbic that can increase the amount of extracted DNA.

The preferential extraction procedure for separating spermatozoa from epithelial cells is always used and in most cases no vaginal DNA was observed on the autoradiograph. However, in cases where a high number of vaginal cells is observed, a mixed profile can be obtained, (Rand 1991). It is in these cases that a control sample is requested from the donor of the swabs. If the DNA is seen to be of good quality on a test gel prepared during the profiling procedure, very low amounts will give results. Our Laboratory has obtained profiles from swabs which yield less than 350 ng. of DNA.

DNA - Profiling
VNTRs probes with SLPs

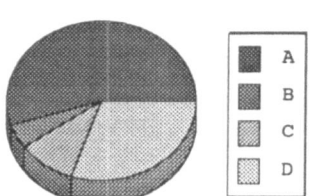

A) Anonymous profiles 55 %
B) Exclusion-suspects 5 %
C) Linked cases 10 %
D) Inclusion-suspects 30 %

Fig. 2. Cases when DNA-profile was obtained (Sexual assaults).

Knickers with semen stains in the cruch and fabric clothing are commonly submitted for DNA profiling and also give a very high success rate. This is an option when there is no semen on washings or vaginal swabs (Greenhalgh 1992). Analysis of these stains is easier now, by the use of Laser Technology, that let us see possible semen stains non visible with the naked eyes. Although stains on fabric are likely to be composed of semen without contaminating vaginal material, the preferential extraction procedure is still performed in some cases. The major problem with this sort of stains is that many fabrics, especially dark colours, are not colour fast and the dyes coextract with the DNA. The most successful method found to overcome this problem is to wash the spermatozoa from the fabric by vortexing in cold water; the fabric is then removed and the cells sedimented by preferential extraction procedure.

Bed linen does not present any particular problem, yielding good results in general (83% success rate). Pollutants that inhibit the restriction process can appear in the papers used to recover semen remains in floors.

Conclusions.

A wide range of semen stained exhibit types is suitable for profiling. The present amount of DNA has some influence on the chances of obtaining a result but it is not the only factor to consider. Small quantities of DNA can give results using SLP analysis if the DNA is undegraded and there are no contaminants present that inhibit the restriction process. If only highly degraded DNA can be isolated it is unlikely that conclusive results will be obtained from SLP analysis. In these cases one possibility is the use of PCR better than SLPs.

References.

Elder JK and Southern EM (1983). Anal. Bioche. 128: 227-231.

Greenhalgh M, Burridge F and Willot G (1992). Experiences with single locus DNA probes in casework. Forensic Science International 57: 29-37.

Rand S, Wiegand P and Brinkmann B (1991). Problems associated with the DNA analysis of stains. Int.J. Leg. Med. 104: 293-297.

PCR-typing of DNA extracted from epidermal particles won by scratching

Sanchez-Hanke, M.[1], Püschel, K.[1], Augustin, C.[1], Wiegand, P.[2], Brinkmann, B.[2]

[1] Institute for Legal Medicine, University of Hamburg, Butenfeld 34, D-22529 Hamburg
[2] Institute for Legal Medicine, Westfälische Wilhelms-University, von Esmarch-Straße 86, D-48149 Münster

INTRODUCTION

In medical emergency examinations and therapy minimal excoriations by violent attacks or abuse are not important, neither to the physican nor to the patient. But such lesions can be essential for the coroner or forensic pathologist concerning the reconstruction of the course of events. Sometimes, the aggressor's skin particles can be found under the victims finger-nails. The conventional serological means of typing scratched epidermal particles are limited. The aim of this study was the application of PCR-based DNA-typing methods to this question.

MATERIALS AND METHODS

The epidermal particles were obtained by two experimental series. In the first experiments four volunteers were scratched by four other volunteers. The epidermal particles attached to the fingernails of the „victims" were preserved.

Subsequently to positive results of this pilot study, different scratches were produced at cadavers in a second experimental series. A special mechanical apparatus was developed for this experiment. On one side of the machine's balance arm a plastic fingernail was fixed. Different weights were applied to regulate force intensity. After every experiment the fingernail was cleaned with a fiberglas plate and preserved.

In both series, epidermal DNA material was isolated using the CHELEX-method and quantified by ACES (Advanced Chemiluminescence Enhancement System; Gibco-BRL, UK; Waye et al.1989). The STR loci HUMACTBP2 (SE 33), HUMTH01 (TC 11) and HUMVWFA31 (VWA) were amplified by PCR according to Wiegand et al.(1993). Alleles were resolved by non-denaturing PAA-gelelectrophoresis according to Wiegand et al.(1993) and visualized by silver staining according to Budowle (1992).

RESULTS

In the first phase of the experiments the skin wounds remained superficial and disappeared within 24 hours. The indices and middle fingers of our victims produced the longest and deepest excoriations so that usually epidermal residues being attached to the fingernails could be seen microscopally. When the attacks were carried out at the neck or the upper arm region, this observation could be made regulary. On the contrary, when the scratch was carried out at forearm positive results could not be obtained.

The serological results of the applied STR systems differed. The findings with the systems TC 11 and SE 33 were coincident; the VWA system showed fewer positive results than the other two systems.

In the second experimental phase the different scratching series exhibited different histological alterations. Only the stratum corneum was affected when applying 200-400g scratching force. At intensities between 400-800g the deeper epidermal layers were affected by the lesion but the basal membrane was always intact. At intensities of 800-1400g the epidermis, in some cases even the dermis lying directly underneath the basement membrane, was destroyed. Intensities above 1400g regulary produced massive morphological alterations, leading to a destruction of almost the complete skin.

The histological results in this second phase were accompanied by the following serological findings: Positive results were regularly obtained by high intensity scratches with all three PCR-systems. Occasionally negative PCR-typing results were found by middle or low force intensities. Sometimes DNA contamination occured in low force intensities. The relationship between the employed force and the quantity of DNA was confirmed by statistical analysis with the Pearson's-correlation test.

DISCUSSION

The possibility to discover epidermal particles under the fingernails used for scratching as reported by Wiegand et al. 1993 could be confirmed in the first experimental phase. The described soft asservation of scratched particles with a small fiberglas plate proved to be an effective method which enabled us to obtain sufficient DNA material for an analysis.

The negative results for the forearm area correlates to the skin's high resistance in this area. The soft skin structure of the neck and upper arm which are quive similar lead to a high percentage of positive and similar results.

In the second phase different force intensities were applied to the upper arms of deceased persons (6-8 hours after death). The subsequent histological findings showed a significant correlation to the acquired amount of DNA.

The DNA quantity gained with forces above 1200g remained constant. This finding can be explained by the micromorphological structure of the dermis which contains few cells and a comparably higher amount of soft tissue which does not contribute to the DNA quantity. In contrast to the dermis, the deep epidermal skin layers contain numerous melanocytes (which led to high amounts of extracted DNA). Subsequently the correlation curve between low scratching intensities and the amount of DNA attached to the fingernails increases logarithmically and remained constant at higher force intensities.

CONCLUSIONS

1) PCR-typing of scratched epidermal particles was sucessfull in about 70% of the cases.

2) A correlation between the quantity of DNA and the employed scratch force could be shown.

3) Force intensities over 1200 g led to levelling of the produced amount of DNA.

4) The interpretation of stain analysis performed by PCR-based VNTR-systems has to be done very carefully with respect to contaminations and conclusions concerning the reconstruction of the kind and timing of contact between the victim and the perpetretor.

REFERENCES

Brinkmann B (1992) The use of STRs in stain analysis. In: Proceedings from the Third International Symposium on Human Identification,357-374. Promega Corporation, Madison (USA)

Budowle B, Chakraborty R, Guisti AM, Eisenberg AJ, Allen R (1991) Analysis of the VNTR locus D1S80 by the PCR followed by High-Resolution-PAGE. Am J Hum Genet 48: 137-144

Waye JS, Presley LA, Budowle B, Shutler GG, Fourney RM (1989) A simple and sensitive method for quantifying human genomic DNA in forensic specimen extracts. Biotechniques 7: 852-855

Wiegand P, Bajanowski T, Brinkmann B (1993) DNA typing of debris from fingernails. Int J Leg Med 106: 81-83

Wiegand P, Budowle B, Rand S, Brinkmann B (1993) Forensic validation of the STR systems SE 33 and TC 11. Int J Leg Med 105: 315-320.

PCR GENOTYPING IN DENTAL PULP FROM OLD HUMAN SKELETAL REMAINS AND FIRE VICTIMS.

SANZ P, PRIETO V, ANDRES MI.

National Institute fo Toxicology. Seville. Spain.

Introduction

The first attempts to recover genetic information from ancient skeletal material was undertaken from an anthropological and palaeontological point of view. Soon after, an ongrowing forensic interest in the possibility of DNA typing of human skeletal remains emerged, thus solving the identification of recent or ancient victims, and specially difficult parentage testing problems. The successful identification of family relationships in three famous cases: the Karen Price case (Hagelberg, 1991), the identification of the skeletal remains of Josef Mengele (Jeffreys, 1992) and of the Romanov family (Gill, 1994) have stimulated the common usage of skeletal remains in forensic questions involving more or less recently dead individuals. Among these skeletal remains, dental pulp, housed in the pulp cavity in the center of the tooth is a rich source of DNA. Moreover teeth endure post-mortem degradation and extreme environmental conditions better than most biological tissues (Sweet, 1995; Cerri, 1994). Here we present the result of PCR genotyping of dental pulp samples obtained from dental surgeon and from casework.

Material and Methods

Control teeth, freshly removed and healthy, were obtained for orthodontic reasons.
Casework teeth:
A.- alleged father (60 years) of a paternity case, exhumed two years after death.
B.- alleged father (20 years) of a paternity case, exhumed four years after death.
C.- Unidentified burnt corpse, victim of a domestic fire (45 years).
D.- Unidentified male corpse (above 40 years) found outdoors; from the decomposition features time after death was estimated at about fifteen to thirty days.

Sample preparation and DNA extraction

Teeth were thoroughly washed in boiling water with the addition of dishwasher machine detergent (Calgonit®), rinsed with distilled water, dried, immersed in liquid nitrogen for at least 24 h, and finely crushed to fine powder with a mortar and pestle. Powdered teeth were decalcified with 0.5M pH EDTA 7.5, according to Hochmeister (1991). The decalcification process took from four to five days. After washing three times in Milli Q sterile water, 2 ml of prewarmed (56°C) extraction buffer containing 10 mM Tris, 10 mM EDTA, 100 mM NaCl, 40 mM DTT and 150 μL of proteinase K (16.2 mg/mL) were added to each pellet and incubated at 56°C overnight. The solutions were extracted three times with phenol-chloroform-isoamyl alcohol (25:24:1), aqueous solutions combined, extracted once with n-butanol to eliminate phenol residues and DNA was concentrated using a Centricon-30 microconcentrator device. Retentates were washed three times with Milli Q water and recovered DNA was stored until use at 4°C or -20°C.

DNA sample analysis

The quantity of human DNA in the samples was determined by slot blot quantification using the QuantiBlot human DNA quantitation Kit (Perkin Elmer®).

The DNA quality was assessed by submarine 0.7% agarose minigel electrophoresis in TBE (0.134M Tris- 75 mM Boric Acid - 2.55 mM Na_2 EDTA, pH 8.8). Lambda Hinf III digested DNA was used as molecular weight ladder and UV visualization carried out after immersion of the gel in an ethidium bromide solution ($0.5\mu g/mL$) for 20 min after the electrophoresis run.

Amplifications and Typing

DQA1: Amplitype HLA DQA1 Forensic DNA amplification and Typing Kit (Perkin Elmer).

PM: Amplitype PM PCR Amplification and Typing Kit (Perkin Elmer).

D1S80: AmpliFLP D1S80 PCR amplification reagent set (Perkin Elmer). PCR products were detected by vertical PAGE (Gene Amp Detection Gel Perkin Elmer) followed by silver staining (Plus One Silver Staining Kit. Pharmacia).

STR: Gene Print STR systems (Promega) were used for TH01, CSF1P0, TPOX, F13A01, FES/FPS and vWF loci. Typing was carried out by poliacrylamide denaturing gel electrophoresis followed by silver staining, according to Promega protocols.

Results

Table 1 DNA recovery.

Sample	Powdered Teeth Weight (g)	DNA recovery ($\mu g/g$)
Control	0.50	2.4
A	1.96	15.9
B	2.18	25.04
C	3.05	295.08
D	1.22	31.96

Dental pulp from the burnt body (C) yielded far more DNA than exhumed specimens. No high molecular weight DNA was recovered in any sample. DQA1 was successfully typed in all the samples. Additionally two STRs were assayed in control teeth (FES/FPS and vWF).

Successful typing of STRs permitted the processing of casework specimens to continue. A set of PCR loci usually amplified in our laboratory was applied. The following results were obtained:

	A	B	C	D
DQA1	+	+	+	+
PM	+	+	+	+
D1S80	+	Undetected	+	+
TH01	+	Spurious bands	+	+
TPOX	+	Spurious bands	+	+
CSF1PO	Faint bands	Spurious bands	+	+
FES/FPS	+	Spurious bands	+	+
vWF	+	Spurious bands	+	+
F13A01	+	+	+	+

+ Successful typing

Comments

Anomalous results or failure in the amplification reaction were obtained only in the tooth sample from the corpse exhumed four years after burial, under the most unfavourable climatic conditions in our region: very high temperatures in summer and a high level of humidity and mild environmental temperatures in winter; moreover the cemetery is located close to the Guadalquivir river.

References

- Cerri N, Mignola R, Papanelli C, De Ferrari F (1994) Genetic identification from dental pulp by using DNA amplification (PCR). Advances in Forensic Haemogenetics 5: 268-270

- Gill P, Ivanov PL, Kimpton C, Piercy R, Benson N, Tully G, Evett I, Hagelberg E, Sullivan K (1994) Identification of the remains of the Romanov family by DNA analysis. Nature Gen 6: 130-135

- Hagelberg E, Cray IC, Jeffreys AJ (1991) Identification of the skeletal remains of a murder victim by DNA analysis. NATURE 352: 427-429

- Hochmeister MN, Budowle B, Borer UV, Eggmann U, Comey CT, Dirnhofer R (1991) Typing of Deoxyribonucleic Acid (DNA) Extracted from Compact Bone from Human Remains.

- Jeffreys AJ, Allen MJ, Hagelberg E, Sonnberg A (1992) Identification of The Skeletal Remains of Josef Mengele by DNA Analysis. For Sci Int 56:65-76

- Sweet DJ, Sweet CHW (1995) DNA Analysis of Dental Pulp to Link Incinerated Remains of Homicide Victim to Crime Scene. JFSCA 40: 310-314

ABO genotyping of the suspects using their sperm DNA.

M Sasaki, K Shimizu, T Fukushima and H Shiono.

Department of Legal Medicine, Asahikawa Medical College, Nishikagura 4,5,3,11. Asahikawa, 078, Hokkaido, JAPAN.

Introduction

In sexual assaults against women, the key to identify the suspect is ABO phenotyping or the typing of other polymorphic markers of the seminal fluid in the victim's vagina. However, ABO phenotyping is frequently unsuccessful, since mixtures of fluids cannot be separated to be subjected to conventional methods for the detection of antibody or antigen material. We therefore studied ABO blood group genotyping of isolated sperm DNA from contaminated vaginal fluid by the polymerase chain reaction-restriction fragment length polymorphism (PCR-RFLP) method [1].

Materials and Methods

10 μ l of post-coital vaginal fluid in 4 sexual assaults were collected from the victim's vaginae with syringes within 24 hr after the crimes. We have examined the two-step extraction procedure for purification of sperm DNA or vaginal epithelial DNA in contaminated specimens by a modification of the NaI method [2,3]. The first step of digestion was to solubilize the non-sperm cells in the mixed fluids. Since sperm nuclei are protected by cross-linked thiol-rich proteins, they remained intact in the first step of digestion without DTT[3]. Thus, the mixed fluids were separated into the sperm heads and the female components by centrifugation. In the second step of digestion, the precipitated sperm heads were solubilized with DTT. And these DNA were then subjected to the PCR-RFLP with a restriction enzyme, Kpn-1 or Msp-1, for each site [1,3]. All specimens were genotyped as shown in Table 1.

ABO genotype	Primer 1f and 1r Kpn-1	Primer 3f and 3r Msp-1
OO	69	140
AA	96	140
AO	96,69	140
BB	96	159
BO	96,69	159,140
AB	96	159,140

(bp)

.e. 1   ABO genotyping by PCR-RFLP

Results

In case 1, only the 69 bp DNA fragment of locus 1 and the 140 bp DNA fragment of locus 3 were found in the digested PCR products of the recovered sperm DNA (lane 2 of Fig 1a, b), whereas the 96 bp DNA fragment of locus 1 and the 140 bp and 159 bp DNA fragments of locus 3 were found in the digested PCR products of the recovered vaginal cell DNA (lane 3 of Fig 1a, b). These findings clearly showed that the genotype of the male suspect was OO and the genotype of the female victim was AB (Table 2). Since the band of the 96 bp DNA fragment of locus 1 and the 159 bp DNA fragment of locus 3 were not found in lane 2 shown in Fig 1a, b. These findings show that sperm DNA extracted by these methods was not contaminated by any female components.

In case 2, the genotype of the male suspect was OO and the genotype of the female victim was BO (Table 2, lane 6 of Fig 1a, b). There was no band of the 96 bp DNA fragment of locus 1 or the 159 bp DNA fragment of locus 3 in the recovered sperm DNA, demonstrating that the sperm DNA did not contain any female components.

In cases 3 and 4, the genotype of the male suspect was AB and the genotype of the female victim was AO (Table 2, lane 6 of Fig 1a, b). There were no bands of the 69 bp DNA fragment of locus 1 in the recovered sperm DNA. These findings indicate that the sperm DNA extracted by these methods did not contain any female components.

Discussion

With this method, mixed samples can be completely separated into the male and female components, and the genotype of the recovered sperm DNA or vaginal epithelial cells can easily be determined. This reliable ABO genotyping method by PCR-RFLP, using separated sperm DNA, should be of value in forensic identification in sexual assaults [3].

References

1. Sasaki, M., Fukushima, T., and Shiono, H. ABO Genotyping of Fingerprints by the PCR-RFLP Method. Japanese Journal of Legal Medicice, Vol. 48, No. 6, 1994, p 428-432.

2. Ishizawa, M., Kobayashi, Y., Miyamura, T. and Matuura, S. Simple procedure of DNA isolation from human serum. Nucleic Acids Research, Vol. 20, 1991, p 5792.

3. Sasaki, M and Shiono, H. ABO genotyping of suspects from sperm DNA isolated from the post-coital samples of sexual crimes. J.Forensic Sci.1996, 41 (3) submitted.

Case	ABO phenotypes of semen-contaminated vaginal fluid	ABO phenotypes of victim	Possible ABO phenotypes of suspect	ABO genotypes of recovered sperm-DNA by PCR-RFLP
1	AB	AB	AB, A, B, O	OO
2	B	B	B, O	OO
3	AB	A	AB, B	AB
4	AB	A	AB, B	AB

Table 2   ABO genotypes of of recovered sperm-DNA by PCR-RFLP from
semen-contaminated vaginal fluid in 4 sexual assaults.

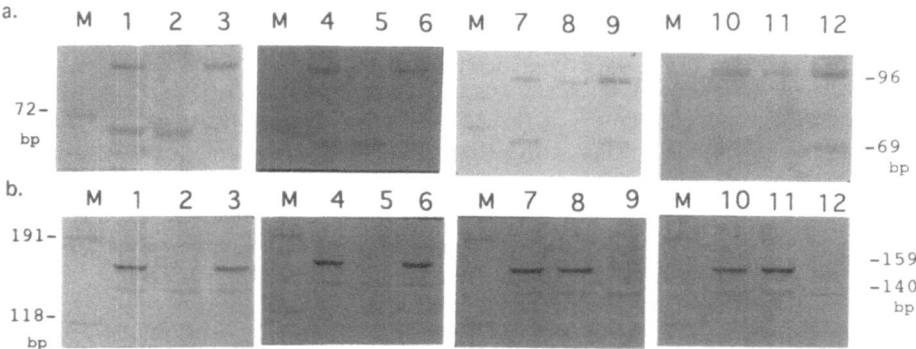

Fig. 1 - Electrophoresis in 10% polyacrylamide gels of each digested PCR product.
a; PCR products of Locus 1 digested with Kpn-1. b; PCR products of Locus 3 digested
with Msp-1. M: φX174/Hae III digest, Lane 1-3; Case 1, Lane 4-6; Case 2, Lane 7-9;
Case 3, Lane 10-12; Case 4. Lane 1, 4, 7, 10; contaminated vaginal fluid, Lane 2, 5,
8, 11; recovered sperm DNAs, Lane 3, 6, 9, 12; recovered vaginal epithelial DNAs.

FORENSIC IDENTIFICATION USING DNA RECOVERED FROM SALIVA ON HUMAN SKIN

D.J. Sweet[1], J.A. Lorente[2], M. Lorente[2], A. Valenzuela[2], E. Villanueva[2]

[1] University of British Columbia, Fac. of Dentistry, Vancouver, Canada
[2] University of Granada, Dept. of Forensic Medicine, Granada, Spain

INTRODUCTION

Bites, suck marks or kisses occur often in crimes of aggression, in self defense and during sexual interactions. Saliva is presumed to be deposited on the skin under these circumstances.

Bite mark analysis using pshysical matching techniques is prone to distortion and subjective interpretation [Rothwell, 1994]. Comparisons depend on measurements of the size and shape of an injury on the skin surface wich is elastic and may be unstable.

Saliva is an adequate source of forensically useful DNA evidence since it contains cells sloughed from the oral epithelium and leukocytes [Raeste and Calonius, 1971; Watanabe et al, 1981; Hochmeister et al, 1991]. Whole saliva mixed body fluid stains containing saliva have been typed and successfully discriminated to their source [Comey and Budowle, 1991]. Salivary evidence is stable over a moderately long postmortem interval [Adams et al, 1991; Walsh et al, 1992].

An experimental protocol was designed to evaluate the amount of DNA wich can be extracted from saliva collected from human skin (of cadavers) and typed using PCR analysis. Stains with a volume of whole saliva equivalent to the amount deposited during a typical bite were studied. The most effective protocol for collecting salivary DNA from skin and avoiding contamination of the sample by DNA from the cadaver were tested.

MATERIALS AND METHODS

Thirty-three sites on the skin of 27 cadavers were divided into 4 quadrants with a surface area of approximately equal to an average adult bite mark (quadrant area = 10.7 cm^2). Expectorated saliva was collected from one male donor and aliquots containing 40 ul of whole saliva were deposited on three out of the four quadrants on the skin of each cadaver. The fourth quadrant remained undisturbed.

Recovery methods were studied to improve the number of nucleated salivary cells wich can be collected from the surface of the skin. A modification of the classical single swab technique was developed. In this method, referred to as the *double swab technique* [Sweet, 1995], a wet swab is used to wash the saliva from the skin. This is followed by a dry swab wich is used to collect the water left on the skin containing rehydrated salivary cells.

A sample was collected from one quadrant after 5 minutes of elapsed time. This was the positive DNA control. Other samples were collected from two other quadrants. one after 24 hours and one after 48 hours. Swabbing was completed on the fourth quadrant where no saliva had been deposited to determine if contamination of the samples occurred. An additional sample was collected from the cadaver as a negative control (blood or tissue).

DNA was extracted using the Chelex-100 extraction method [Walsh et al, 1991] with several modifications. These included: a) washing the cotton swab tips with a solution of distilled water and proteinase K (1 mg/ml); b) incubation at 56°C and at 100°C (8 minutes) prior to addition of Chelex-100; c) micro-concentration using Microcon-100™ tubes. DNA yield was quantified using a slot-blot apparatus and amplified using the short tandem repeats (STR) loci HUMTH01 and HUMVWA.

RESULTS

Using the classic single wet swab recovery technique, $33.5 \pm 4.8\%$ of the saliva deposited on the skin was recovered. Using the double swab method saliva recovery was improved to $44.6 \pm 6.4\%$ of the total amount of saliva deposited.

Following the classic Chelex-100 extraction method, $31.9 \pm 4.2\%$ of the DNA present in a solution with a known concentration was extracted. After incubation in a wash solution containing proteinase K, incubation at 56°C and at 100°C, and micro-concentration with Microcon-100 tubes, DNA yield was increased to $47.7 \pm 6.9\%$

Positive PCR amplification results were obtained at locus HUMTH01 for 78.8% of the samples collected after 5 minutes, 75.8% of those recovered after 24 hours, and 69.7% of those recovered at 48 hours. Results were similar for the HUMVWA locus since 78.8% positive amplifications resulted after 5 minutes, 66.7% after 24 hours, and 57.6% after 48 hours.

DISCUSSION & CONCLUSSIONS

Extraction of DNA from saliva using Chelex-100 resin is improved if the samples ares ubmitted to pre-extraction treatment consisting on incubation in proteinase K and filtration with Microcon-100. The concentration of DNA in saliva recovered from skin varies as a function of time since deposition. There is a significant decrease in concentration in the first 24 hours, but the concentration remains stable from 24 to 48 hours.

In the majority of cases, positive PCR amplifications were obtained for STR loci HUMTH01 and HUMVWA from saliva deposited on the skin of cadavers. Amplification success is independent of time since deposition or concentration of DNA in the saliva sample. Contamination from the skin of the cadaver was not found in any of the cases studied.

These results indicate that forensic analysis of DNA from saliva recovered from human skin may be a valuable identification tool in cases involving bite marks or suck-marks, or in any case where saliva trace evidence is discovered.

REFERENCES

Adams DE, Presley LA, Baumstark AL, Hensley KW, Campbell PA, McLauglin CM, Budowle B, Giusti AM, Smerick JB, Baechtel FS (1991) Deoxyribonucleic acid (DNA) analysis by restriction fragment length polymorphisms of blood and other body fluids stains subjected to contamination and environmental insults. J Forensic Sci 36: 1284-1298

Auvdel MJ (1988) Comparison of laser and high-intensity qaurtz arc tubes in the detection of body secretions. J Forensic Sci 33: 929-945

Comey CT, Budowle B (1991) Validation studies on the analisis of the HLA DQx locus using the polymerase chain reaction. J Forensic Sci 36: 1633-1648

Hochmeister MN, Budowle B, Jung J, Borer UV, Comey CT, Dirnhofer R (1991) PCR-based typing of DNA extracted from cigarette butts. Int J Legal Med 104: 229-233

Raeste AM, Calonius PEB (1971) The modified Millipore technique for the study of oral leukocytes. Scand J Dental Res 79: 327-332

Rothwell BR (1994) Bite marks in forensic odontology: fact or fiction?. In: Worthington P, Evans JR (ed) W.B.Saunders Co., Philadelphia pp: 588-600 (Controversies in Oral & Maxillofacial Surgery)

Sweet DJ (1995) Identification of stains in human saliva using forensic DNA analysis. Doctoral Thesis, University of Granada, Spain.

Walsh DJ, Corey AC, Cotton RW, Forman L, Herrin GL, Word CJ, Garner DD (1992) Isolation of deoxyribonucleic acid (DNA) from saliva and forensic science samples containing saliva. J Forensic Sci 37: 387-395

Walsh PS, Metzger DA, Higuchi R (1991) Chelex-100 as a medium for simple extraction of DNA for PCR-based typing from forensic material. BioTechniques 10: 506-513

Watanabe T, Ohata N, Morishita M, Iwamoto Y (1981) Correlation between the protease activities and the number of epithelial cells in human saliva. J Dental Res 60: 1039-1044

This work was supported by a grant from the Ministry of education and Science, Spain, and by the Dentistry Canada Fund/Warner Lambert Foundation, Ottawa, Canada.

ANALYSIS OF STR LOCI IN OLD BLOOD STAINS USING AUTOMATED AND MANUAL GENOTYPING SYSTEMS

J. Thomson, C. Phillips, D. Beckett, O. Summerfield and P. Lincoln.

Department of Haematology, London Hospital Medical College, London, UK.

INTRODUCTION

PCR based analysis of polymorphic short tandem repeat (STR) loci is becoming widely used in forensic identity testing (Lygo *et al.*1994). These systems offer a number of important advantages over the Southern blot analysis of VNTR loci using single locus probes; the technique which has been predominantly used over the past decade. These advantages are principally,(1) increased sensitivity; (2) the ability to analyse highly degraded DNA; and (3) the ability to co-amplify a number of loci simultaneously, so reducing the overall time for the analysis.

Various methodologies have been developed for the identification of the different length alleles amplified by PCR. These have included high sieving agarose with ethidium bromide staining; polyacrylamide electrophoresis under both denaturing and non-denaturing conditions combined with ethidium bromide or silver staining; capillary electrophoresis; and detection of fluorescently labelled PCR products using an automated DNA sequencing apparatus and appropriate analysis software.

This study investigates the suitability for STR typing of aged blood stains, dating from 1968 to 1994, from four individuals. The STR locus chosen for this analysis was humTH01. The aim of the study was threefold. To investigate the effect of increasing age of blood stain on STR profiles from the same individual; to investigate the relationship between the size of the blood stain and the STR profile obtained; and finally to assess the relative suitability of manual MetaPhor agarose electrophoresis and an automated fluorescent detection system in genotyping these old and small stains.

MATERIALS AND METHODS

Samples: Three blood stains on cotton cloth from each of four individuals dating from 1968, 1975 and 1994. Two further fresh blood stains on cotton cloth from staff members. DNA was extracted using a 5% chelating resin (Lareu *et al.* 1994). Samples of the stained material 3mmx3mm were used in the investigation of increasing age of stain. To investigate the suitability of small stains, single cotton threads were removed from the stained material and lengths of thread of 0.5mm, 1mm, 4mm and 12mm were used as starting material.

PCR: PCR was carried out in 20µL reaction volumes with 8µL of DNA extract , 200mM dNTP, 0.25µM of each primer and 0.4U of Taq polymerase. PCR conditions were 94°C x 45 secs; 54°C x 60 secs; 72°C x 60 secs for 26 cycles.

Automated fluorescent detection: 1µL of PCR product was mixed together with 2µL of formamide/dextran blue and 0.3µL of internal size standard GS2500 (labelled with 6-carboxy-X-rhodamine [ROX] dye). Samples were denatured at 95°C for 5 min before loading into a 36 well 6% polyacrylamide, 8M urea denaturing gel (Sequagel-6, National Diagnostics). Electrophoresis was carried out in an ABI 373 DNA Sequencer at 30W for 3 hours. Fragment sizes were analysed automatically using the 672 GeneScan software.

Agarose / ethidium bromide detection: 20µL of each PCR product were run in 4.5% MetaPhor agarose (FMC) gels as previously described (Lareu *et al.* 1994). Gels were visualised and photographed under UV

RESULTS

Automated fluorescent detection

1. Increasing age of stain. Samples from four individuals dating from 1968, 1975 and 1994 were typed for TH01 by automated fluorescent detection. TH01 was successfully typed for all ages of stain in at least three of the four individuals. The results of this typing are summarised in table 1.

Sample	Fluorescence Peak Height		
	27 years	20 years	1 year
PL	60	150	3500
SW	50	0	2100
BD	0	240	6100
MW	40	160	3900

Table 1. Mean peak height fluorescence for TH01 alleles detected in blood stain material of varying age.

2. Decreasing size of stain. Single bloodstained cotton threads of 12mm, 4mm, 1mm and 0.5mm from four individuals were typed for TH01. Control stains of 3mmx3mm were also typed. The 0.5mm threads gave no visible product for any of the samples. However, threads of 1mm, 4mm and 12mm were all typed successfully in at least two of the individuals. These results are summarised in table 2.

Sample	Fluorescence Peak Height				
	0.5mm thread	1mm thread	4mm thread	12mm thread	3x3mm control
DB fresh	0	100	150	200	2500
JT fresh	0	50	40	280	1500
BD 1 yr old	0	0	0	210	4700
MW 1 yr old	0	0	140	450	1400

Table 2. Mean peak height fluorescence for TH01 alleles detected in varying lengths of blood stained thread from four individuals

MetaPhor agarose / ethidium bromide detection

PCR product from TH01 typing of both the old and small stains was also analysed using MetaPhor agarose and ethidium bromide staining. Photographs of these analyses are shown in fig. 1.

From these results it is evident that ethidium bromide staining will reliably provide results only for recent (one year old) stains, although some signal is visible in one of the 1975 stains (lane 8) and possibly in one of the 1967 stains (lane 4). The minimum stain size giving a readable result is the 4mm thread for the one individual analysed.

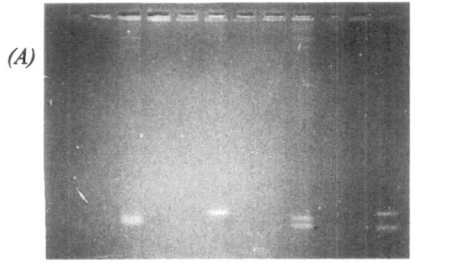
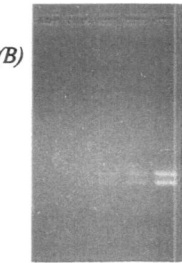

Fig.1. Results of 4.5% MetaPhor agarose / ethidium bromide typing of (A) old stains from four individuals (MW, BD, SW, PL) and (B) varying sized stains from one individual. (A):Lane1:MW 27yrs old; 2:MW 20yr; 3:MW 1yr; 4:BD 27yrs; 5:BD 20yrs; 6:BD 1yr; 7:SW 27yrs; 8: SW 20yrs; 9: SW 1yr; 10:PL 27yrs; 11: pl 20yrs; 12: PL 1yr. (B): Lane 1:JT 0.5mm; 2: JT 1.0mm; 3: JT 4mm; 4: JT 12mm; 5: JT 3mmx3mm control.

DISCUSSION

This study helps to confirm the advantages of using STR analysis combined with an automated fluorescent detection system in forensic analyses.

The availability of stains dating back to 1967 from four different individuals, prepared and stored under identical conditions allows the effect of ageing to be studied in isolation from any other environmental factors. The results show clear quantitative trends, even between the 20 year old stains and the 27 year old stains, indicating that DNA quality continues to decrease over a long period of time. Despite this, successful typing of 3mmx3mm samples of three of the four 27 year old stains confirm the important potential of this technique in investigations involving aged materials.

The sensitivity of PCR based systems are central to their widespread adoption in forensic science. The experiment using short lengths of stained cotton thread confirms that samples previously untypable using Southern blot techniques are now viable substrates for STR analysis. 1mm of thread removed from a stain corresponds to approximately $0.025\mu L$ of whole blood. This represents about 125-200 white cells which theoretically contain approximately 0.6-1ng of DNA. The amount of DNA recovered from these stains was not measured in this study but this theoretical yield corresponds closely with the minimum quantities of 0.5-1ng reported previously (Lygo *et al.* 1994).

The results from the agarose gel analysis of the same PCR products confirm that this form of manual electrophoretic analysis is only useful in cases where a relatively large quantity of PCR product can be produced. In this study, this is limited to stains up to one year old of 3mmx3mm in size, or fresh stains down to 4mm of thread. In cases where sample size or condition are not limiting, MetaPhor agarose analysis could offer a viable alternative to automated fluorescent detection.

REFERENCES

Lareu MV, Phillips CP, Carracedo A, Lincoln PJ, Syndercombe Court DS and Thomson JA. (1994) Investigation of the STR locus humTH01 using PCR and two electrophoretic formats: UK and Galician caucasian population surveys and usefulness in paternity investigations. *For. Sci. Int.* **66** 41-52.

Lygo JE, Johnson PE, Holdaway DJ, Woodroffe S, Whitaker JP, Clayton TM, Kimpton CP and Gill P. The validation of short tandem repeat loci for use in forensic casework. *Int. J. Leg. Med.* (1994) **107** 77-89

MICROSATELLITE DNA POLYMORPHISM ANALYSIS IN A CASE OF ILLEGAL CATTLE PURCHASE

D. Beamonte; E. Valverde; A. Guerra; B. Ruíz and J. Alemany
PharmaGen s.a., c/ de la Calera 3, Tres Cantos, 28760 Madrid, SPAIN

INTRODUCTION

Traditionally, illegal animal purchasing has been difficult to prove, especially in two cases: Young animals not-registered yet in the official genealogical book, and those animals not registered because they don´t belong to any pure breed. Microsatellite Short Tandem Repeat (STR) DNA polymorphism is currently used in human forensic medicine as a powerful tool to solve criminal cases with a high degree of accuracy in a short period of time. However, this practice is not common in criminal cases affecting animals of different species.

Polymorphic STR loci have been described for cattle [1,2], horses [3], swine [4-6], sheep [7,8], or dogs [9]. Specifically, more than 300 polymorphic loci have been described in cattle [2], with the aim of constructing the Bovine genomic map. These loci are currently used in the detection of Quantitative Trait Loci (QTL) [10-12] or pedigree analysis [13]. In the present paper a case of illegal cattle purchase has been proven through maternal testing by using polymorphic DNA microsatellites.

CASE HISTORY

Basque country police (Ertzaintza) were requested to investigate a case of alleged illegal cattle purchase from a farm located in Carranza (Bizkaia, Spain). The animals were an outcross of Charolais and the Spanish Monchina breed. Three recently dead animals were identified as the alleged stolen calves. The Ertzaintza forwarded to our laboratory six blood samples (three from the putative mothers and three from the alleged stolen calves) for analysis to stablish the possible parental linkage.

LABORATORY PROCEDURES

SAMPLE COLLECTION AND DNA EXTRACTION: 5 ml of blood from each of the three alleged stolen animals and the three putative mothers were submitted to the laboratory. 300 µl of blood were centrifuged and the pellet resuspended in TE/NaCl buffer and digested with SDS/proteinase K. The DNA was obtained with a phenol:chloroform extraction procedure.

PCR AMPLIFICATION: The four loci analyzed were: BoLA DRBIII (BoLA) [14], ILSTS002 (IL2) [15], Bovine brain ribonuclease gene (BBR) [16,17], and Bovine TAU gene (TAU) [18,19]. BoLA/IL2 and BBR/TAU loci were coamplified. Oligonucleotide primers sequence for IL2, BBR and TAU were as described [15-19]. The primer sequences for the BoLA locus were designed from the GeneBank. One of each pair of primers was end labelled with ^{32}P-γ- ATP. 4 μl of the amplification product were electrophoresed in a 5% polyacrilamide sequencing electrophoresis gel under denaturing conditions, and exposed to an x-ray film after drying (Fig 1). Samples of known size (previously compared to a sequencing reaction) were used as allele size markers.

RESULTS AND DISCUSSION

The summary of the results obtained are presented in Table I. These data indicate that dams A, B and C can be the mothers of the stolen calves. As can be inferred by the allele combination of the different samples, the only possible parentage match is: dam A/Calf 3, dam B/calf 1 and dam C/calf 2. For instance, looking at the BoLA locus, calf 3 received allele 147 bp from dam A, calf 2 received allele 161 bp from dam C and calf 1 received allele 175 bp from dam B. Any other dam/calf combination is excluded.

TABLE I

ANIMAL	BBR alleles (bp)	BoLA alleles (bp)	IL2 alleles (bp)	TAU alleles (bp)
Dam A	128/**140**	**147**/151	**123/125**	**88/94**
Calf 3	**140/140**	**147**/147	115/**123**	**88/94**
Dam B	130/**132**	159/**175**	**129/129**	88/96
Calf 1	128/**132**	119/**175**	115/**129**	94/96
Dam C	**128**/142	125/**161**	**125/131**	**94/94**
Calf 2	**128**/130	135/**161**	**125/131**	**94/94**

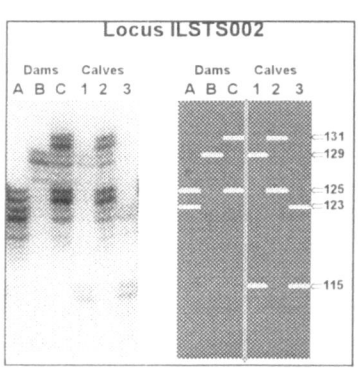

Locus ILSTS002

The calculation of the Probability of Paternity (W) and the Paternity Index (PI) was performed following the Bayesian approach. One of the main problems found with this approach is in the definition of the specific population database to be applied. In Spain alone, more than 50 native cattle breeds have been described. The animals under investigation were not pure breed, but an outcross of Charolais and Monchina. In our laboratory, we have analyzed the allele frequency distribution of 4 native Spanish breeds and of the Holstein-Fresian and Charolais races [20]. These databases have been constructed using samples from pure unrelated individuals. In all cases the populations are in Hardy-Weinberg equilibrium. Based in these data, two W were calculated (Table II): The first one used Charolais database, and the second was the mean of the other 5 databases available. In both cases there were not significant difference in the estimate of W. W values expressed as Hummel´s Verbal Predicates indicate that dam A is "very probable" the mother of calf 3, and maternity of damB/calf1 and damC/cald3 are "practically proven".

TABLE II
PROBABILITY OF PATERNITY

DAM/CALF COMBINATION	W (Charolais)	W (Mean 5 breeds)
Dam A/Calf 3	0.9886	0.9647
Dam B/Calf 1	0.9999	0.9994
Dam C/Calf 2	0.9926	0.9984

This type of analysis can be applied to other animal species as swine, horses, sheep or dogs. For instance, another case of illegal purchasing, this time in dogs, was submitted by the Ertzaintza to our laboratory. We used four loci and excluded the alleged mother.

REFERENCES

[1] Fries, R. et al. *Genomics*, Vol 8, 1990, pp. 403-406.

[2] Fries, R. et al. *Mammalian Genome,* Vol. 4, 1993, pp. 405-428.

[3] Ellegren, H. et al. *Animal Genetics*, Vol. 23, 1992, pp. 133-142.

[4] Coppieters, W. et al. *Animal* Genetics, Vol. 24, 1993, pp.163-70.

[5] Moran, C. *J. Hered*, Vol 84, 1993, pp. 274-80.

[6] Ellegren, H. et al. *Genomics*, Vol.16, 1993, pp. 431-439.

[7] Dietz, A.B. et al. *Animal Genetics*, Vol. 24, 1993, pp. 433-436.

[8] Crawford, A.M. et al. *Animal Genetics*, Vol 21, 1990, pp. 433-434.

[9] Ostrander, A.,E. et al. *Genomics*, Vol. 16, 1993, pp. 207-213.

[10] Hines, H.C. et al. *Dairy Sciences*, Vol. 64, 1981, pp 71-76.

[11] Harley, C.,S. *Animal Genetics*, Vol. 22, 1991, pp. 259-277.

[12] Morris, S. *J. Dairy Sciences*, Vol. 73, 1990, pp. 2628-2646.

[13] Trommelen, J.M. et al. *Journal of Dairy Sciences*, Vol, 76, 1993, pp. 1403-1411.

[14] Groenen, M.A. et al. *Immunogenetics,* Vol. 31, 1990, pp.37-44.

[15] Kemp, S.J. et al. *Animal Genetics,* Vol. 23, 1992, pp.184-184.

[16] Sasso, M.P. et al. *Nucleics Acids Res.* Vol. 19, 1991, pp. 6469-6474.

[17] Moore, S.S. and Byrne, K. *Animal Genetics.* Vol. 23, 1992, p. 574.

[18] Moore, S.S. et al. *Animal Genetics*, Vol. 23, 1992, pp. 463-467.

[19] Himmler, A. et al. *Molecullar and Cellular Biology*, Vol. 9. 1989, pp. 1381-1388.

[20] Beamonte D. et al. (submitted).

DISASTER VICTIMS IDENTIFICATION BY USING THE DNA TECHNOLOGY ON DENTAL PULP: preliminary results.

A. MARCOTTE*, B. HOSTE*, M. FAYS*, E. DE VALCK** & A. LERICHE*

* Institut National de Criminalistique et de Criminologie, Chaussée de Vilvorde, 98-100, 1120 Brussels, Belgium
** Forensic Odontologist, Parklaan, 10, 1852 Beigem, Belgium

INTRODUCTION

On March 31st, 1995 a Roumanian Airbus A310 flying to Brussels crashed in Balotesti near Bucarest. The Disaster Victims Identification (DVI) teams identified 52 of the 60 victims. We were requested to identify 8 victims by DNA typing for which insufficient morphological data was available.

The human tooth plays an important role in victim identification when the corpse is extremely decomposed, as dentine and enamel provide a protective enclosure for genomic and mitochondrial DNA. DNA typing assays were first performed on selected clinical samples obtained through both the conservative (by sampling of dental pulp) and destructive (by crushing the entire tooth) approaches. 26 unidentified jaw fragments were then submitted to analyses.

MATERIALS & METHODS

- 4 undiseased teeth from 3 patients from the dental clinic, with a bloodstain from each patient.
- 15 unidentified jaw fragments were taken during the week after the aircraft disaster (A series) They were stored in non hermetically closed plastic bags during 6 weeks at 0 - 10 ° C, mixed with unidentified corpse fragments, then at -20 ° C in our laboratory.
- A second series (B series) of 11 jaw fragments were found 6 weeks later on the site of the accident, then kept at -20 ° C in our laboratory.
- Blood samples on EDTA or bloodstains from 18 relatives of 6 victims were collected.

DNA Extraction
- For the clinical teeth, the pulp was sampled immediately after extraction, the teeth without pulp were kept during a week at room temperature.
- 2 clinical teeth without pulp were crushed in fine power with a mixer mill type MM 2000 (Retsch, Germany) and recovered with 1,5 ml 8 M Urea - 300 mM NaCl - 10 mM Tris-HCl, pH 8 - 5 mM EDTA, pH8 - 2 % SDS. Organic extraction was done and the extracted DNA resuspended in 300µl 10 mM Tris-HCl, pH 7,5 - 1 mM EDTA, pH 8 ($T_{10}E_1$).
- The dental pulp of 51 teeth from the 26 jaw fragments was sampled after selection by radiographic examination by the odontologist. The pulp was extirpated from the coronal pulp chamber and radicular canals, after horizontal section of the tooth at the cementoenamel junction (Smith et al. 1993).

These pulpes were put either in 700 µl homogenization solution with urea (remaining non dissolved fragments were further digested with Proteinase K), either in 700 µl 10 mM Tris-HCl, pH 8 - 10 mM EDTA, pH 8 - 100 mM NaCl - 0.5 % SDS with 20 µl of Proteinase K (10 mg/ml) and 10 µl of β-Mercaptoethanol. After over night incubation room temperature (urea) or at 50 ° C (Proteinase K), organic extraction was performed and the extracted DNA resuspended in 50 to 150 µl $T_{10} E_1$ or 10 mM Tris-HCl, pH 7,5 - 0.1 mM EDTA, pH 8 ($T_{10} E_{0.1}$).

DNA Quantification
- *Dental pulp and crushed teeth*: First the quantity and quality of total DNA was estimated by loading 1/30 to 1/10 of the resuspended DNA on 0.8 % agarose gels, followed by ethidium bromide staining. A more accurate estimate of the amount of human DNA was then obtained by using the "human DNA quantitation system" (GIBCO BRL, USA) based on the hybridization

to the human D17Z1 probe (Waye et al. 1989).

- *Blood Samples*: the DNA yield was determined by U.V. absorption at 260, 270 and 280 nm and by hybridization with the D17Z1 probe.

Analysis methods: By RFLPs and by PCR amplification

RFLPs method:

Briefly, DNA from blood samples and teeth were restricted by HinfI, then loaded on 1 % agarose gels in 40 mM Tris acetate - 1 mM EDTA buffer (60 volts - 20 hours) . After transfer on nitrocellulose membranes, the samples were successively hybridized with the radioactive probes pH30 and pLH1 (GIBCO BRL, USA) (Milner et al. 1990, Eisenberg et al. 1993). Radiographies were obtained with intensifying screens at - 70 ° C.

PCR methods:

Amplification conditions:

- *D1S80 locus* (AmpliFLP™ D1S80, PCR amplification kit, Perkin Elmer, USA) (Kasai et al. 1990, Budowle et al. 1991)

The amplification reaction occured in a total volume of 50 μl (20 μl mix with AmpliTaq DNA Polymerase, 10 μl 5 mM Mg Cl and 20 μl of a 0.5ng/μl DNA dilution.

96 °C - 3 min; 29 cycles [95 °C - 15 sec, 66 ° C - 15 sec, 72 ° C - 40 sec]; 72 ° C - 10 min (GeneAmp PCR System 9600, Perkin Elmer, USA).

- *HUMTHO1 locus* (Geneprint™ STR THO1 System, Promega, USA) (Polymeropoulos et al. 1991, Edwards et al. 1992)

The amplification reaction occured in a total volume of 25 μl (22.5 μl mix (with Taq DNA Polymerase (Promega), and 2.5 μl of a 10 ng/μl DNA dilution.

96 ° C - 3 min; 28 cycles [95 ° C - 60 sec, ramp to 60 ° C - 120 sec, 60 ° C - 60 sec]; 72 ° C - 10 min (GeneAmp PCR System 9600, Perkin Elmer, USA).

Electrophoretical separation of amplified fragments:

It was realised on gels 32 cm long, for both loci (GIBCO BRL Model SA-32).

- *D1S80 locus*: instructions of manual from the kit (Perkin Elmer) were strictly followed.

- *HUMTHO1 locus*: the separation of the amplified products was done on denaturing 6% Hydrolink Long Ranger gels (FMC, USA).

The visualisation of the bands was performed by *silver staining* according to the given instructions of the two kits, respectively.

RESULTS AND DISCUSSION

Fig. 1 : agarose electrophoresis + ethidium bromide staining. Sample 1 : pBR322 DNA ladder; 2,3 : "clinical" pulps; 4,5 : "clinical" crushed teeth; 6,7,8: B-series pulps; 9 : 50 ng λ DNA

For the clinical teeth, high amounts of intact DNA (from 900 to 2000 ng, mean 1570 ng) were obtained from the pulps. The powdered remaining teeth yielded higher amounts of DNA (6000 ng), but it was much more degraded (Fig. 1). This confirms the observations of Smith et al. (1993).

For the aircraft samples, 2 or 3 teeth per jaw fragment were analysed, except for 3 of the 26 fragments which contained only 1 tooth. Each tooth of the same fragment gave similar DNA yield, except for 3 of the 23 fragments.

For all the B series samples, the amount of DNA extracted from the pulp was high (from 100 to 10000 ng, mean 3500 ng) and only partially degraded (Fig. 1). This result was obtained for only 5 jaw fragments of the A series (from 0 to 4800 ng, mean 1880 ng); all other A fragments yielded hardly any DNA (from 0 to 60 ng, mean 14 ng).

The quality of the DNA recovered from the clinical teeth, the 11 aircraft B-teeth analysed and only 3 of the 15 jaw fragments of the A series was sufficient to use the RFLP typing method with success. These results show that although teeth provide a protective environment, storage conditions still remain important. However, air dried storage seems to be a simple and efficient procedure to keep relatively intact DNA containing source.

The RFLP results were confirmed by D1S80 and HumTHO1 typing for the clinal teeth and for 11 jaw fragments. We never observed more than 2 alleles per sample, which indicate that we do not seem to have contamination problems. At this stage of the study, compared to the RFLP technology, the PCR methods has not allowed us to type more degraded samples. And we have not obtained more results for STR (HUMTHO1) typing than for VNTR (D1S80) typing, as could be expected from the size difference between these markers. However, the amplifications should be repeated after purification of the DNA by Microcon 100 microconcentrator. Several dilutions of DNA template should also be tried, indeed the amount of human DNA could be underevaluated for severely degraded samples (Prinz et al. 1993).

We were able to determine the genetic profile of jaw fragments from 14 different persons and 4 of these jaws correspond to 4 of the missing victims.

REFERENCES

Budowle B, Chakraborty R, Giusti AM, Eisenberg AJ, Allen RC (1991) Analysis of the VNTR Locus D1S80 by the PCR followed by high resolution PAGE. Am J Hum Genet 48: 137-144

Edwards A, Hammond HA,Jin L, Caskey CT, Chakraborty R (1992) Genetic Variation at Five Trimeric and Tetrameric Tandem Repeat Loci in Four Human Population Groups. Genomics 12: 241-253

Eisenberg AJ, Clement M, Gaskill ME, Carlson DP, Klevan L (1993) Characterisation of a new single-locus VNTR Probe for RFLP Analysis: LH1 (D5S110). Second Int Symp on the forensic aspects of DNA analysis, FBI, USA

Kasai K, Nakamura Y, White R (1990) Amplification of a Variable Number of Tandem Repeats (VNTR) Locus (pMCT118) by the Polymerase Chain Reaction (PCR) and its Application to Forensic Science. J Forensic Sci 35: 1196-1200

Milner ECB, Lotshaw CL, Willems van Dijk K, Charmley P, Concannon P, Schroeder JHW (1989) Isolation and mapping of a polymorphic DNA sequence pH30 on chromosome 4 D4S139. Nucl Acids Res 17: 4002

Polymeropoulos MH, Xiao H, Rath DS, Merril CR (1991) Tetranucleotide Repeat Polymorphism at the Human Tyrosine Hydroxylase Gene (TH). Nucl Acids Res 19: 3753

Prinz M., Schmitt C. (1993) Effect of degradation on PCR based DNA typing. Advances in Forensic Haemogenetics 5: 375-378

Smith BC, Fisher DL, Weedn VW, Warnock GR, Holland MM (1993) A Systematic Approach to the Sampling of Dental DNA. J Forensic Sci 38: 5: 1194-1209

Waye JS, Presley LA, Budowle B, Shutler GG, Fourney RM (1989) A Simple and Sensitive Method for Quantifying Human Genomic DNA in Forensic Specimen Extracts. Biotechniques 7: 8: 852-855

Combined STR VNTR and MVR Typing and mtDNA Sequencing, led to the Identification of Human Remains Emergent from the AMIA Explosion in Buenos Aires

Corach, D[1.]; Sala, A[1.].; Penacino, G[1.]. and Sotelo, A[2.]..
1-Servicio. de Huellas Digitales Genéticas, Fac. de Farm. y Bioq. UBA.
2- Cuerpo Médico Forense de la Justicia Nacional.

Introduction

On July 18t[th], 1994, the building of a Jewish Association (AMIA) was blown by a bomb in Buenos Aires. The attack resulted in more than 90 fatal and over 300 injured victims and the complete destruction of the building. A high number of fragmentary human remains were found. National authorities required us to characterize over 80 human remains and to identify victims by comparison with family groups searching for missing relatives.

Combined molecular typing approaches, including seven STRs, four VNTR and PCR-MVR, were used, supplemented with mtDNA sequencing. The strategy employed sped up the identification process. The high efficiency of sample handling and molecular typing systems employed is due in part to a previous experience, the bombing attack against the Israeli Embassy occurred in 1992, after which our laboratory also contributed to the identification of remains (Corach et al.,1994).

Materials and Methods

Strategy.

1-DNA was extracted from samples inmmediately after receiving them from the morgue.

2-A set of seven microsatellite systems were typed, including two sex chromosome specific-STRs that additionally allowed rapid gender determination.

3- All samples displaying identical STR genotypes were further analyzed by means of typing with four minisatellites.

4- Samples that could not be typed with minisatellites due to degradation (absence of signal) or severe mismatch were then typed by means of PCR-MVR.

5- Some remains, discovered several months after the disaster, required to be analyzed by mtDNA control region sequencing .

DNA Extraction: CTAB extraction protocol (Corach et al., 1995) was used.

STR Analyses. The following STRs were employed: HUMTHO-1, HUMFABP, HUMRENA4 and HUMHPRTB (Edwards et al.,1992) HUMVWA (Kimpton et al., 1992), HUMFES/FPS (Polymeropoulus et al., 1991) and the Y specific STR Y27H39 (Roewer et al., 1992). PCR reactions were carried out in a Perkin Elmer Thermal Cycler. A triplex comprising variable sex chromosome-specific sequences HUMHPRTB / Y27H39 and a monomorphic Y specific sequence located at Yq12qter (Kogan·et al., 1992) allowed typing and gender determination. All reaction mixtures included a 0.02 mCi/sample α-P32-dATP. Reaction volume was 30 μl.

Amplicon Evaluation by PAGE. Amplicons were separated in denaturing 5% Acrylamide:Bisacrylamide (38:2) gel in an S2 sequencing electrophoretic apparatus (BRL LifeTechnologies, USA). Gels were run at 1,500 Volts (constant voltage). After electrophoresis, gels were exposed overnight to radiographic film at -70°C .

VNTR Analyses. Remains displaying identical STR genotypes were Hae III-digested, analyzed by means of Southern Blot and probed sequentially with four minisatellites :YNH-24 (D2S44), PH-30 (D4S139), MS-1 (D1S7) and LH-1 (D5S110). The first was radiolabeled with α-dATP P³² by random priming, and the other three were chemiluminiscent Alkaline Phospatase-linked oligo probes. Detection of signals was by autoradiography and by ACES (LifeTechnologies, BRL) respectively.

MVR Analyses. Samples showing identical STR genotypes and similar VNTR patterns denoting single band or complete profile shifts, or that could not be VNTR typed due to severe degradation, were selected for MVR evaluation. An MVR Kit was kindly provided by Dr. Alec Jeffreys and CellMark Diagnostics. Samples were PCR–amplified, Southern blotted, probed and detected according to the protocol supplied. Interpretation of results was based on Jeffreys et al.,(1991).

mtDNA Sequencing· Samples recovered several months after the explosion, were initially typed with all STRs and compared with the samples typed previously. Samples displaying identitical STR genotypes were chosen for amplification of mtDNA control regions 1 and 2(Orrego and King,1991). Sequencing was performed by using DS DNA Cycle Sequencing System (BRL, LifeTechonologies,U.S.A)

Results and Discussion

STR typing was attained, at least partially, in 100% of the samples analyzed. However, a 77% were completely typed; the remainder 23% failed to be fully evaluable. Under identical PCR conditions, some STRs were more efficient than others as regards amplification.

Combined sex chromosome microsatellites allowed to getting a two-fold purpose in order to contribute, on the one hand, with to the typing of the remains and, on the other, with to gender determination. This procedure showed that 25% of the samples belonged to females, 69% to males and 6% remained undetermined on account of partial typing. Genotype comparison allowed grouping the remains according to the number of samples displaying identity. Genotypes were loaded on a Fox Pro-based program in order to establish identity and detect kinship with potential relatives. These and victims that shared STR alleles were then investigated by VNTR analysis. In some cases, inclusions were further confirmed by mtDNA sequencing of putative mothers and the remains of their offsprings. However, in some others, inclusion based on STR typing were shown to be excluded by VNTR typing. In addition, genotype identity allowed us to correlate remains previously identified by conventional means with unidentified ones. This permitted confirm the identity of 14 remains. In order to evaluate the STR applicability for identification in complex forensic case work, confirmation of the above results was performed by means of minisatellite VNTR evaluation of those remains displaying identical STR genotypes. Most samples tested with four different probes agreed with STR information. Nevertheless, absence of bands as well as a band or profile shift was observed. Such results may be expected when dealing with DNA obtained from decomposed cadaveric material. PCR-MVR typing and mtDNA sequencing evaluation were applied to these samples so as to verify their genetic identity. In all instances in which VNTR typing failed in confirming STR data, those approaches permitted confirmation of the results. Multiplex reactions, which sped up the typing process, and the combination of sex chromosome specific sequences, also contributed to the molecular determination of sex and to the identification of fragmentary human remains (Corach et al.,1995). The identification potential of STR systems will be correlated with the number of systems to be employed. Since the aim of this paper is the evaluation of STR systems in a complex forensic case work, conventional VNTR analyses, mtDNA sequencing and the novel MVR-PCR systems were used as verification approaches. A remarkable result arose as a by-product of the STR confirmation: the high efficiency of MVR-PCR typing. Two simultaneous amplifications, a southern blot and probing can generate as much information as that provided by many STR systems put together. As the analytical range of this system is 300 bp to 2 kb and a high number of hypervariable alleles can be scored, its applicability to forensic sample analysis should be considered.

Acknowledgements: This investigation was supported in part by a grant from UBACyT FA131.
All Correspondence must be addressed to Dr.D.Corach, Servicio de Huellas Digitales Genéticas, Facultad de Farmacia y Bioquímica-UBA, Junín 956, 1113-Buenos Aires, ARGENTINA. Fax 54 1 964 0224.

References:
Corach D, Penacino G and Sotelo A.(1994).Dealing with Human Remains Sampled in Disaster Areas. The Case of the Israeli Embassy Explotion Ocurred in Buenos Aires. Advances in Forensic Haemogenetics 5259-261.
Corach D., Penacino G. and Sala A.Cadaveric DNA Extraction Protocol Based on Cetyl Trimethyl Amonium Bromide(CTAB). Medinae Legalis 1994 (In Press). Springer Verlag.
Corach D., Sala A, Penacino G and Sotelo A.(1995). Mass disasters: rapid molecular screening of human remains by means of short tandem repeats typing. Electrophoresis, (in press).
Edwards A., Hammond H., Jin L., Caskey CT., Chakraborty R (1992). Genetic variation at five trimeric and tetrameric tandem repeat loci in four human population groups. Genomics 12: 241-253
Jeffreys A.J., MacLeod A.,Tamaki K., Neil D. and Monckton D.(1991). Minisatellite repeat coding as a digital approach to DNA typing. Nature 354: 204-209..
Kimpton C., Walton A. and Gill P. (1992).A Futher Tetranucleotide Repeat Polymorphism in the vWF Gene. Hum. Molec. Genet. 1(4): 287.
Kogan S.G., Doherty M. and Gitschier J. (1992). An improved method for pregnatal diagnosis of genetics diseases by analysis of amplified DNA sequences. Applications to Hemophilia A, N. Engl. J. Med. 317: 985-990.
Orrego, C. and King, M.C. (1991)Determination of Familial Relationships. In: PCR Protocols. Edited by M.A. Innis, D.H. Gelfand, J.J. Sninsky and T.J. White. Academic Press, New York, pp.416-426.
Polymeropoulos MH., Rath DS., Xiao H. Merril CR. (1991) Tetranucleotide repeat polymorphism at the human c-fes/fps proto-oncogene (FES). Nucleic Acids Res 19: 4018.
Roewer L., Armemann J., Spurr Grzeschik K.H., Epplen J.T. (1992).Simple Repeat Sequences on the Human Y Chromosome are Equally Polymorphic as Their Autosomal Counterparts. Hum. Genet. 89: 389- 394

6 Methodology

RAPID SEX-TYPING BY FLUORESCENT BASED PCR OF THE X-Y HOMOLOGOUS AMELOGENIN GENE AND ANALYSIS BY CGE

AD Kloosterman, MJ Schans van der*, HJT Janssen and FM Everaerts*

Forensic Science Laboratory of the Ministry of Justice, Rijswijk, NL
*Lab of Instrumental Analysis, Eindhoven University of Technology, NL

Summary

Sexing of human DNA in biological stains can be performed by amplifying a fragment of the X-Y homologous amelogenin gene. We analysed the fluorescent X and Y specific PCR-fragments by capillary gel electrophoresis (CGE) with laser induced fluorescent (LIF) detection. The CGE-procedure was optimised with respect to separation and analysis-time. We validated the CGE-LIF procedure by comparing the obtained XY-sextyping results with the typing results obtained by denaturing Polyacryl-amide gelelectrophoresis with automated detection of the alleles using an ABI 373A automated sequencer. It was found that fluorescence-based PCR together with CGE and LIF detection provided a reliable sex-typing procedure. Besides, extremely fast run times (3 minutes) were possible using replaceable gelmedia and pressure injection.

Introduction

Sex-determination has become a valuable tool in forensic identity testing. A rapid and simple sex determination assay can give valuable information on the origin of biological stains and on the gender of unidentified human remains. Sexing of human DNA in biological stains can be performed by amplifying a fragment of the X-Y homologous amelogenin gene. According to Sullivan et al [1] we used a single pair of primers spanning part of the first intron of the amelogenin gene which generates different length products from the X- (106 bp) and Y-homologues (112 bp). The electrophoretic analysis of the X-Y PCR-products can be automated by the fluorescent tagging of the PCR-products. While conventional gel electrophoresis with automated detection of the alleles has proved to be a reliable technique for many years, the preparation of the gels and of the PCR-products remains labour-intensive and is difficult to fully automate. Capillary gel electrophoresis (CGE) is a new and fast high-resolution tool for the analysis of PCR products[2].
We analysed the fluorescent X and Y specific PCR-fragments by capillary gel electro-phoresis (CGE) with laser induced fluorescent (LIF) detection. We validated the CGE-LIF procedure by comparing the obtained XY-sextyping results with the typing results obtai-ned by denaturing Polyacrylamide gelelectrophoresis with automated detection of the alleles using an ABI 373A automated sequencer.

Materials and methods

Amplification conditions and gel-electrophoresis

The amplification reaction parameters of the X-Y homologous amelogenin gene and the sequences of the FAM-labeled forward primer and the unlabeled reverse primer, were according to Sullivan et al [1].

Gel-electrophoresis and typing of the amplified DNA-samples, using the automated fluorescent detection system on an ABI373A DNA-sequencer was carried out onto standard 6% Polyacrylamide denaturing sequencing gels (12 cm well to read). The length of the amplified fragments were determined from the internal lane standard Genescan-350 ROX (Perkin Elmer). Fragments were sized automatically by the Southern Local method using Genescan PCR Analysis software (Genescan 1.2.2-1, ABI).

Capillary Electrophoresis

Capillary electrophoresis experiments were performed on a P/ACE 2200 capillary electrophoresis instrument from Beckman Instruments (Fullerton, CA, USA). Detection was performed by Laser Induced Fluorescence (LIF) using an Argon Ion laser from Beckman Instruments. Excitation wavelength was 488 nm and emission wavelength was 520 nm. Running temperature was kept at 40 °C. The length of the coated capillary was 27 cm (effective length to detector was 20 cm). The capillary was rinsed with gel buffer for 3 minutes before each injection. Fused silica capillaries with an i.d. of 50 mm were coated with polyacrylamide as described previously [3].

Linear polyacrylamide gel buffers were prepared by polymerisation of 8% acrylamide in 0.1 M Tris borate (pH 8.3) containing 0.5 % TEMED and 0.08% ammonium persulphate for 24 h at 4°C [4]. Then the buffer was diluted with a concentrated urea solution to a final concentration of 4% polyacrylamide and 7M urea .

PCR samples were mixed with formamide to a final concentration of 50% formamide. Samples were heated for 3 minutes at 95°C and snap cooled in water-ice for 3 minutes. After this denaturing step samples were placed in the CE instrument and analysed. Sample introduction took place by pressure injection of 40 seconds. Separation voltage was 16.2 kV (600V/cm) applied in the reversed mode (cathode on the injection side).

Results

Gel-electrophoresis with automated fluorescence analysis

Correct XY-typing results were obtained from all male and female DNA-samples. Using the internal lane standard Genescan-350 ROX the X-specific fragment was sized to an average product length of 108.56 bp with an accuracy of 0.111 bp (1SD) and the Y-specific fragment was sized to an average product length of 114.34 (±0.107) bp. Amplification of minimal diluted DNA-samples showed that PCR-products generated from as little as 120 pg of genomic template-DNA could still be detected with this technology.

Capillary gel electrophoresis

Figure 1 shows two electropherograms representing the PCR products from male (XY) and female (XX) genomic DNA samples. Good resolution is achieved within three minutes between the X and Y specific fragments. The PCR products were sized using the FAM labelled 50-500 DNA sizer from Pharmacia as internal standard. The X - and Y specific fragments were detected very close to their theoretical value (106.2 and 111.8 bp resp.). Approximately 6 nl of the sample is actually injected into the capillary. This very low amount of DNA can be detected with a signal to noise ratio wide above the detection limit.

Discussion

It was found that fluorescence based PCR together with CGE and LIF detection provides a reliable and rapid sex typing procedure. Good agreement in typing 100 samples was obtained between CGE and conventional slab gel electrophoresis. The big advantage of CGE over slab gel electrophoresis is the rapid analysis. Nine samples can be analysed in one hour. The ABI 373A sequencer can handle as much as 36 samples in 5 hours (including gel pouring, separation and analysis). However CGE is a ready to use technique that produces results in 10 minutes. This is of great advantage in those cases where a limited amount of samples have to be analysed in the shortest possible period of time. However, inherent to CGE is the low sample amount which can be loaded into the capillary. This may result in lower sensitivity.

References

1 K.M. Sullivan, A. Mannucci, C.P. Kimpton, P. Gill,   Biotechniques 15 (1993) 636
2 P.E. Williams, M.A. Marino, S.A. Del Rio, L.A. Turni, J.M. Devayney, J. Chromatogr 680 (1994) 525.
3 M.J. van der Schans, J.L. Beckers, M.C. Molling, F.M. Everaerts, J. Chromatogr. A, in press
4 Y.F. Pariat, J. Berka, D.N. Heiger, T. Schmitt, M. Vilenchik, A.S. Cohen, F. Foret and B.L. Karger, J. Chromatogr. A, 652 (1993) 57

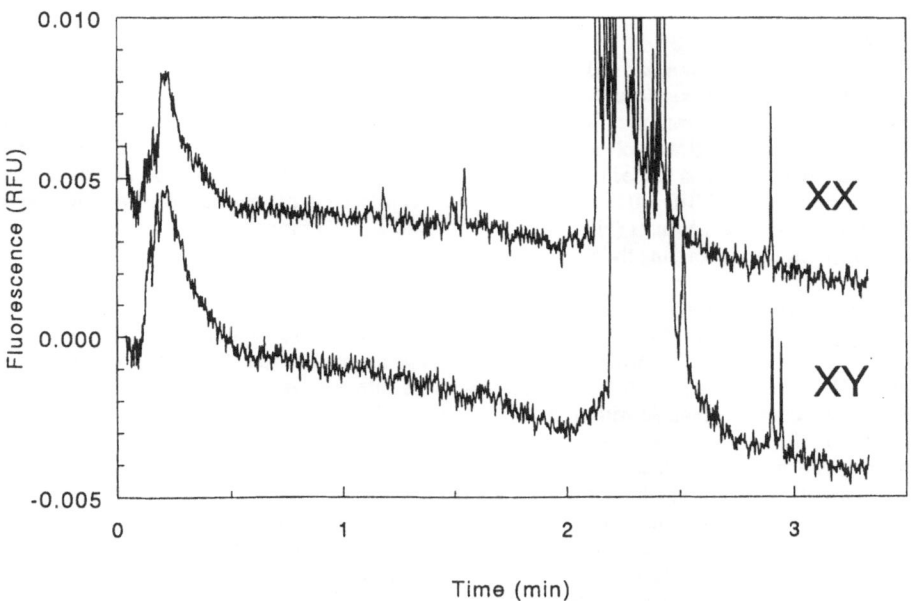

Fig 1 Separation of the XX and XY specific DNA-fragments with CGE. Injection: 40 sec by pressure; Voltage: 16.2 kV; Capillary: 50 μm 20/27 cm

HETERODUPLEX ANALYSIS IS A RAPID METHOD FOR THE DETECTION OF SUBALLELES CAUSED BY MIXED LENGTH AND SEQUENCE VARIABILITY IN SHORT TANDEM REPEAT SYSTEMS

R. Szibor, I. Plate and D. Krause

Institut für Rechtsmedizin der Otto von Guericke Universität Magdeburg, Leipziger Strasse 44, 39120 Magdeburg, Germany

INTRODUCTION

STR polymorphisms differ in the number of the tandem repeats. However, in addition, a microheterogenity, as far as the sequence variation is concerned, has been detected in some systems (HumVWA and others) (Möller 1994). The aim of our paper is to demonstrate the usefulness of the heteroduplex (HD) analysis (HDA) for the detection of suballeles in DNA systems such as HumVWA (Kimpton 1992), HumCD4 (Edwards 1991) and Hum Dys19 (Roewer 1992). The HDA is a well-established technique (Wilkin 1993) but, to our knowledge, HDA is not usual in forensic application. During PCR amplification, the DNA products are submitted to a melting and a reassociation process. In case of a homozygous genotype, the reassociation produces only homoduplexes. However, if there are DNA fragments with different numbers of repeats and / or significant differences concerning the sequence, the reciprocal association produces two or more types of HDs in addition to homoduplexes. On dependency on the extension of the missmatch area, the HDs migrate noticeably slower than homoduplexes in the nativePAGE. Thus, HD can provide several pieces of information which remain hidden, if only measurements of the length are performed.

Y-chomosomal markers occur in hemizygous state, that means that natural HDs are not existent. We show that the construction of artficial heterozygous genotypes makes the STR Dys 19 accessible to HDA.

MATERIAL and METHODS

During routine work using VWA and CD4, our attention was focused on the allele length assessment and the HD variabillity as well. Conspicous HD variants were checked by an electrophoretic site-to-site comparison with well studied samples (Fig 1). If a special genotype produces an atypical HD, sequencing can clarify which of the 2 alleles involved carries a sequence variation. For this purpose, the stained bands were dissected, reamplified and read using the A373 sequencer in combination with the Taq cycle sequencing technique (APPLIED BIOSYSTEMS). For the construction of artificial genotypes, we mixed the reamplified single allele products (Fig 2) in new combinations. HD formation occurs if the mixture is submitted to 5 PCR cycles omitting the enzyme.

RESULTS and DISCUSSION

HDA in VWA: The gel depicted in Fig. 1 shows natural VWA genotyps containing the allel 17 in combination with the other alleles. Obviously, homozygous genotypes such as 17 / 17 do not produce considerable HDs. In addition, the alleles 14, when combined with other ones, tend to make no or only weak HDs. HDs which are mutated with regard to the distances between the bands (but less with regard to the intensity) reflect the sequence deviations in one of the alleles.

The Fig.3 shows a gels with artificial arrangements of interesting allele products. Several fragments chosen from genotypes with common and conspicous HDs as well were combined with a common and a variant allel 17 fragment. Some pieces of information can been drawn from this gel:

1.: In spite of the fact, that the common allel 17 was mixed with its variant counterpart, a formation of HDs in the mixed 17 common and 17 variant is only very weak. This indicates that the sequence heterogenity is not compellingly conspicuous by HD formation.

2.: Despite the fact that the combination of the different allel 16 with the common allel 17 reveals a gross HD difference, the combination with the variant allele 17 variant shows only a discrete band distance deviation.

3.: The combination of 17 common and 15 variant alleles produces HDs which are similar to those of the reciprocal situation 17 variant and 15 common.

4.: Leaving aside the situation in homozygous genotypes with regard to the length there is a good chance of detecting the sequence variants investigated here, since all combinations of the allele 17 variant differ from the combinations with the allele 17 common with regard to the HD band distances. In principle results in experiments using other alleles confirm these statements (not shown).

In the VWA System, we have found a considerable variability in the alleles 15, 16, and 17, and low or no variability in the alleles 14 , 18, 19 and 20 up to now.

HDA in CD4: Fig.4 shows an arrangement of natural genotypes. Only within the genotypes 108/ 88 bp, there are some intensive variations but no distance mutations. Sequence analysis and the construction of artificial genotypes as well (not shown) revealed that variability in HD intensity does not definitively reflect the existence of sequence variations. Thus, our study into 400 alleles from European population and 50 Asian alleles could not detect any suballeles in CD4.

HDA in Dys 19: Artificial combinations of the allele D with all further frequent alleles can reveal that there is no variability in the HDs formation.(Fig 5). This investigation has been conducted on more than 100 alleles. Therefore, we are strongly convinced that in DYS 19 the occurrence of suballeles is a rare event.

Paternity testing: In the pedigree of Fig.6. VWA allele lenght assessment includes the putative father for both children as the possible true father. By HDA the putative father is excluded to be the true father for one of them due to the fathers' common HD type and the rare HD in the 2nd child (lane 4). This has been confirmed by sequencing data and by exclusions in further systems.

Symbols used in the figures: = > homoduplexes; ∗ HDs; C= common HD type; R= rare HD type

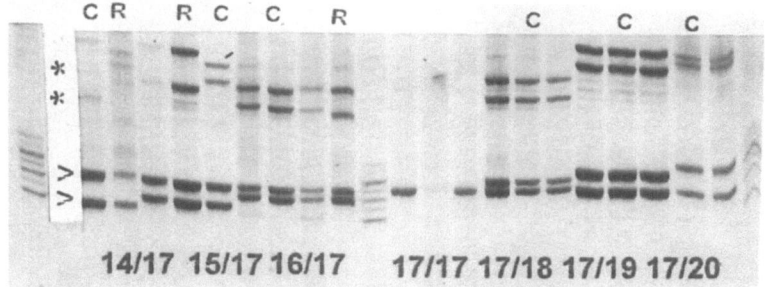

Fig.1: VWA genotypes involving allel 17 with common (C) and rare (R) HD types.

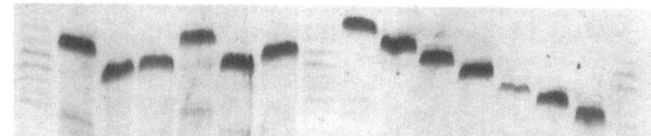

Fig.2: Sinlge VWA allele fragments produced by reamplification of chosen bands from probands with common and rare HD type.

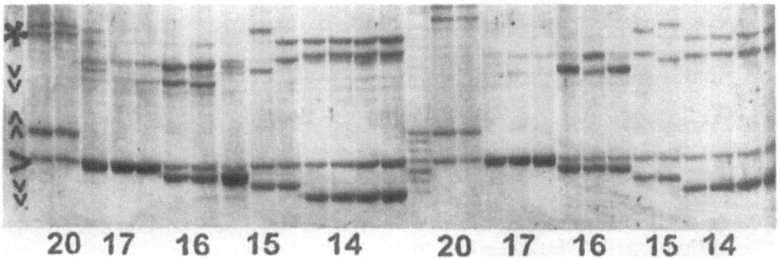

Fig. 3: Artificial genotypes in VWA established by mixing a common (left) and a rare (right) variant of the allele 17 with an ensemble of common and rare alleles.14-20.
Allele 17: TCTA (TCTG)$_4$ TCTA$_{11}$; Allele 17 var: TCTA (TCTG)$_3$TCTA $_{12}$

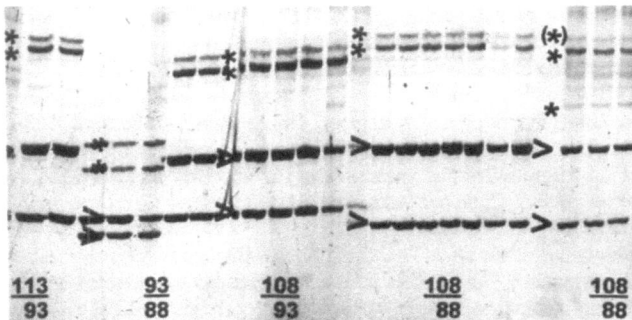

Fig. 4: Natural genotypes of the STR CD4 chosen from routine work

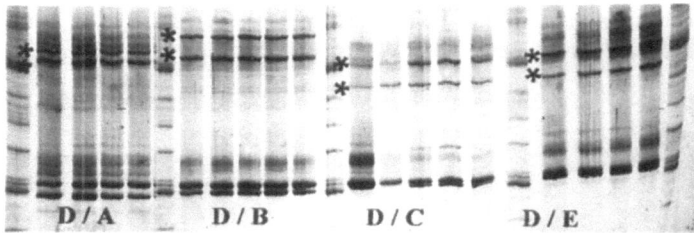

Fig. 5: Artifcial genotypes in Dys 19 including the alleles A-D are lacking HD variabillitiy

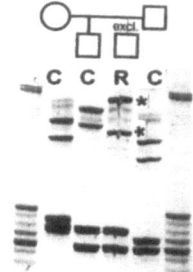

Fig. 6:
HDA in VWA paternity testing: Paternity exclusion cannot
be drawn in length assessment but in HDA and by sequencing
Allele 16 (C): TCTA (TCTG)$_4$ TCTA $_{11}$
Allele 16 (R): TCTA (TCTG)$_3$ TCTA $_{12}$

Conclusions:

1.: HDA helps to detect the most of the existing suballeles within alleles of equal length.

2.: As work and material do not cause high costs, HDA is highly recommended if extended population genetic studies of variability have to be made within the main alleles.

3.: HDA can provide increased information in routine work without additional expenditure of work and material. However, the inclusion of HD information into the expertise requires a detailed investigation into the suballele.

References

Edwards A, Clemems PR, Tristan M, Pizzuti A, Gibbs RA (1991) Pentanucleotide repeat length polymorphism at the human CD4 locus. Nucleic Acids Res 19: 4791.

Kimpton C, Walton A, Gill P (1992) A further tetranucleotide repeat polymorphism in the vWF gene. Hum Mol Gen 1: 287.

Möller A, Meyer E, Brinkmann B (1994) Different types of structural variation in STRs: HumFES/FPS, Hum VWA and Hum D21S11. Int J Leg Med 106; 319.

Roewer L, Arnemann J, Spurr NK, Grzeschik KH, Epplen JT (1992) Simple repeat sequence on the human Y chromosome are equally polymorphic as their autosomal counterparts. Hum Genet 89:389.

Wilkin DJ, Koprivnikar KE, Cohn DH(1993) Heteroduplex analysis can increase the informativeness of PCR-amplified VNTR markers: application using a marker tightly linked to the COL2A1 gene. Genomics. 15:372.

Use of CDP-STAR in a fast and highly sensitive chemiluminescent detection procedure for VNTR loci with neutral and charged membranes.

S. L. Leary, J. Victor and I. Balazs

Lifecodes Corporation, Stamford CT 06902, USA

INTRODUCTION

The use of directly labeled alkaline phosphatase oligonucleotides (AP-probes) and chemiluminescent substrates for the analysis of VNTR loci has proven to be a simple, rapid and convenient format for DNA typing(Baum, 1990, Neuweiler 1992, Balazs 1994 and Baird 1994). The advent of new and more sensitive chemiluminescent substrates for alkaline phosphatase has provided the identity laboratory with even more powerful chemiluminescent probes for DNA typing. This paper discusses the development of a protocol for the use of a new, highly-sensitive alkaline phosphatase substrate, CDP-Star™ (Tropix Inc., Bedford, MA) with a number of AP-probes and with either charged or neutral membranes.

MATERIALS AND METHODS

VNTR probes were conjugated to alkaline phosphatase using the NICE™ method (Cellmark Diagnostics, Abingdon UK). They included; D1S7, D1S339, D2S44, D4S163, D5S110, D6S132, D7S467, D10S28, D17S26 and D17S79. Duplicate membranes were prepared using different amounts of Hae III digested DNA that was isolated, digested, electrophoresed and transferred to either Pall Biodyne B (charged) or MSI Magna (neutral) membranes as described (Balazs 1994). Charged membranes were baked after Southern Transfer and neutral membranes were baked and U.V cross-linked. NICE-labeled VNTR probes, QUICK-LIGHT™ hybridization solution and Buffers were supplied by LIFECODES CORPORATION.

1X QUICK-LIGHT Buffer, Wash I and Wash II were prepared according to manufacturer's instructions. CDP-Star was brought to room temperature and hybridization solution, Wash I and Wash II were equilibrated to 55°C for at least 90 minutes. Membranes to be hybridized were placed into an appropriate sized container containing pre-warmed Wash II (0.125 mL Wash II/cm² membrane) for 5 to 10 minutes. 0.5 - 1.0 µL NICE probe was added per mL of 55°C pre-warmed hybridization solution (hybridization solution volume = 0.0375 mL/cm² membrane). Wash II Solution was decanted and the NICE Probe/Hybridization solution was added. The membranes were incubated with the probe/hybridization solution for 20 - 30 minutes at 55°C with shaking. The membranes were then washed two times with pre-warmed Wash I solution (0.375 mL per cm² membrane) for 10 minutes at 55°C with shaking. The membranes were then washed two times with pre-warmed Wash II solution (0.375 mL per cm² membrane) for 10 minutes at 55°C with shaking. After the last Wash II solution was decanted, 0.125 mL/ cm² membrane of 1X QUICK-LIGHT Buffer was added to the container. The container is then covered and gently shaken. Using forceps, each membrane is carefully separated to allow complete wetting, the QUICK-LIGHT solution was decanted and this step was repeated three times. The membranes were left in the last QUICK-LIGHT rinse and one-by-one were transferred, first allowing excess buffer to drain off, to a clean, container with CDP-Star (0.025 mL CDP-Star per cm² membrane). The excess CDP-Star was drained off and the membranes were placed in an open

Development Folder (LIFECODES). The folder was heat-sealed after the removal of air bubbles and excess CDP-Star. The surface of the folder was wiped dry and the folder was then placed into an X-ray cassette and exposed to Kodak XAR or Fuji RX film for up to 3 hours and overnight at room temperature. Prior to re-hybridization to other probes, membranes were incubated in Wash I for at least 30 minutes at 65°C with shaking to inactivate the AP-probe on the membrane. Membranes were air- dried for storage.

RESULTS AND DISCUSSION

CDP-Star, a 1,2-dioxetane, provides rapid, high intensity and prolonged light emission which permits the detection of 25-50 ng of genomic DNA bound to charged or neutral membranes in an exposure time of a few hours or less. The probes tested fell into three general groups based upon their sensitivity (Table 1). The first group consisted of D1S7, D1S339, D2S44 and D7S467, all of which gave strong signal with minimal noise. The second group consisted of D6S132, D17S79, D4S163 and D5S110 which gave good signal with minimal background and the third group consisting of D17S26 and D10S28 which gave adequate signal with minimal background. Additionally, D17S26 displayed a significant difference in allele signal intensity, with the lower allele of K562 DNA being much lighter than the upper allele which complicated the sensitivity determination.

Table 1. Sensitivity of NICE Probes using CDP-Star

Probe/Exposure	≤ 1 hour	≤ 3 hours	overnight
Group I D1S7, D1S339 D2S44, D7S467	<500ng	< 50ng	< 10ng
Group II D4S163, D5S110, D6S132, D17S79	500ng	50ng	< 50ng
Group III D10S28, D17S26	500ng	50-100ng	50ng

The results of Table 1 show that the VNTR probes in Group I provide sensitivity of less than 10ng of DNA after an overnight exposure using CDP-Star making them extremely valuable when the amount of DNA is limited.

An additional major advantage is CDP-Star's ability to be used with both neutral and charged membranes. This is due to CDP-Star's compatibility with SDS-detergent based hybridization/wash systems such as QUICK-LIGHT reagents. Another second-generation dioxetane/enhancer system, Lumi-Phos® Plus (Lumigen Inc. Detroit, MI) is incompatible with SDS-systems because the SDS quenches the enhanced chemiluminescence by interacting with enhancer (Price, in press). Such systems are precluded from using charged membranes because Tween-based systems cannot prevent non-specific binding of AP-probes to charged membranes. In this study, charged membranes gave slightly higher background but displayed better sensitivity than neutral membranes, especially with small allele sizes (Fig. 1).

Repeated stripping and rehybridization showed some loss of sensitivity which could be corrected by longer exposure times. For example, a Pall Biodyne B membrane stripped 4 times still yielded 100ng sensitivity after an overnight exposure when probed with D17S79 (data not shown).

The appearance of relatively weak artifact bands after overnight exposure, with more than 50 ng of genomic DNA, when using the more sensitive alkaline phosphatase substrates, has been previously reported (Price). Such bands were noted when membranes probed with D2S44, D6S132, D7S467 (Fig. 1) and D17S79 were over-exposed. These extra bands can be eliminated by reducing the amount of probe added to the hybridization solution. Such bands may be more evident in Tween-based systems due in part to the lower wash and hybridization stringencies. CDP-Star added sensitivity does require added care when preparing and performing hybridizations. Increased background due to contamination is more common, manifesting itself as heavy speckling all over the developed film. Using clean containers for the CDP-Star incubations as well as using freshly prepared reagents can eliminate background spots.

In summary, we have examined 10 NICE-labeled VNTR AP-probes using CDP-Star as the substrate and have found it provides sensitive detection, rapid turn-around times and allows the use of charged membranes in VNTR loci analysis.

D7S467 Hybridized to Uncharged and Charged Membranes

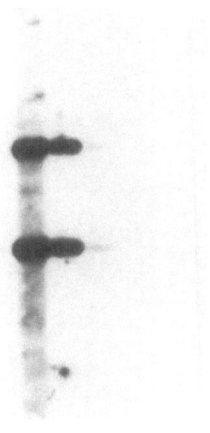
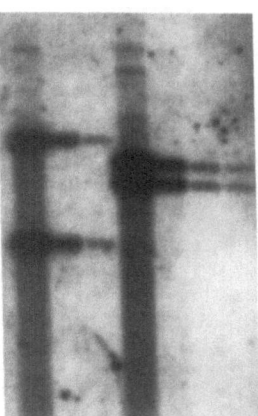

Figure 1. Left: Uncharged membrane containing 500ng, 50ng and 10ng of Hae III digested K562 genomic DNA. Right: Charged membrane containing 500ng, 50ng, 10ng Hae III digested K562 genomic DNA and 500ng, 50ng, 10ng, 5ng Hae III digested male genomic DNA. Both membranes were hybridized to NICE-labeled D7S467, incubated with CDP-Star and exposed overnight at room temperature.

REFERENCES:

Baird M, Galbreath L, Cunningham R, Lastella J, Balazs I (1994) Use of chemiluminescent labeled probes for forensic and paternity determinations. In: Bar W and Rossi U (eds) Advances in Forensic Haemogenetics, vol 5. Springer-Verlag, Berlin Heidelberg, p 130.

Balazs I, Neuweiler J, Kowalski K, Victor J (1994) Streamlining VNTR analysis. A fast procedure for non-isotopic DNA profiling. In: Bar W and Rossi U (eds) Advances in Forensic Haemogenetics, vol 5. Springer-Verlag, Berlin Heidelberg, p 112.

Baum HJ, Fitz-Charles H, McKee R (1990) A non-isotopic DNA detection system with the sensitivity of P^{32}: Applications for paternity and forensic identifications. In: Polesky HF and Mayr WR (eds) Advances in Forensic Haemogenetics, vol 3. Springer-Verlag, Berlin Heidelberg, p 37.

Neuweiler J, Venturini J, Balazs I, Komher S, Hintz D, Victor, J (1992) The use of a chemiluminescent detection system for paternity and forensic testing. Verification of the reliability of the oligonucleotide-probes used for genetic analysis. In: Rittner C and Schneider PM (eds) Advances in Forensic Haemogenetics, vol 4. Springer-Verlag, Berlin Heidelberg, p 132.

Price DC Chemiluminescent substrates for detection of restriction fragment length polymorphism. Journal Forensic Science Society, in press.

EVALUATION OF PRIMER EXTENSION PREAMPLIFICATION (PEP) IN FORENSIC STUDIES

Y. Itoh and R. Kobayashi

Department of Forensic Medicine, Juntendo University School of Medicine, Tokyo, Japan

INTRODUCTION

The content of DNA in hairs is usually limited. Hair root with or without surrounding sheath cells may contain less than 375 ng DNA. The sensitivity of the polymerase chain reaction (PCR) is sufficient to permit the analysis of DNA in a single hair (Higuchi 1988). An efficient method called primer extension preamplification (PEP) has been developed using a random 15-mer oligonucleotide primer (Zhang 1992). This method makes it possible to generate enough template DNA for several PCR-reactions in case the amount of DNA is limited (Huber 1993). The purpose of this study is to evaluate PEP-PCR analysis in forensic studies.

MATERIALS AND METHODS

1. PEP: Template DNA samples were subjected to amplification in a final volume of 60 µl containing 33.33 µM random 15-mer oligonucleotide primer (Operon Technologies, Alameda, CA), 10 mM Tris-HCl (pH 8.3), 50 mM KCl, 0.01% gelatin, 1.5 mM $MgCl_2$, 0.1 mM dNTPs and 5 unit AmpliTaq DNA polymerase (Cetus, Emeryville, CA). This was followed by fifty cycles of 1 min at 92 °C, 2 min at 37 °C, 3 min transition at 37-55 °C, and 4 min extension at 55°C.

2. PEP-PCR: Aliquots of the PEP products were further subjected to reamplification with two specific sequences, including VNTR (COL2A1), STR (ACTBP2, TH01) and sex determining primers (Kogan 1987; Witt 1989). Positive and negative controls were always included in each PCR run. The amplified products were analyzed using agarose gel electrophoresis or polyacrylamide gel electrophoresis, then visualized and photographed under ultra-violet light or silver staining.

3. Sequencing of PCR and PEP-PCR products: Subcloning of PCR and PEP-PCR products was performed using the Original TA Cloning Kit (Invitrogen, San Diego, CA). PCR and PEP-PCR products were ligated into plasmid pCR[TM]II and transformed into One Shot[TM] competent cells. The presence of cloned PCR and PEP-PCR products was verified to analyze minipreparations of plasmid DNA. The nucleotide sequence of these PCR cloned products was determined by using a Taq DyeDeoxy[TM] Terminator Cycle Sequencing Kit

(Applied Biosystems, Inc. CA.) and Taq Dye Primer Cycle Sequencing Kit (Applied Biosystems, Inc. CA.).

RESULTS AND DISCUSSION

1. Both products of PEP-PCR and PCR alone showed identical electrophoretic mobility of the allelic state at the loci of VNTR, and STR and determination of sex. The bands of identical mobility were further used to examine their nucleotide sequences. In our ACTBP2 bands, both products showed identical nucleotide sequences, including the 12-base deletion, compared with the data base (Fig.1). Allelic dropout or mutation caused by the PEP method was not observed.

2. In the COL2A1 locus, 75 pg of template DNA was detected by PEP-PCR, whereas 7.5 ng of template DNA was detected by PCR alone (Fig. 2). The quantities of DNA were calculated before the PEP reaction. This data mean that PEP method enables 10-100 copies of template DNA to be generated for subsequent PCR analyses. These amplified sizes were less than 660 base pairs long. In the ACTBP2, X1 and Y1 loci, the PEP method permits 100 to 1000 copies of template DNA to be generated. These were under 310 base pairs long. The effectiveness of the PEP method was closely related to the primers used for subsequent PCR analyses. The efficiency of PEP-PCR was remarkable in STR primers and sex determining primers.

3. It was possible to analyze PEP products from a single hair using COL2A1, ACTBP2, TH01 and sex determining primers. Thus PEP-PCR was an effective tool for discrimining single hairs. Its use in personal identification from a single hair may be expected.

CONCLUSION

This is the first study to demonstrate identical nucleotide sequences between the products of PEP-PCR and PCR alone. The PEP method permits more copied template DNA to be generated for subsequent locus-specific amplification by PCR. PEP-PCR proved to be an effective tool in forensic science investigation.

REFERENCES

Higuchi R, von Beroldingen CH, Sensabaugh GF, Erlich HA (1988) DNA typing from single hairs. Nature 332: 543-546

Huber P, Holtz J (1993) Random priming and multiplex PCR with three short tandem repeats in forensic caseworks. Advance in Forensic Haemogenetics 5: 363-365

Kogan SG, Doherty M, Gitschier J (1987) An improved method for prenatal diagnosis of genetic diseases by analysis of amplified DNA sequences, Applications to Hemophilia A. N Engl J Med 317: 985-990

Witt M, Erikson RP (1989) A rapid method for detection of Y-chromosomal DNA from dried blood specimens by the polymerase chain reaction. Hum Genet 82: 271-274

Zhang L, Cui X, Schmitt K, Hubert R, Navidi W, Arnheim N (1992) Whole genome amplification from a single cell: Implications for genetic analysis. Proc Natl Acad Sci 89: 5847-5851

```
HSAC04    1' CTACAGTGAGCCGAGGTCATGCCATTGCACTCCAATCTGGGCGACAAGAGTGAAACTCCG
PCR-alone                                 *************************
PEP-PCR                                    *************************

HSAC04   61' TCAAAAGAAAGAAAGAAAGAGACAAAGAGAGTTAGAAAGAAAGAAAGAGAGAGAGAGAGA
PCR-alone    ************************************************************
PEP-PCR      ************************************************************

HSAC04  121' AAGGAAGGAAGGAAGAAAAAGAAAGAAAAAGAAAGAAAGAGAAAGAAAGAAAGAGAAAGA
PCR-alone    ********************************************************----*
PEP-PCR      ********************************************************----*

HSAC04  181' AAGAAAGAAAGAAAGAAAGAAAGAAAGAAAGAAAGAAAGAAAAAGAAAGAAAGAAAGAAA
PCR-alone    ************************************************************
PEP-PCR      ************************************************************

HSAC04  241' GAAAGAAAGAAAGAAAGAAAGAAAGAAAGAAAGAAAGAAAGGAAGGAAAGAAAGAGCAAG
PCR-alone    ****_____*********************************************
PEP-PCR      ****_____*********************************************

HSAC04  301' TTACTATAGCGGTAGGGGAGATGTTGTAGAAATATATATAAACCTCCTTACACCGCGGAG
PCR-alone    **********************
PEP-PCR      **********************
```

Fig. 1 Nucleotide sequences of the PCR and PEP-PCR products in the ACTBP2 locus. HSA04: Data base (V00481), Underline shows PCR primers.

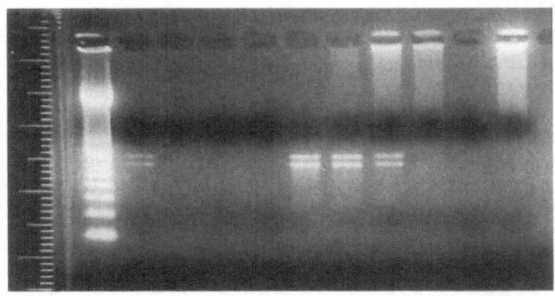

Fig. 2. Electrophoresis of the PCR or PEP-PCR products in the COL2A1 locus.
The quantities of DNA were calculated before the PEP reaction. Lane 1: 100 Base-Pair Ladder Marker; lanes 2 and 6: 7.5 ng of DNA; lanes 3 and 7: 750pg of DNA; lanes 4 and 8: 75pg of DNA; lanes 5 and 9: 7.5 pg of DNA; lanes 10 and 11: No DNA was added. Different concentrations of human genomic DNA with or without PEP reaction were analyzed by PEP-PCR (lane 6-9, 11) or PCR alone (lane 2-5, 10).

SEQUENTIAL MULTIPLEX AMPLIFICATION (SMA) IN CASES WITH MINIMAL AMOUNTS OF DNA

M. Lorente[1], J.A. Lorente[1], J.A. Alvarez[1], B. Budowle[2], &
E. Villanueva[1]

[1]University of Granada, Dept. of Forensic Medicine, Granada, Spain

[2]FSRTC - Research Unit. Laboratory Division. FBI Academy, Quantico, Va, USA

INTRODUCTION

Typing polymorphic loci at the DNA level has become a routine procedure in the identity testing field. DNA samples are usually amplified by PCR and subsequently typed; the remainder of the untyped PCR is generally not used or discarded.

To obtain more genetic information from a sample several distinct loci can be amplified in one PCR simultaneously by a process known as multiplex PCR (Edwards et al. 1992).

We proposed an alternate multiplex approach called *SEQUENTIAL MULTIPLEX AMPLIFICATION (SMA)*. SMA enables the typing of several loci using only one DNA sample without requiring all the loci to be amplified under one set of PCR conditions (Lorente et al, 1994a).

MATERIALS AND METHODS

The *general procedure* for SMA typing is as follows:

1. Extract DNA (organic or chelex).

2. Determine the quantity of the DNA with a slot-blot procedure using a human specific alphoid probe.

3. Amplify and type DNA for the D1S80 locus according to the method of Budowle et al (1991).

4. Recover the genomic DNA from the remaining D1S80 PCR solution by filtration through a Microcon-100 (Amicon, Beverly, Ma).

5. Amplify and type the recovered DNA for the HUMTH01 locus (Lorente et al. 1994b).

6. Repeat step 4 and amplify and type for HUMVWA (Lorente et al. 1994c).

7. Repeat step 4 and amplify and type for HLA-DQx (Saiki et al. 1989).

Following the SMA procedure, we have reconsidered 62 cases (44 from previous research programs; 18 from casework samples) that were studied (PCR-based technology) in our Laboratory between 1989 and 1995. In all cases, only one locus could be amplified at that time (usually D1S80 or HLA-DQA1), because the amount of DNA was not enough to try further loci.

The 62 samples considered came from blood-stains (24), semen-stains (8), hairs (11), cigarette butts (9), stamps or envelopes (5), and bones (5).

All of these samples had been frozen at -40°C during the last 1 to 6 years, and for this study were thawed in the refrigerator(+4°C). Since the whole genomic DNA extracted were used for the amplifications performed some years ago, SMA procedure started by step #4 of the Materials & Methods.

RESULTS and DISCUSSION

SMA has enabled amplification of further loci up to 6 years after the extraction and initial amplification. Therefore, a higher degree of discrimination was thus obtained from a small quantity of sample.

Out of 62 samples, 60 (96.7%) could be positively amplified after SMA for a second locus; for a third locus, positive amplification and correct typing was possible in 32 (53.3%) out of the 60 cases that yielded a positive third amplification; furtherly, 12 (32.5%) samples out of 32 were amplified for an additional fourth locus or set of loci, as Polymarker^R (Perkin Elmer Corporation, Norwalk, CT).

As an average, the probability of discrimination increased from 0.934 (HLA-DQA1), 0.921 (D1S80), 0.933 (HUMTH01) or 0.995 (Polymarker^R) to 0.9995, considering all the loci together. Considering a database of the Spanish population, probabilities can be increased from 1 in 2.500 to 1 in 3.000.000, depending on the allele frequencies in each case.

When using the SMA procedure with the Perkin-Elmer-Cetus's Polymarker or HLA-DQA1 kits, special attention should be given to the interpretation of the *control-dots* if the same sample had been previously analyzed with any of these kits, since the controls appear more intense as regularly. This usually happens with old samples that had been previously submitted to HLA-DQA1 analysis and now can be processed through SMA and be ready for Polymarker^R. (Hochmeister et al, J Forensic Sci, July 1995)

In any case, the SMA procedure can be useful for situations where the quantity of template DNA is limited or to amplify additional loci from DNA templates that have been previously used and that were adequately frozen or refrigerated.

With this procedure it is also possible to recover template DNA from PCR tubes that yielded no amplification product (e.g. DNA from evidentiary samples that might be degraded for a given locus, but that could be amplified for some other loci).

The SMA approach is compatible with any of the multiplex amplification approach, and we've got good results by using the Promega^R Triplex (CSF, TH01, TPOX) after a D1S80 amplification and just before using the HLA-DQA1 kit.

Special care should also be taken during the SMA procedure, since amplified materials are handled; we strongly recommend to proceed in post-amplification rooms and using specific set of primers, dNTP's and Taq, following the same rules and cautions that are usual when re-amplifying allelic ladders.

As a general rule, it is recommended that amplification should proceed as follows: length polymorphisms first, in descending order by size, followed by sequence polymorphisms (currently detected by sequence-specific oligonucleotide probes).

REFERENCES

Budowle B, Chakraborty R, Giusti AM, Eisenberg AJ, Allen RC (1991) Analysis of the VNTR locus D1S80 by the PCR followed by high-resolution PAGE. Am J Hum Genet 48: 137-144

Edwards A, Civitello A, Hammond HA, Caskey CT (1991) DNA typing and genetic mapping with trimeric and tetrameric tandem repeats. Am J Hum Genet 49: 746-756

Lorente JA, Lorente M, Wilson MR, Budowle B, Villanueva E (1994a) Sequential Multiplex Amplification (SMA) of genetic loci: a method for recovering DNA for susequent analysis of additional loci. Int J Legal Med 107: 156-158

Lorente JA, Lorente M, Budowle B, Wilson MR, Villanueva E (1994b) Analysis of the HUMTH01 allele frequencies in the Spanish population. J Forensic Sci 39: 1270-74

Lorente JA, Lorente M, Budowle B, Wilson MR, Villanueva E (1994c) Analysis of the Short Tandem Repeat (STR) HUMVWA in the Spanish population. Forensic Sci Int 65: 169-175

Saiki RK, Scharf S, Faloona T, Mullis KB, Hoen GT, Erlich HA, Arnheim N (1985) Enzymatic amplification of beta-globin genomic sequences and restriction analysis for diagnosis of sickle cell anemia. Science 230: 1350-1354

This work was supported by a grant of the Spanish Ministry of Education and Science (DGCYT) PB93-1155.

DETECTION OF SINGLE BASE CHANGES IN PCR-AMPLIFIED DNA USING DOUBLE AND SINGLE STRAND CONFORMATIONAL POLYMORPHISMS (SSCP AND DSCP)

F. Barros, M.S. Rodriguez-Calvo, I. Muñoz, C. Pestoni, M.V. Lareu and A. Carracedo

Institute of Legal Medicine, Faculty of Medicine, 15705 Santiago de Compostela. Spain.

Among the methods to detect single base changes (without sequencing) DSCP (Barros, 1991), also known as HA, is, together with SSCP (Orita, 1989), one of the more widely used.

The application of DSCP and SSCP in Forensic Genetics is investigated through the study of variation in coding DNA (HLA-Class II loci), the analysis of sequence variation in STRs and the analysis of mt-DNA

METHODS

PCR amplification:

System	Primer	PCR mixture
HLA-DQA1	5' GTGCTGCAGGTGTAAACTTGTACCAG 3' 5' CACGGATCCGGTAGCAGCGGTAGAGTTG 3'	A
HLA-DPB1	5' CAGGTACCCGCAGAGAATTAC 3' 5' CCCTCACTCACCTCGGCG 3'	A
HUMTH01	5' GTGGGCTGAAAAGCTCCCGATTAT 3' 5' ATTCAAAGGGTATCTGGGTCTTGG 3'	B
mtDNA	5' CACCATTAGCACCCAAAG 3' 5' AGGGGGGGTTTGGTGGAAATTT 3'	C

Mixture A: 1 - 10 ng DNA, 10 mM Tris-CLH (ph 8.3), 2.5 mM $MgCl_2$, 50 mM Kcl, 0.01% gelatin, 200 µM of each dNTP, 0.2 µM of each primer and 2.5 units of AmpliTaq DNA Polymerase (Cetus, Emeryville, USA).

Mixture B: 5 - 25 ng DNA, 10 mM Tris-CLH (ph 8.3), 1.5 mM $MgCl_2$, 50 mM Kcl, 0.01% gelatin, 200 µM of each dNTP, 0.25 µM of each primer and 1.25 units of AmpliTaq DNA Polymerase.

Mixture C: 5 - 25 ng DNA, 10 mM Tris-CLH (ph 8.3), 1.5 mM $MgCl_2$, 50 mM Kcl, 0.01% gelatin, 200 µM of each dNTP, 0.2 µM of each primer and 5 units of AmpliTaq DNA Polymerase.

Amplification conditions:

Loci	Denaturation	Annealing	Extension	Cycles
HLA-DQA1	94°C, 1 min	60°C, 30 sec	72°C, 30 sec	32
HLA-DPB1	95°C, 1 min	55°C, 1 min	72°C, 90 sec	32
HUMTH01	94°C, 45 sec	54°C, 1 min	72°C, 1 min	30
mtDNA	95°C, 10 sec	55°C, 20 sec	72°C, 1 min	32

SSCP and DSCP analysis:

SSCP: denaturing the PCR reaction mixture after amplification at 95°C for 8 mins with 95 % formamide and 20 mM EDTA (1:1). The denatured product was immediately frozen on ice.

DSCP: heating the PCR product at 95°C for 8 mins. The product was immediately frozen on ice and finally heated at 40°C for 10 mins.

The mtDNA fragments were previously cut with the restriction enzyme Dde I.

PAGE and SDS-PAGE:

PAGE was carried out in PhastGels (Pharmacia Biotech, Uppsala, Sweden) Homogeneus T = 20 % and SDS-PAGE in PhastGels Gradient T = 8-25 %. Buffer systems, electrode strips and electrophoretic conditions used were as descrited in Barros 1994.

RESULTS AND DISCUSSION

1. PCR conditions for DSCP and SSCP analysis

SSCP: Single strand DNA was made by denaturing the amplified DNA fragment at 95°C with formamide (Fig. 1.A).
DSCP: Heteroduplexes are created only after a denaturation / renaturation cycle. The optimal conditions for creating heteroduplexes are first to form single-strand DNA without formamide, to freeze the sample on ice, and then to heat the sample at a temperature below the melting domain for heteroduplexes (Fig. 1.B).
Conditions can be designed to obtain homoduplexes, heteroduplexes and single-strand DNA in the same gel (Fig 1.C)

2. Electrophoretic conditions

SSCP and DSCP patterns were analyzed in miniaturized polyacrilamide gels. The best type of gels using PhastGels are:
    For SSCP   T = 20 % (homogeneus)
    For DSCP   T = 8 - 25 % (gradient)

3. Analysis of mutations in coding DNA

Single base mutations can be distinguished in the two HLA-Class II loci studied (HLA-DQA1 and HLA-DPB) (Fig 1) using both SSCP and DSCP. SSCP has advantages over DSCP in typing systems with high number of alleles, because it is not necessary to have a diagram of all possible combinations of the alleles (Barros, 1994).

4. Analysis of mutations in mt-DNA

Most mtDNA variation is within the non-coding region which contains the origen of replication for H strand, both origins of transcription and the D-loop region (Anderson, 1981). A 902 bp fragment was amplified and subsequently cut with Dde I. So three fragments are obtained, two of them available for SSCP and DSCP analysis (Fig. 2).

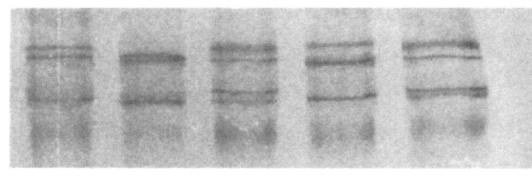

Figure 1A. SSCP patterns of HLA-DPB1 alleles in PhastGel T = 20 %. From left to right: lane (1) *0201-0402*, (2) *0401-0402*, (3) *0201-0401*, (4) *0201-0901*, (5) *0202-0401*.

Figure 1B. DSCP patterns of HLA-DQA1 alleles in PhastGel T = 8-25 %. From left to right: 123 bp ladder marker, lane (1) 1.2-4, (2) 1.1-2, (3) 1.2-4, (4) 1.1-4, (5) 2-3, (6) 4-4, (7) 3-4.

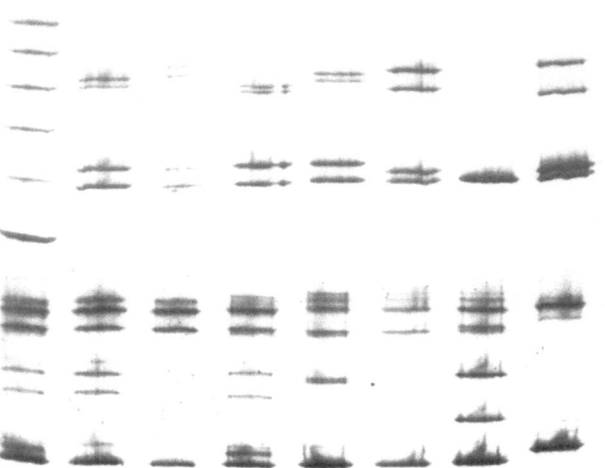

Figure 1C. SSCP and DSCP patterns of HLA-DQA1 alleles. From left to right: lane (1) 3-4, (2) 1.1-4, (3) 2-2, (4) 2-3, (5) 1.1-2, (6) 2-2, (7) 2-4, (8) 3-3.

The SSCP patterns of seven samples, with three variants, are shown in Figure 3. In the used conditions SSCP seems to be advantageous for detecting mutations and the analysis and lecture of the patterns is considerably easier.

5. Analysis of sequence variations in STRs

Single base substitutions or one base deletions in the repeating unit of STRs can be investigated through DSCP and SSCP analysis. One example is shown in the Figure 4 , where HUMTH01 9.3 - 10 heterozygote is detected in miniaturized gels using DSCP. HUMTH01 10 is a rare allele and can be confused with the 9.3 allele, since both fragments differ in a single base. DSCP offers, in this case, a fast and useful method to detect hidden variation in STRs.

This work was supported by grants from DGICYT (PB92-0371) and FISS (94/1053)

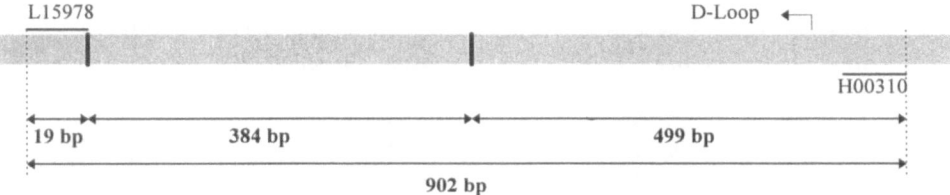

Figure 2. Diagram of the non-coding mtDNA fragment amplified with the Dde I restriction sites.

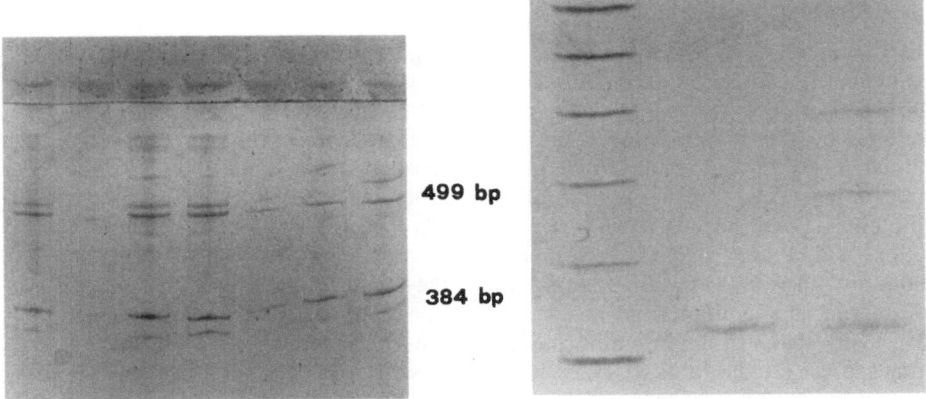

499 bp

384 bp

Figure 3. SSCP patterns of 384 bp and 499 bp mtDNA fragments in PhastGel T = 20 %.

Figure 4. DSCP patterns of HUMTH01 alleles in PhastGel T = 8-25 %. From left to right: 123 bp ladder marker, lane (1) 9.3-9.3, (2) 9.3-10.

References

Anderson, S.; Bankier, A.T.; Barrell, B.G.; deBrujin, M.H.L.; Coulson, A.R.; Drouin, J.; Eperon, I.C.; Nierlich, D.P.; Roe, B.A.; Sanger, F.; Schreier, P.H.; Smith, A.J.H.; Staden, R. and Young, I.G. (1981) Sequence and organisation of the human mitochondrial genome. Nature 290:457-465.
Barros, F.; Carracedo, A.; Lareu, M.V. and Rodriguez-Calvo, M.S. (1991) Electrophoretic human leukocyte antigen HLA-DQA1 DNA typing after polymerase chain reaction amplification. Electrophoresis 12:1041-1045.
Barros, F. ; Muñoz-Barús, I.; Lareu, M.V.; Rodriguez-Calvo, M.S. and Carracedo, A. (1994) Double- and single-strand conformation polymorphism analysis of point mutations and short tandem repeats. Electrophoresis 15:566-571.
Orita, M.; Iwahana, H.; Kanazawa, H.; Hayashi, K. and Sekiya, T. (1989) Detection of polymorphisms of human DNA by gel electrophoresis as single-strand conformation polymorphisms. Proc. Natl. Acad. Sci. U.S.A. 86:2766-2770.

EVALUATION OF HYBRIDISATION EQUIPMENT FOR USE WITH NON ISOTOPICALLY LABELLED PROBES

W P Childs and G Rysiecki

Cellmark Diagnostics, Blacklands Way, Abingdon Business Park, Abingdon, Oxfordshire, OX14 1DY, UK.

INTRODUCTION

One of the most critical stages in producing a DNA fingerprint or DNA profile is hybridisation of the membrane-bound DNA samples to a labelled multilocus or single locus (VNTR) probe. Until the early 1990's the probes used were usually prepared by radioactive labelling of purified plasmid inserts. More recently non-isotopic labelling systems have become available and probes for DNA fingerprinting and DNA profiling can now be purchased labelled and ready to use eg, NICE™ probes (Cellmark). Apart from their obvious safety and environmental advantages, non-isotopic probes allow reduced labour costs and more reproducible, high quality results and have therefore been very widely adopted (Ref. 1).

Non-isotopic probes are usually enzyme-labelled oligonucleotides. The high concentration of the oligonucleotide allows very rapid hybridisation when compared with radioactively labelled insert probes, typically 20-30 minutes at 50°C compared with overnight at 65°C. Because the hybridisation reaction is so short, there is insufficient time for temperature equilibration and this can result in incorrect hybridisation temperatures and therefore incorrect stringencies. If probe hybridisation is carried out at too low a stringency, non-specific binding and secondary bands will occur. At too high a temperature the reaction conditions will be too stringent, resulting in loss of sensitivity. It is essential that all solutions are pre-warmed to 50°C, but even then they can cool rapidly as they are transferred into the hybridisation apparatus so that correct hybridisation conditions are never actually achieved, leading to inconsistent quality. To avoid these problems it is important to use a hybridisation system which allows temperature to be maintained exactly throughout the process. A wide variety of hybridisation equipment is now available and several systems were assessed for use with NICE™ probes.

METHODS

The following equipment was evaluated: Hybritube™ (Life Technologies Inc), rotisserie hybridisation oven (Hybridiser 600 Stratagene), NICE™ chamber (Cellmark), sandwich boxes or perspex hybridisation chambers in either waterbaths or dry incubators. Membranes (Hybond-N, Amersham) containing human genomic DNA digested with HinfI were hybridised with NICE™ probes (Cellmark) using recommended conditions. Membranes were sprayed with Lumi-Phos® 530 (Lumigen Inc) and exposed to X-ray film (Hyperfilm, Amersham).

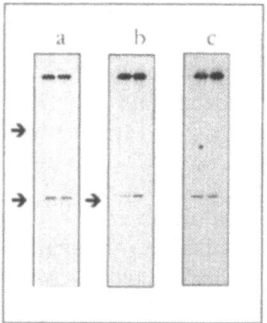

Figure 1
Three identical membranes containing 2 μg K562 DNA digested with HinfI and probed with NICE™ G3. Hybridisation and washing were carried out at a) 40 °C, b) 45 °C and c) 50 °C (recommended temperature). Exposures were for 3 hours at 30 °C.

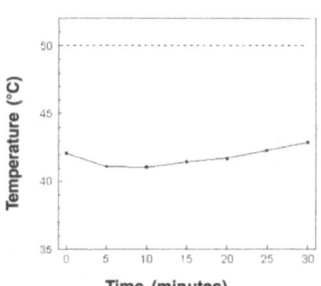

Figure 2
Temperature drift in a hybridisation reaction. Hybridisation solution was pre-warmed to 50 °C then poured into a perspex hybridisation chamber containing membranes and incubated in a 50 °C dry incubator for 30 minutes. The temperature of the solution was recorded with a Squirrel Data Logger (Grant Instruments).

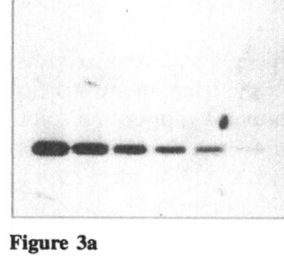

Figure 3a

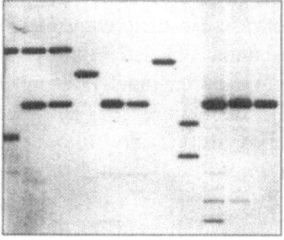

Figure 3b

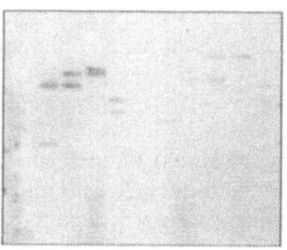

Figure 3c

Figure 3a-c
Membranes hybridised and washed in a rotisserie oven set at 50 °C (a and b) and a Hybritube™ incubated in a waterbath set at 50 °C (c).
a Concentration gradient of HinfI digested K562 DNA probed with NICE™ MS8, 3 hour exposure.
b Human genomic DNA (approximately 1-4 μg per track) digested with HinfI and probed with NICE™ MS8, 3 hour exposure.
c Human genomic DNA (approximately 1-4 μg per track) digested with HinfI and probed with NICE™ MS205 and MW100, overnight exposure.

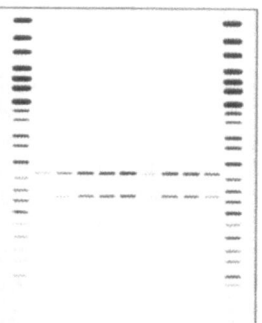

Figure 4
Mebrane containing HinfI digested K562 DNA (2 μg per track) and DNA Analysis Marker Ladder (LTI) hybridised in NICE™ chamber at 50 °C to MS205 and MW100, 3 hour exposure.

RESULTS

Figure 1 shows the effect of deliberately varying hybridisation and washing temperature. Secondary bands are visible when the temperature is below the recommended level. Figure 2 shows how even pre-warmed hybridisation solutions can cool rapidly, leading to hybridisation at temperatures below those intended. Hybridisation temperature fell as low as 41°C reaching a maximum of only 42.9°C after 30 minutes. Figures 3 and 4 show results using various hybridisation equipment. Figures 3a and 3b show membranes hybridised and washed in a rotisserie oven with poor results due to insufficient washing. In Figure 3a the membrane had overlapped and stuck to itself in the roller preventing wash solutions from reaching all areas. Figure 3b shows the middle membrane of three which were hybridised in a single roller. Again efficiency of washing was very poor resulting in high background and secondary bands. The membrane in Figure 3c was hybridised and washed in a Hybritube™ (diameter approximately 20 mm). The results are very patchy with secondary bands and poorly washed areas. The membrane must be rolled quite tightly before insertion into the Hybritube™ and this resulted in poor access for the probe and wash solutions due to the membrane sticking to itself. The membrane in Figure 4 was hybridised and washed in a NICE™ chamber which is specially designed for use with alkaline phosphatase labelled probes. The hybridisation reaction and washing steps occur in a chamber which is surrounded by a waterjacket, allowing very accurate maintenance of temperature throughout the process. Membranes are laid flat in the chamber which is placed on a shaking platform, allowing thorough agitation and ensuring that the probe and wash solutions are in good contact with all areas of the membrane.

DISCUSSION

In order to achieve consistently good results with alkaline phosphatase-labelled oligonucleotides probes it is essential to maintain the correct temperature in the actual hybridisation reaction and subsequent wash steps and to agitate the membranes to prevent sticking and allow thorough washing. Rotisserie ovens are convenient when probing only one or two membranes, but care must be taken to avoid membranes sticking together and to ensure that the solutions do not cool below the recommended temperatures at any stage. Artifacts can be avoided by increasing the amount of mixing, the volume of solution and the diameter of the roller. Significant problems can be encountered when incubating sandwich boxes in dry ovens due to poor heat exchange and cooling of pre-warmed solutions. Results are generally better when incubation is in a shaking waterbath. The most consistent results were obtained using the NICE™ chamber. This system is ideal for probing up to ten membranes simultaneously but probably less appropriate for small-scale hybridisations.

REFERENCES

1. A F Giles, K J Booth, J R Parker, A J Garman, D T Carrick, H Akhavan, A P Schaap. Rapid, simple Non-Isotopic Probing of Southern Blots for DNA Fingerprinting. In Advances in Forensic Haemogenetics 3. Eds H F Polesky and W R Mayr. Springer-Verlag Berlin Heidelberg 1990.

CDP-STAR™ AS A CHEMILUMINESCENT SUBSTRATE FOR USE WITH ALKALINE PHOSPHATASE LABELLED PROBES

W P Childs, G Rysiecki, P Elsmore

Cellmark Diagnostics, Blacklands Way, Abingdon Business Park, Abingdon, Oxfordshire OX14 1DY, UK.

INTRODUCTION

In the last five years alkaline phosphatase-labelled probes have been widely adopted for use in DNA fingerprinting and DNA profiling eg NICE™ probes (Cellmark) (Ref. 1). Apart from the obvious operational advantages of using non-radioactive systems, hybridisation with alkaline phosphatase-labelled probes is far more rapid than with traditional systems. Typically membranes can be hybridised and autoradiographs produced within seven hours. Hybridisation is detected by the application of a chemiluminescent substrate to the membrane. The substrate is activated by the alkaline phosphatase label on the probe resulting in emission of visible light which is recorded on X-ray film. One of the slowest parts of the procedure is exposure of hybridised membranes to X-ray film, which takes 3-4 hours or more. In an effort to shorten exposures and reduce the overall length of the DNA profiling process, we examined the performance of two different chemiluminescent substrates, Lumi-Phos® 530 (Lumigen Inc, Ref. 2) and CDP-Star™ (Tropix Inc, Ref. 3) which is reported to give shorter exposure times.

METHODS

Membranes (Hybond-N, Amersham) containing HinfI digested human DNA were hybridised to various NICE™ probes (Cellmark) following recommended conditions. These were either standard membranes containing concentration gradients of K562 DNA (Fig. 1 and 3) or samples from paternity casework at approximately 1-4 µg per track (Fig. 2). Following hybridisation and washing, membranes were either sprayed evenly with Lumi-Phos® 530 or incubated in CDP-Star™ for 5 minutes at room temperature. Each membrane was then sandwiched between two polyester sheets and excess chemiluminescent substrate gently squeezed out. Exposure to X-ray film (Hyperfilm, Amersham) was carried out at 30°C for various lengths of time.

RESULTS

Figure 1 shows two identical membranes containing HinfI-digested K562 genomic DNA and probed with MS31. The membrane in Fig 1a was treated with CDP-Star™ and exposed to X-ray film for 1 hour while that in Fig 1b was treated with Lumi-Phos® 530 and exposed to X-ray film for 1 hour. After a 1 hour exposure, 10ng of DNA was clearly visible on the CDP-Star™ treated membrane, while on the Lumi-Phos® 530 treated

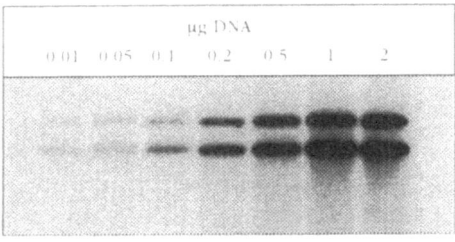

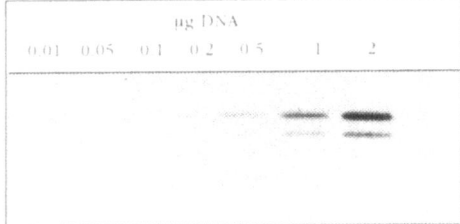

Figure 1a, b
Gradients of HinfI digested K562 DNA probed with MS31.
a CDP-*Star*™ treated and exposed to X-ray film at 30 °C for 1 hour.
b Lumi-Phos® 530 treated and exposed to X-ray film at 30 °C for 1 hour.

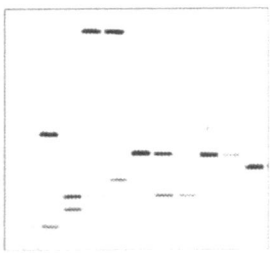

Figure 2a

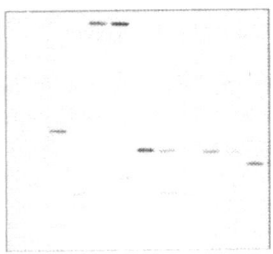

Figure 2b

Figure 2a,b
Human DNA samples digested with HinfI, probed with MS205 and exposed to X-ray film for 30 minutes at 30 °C.
a 4 hours after CDP-Star™ treatment.
b 2 days after CDP-Star™ treatment.

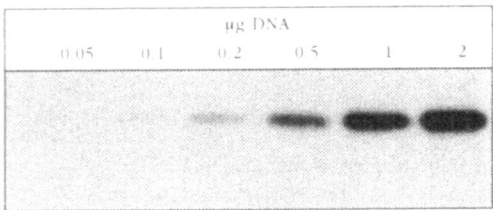

Figure 3
Membrane containig a gradient of HinfI digested K562 DNA, probed with G3 and treated with CDP-*Star*™ which had been used on the previous 3 days. Exposure was for 1 hour at 30 °C.

membrane 200 ng could be detected.

In order to examine the flexibility of using CDP-Star™, a membrane containing paternity casework samples (approximately 1-4 µg DNA per track) was treated with CDP-Star™ and exposed to X-ray film after 4 hours (Fig. 2a), and then again 2 days after CDP-Star application (Fig. 2b). Chemiluminescence of CDP-Star™ continues over a period of several days and although sensitivity of detection does decrease with time, several exposures of a membrane can be taken without the necessity of reprobing or reapplication of chemiluminescent substrate.

The potential for reuse of CDP-Star solutions is shown in Figure 3. A membrane containing a concentration gradient of K562 DNA was hybridised with NICE™ probe G3 and incubated in CDP-Star™ which had already been used on the three preceding days and stored at 4°C. Following a 1 hour exposure, 100 ng of K562 DNA is still clearly visible.

DISCUSSION

Various chemiluminescent substrates are now available for use with alkaline phosphatase labelled probes, all offering major advantages over the traditional radioactive systems. This study compares the performance of CDP-Star™ and Lumi-Phos® 530 in DNA Profiling. Whilst the overall sensitivity (ie total chemiluminescence) of both substrates is very similar, the use of CDP-Star™ reduces film exposure time significantly. This offers clear advantages in DNA profiling as sequential hybridisation with several probes can take several days to accomplish. It is also important in forensic applications where very small DNA samples can often only be visualised after lengthy exposures.

REFERENCES

1.   A F Giles, K J Booth, J R Parker, A J Garman, D T Carrick, H Akhavan and A P Schaap. Rapid, Simple, Non-Isotopic Probing of Southern Blots for DNA Fingerprinting. In: Advances in Forensic Haemogenetics 3, Eds H F Polesky and W R Mayr. Springer-Verlag, Berlin Heidelberg 1990.

2.   A P Schaap, H Akhavan and L Romano (1989). Chemiluminescent Substrates for Alkaline Phosphatase. Clin. Chem. 35, 1863-1864.

3.   H Hoeltke, S Schneider, I Ettl, R Binsack, I Obermaier, M Seller and G Sanger. (1995) Rapid, Highly Sensitive Detection of Digoxigenin-labelled Nucleic Acids by Improved Chemiluminescent Alkaline Phosphatase Substrates. Biochemica, 1, 17-20.

The single locus probes discovered by Professor Alec Jeffreys are claimed in UK Patent No 2188323 and corresponding worldwide patent applications. Lumi-Phos® 530 is a proprietary product of Lumigen Inc and is a subject of European Patent Numbers 254051B1 and 352712B1 and corresponding worldwide patents. CDP-Star™ is a proprietary product developed and produced exclusively by Tropix Inc and is a subject of US Patent Number 5326882 and corresponding worldwide patents.

SIMPLE AND RAPID TYPING OF STRs ON AN AUTOMATED DNA SEQUENCER

R. Decorte and J.-J. Cassiman

Center for Human Genetics, K.U.Leuven, Herestraat 49, B-3000 Leuven, Belgium

INTRODUCTION

Short Tandem Repeat (STR) loci are very abundant in the human genome: di-nucleotide repeats occur approximately every 6 kb while tri- and tetra-nucleotide repeats every 300 to 500 kb (Edwards 1991). The lower size of the polymorphic region increases the sensitivity for typing of small amounts of degraded DNA which is in contrast to VNTRs. It is therefore not surprising that STR loci have become the principal polymorphic markers in forensic DNA typing. Whereas, initially the analysis of the PCR products relied on radioactive procedures, it is now possible to type STR alleles in a non-radioactive manner either by silver staining or by electrophoresis of fluorescent PCR products on an automated DNA sequencer.

We have previously reported about the accuracy for sizing fluorescent-labelled VNTR alleles (APOB) on the A.L.F. DNA sequencer (Decorte 1993). In this paper, we evaluated the A.L.F. DNA sequencer for separating 4 STR loci simultaneously at high speed and with a high throughput. Furthermore, a population study was performed on 122 unrelated Caucasians of Belgian descent.

MATERIALS AND METHODS

Genomic DNA was extracted from venous blood samples according to standard procedures. Amplification of the STR loci HUMvWF, D21S11, HUMTHO1 and HPRT was done as described by Frégeau and Fourney (1993). The PCR primers have been reported by Frégeau and Fourney (1993) and the forward primers were labelled with fluorescein. In total 28 cycles were done on a GeneAmp 2400 or 9600 Cycler (Perkin-Elmer) in a reaction volume of 25 µl. PCR products were diluted five fold after quality control on 6% polyacrylamide gels. The diluted PCR products for the 4 STR loci were mixed together and 4 µl was applied to 4 µl of stop-mix (95% formamide, 5 mg/ml dextran blue and fluorescein-labelled PCR products of 123 and 375 bp). The PCR products were loaded on gel after 3 min. denaturation at 85°C. A.L.F. gels with a well-to-laser distance of 19 cm and spacers of 0.35 mm contained 6% Hydrolink Long Ranger (J.T. Baker), 7M Urea (BRL) and a running buffer of 0.6xTBE (53.4 mM Tris, 64.2 mM boric acid and 1.2 mM EDTA). Running conditions were 2000 V, 70 mA, 45 W and 50°C, 1.5 sec. sampling interval for 140 min. The same gel was reloaded with other samples without a pre-run of 10 min. Each run included two lanes with a combination of allele markers for each locus (Fig.1).

RESULTS AND DISCUSSION

The STR loci D21S11, HUMvWF, HUMTHO1 and HPRT were selected on the basis of non-overlapping allele size distributions (Table 1) and identical annealing conditions in the PCR (D21S11 and HUMvWF: 64°C; HUMTHO1 and HPRT: 60°C). Initially, we evaluated an A.L.F. gel with a laser-to-well distance of 10 cm and a 8% Hydrolink Long Ranger - 7M Urea gel. This way, it was possible to separate the STR alleles in a run of 75 min. The accuracy of the size estimates was high (average of 99.92%) when two internal markers (123 and 375 bp) were included in each lane to compensate for any lane-to-lane differences. An average accuracy of 99.16% was obtained when no internal markers were used.

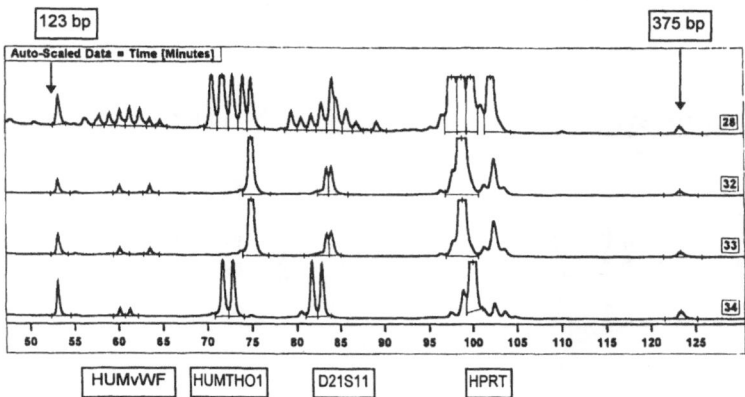

Figure 1: Multiplex analysis of 4 STR loci on the A.L.F. DNA sequencer.
Lane 28 contains the 4 allelic markers, Lane 32 and 33 are DNA samples from a twin and lane 34 is a positive control. The results are displayed in function of the running time.

During a population study for HUMTHO1, one allele was observed which showed a dif-ference of 1 bp (allele 10: 199 bp) with the preceding allele (9.3: 198 bp). However, exact sizing of this allele on the short gels was problematic: one of the 4 times that the sample was loaded on a short gel, resulted in a classification of the allele as a 9.3 allele. This could be overcome when the distance between the two alleles in a heterozygous DNA sample was taken into account. To avoid this complication, we developed a high speed sizing protocol on a regular A.L.F. gel (well-to-laser distance of 19 cm) as described in the materials and methods section. The run time increased from 75 min. to 125 min. without a significant decrease of the average accuracy (99.91%) compared to a 10 cm gel, although a 6% Hydrolink gel was used instead of a 8% (Fig. 1). The gels could be reloaded again and there was no difference in the accuracy of the size

Table 1: Summary of the results for the 4 STR loci in the Belgian population

Locus	Number of chromosomes	Size range (bp)	Heterozygo-sity (%)	Probability of paternity exclusion	Match probability
HUMvWF	244	138-162	80.9	0.621	0.064
HUMTHO1	204	179-199	78.9	0.582	0.077
D21S11	236	209-249	85.3	0.709	0.038
HPRT	149	275-299	73.2	0.345	0.114
			Cumulative:	**0.970**	**0.000021**

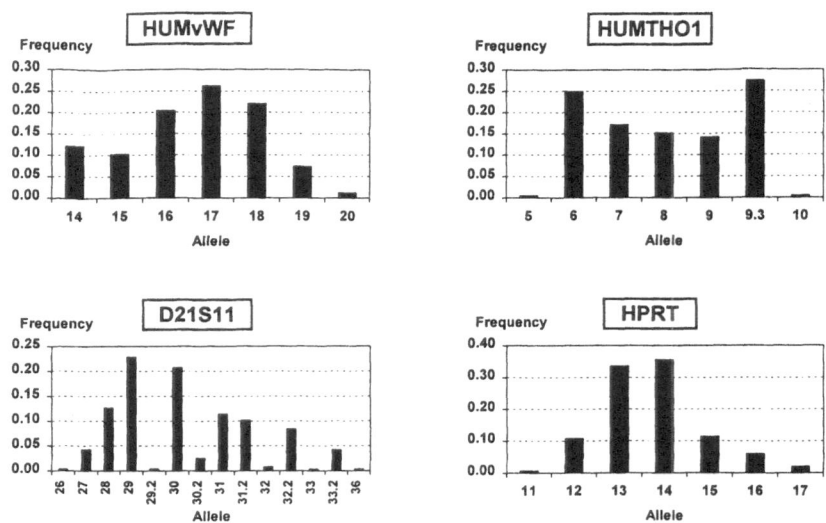

Figure 2: Frequency distribution of the STR alleles in the Belgian population. Alleles indicate the number of repeats present in the PCR product according to the nomenclature recommended by the DNA commission of the ISFH.

estimates between the first (99.93%) and the second run (99.88%). This way, a throughput was obtained of 76 DNA samples for 4 loci in one working day.

The 4 STR loci were studied in a population of 122 unrelated Caucasian individuals. Seven alleles were observed for HUMvWF, HUMTHO1 and HPRT, and 14 alleles for D21S11 (Fig. 2). The expected heterozygosity for the four STR loci ranged between 85.3% (D21S11) and 73.2% (HPRT). The genotype distributions for all the four loci were in Hardy-Weinberg equilibrium. The combined match probability for forensic identity testing was 2.1×10^5 while the combined probability of paternity exclusion was 0.97 (Table 1). In combination with 3 highly polymorphic AMP-FLPs (D1S111, D17S5 and DXYS17), the match probability increased to 2.8×10^9 and the probability of paternity exclusion to 0.9988. Therefore, this highly discri-minating system can be used as a rapid and efficient method in the analysis of forensic evidence samples and for paternity determinations.

REFERENCES

Decorte R, Marynen P, Cassiman JJ (1993) High-speed automated detection of PCR-amplified VNTR alleles: application to the apolipoprotein B 3' hypervariable region. Science Tools 37:1-4
Edwards A, Civitello A, Hammond HA, Caskey CT (1991) DNA typing and genetic mapping with trimeric and tetrameric tandem repeats. Am. J. Hum. Genet. 49: 746-756
Frégeau CJ, Fourney RM (1993) DNA typing with fluorescently tagged short tandem repeats: A sensitive and accurate approach to human identification. BioTechniques 15: 100-119.

A MODIFICATION TO THE "CHELEX" DNA EXTRACTION METHOD FOR CASEWORK SAMPLES.

M.J.Greenhalgh

Metropolitan Police Forensic Science Laboratory,
109, Lambeth Road,
London SE1 7LP
United Kingdom.

Introduction.

DNA profiling using multiplex amplification of four tetrameric STR loci is routinely used in casework at the Metropolitan Police Laboratory.

The loci used are:	HUMVWA31
(Kimpton et al.1994)	HUMTHO1
	HUMF13A1
	HUMFES

DNA is extracted from stain material using "Chelex 100" as described by Walsh et al. (1991). The problem encountered at the Metropolitan Police Lab was that the DNA from a significant number of stains, extracted using this method would not amplify. This was especially noticeable with semen and saliva staining. Organic extraction can be useful but it is a lengthy process and involves the use of hazardous reagents. One of the advantages of "Chelex" is that it is an extremely rapid method. Any solution to the problem could not be allowed to increase the extraction time significantly.

A method has now been introduced which filters the aqueous DNA extract produced by the "Chelex" method using a microconcentrator with a molecular weight cut off of 30,000 Daltons. This retains the majority of the DNA whilst allowing low molecular weight inhibitors of PCR to pass through. The DNA can then be rehydrated and the PCR process repeated. The "Microcon" range of miniconcentrators have been used though similar devices are available from other manufacturers.

Description of the Microcon Device:

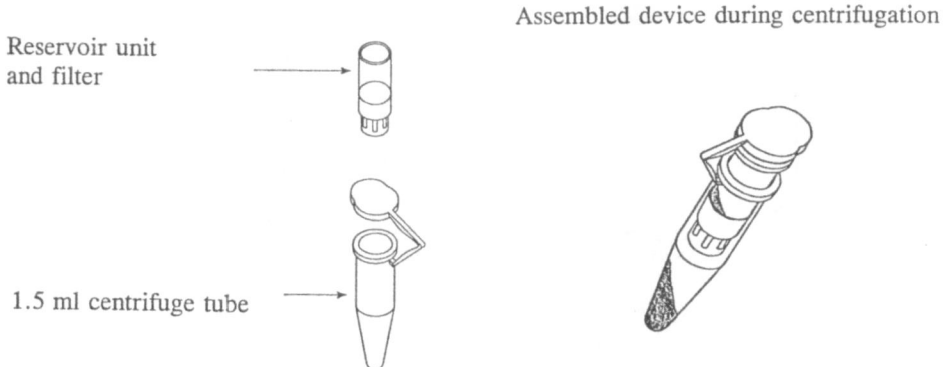

Reservoir unit and filter

1.5 ml centrifuge tube

Assembled device during centrifugation

The Microcon miniconcentrator consists of a sample reservoir with an integral filter which connects to a 1.5 ml microcentrifuge tube. The membranes are available in a range of pore sizes. The reservoir can accept a maximum volume of 500 μl.

MPFSL Microcon Protocol:

This method is used on DNA solutions produced by the "Chelex" extraction method which should have sufficient DNA to give a result yet have produced no profile.

1)   Assemble the filter unit in the microcentrifuge tube provided and label with the appropriate identifier.

2)   Load the sample (max vol 500 μl) into the reservoir and close the cap.

3)   Centrifuge at 14,000 g for 12 minutes. (the majority of the solution passes through the filter into the lower tube).

4)   Add 300μl of TE buffer to the reservoir and centrifuge again as above.

5)   Add 75μl of TE buffer to the reservoir, mix by pipetting up and down 2-3 times and then pipette all the solution from the reservoir into a sterile tube.

6)   This sample is assayed and the PCR reaction repeated using 1-3 ng of target DNA.

An example of results following Microcon treatment.

This item was vaginal swab stained with semen. A preferential extraction was performed and 3ng of DNA amplified. The initial result was negative. Following the use of the Microcon, the profile below was obtained.

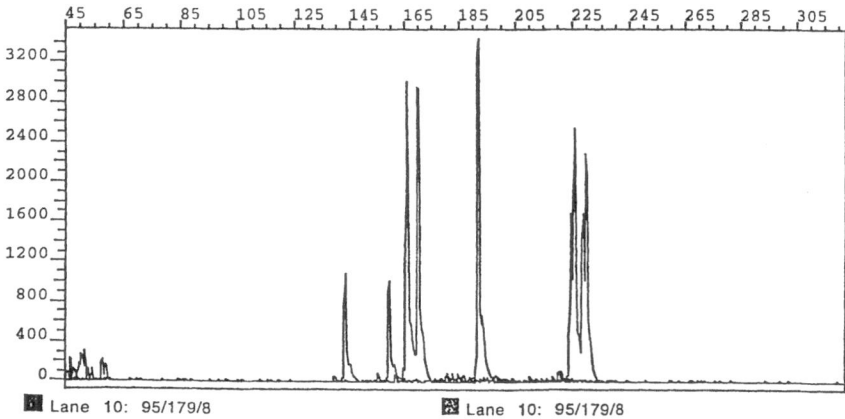

Discussion:

Initially the Microcon procedure was used on samples that contained DNA yet which failed to amplify. Approximately 40% of these samples gave a full or partial profile when repeated. A significant proportion of these samples were semen or saliva stains and now all these types of stain are given the treatment as routine. It is inevitable that some of the DNA cannot be recovered from the device and it advisable to perform an assay before proceeding to the PCR stage.

The manufacturers recommend that after the filtration spin, the unit is inverted into a fresh tube and spun briefly to remove the retentate. Unfortunately after a 12 minute spin at high speed the two parts are firmly wedged together. Separating them requires some force and runs the risk of contaminating the operator's gloves with DNA or creating an aerosol of DNA solution. This DNA is concentrated and pure - An ideal substrate for PCR and therefore a possible contamination risk. At the Metropolitan Police Lab the procedure has been modified to avoid this. Buffer is added to the upper chamber, mixed and then pipetted into a fresh tube.

Conclusion:

Microconcentrators are a useful tool for additional purification of DNA extracts prior to PCR. They are quick to use and make a significant difference to the success rate of DNA STR profiling.

References:

Kimpton et al. Evaluation of an automated DNA profiling system employing multiplex amplification of four tetrameric STR loci. Int J Leg Med. (1994) 106:302-311

Walsh et al. Chelex 100 as a medium for the simple extraction of DNA for PCR based typing from forensic material. Biotechniques 1:91-98.

APPLICATION OF HLA-DR TYPING BY PCR-SSP TO FORENSIC SAMPLES

M. Ota, Y. Katsuyama, Y. Hama, N. Harashima, CY. Liu and H. Fukushima

Department of Legal Medicine, Shinshu University, Matsumoto, Japan

INTRODUCTION

An anlysis of the HLA complex by molecular methods has revealed an extensive degree of polymorphism. These genes are one of useful human genetic markers in forensic investigations. Class II HLA polymorphisms have been defined at the DNA level, due to the availability of allelic nucleotide sequences in this region as well as the successful application of molecular typing techniques. Various PCR based HLA class II DNA typing methods have been developed and applied. To date, one commercial kit for HLA-DQA1 typing has been validated for forensic investigations, and is used routinely in many laboratories. Among HLA class II genes, the DRB1 gene is one of the most useful in forensic genetics. In this study we have investigated the applicability of HLA-DR "low-resolution" typing by PCR-SSP (sequence specific primers) to forensic practice.

MATERIALS and METHODS

To define HLA-DR1 to DR10 by PCR-SSP, we designed 9 forward primers and 9 reverse primers (Table 1), which were created with a little modification in previous publications (1, 2).

DNA for investigation

This study uses twenty randomly selected healthy individuals who have been serologically DR typed. DNA was prepared by phenol/chloroform extraction. DNA from homozygous cells of 10th International Histocompatibility Workshop was used to verify primer specificities. The cell lines represented the following DRB1 alleles: 0101, 0102, 1501, 1502, 1601, 1602, 0301, 0401, 0402, 0404, 0405, 1101, 1102, 1103, 1201, 1301, 1302, 1401, 0701, 0801, 0802, 0803, 0901.

Amplification conditions

The PCR reactions were carried out in 25 µl volumes, which contained genomic DNA template, 10 pmol of each sequence-specific primer, 200 µM of each dNTP, 2 units of Taq DNA polymerase, 1.5 mM $MgCl_2$ 10 mM Tris-HCl, 50 mM KCl, and 0.1% Triton-X. Samples were amplified after initial denaturation at 94 °C for 3 minutes, followed by 30 cycles of 94 °C denaturation for 60 seconds, 60 °C annealing for 90 seconds, 72 °C for extension for 60 seconds and a final 72 °C extension for 5 minutes, using a thermal sequence TSR-300 (Iwaki Glass Co., Japan)

Nested PCR

For typing from extremely small amounts of DNA, we applied the nested PCR method to increase amplification sensitivity. Generic primers were generated from outside sequences to the nested primers used for PCR-SSP(table 1). After performing the first round of PCR using generic primers, the amplification mixture was purified by Centri-Sep column (Princeton Separations, Inc. NJ USA) to remove excess primers and dNTPs. An appropriate volume (usually 1μl) of purified DNA was subjected to a second round of PCR. The second PCR was performed under the following conditions: 1μl of the first amplification product was used as the template in 100μl of reaction mixture. Constituents and concentrations of the reaction buffer and reaction thermocycles were the same as in the first round of PCR, except that the number of cycles was reduced to 20.
  We applied this method to determine the HLA-DR type of a DNA sample extracted from hair and left at 4 °C for 3 years.

RESULTS and DISCUSSION

The PCR-SSP method could type DR1 to DR10 specifically (DR1, DR2, DR3, DR4, DR11, DR12, DR13, DR14, DR7, DR8, DR9, DR10) for the DNA samples obtained from cells from randomly selected healthy individuals and from 10th International Histocompatibility Workshop. Furthermore, when combined with the PCR-RFLP method(2), this method is able to determine the sub-allelic types of DR2, DR4 and DR8, which have relatively high gene frequencies in Japanese (0.182, 0.228 and 0.133).
We could determine DR types with as little as 10ng DNA. Moreover, when we used the nested PCR method, it was possible to determine the DR type using only 10pg of DNA. This nested PCR method made it possible to conduct typing using only 0.2ng of DNA extracted from hair (Figure 1). This system yielded a 0.90 power of discrimination and a 0.71 chance of exclusion. This method promises to be a useful tool for forensic investigations.

REFERENCES
1) O. Oleraup and H, Zetterquist, Tissue Antigens, 1992:39:225-235.
2) M. Ota et al., Tissue Antigens, 1992: 39:187-202.

Table 1. Primer pairs for identification of DR1-DR10 specificities
by PCR-SSP technique

```
---------------------------------------------------------------------------------------
G.P.                        5' primer                                3' primer
            DRBF:5'-CCGGATCCTTCGTGTCCCCACAGCACG       DRBR:5'-CCGCTGCACTGTGAAGCTCT

SSP
DR1      5'R1:     5'-GGTTGCTGGAAAGATGCATCT        DRBR:    5'-CCGCTGCACTGTGAAGCTCT
DR2      5'R2:     5'-TTCCTGTGGCAGCCTAAGAGG        DRBR:    5'-CCGCTGCACTGTGAAGCTCT
DR3      5'R3:     5'-TACTTCCATAACCAGGAGGAGA       3'R3:    5'-AGTAGTTGTCCACCCGGC
DR4      5'R4:     5'-GTTTCTTGGAGCAGGTTAAAC        DRBR:    5'-CCGCTGCACTGTGAAGCTCT
DR11     5'R3568:5'-ACGTTTCTTGGAGTACTCTACG         3'R11:   5'-CTGGCTGTTCCAGTACTCCT
DR12     5'R12:    5'-AGTACTCTACGGGTGAGTGTT        3'R12:   5'-CACTGTGAAGCTCTCCACAG
DR13.1   5'R3568:5'-ACGTTTCTTGGAGTACTCTACG         3'R13-1:5'-CCCGCTCGTCTTCCAGGAT
DR13.2   5'R3568:5'-ACGTTTCTTGGAGTACTCTACG         3'R13-2:5'-TGTTCCAGTACTCGGCGCT
DR14.1   5'R3568:5'-ACGTTTCTTGGAGTACTCTACG         3'R14-1:5'-TCTGCAATAGGTGTCCACCT
DR14.2   5'R3568:5'-ACGTTTCTTGGAGTACTCTACG         3'R14-2:5'-TCCACCGCGGCCCGCCT
DR7      5'R7:     5'-AGTTCCTGGAAAGACTCTTCT        DRBR:    5'-CCGCTGCACTGTGAAGCTCT
DR8      5'R3568:5'-ACGTTTCTTGGAGTACTCTACG         3'R8:    5'-CTGCAGTAGGTGTCCACCAG
DR9      5'R9:     5'-GAAGCAGGATAAGTTTGAGTG        DRBR:    5'-CCGCTGCACTGTGAAGCTCT
DR10     5'R10:    5'-GGTTGCTGGAAAGACGCGTCC        DRBR:    5'-CCGCTGCACTGTGAAGCTCT
---------------------------------------------------------------------------------------
G.P. Generic Primers, SSP: Sequence Specific Primers
```

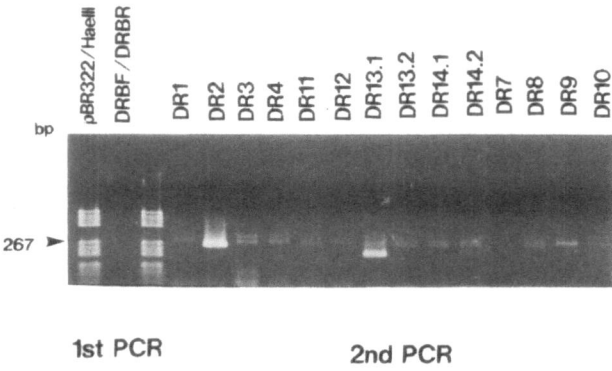

Figure 1.
HLA-DR"low-resolution"PCR-SSP typing of a DNA sample extracted
from hair (3 cm length with a root) and left at 4 °C for 3 years. First PCR
with primers DRBF and DRBR. Second PCR was perfomed by using 1 µl of
first PCR product and each sequence specific primers(SSP). By second
PCR using SSP typing method the sample could be typed DR2 and DR13.2
heterozygotes.

THE MVR-PCR APPROACH FOR THE TYPING OF THE MS32 LOCUS: USEFULNESS AND TECHNICAL PROBLEMS

M.S. Rodríguez-Calvo, S. Bellas, M.V. Lareu, J.I. Muñoz, C. Pestoni, F. Barros, A. Carracedo.

Institute of Legal Medicine. University of Medicine. Santiago de Compostela, Spain

INTRODUCTION

The analysis of the interspersion pattern of variant repeat units along minisatellite alleles using PCR (MVR-PCR, Minisatellite Variant Repeat mapping) is a new approach to assessing individual variation in DNA. This method was developed by Jeffreys et al. in 1991 [1] and has been successfully applied to the hypervariable human minisatellite MS32 (locus D1S8).
One such minisatellite, D1S8 (MS32) consists of a 29 bp repeat unit showing two major classes of Minisatellite Variant Repeat (MVR) [designated a-type and t-type], which differ by a single base substitution [2] and show highly diverse dispersion patterns within alleles [3].
Using MVR specific amplimers and a specific primer located in the DNA flanking the minisatellite it is possible to generate a ladder of PCR products corresponding to the position of each a-type and t-type repeat.
In this study, our experiences in the analysis of D1S8 locus (MS32) using conventional agarose gels and non-radioactive hybridization as well as automatic detection of fluorescent labelled alleles are described.

MATERIALS AND METHODS

SAMPLES

Blood samples were obtained from healthy individuals of the Galician population. DNA was extracted using the phenol-chloroform method [4] and quantified with a spectrophotometer (Perkin-Elmer).

MVR-PCR

Primers (Provided by Cellmark)

32-OR	5' GAGTAGTTTGGAAGGGTGGT 3'
TAG	5' TCATGCGTCCATGGTCCGGA 3'
32-TAG-A	5'TCATGCGTCCATGGTCCGGA**CATTCTGAGTCACCCCTGGC**3'
32-TAG-T	5'TCATGCGTCCATGGTCCGGA**CATTCTGAGTCACCCCTGGT**3'

Amplification conditions

1.-Reaction Volume: 28 µl
   DNA: 100 ng.
   Primers: 10 µM 32-OR, 10 µM TAG, 0.1 µM 32-TAG-A, 0.2 µM 32-TAG-T
   Buffer: 4.5 mM Tris-HCl (pH 8.8), 11 mM ammonium sulfate, 4.5 mM $MgCl_2$, 6.7 mM 2-mercaptoethanol, 4 µM EDTA, 1 mM dNTPs, BSA 113 µg/ml.
   AmplyTaq DNA Polymerase: 0.3 U.
   Cycles: **a.**- Pre-soak for 5 min at 94°C; 1.2 min at 94°C, 1 min at 66°C and 2 min at 70°C, for 19 cycles.
         b.- 1.3 min at 96°C, 1 min at 68°C and 5 min at 70°C for 30 cycles, followed by a chase for 10 min at 67°C, 5 min at 70°C for 2 cycles [5].

2.-Reaction Volume: 50 µl
   DNA: 1 µg
   Primers: 10 pmol 32-OR, 10 pmol TAG, 0.01 pmol 32-TAG-A, 0.02 pmol 32-TAG-T
   Buffer: 200 µM dNTPs, 1.5 mM $MgCl_2$, 50 mM KCl, 10 mM Tris-HCl and 0.1 % Triton X-100.
   AmplyTaq DNA Polymerase: 0.25 U.
   Cycles: Pre-soak for 5 min at 94°C; 1.3 min at 94°C, 1 min at 68°C, 5 min at 70°C for 25 cycles followed by a chase for 1 min at 67°C for 2 cycles [6].

378

Detection of amplified products

a.- The ladder of PCR products was separated by electrophoresis on 2% Nusieve 3:1 agarose gels (20 x 25 cm) in 1 x TBE buffer (44.5 mM Tris-borate, 1mM EDTA) until bromophenol blue dye had reached 1 cm from the end of the gel (at 150V for 6 hours). Hybridization with non-radioactive labelled MS32 probe was carried out according to the manufacturer's protocol (NICE™ probes, Cellmark Diagnostics). Luminography was carried out for 3 h at 37°C.

b.- Automated Fluorescent Detection
PCR products were electrophoresed through a 6% (w/v) polyacrylamide gel in TBE (100 mM Tris-borate, 1mM EDTA Na$_2$, pH 8.3), with 6 M urea. Electrophoresis was carried out at 1600 V, 45 W and 38 mA for 540 min.

RESULTS AND DISCUSSION

MVR-PCR distinguishes three types of repeat unit: a-type (detected in the A track), t-type (detected in the T track) and rare unamplified null or 0-type repeats. MVR-PCR of total genomic DNA produces a profile of both alleles superimposed to generate six different types for each "rung" of the ladder: code 1 (an intense band in the A track, aa), code 2 (an intese band in the T track, tt), code 3 (a faint band in the A track with a faint band in the T track, at), code 4 (a faint band in the A track, a0), code 5 (a faint band in the T track ,t0), code 6 (no band in either A or T track, 00).

When band intensity information is removed, quaternary codes (1, 2, 3 and 6) are generated and are still highly discriminatory [1]. In this study, quaternary codes were used for the interpretation of MVR patterns.

Fig. 1 shows the results of a MVR-PCR from different samples obtained after agarose gel electrophoresis and non-radioactive hybridization with a MS32 probe. The a- and t-type MVR products for each person were electrophoresed adjacent to each other . Lanes 1-6 correspond to the amplification of 3 samples with the conditions described in paragraph 1.a of Materials & Methods. Samples in lanes 9-14 were amplified with the conditions described in paragrahp 1.b of Materials & Methods. As can be seen, the best results were obtained with the former conditions (1.a); the patterns were more uniform in the different samples and more code positions could be identified. MVR-PCR patterns were reliable and 30 or more code positions could be detected.

Lane 1: 313113133121323311112111211213
Lane 2: 133111113121131323213111311111
Lane 3: 133222323333323333322321331233

Fig. 2 shows MVR-PCR patterns after non-radioactive hybridization of an agarose gel; in this case, the amplification condition number 2 of Materials & Methods were used. Patterns are clear and uniform, but the amount of DNA was 10 times more than in Fig.1.

Fig. 3 shows a fragment of a MVR-PCR pattern obtained after polyacrylamide electrophoresis and automatic detection. The 32-OR fluorescent-labelled primer was used.

We have also produced MVR patterns using TAG fluorescent labelled primer, and using 32-OR and TAG fluorescent-labelled primers, but the patterns were poorer than using the 32-OR labelled primer.

Ease of interpretation and of recording the high number of potential alleles makes automated detection using fluorescent tagged alleles ideal for MVRs.

MVR-PCR provides a new and powerful method for individual identification from human DNA. The choice of method (agarose gels and hybridization or automatic detection) will depend on the characteristics of the sample and the capabilities of the laboratory.

REFERENCES

1. Jeffreys, A.J., MacLeod, A., Tamaki, K., Neil, D.L and Monckton, K.G. (1991) *Nature*, 354, 204-209.
2. Wong, Z., Wilson, V., Patel, I., Povey, S. and Jeffreys, A.J. (1987) *Ann. Hum. Genet.*, 51, 269-288.
3. Jeffreys, A.J., Neumann, R. and Wilson, V. (1990) *Cell*, 60, 473-485.
4. Valverde, E., Cabrero, C., Cao, R., Rodríguez-Calvo, M.S., Díez, A., Barros, F., Alemany, J., and Carracedo, A., (1992) *Inter. Jour of Legal Medicine* 105, 251-256.
5. Tamaki, K., Monckton, D.G., MacLeod, A., Neil, D.L, Allen, M., and Jeffreys, A.J., (1992) *Hum. Mol. Genet.*, 6, 401-406.
6. Hinney, A., Luckenbach, C. Dür, C., Rodewyk, S., Pöltl, R., and Ritter, H. (1994) *Advances in Forensic Haemogenetics*, 5, 115-117.

This work was supported by grants form DGICYT (PB92-0371) and FISS (94/1053)

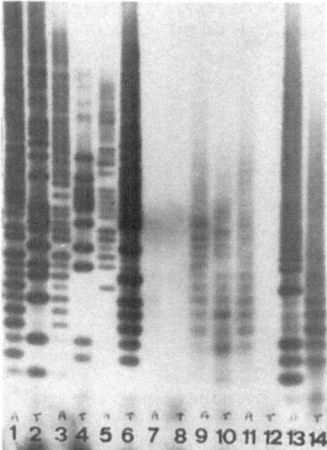

Fig. 1.- MVR-PCR from different samples obtained after agarose gel electrophoresis and non-radioactive hybridization with a MS32 probe. Lanes 1-6 correspond to the amplification of 3 samples with the conditions described in paragraph **1.a** of Materials & Methods. Samples in lanes 9-14 were amplified with the conditions described in paragraph **1.b** of Materials & Methods.

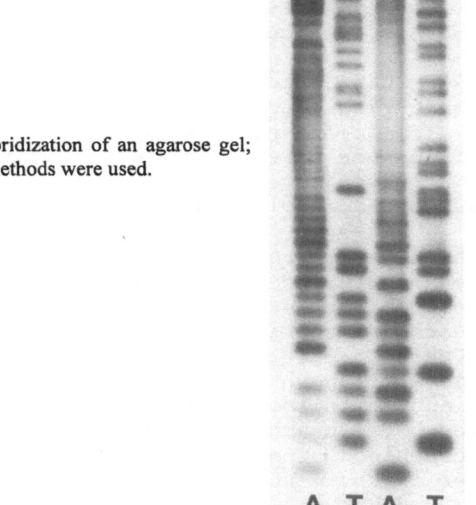

Fig. 2.- MVR-PCR patterns after non-radioactive hybridization of an agarose gel; the amplification condition number **2** of Materials & Methods were used.

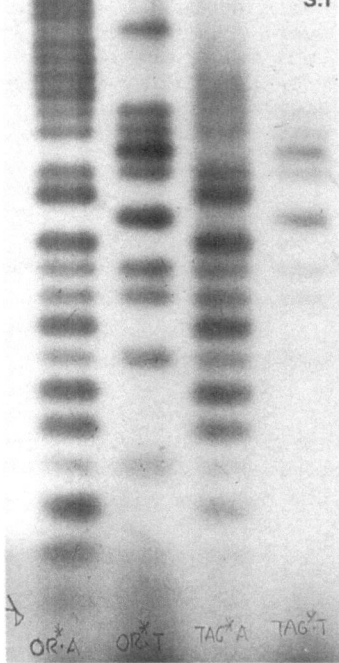

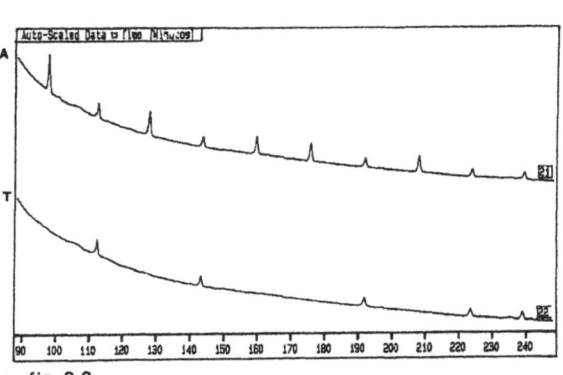

fig. 3.2

Fig. 3.- A fragment of a MVR-PCR pattern obtained after agarose gel electrophoresis and non radioactive hybridization with a MS32 probe (Fig. 3.1), and after polyacrylamide electrophoresis and automatic detection (Fig. 3.2).

Introduction of Two New Electrophoresis Gel Systems for Screening and
High Resolution Identification of STRs under Native Conditions

HP. Schickle, and R. Westermeier

ETC Elektrophorese-Technik, Bahnhofstr. 26,
D-72138 Kirchentellinsfurt, F.R.G.

INTRODUCTION

When polyacrylamide gels are employed for electrophoresis of DNA fragments, the mobilities are not only dependent on the fragment length,
but also on the base sequence. Single strand conformation polymorphism
SSCP and double strand conformation polymorphism DSCP (Barros et al.
1992) can be detected in these gels. However, when they are run under
denaturing conditions, in the presence of high concentrations of urea
or formamide and at elevated temperature (50 °C and higher), the mobilities are directly proportional to the sizes. This is the method for
DNA sequencing, because under these conditions it is no problem to
achieve a resolution of Δ 1 base.

Short tandem repeats (STR) analysis is performed in denaturing and in
non-denaturing gels. In both cases, the assignment of alleles with
well-defined (sequenced) allelic ladders of the respective STR locus,
which are run in the same gel, proved to be the most reliable method
(Puers et al. 1993; Möller et al. 1994). However, additionally to the
regular length variation types, in some STR loci there are sequence variants existing, which can only be identified by sequencing the fragments or running them on non-denaturing polyacrylamide gels. For
screening purposes and allel identification in the daily work, the latter is the method of choice.

Conventional native gels exhibit less resolution than denaturing gels.
In the following contribution, two new electrophoresis gel systems are
presented for screening and identification of STR alleles with adequate resolving power under native conditions.

MATERIAL AND METHODS

Samples: DNA was extracted according to Brinkmann et al. (1991); PCR[1]
amplification was performed according to Möller et al. (1994a,1994b).
4 — 7 µL of each sample were directly after the PCR reaction applied
to the electrophoresis gel.

---

[1] The PCR process is covered by U.S. patents 4,683,195 and 4,683,302
owned by Hoffman-La Roche Inc. Use of the PCR process requires a licen-
se.

<u>Gels and electrophoresis</u>: *Short gels*: CleanGel HyRes (25 × 11 cm, 430 μm thickness) for 48 samples of 7 μL, 9 cm separation distance; wicks: 5.0 × 25.3 cm special thick filter paper.
Long gels: CleanGels Long-Hyres (25 × 11 cm, 650 μm thickness) for 22 samples of 7 μL, 18 cm separation distance long direction, strips 1.8 × 11.7 cm special thick filter paper.

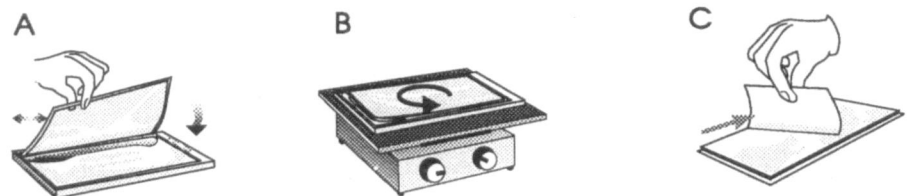

A   B   C

<u>Fig. 1:</u> Equilibration of the Cleangels HyRes in the gel buffer, and removing the excess buffer from the surface.

A GelPool is layed on a rotating platform; 50 mL equilibration solution is pipetted into the chamber. The gel-film — with the gel surface facing down — is layed into the rehydration buffer (fig. 1A) It is equilibrated for 1 hour 30 min (fig. 1B).After equilibration, excess buffer is removed with filter paper (fig. 1C).
The gels are laid on the center of the cooling plate of an horizontal electrophoresis apparatus. Special filter paper strips are soaked in the running buffer and applied over the gel edges. The gels are run at 15 °C; the short gel for 3 hours, the long gel for 3 hours 50 minutes. For *double loading*, the separation is interrupted after 1 hour 30 min, the wells are dried out with filter paper, and 48 more samples are loaded, electrophoresis is continued for another 1 hour 30 min.

<u>Silver staining:</u> The method according to Bassam et al. (1991) had to be modified for higher crosslinked gels: Fixing for 45 minutes with 15 % ethanol and 5 % acetic acid at 40 °C gives a lighter background; the times for all steps have to be doubled. The gels are preserved by impregnating them in 15 % glycerol and 15 % monoethylenglycol(v/v)for 30 minutes, drying at room temperature for 2 hours, then covering the surface with a polyester film, and storing the gels in a plastic bag.

RESULTS

CleanGel HyRes 48 S combined with the LongRun buffer system provide a resolution of down to less than $\Delta 4$ bp under native conditions (double strands) within a separation distance of 9 cm; the optimal separation is achieved between 50 and 200 bp. Up to 96 samples can be separated in one gel within a separation time of 3 hours by double loading (see fig. 2). With these gels, high sample throughput, good reproducibility, and high resolution for all these STR systems can be achieved.
Thus, these gels are very useful for screening purposes. Figure 3 shows a complete gel with single loaded samples of the HumVWA and Hum THO1systems.
The "high-resolution gel" has the same size, however it is run along the long distance for 4 hours. In this gel a resolution of down to $\Delta 1$ bp is obtained under non-denaturing conditions, even a complete separation down to the baseline between allel 9.3 and 10 of the HumTHO1 allelic ladder (see fig. 4).
The gels shown also demonstrate the usefulness of running well-defined allelic ladders parallelly to the samples for allel identification.

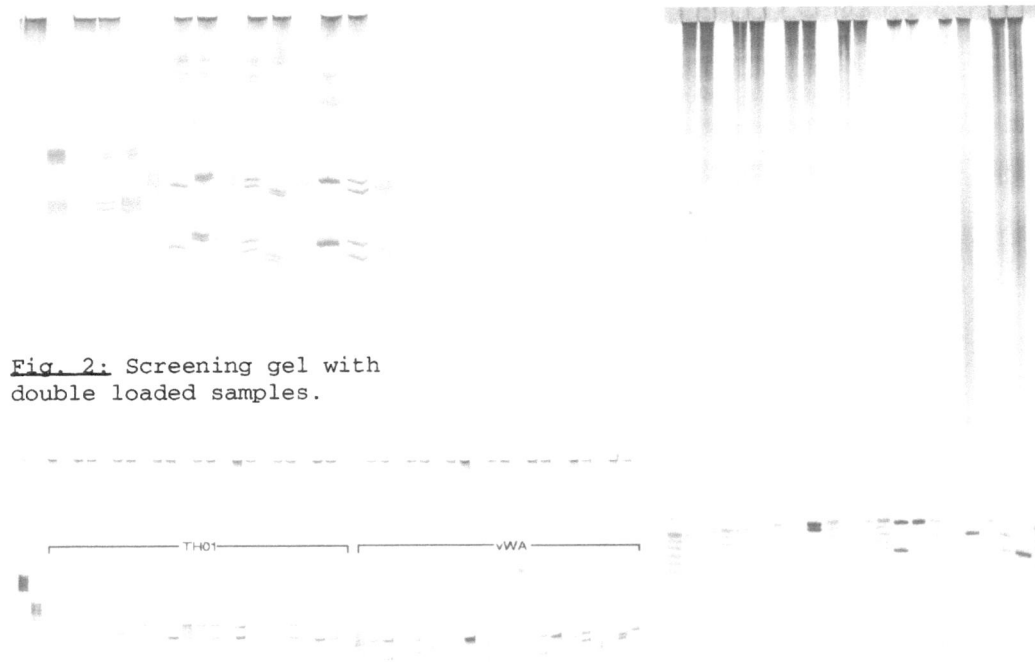

Fig. 2: Screening gel with
double loaded samples.

Fig. 3: Screening gel with separations of   Fig. 4: High resolution gel
VWA and TH01 samples.   with TH01 samples.

REFERENCES:

Barros F, Muños-Barús, Lareu MV, Rodriguez-Calvo MS, Carracedo A
(1994) Double- and single-strand conformation polymorphism analysis of
point mutations and and short tandem repeats. Electrophoresis 15:566-
571
Bassam BJ, Caetano-Annollés G, Gresshoff PM (1991) Fast and sensitive
silver staining of DNA in polyacrylamide gels. Anal Biochem 80:81-84
Brinkmann B, Rand S, Wiegand P (1991)Population and and family data of
RFLPs using selected single- and multi-locus systems. Int J Leg Med
104:81-86.
Möller A, Meyer E, Brinkmann B (1994a) Different types of structural
variation in STRs: HumFES/FPS, HumVWA and HumD21S11. Int J Leg Med
106:319-323
Möller A, Wiegand P, Grüschow C, Seuchter SA, Baur MP, Brinkmann B
(1994b) Population data and forensic efficiency values for the STR systems HumVWA, HumMBP and HumFABP. Int J Leg Med 106:183-189
Puers C, Hammond HA, Jin L, Caskey CT, Schumm JW (1993) Identification
of repeat sequence heterogeneity at the polymorphic short tandem repeat locus HUMTH01[AATG]n and reassignment of allels in population analysis by using a locus-specific allelic ladder. Am J Hum Genet
53:953-958.

Oligo-AP probes and chemiluminescence: sensitivity for stains analysis

A. Teyssier

Institut Universitaire de Médecine Légale, Geneva, Switzerland

SUMMARY

The sensitivity of the oligo-AP probes (alkaline phosphatase labelled oligonucleotides) MS1 and YNH 24 (Cellmark Diagnostic) is studied on stains with respect to white cell counts for blood stains, sperm count for semen stains, and for volumes varying from 1 to 5o ul.

INTRODUCTION

DNA profiling with single locus probes (SLP) detects VNTR loci of high variability and can provide highly discriminating identification.

The NICE (Non Isotopic Chemiluminescent Enhanced) probes system from Cellmark Diagnostic presents a high sensitivity and is rapid, reliable and safe. It also enables the analysis of small or mixed samples.

In the case of blood or sperm stains, the sensitivity of the analysis can also depend upon the white cell count and the sperm count respectively.

BLOOD: the normal white cell values vary between 4.000 and 10.000 cells per mm3, but in the presence of illness or ethnical differences, it can be lower.

SEMEN: the normal sperm count is higher than 20×10^6 sp/ml. In many cases it can be lower: alcohol, drugs, tobacco and medicaments abuses, infections, traumatisms, obstructions, hormonal deficits, illness, hereditary anomalies, exposition to toxics etc.

The aim of this study is to evaluate the sensitivity of the oligo-AP probes and chemiluminescence technique with respect to the volumes of stains and to determinate the influence of the cell count (white blood cells or sperms) on this sensitivity.

MATERIAL and METHOD

STAINS

BLOOD: blood samples were provided by the Central Laboratory of Haematology (Cantonal Hospital Geneva)
White cells counts: 2.000, 5.000 and 10.000 white cells/mm^3
Stains volumes: 5, 10, 20 and 50 ul.

SEMEN: semen samples were provided by the Andrology Laboratory (Geneva).
Sperm counts: $0,7 \times 10^6$, 10×10^6 and 40×10^6 sp/ml.
Stains volumes: 1, 2, 5 and 10 ul.

Stains were made on white cotton, air dried, stored at room temperature and analysed after 5 days and after one month.

EXTRACTION

Stain material was incubated overnight at 37°C in 600 ul extraction buffer (0.01M TrisHCl pH 7.6, 0.01M EDTA pH8, 0.1M NaCl, 2% SDS, and for semen samples, 0.04M DTT) plus 40ul each of proteinase K(20 mg/ml) .

DNA was extracted from samples by a conventional phenol-chloroform method (phenol / phenol-chloroform / chloroform-isoamyl alcohol) followed by ethanol precipitation. The pellet was dissolved in 20 ul Tris-EDTA buffer.

A second series of stains was incubated under the same conditions and then extracted with the QIAamp Blood extraction Kit (QIAGEN) following the manufacturers' instructions (including a 10 minutes at 70°C step before the elution).

QUANTIFICATION

Extracted DNA were quantified by hybridisation with the probe D17Z1 using the ACES Human DNA Quantitation System and the Convertible slot-blot apparatus from Gibco-BRL (with modifications).

1 ul of each sample was denatured in 500 ul alkaline solution, and then blotted onto a positively charged nylon membrane (Boehringer-Mannheim) using the slot-blot apparatus.

The membrane was neutralized and while it was still damp, the DNA was fixed by UV cross-linking (2 minutes at 302 nm). The membrane was then air dried during two hours (or alternatively baked for 15 minutes at 120°C) and hybridized to the D17Z1 probe (3 ul in 6 ml NICE hybridisation solution) following the same technique as for the NICE probes (see thereafter).

DIGESTION

All samples were subsequently digested with Hinf 1 (5u/ug) for 16 hours at 37°C and the quality of the digestion was checked by minigel electrophoresis.

SOUTHERN blot analysis

Fragments were separated by agarose gel (0,8% in TBE) electrophoresis (40V, 22 hours) and transferred onto a positively charged nylon membrane (Boehringer-Mannheim) by capillary blotting in 10x SSC for 16 hours. The DNA was then fixed by UV cross-linking (2 minutes at 302nm), followed by baking at 120°C for 15 minutes.

PREHYBRYDISATION

The membrane was placed in a plastic bag, for 30 minutes at 50°, in 30 ml hybridisation solution (0,5M Na_2HPO_4 pH 7,2, 0,1% SDS, and with 1% blocking reagent (Boehringer-Mannheim).

HYBRIDISATION

The blot was then probed with 10 ul MS1 in 16 ml hybridisation solution for 45 minutes at 50°C with agitation (or with 10 ul YNH24 after stripping). The blot was then washed twice for 10 minutes at 50°C in 0,01 M Na_2HPO_4pH 7,2, 0,1% SDS and twice for 5 minutes at room temperature in 1xSSC.

CHEMILUMINESCENT DETECTION

The membrane was equilibrated 5 minutes in a carbonate buffer (50 mM $NaHCO_3$ titrated to pH 9,6 with 50 mM Na_2CO_3, 1mM $MgCl_2$) and then incubated during 5 minutes in CSPD (Tropix) 1% in carbonate buffer. The membrane was then exposed for 6 hours and for 16 hours (or more) on X-ray film (Hyperfilm MP Amersham) at 37°C.

STRIPPING

Was performed in 0,1% SDS for 15 minutes at 80°C, followed by a rinse in 1xSSC.

SENSITIVITY

The sensitivity of this technique was tested using dilutions of K562 cell line DNA (1 ug to 7 ng).

RESULTS

SENSITIVITY

After an expoxure of 16 hours, it was possible to detect 7 ng of K562 DNA.

QUANTIFICATION

A better DNA yield is observed with the classical phenol-chloroform extraction. The DNA quantities obtained with the QIAamp Kit were lower; this was confirmed by subsequent Southern blot and hybridisation with MS1 (data not shown).

It is difficult to evalue with precision the exact quantities of DNA using the slot blot method. But by comparing these results and the results of the Southern blot to the theoretical quantities of DNA in each stain, we can evaluate that the phenol-chloroform extraction yields about 30% of the total DNA in semen stains, and 10 to 20% in blood stains. The quantities obtained by the QIAamp Kit are around 75% of those obtained by phenol-chloroform extraction.

HYBRIDISATION with MS1 and YNH24

(see DISCUSSION)

DISCUSSION

The oligo-AP probes (NICE probes Cellmark) and chemiluminescence detection are a powerful technique that enables the detection of a profile with DNA amounts down to about 7 ng.
The sensitivity of the test depends not only upon the volume of the stains but also upon the white cell count for blood stains and the sperm count for semen stains.
In the case of blood stains, it was possible to detect a profile with the probe MS1 for all 5 days old stains (2.000, 5.000, 10.000 wc/mm^3, and for all volumes (5, 10, 20, and 50 ul). For the one month old stains, the profile with the lower volumes (5 and 10 ul) and the lower white cells count (2.000 and 5.000 wc) was too faint to be useful.
In the case of semen stains, it was possible to detect a profile with MS1 for the 5 days old normospermic stains and for all of the volumes analysed (1, 2, 5, 10 ul). For the oligospermic stains ($10x10^6$ sp/ml) the profile was clear for the higher volumes (5 and 10 ul) after 16 h. of exposure. For the very low oligospermic stains ($0,7x10^6$ sp/ml) no profile was clear enough.
For the one month old stains, only the higher volumes (5 and 10 ul) of the normospermic stains are useful.
After stripping and reprobing with YNH24, and after an exposure of 16 hours, all profiles for all blood stains can be interpreted.

In conclusion, oligo-AP probes and chemiluminescence enable the analysis of small good quality stains with a high degree of sensitivity.With blood or semen stains of variable cell or sperm counts, and for various ages, there is good consistency of the results.

REFERENCES

Baird M, Galbreath L, Cunningham J, Lastella J and Balazs I (1994) Use of chemiluminescent labeled probes for forensic and paternity determinations.In: Poleski HF and Mayr WR (eds) Advances in Forensic Haemogenetics 5. Springer-Verlag Berlin Heidelberg, 130-132.

Baum HJ, Fitz-Charles H and McKee R (1990) A non isotopic DNA Detection System with the sensitivity of ^{32}P: applications for paternity and forensic identifications. In: Poleski HF and Mayr WR (eds) Advances in Forensic Haemogenetics 3. Springer-Verlag Berlin Heidelberg, 37-39.

Budowle B, Klevan L and Eisenberg AJ (1994) RFLP typing: a new highly polymorphic VNTR locus and chemiluminescent detection. In: Poleski HF and Mayr WR (eds) Advances in Forensic Haemogenetics 5. Springer-Verlag Berlin Heidelberg, 245-251.

Comey CT, Koons BW, Prestley KW, Smerick JB, Sobieralski CA, Stanley DM and Baechtel FS (1994) DNA extraction strategies for amplified fragment length polymorphism analysis. J Forensic Sciences 39(5):1254-1269.

Dimo-Simonin N, Brandt-Casadevall C and Gujer HR (1992) Chemiluminescent DNA probes: evaluation and usefulness in forensic cases. Forensic Sci Int 57: 119-127.

Neuweiler J, Venturini J, Balazs I, Kornher S, Hintz D, Victor J (1992) The use of a cheniluminescent detection system for paternity and forensic testing, verification of the reliability of the oligonucleotide-probes used for genetic analysis. In Poleski HF and Mayr WR (eds) Advances in forensic haemogenetics 4. Springer-Verlag Berlin Heidelberg, 132-136.

Walsh PS, Varlaro J and Reynolds R (1992) A rapid chemiluminescent method for quantitation of human DNA.Nucl Ac Res 20(19):5061-5065.

Waye JS, Michaud D, Bowen JH and Fourney RM (1991) Sensitive and specific quantification of human genomic deoxyribonucleic acid (DNA) in forensic science specimens: casework examples. J Forensic Sciences 36(4):1198-1203.

ACKNOWLEDGEMENTS

I am grateful to R.Coquoz, G.Lawrence and J.Teyssier for their helpful assistance.

AUTOMATION OF *IN SITU* DNA SAMPLE PREPARATION FOR PCR USING THE FTA™ DNA COLLECTION SYSTEM AND THE ROSYS LABORATORY WORKSTATION

P. Williams, S. Seim, L. Wiessner, P. Stover, H. Polesky, E. Heath and L. Hammer

Fitzco Inc., 5600 Pioneer Creek Drive, Maple Plain, MN 55359

INTRODUCTION

The development of dried blood stain technology has greatly facilitated the collection, transport, and isolation of DNA from blood samples. Blood stain cards are currently being used in clinical screening programs for Cystic Fibrosis (Audrezet and Costes, 1993; Raskin, 1992) and Human Immunodeficiency Virus (HIV) (Nyambi, 1994; Cassol, 1991). Within the forensic community, blood stain cards are being used to collect DNA samples from convicted felons and/or sex offenders, as military reference samples (Williams et al., 1994), and for parentage testing. Current blood stain technology, which is based on the use of filter paper cards, has provided a simple system for the collection, transport, and storage of whole blood DNA samples. However, the DNA must be extracted from the blood stain card prior to amplification and analysis.

The FTA DNA collection system provides a new and integrated approach to blood stain technology. The FTA system begins with a blood stain card which is chemically impregnated to kill any existing pathogens in the collected blood sample and to protect against bacterial and environmental degradation of the DNA.

Current protocols for PCR based analysis of DNA from blood stain cards require that the DNA be extracted from the card prior to amplification, or the protocols contain steps which liberate the DNA from the card as part of the amplification process (McCabe 1987; Carducci et al., 1992; Gregory et al., 1995; Harvey et al., 1995). Methods for the micro-extraction of DNA, particularly those using ion exchange resins or cards treated with chaotropic agents, are time consuming and/or labor intensive. These extraction methods are not amenable to automation since they require vortexing, centrifugation, and in some cases boiling of the sample. To overcome these obstacles to high through-put DNA sample preparation, a novel, integrated system for DNA collection and purification has been developed. This new method uses a single reagent, is fast, truly automatable, involves no manipulation of the sample during processing, and permits amplification of the sample directly from the card (Figure 1.). The Rosys laboratory workstation used in this method can also be used to set-up PCR reactions following sample preparation.

MATERIALS AND METHODS

FTA and S&S 903 blood stain cards were spotted with anticoagulated whole blood and allowed to dry. The blood stain cards were then placed in vapor barrier bags and stored at -20°C. For sample processing, a 2mm^2 or 3mm circular punch was taken from either the FTA or S&S card. Samples were then placed into tubes and/or 96-well plates as appropriate for the experiments.

In Situ Sample Preparation

In Situ sample preparation was performed using various reagent protocols: Phenol/Chloroform/Isoamyl Alcohol; Proteinase K; Wizard™ Genomic DNA Purification Kit (Promega Inc., Madison, WI); and One-Step DNA purification reagent (Fitzco, Inc. Maple Plain, MN) and the Rosys 3300 robotic workstation (Rosys, Wilmington, DE).

Phenol/Chloroform/Isoamyl Alcohol

200 µl of buffered phenol/chloroform/isoamyl alcohol was added to each well and the plate was incubated for 30 minutes at 50°C. The samples were then washed once with 200 µl of the phenol solution, and three times with 200 µl of isopropanol/0.1M potassium acetate (75%/25%, v/v, pH 7.8). Samples were then incubated for 20 minutes with 200 µl of isopropanol/0.01M magnesium acetate (75%/25%, v/v, pH 7.8) at room temperature, washed with 100 µl of pure isopropanol, and dried for 10 minutes at 50°C.

Proteinase K

200 µl of cell lysis buffer was added to each well and the plate was incubated for 15 minutes at 27°C. Incubation in fresh cell lysis buffer was repeated for a total of three times. Samples were then incubated for two hours at 60°C in 200 µl of Proteinase K digestion buffer (10 mM Tris-HCL, 400 mM NaCl, 2 mM Na₂EDTA, 1% SDS, Proteinase K (20 mg/ml) and 0.1% B-mercaptoethanol). Samples were then washed three times with 200 µl of isopropanol/0.1M potassium acetate, incubated for twenty minutes in 200 µl of isopropanol/0.01M magnesium acetate at RT (22°C), washed with 200 µl of pure isopropanol, and dried for 10 minutes at 50°C.

Wizard Genomic Purification Kit
200 µl of cell lysis buffer was added to each well and the plate was incubated for 15 minutes at 27°C. Incubation in fresh cell lysis buffer was repeated for a total of two times. Samples were then incubated for 15 minutes in 200 µl of nuclei lysis buffer at 27°C, washed with 200 µl of isopropanol/0.01M magnesium acetate, 200 µl of pure isopropanol, and dried for 10 minutes at 50°C.

One-Step™ DNA Purification
200 µl of One-Step reagent was added to each well and the plate was incubated for 15 minutes at 27°C. Incubation in fresh One-Step was repeated for a total of three times. Samples were then washed with 200 µl of pure isopropanol and dried for 10 minutes at 50°C.

Samples from this study were analyzed using the DQ-α typing system and/or a STR system (D1S80, F13B, or CSF1PO).

PCR amplification and analysis
All PCR reactions were carried out in a Perkin Elmer DNA Thermal Cycler (Foster City, CA). The reverse dot blot system, Amplitype HLA DQ-α (Perkin Elmer, Foster City, CA) was amplified and analyzed in accordance with the manufacturer's instructions. STR systems (F13B and CSF1PO) (Promega, Madison, WI) and D1S80 (Perkin Elmer, Foster City, CA) were amplified in accordance with the manufactures instructions. Amplification products were analyzed on yield gels, 2% agarose containing 0.125 µg/ml ethidium bromide. The amplification products were run at 80 volts for 45 minutes and photographed on a UV transilluminator.

Vertical gel electrophoresis was performed using 40 µm, 6% polyacrylamide denaturing gels. Samples, ladders, and sizing markers were loaded using STR 2X Loading solution (Promega, Madison, WI) and run at a constant current of 1.3watts/cm. Following electrophoresis, the samples were silver stained using the Promega DNA Silver Staining System.

Comparison of FTA and S&S 903 Blood Stain Cards
3 mm punches of spotted FTA and S&S 903 cards were placed into a 96-well plate and processed using One-Step DNA purification reagent. Following sample preparation, DNA was amplified using the D1S80 primer set according to manufacturer's guidelines. Amplification products were analyzed on a 2% agarose gel as described.

Contamination Study
Samples of spotted FTA cards were processed in two ways: First, samples of two individuals were placed in a 96-well plate, with every fourth well containing both of the samples. Following processing with One-Step DNA reagent, the samples were amplified individually using the Amplitype DQ-α typing system. Second, six samples each from two individuals were placed in the same tube (total of twelve punches), processed using One-Step DNA reagent and amplified individually using the D1S80 typing system.

SUMMARY
1. An evaluation of various reagent systems for the automated pre-amplification sample preparation of DNA from FTA blood stain cards was performed. Fitzpak One-Step™ DNA purification reagent proved to be more effective than phenol/chloroform/isoamyl alcohol or the Wizard reagent system. Amplification of DNA following sample preparation with One-Step resulted in robust amplification products and typable results. the proteinase K protocol used in this study was not effective and resulted in poor amplification signal.

2. An evaluation of amplification from FTA and S&S 903 blood stain cards was performed. Following sample preparation with One-Step DNA purification reagent, the FTA blood stain card proved to be a superior matrix for the direct amplification of DNA and routinely produced typable results.

3. Cross-contamination studies indicate that there is no migration of the DNA during any of the sample preparation protocols. The FTA matrix tightly binds the DNA while releasing PCR inhibitors and cellular debris.

TRADITIONAL DNA EXTRACTION

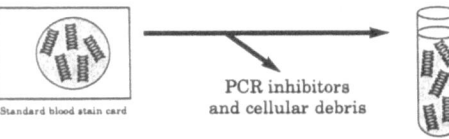

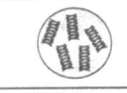

PCR inhibitors
and cellular debris

Standard blood stain card

IN SITU DNA PURIFICATION

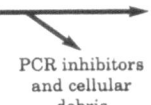

FTA blood stain card

PCR inhibitors
and cellular
debris

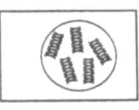

Figure 1. Schematic diagram of traditional DNA extractions from blood stain cards and in situ DNA purification using the FTA blood stain card. In traditional extraction procedures, which can include vortexing, centrifugation, and boiling, the DNA is removed from the card, purified from PCR inhibitors, and then concentrated in a tube. The FTA DNA system removes PCR inhibitors from the card and leaves the purified DNA on the card. This DNA is now ready for PCR amplification.

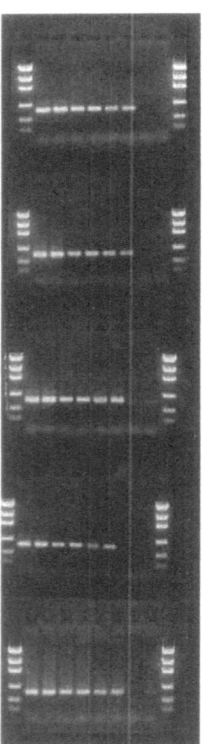

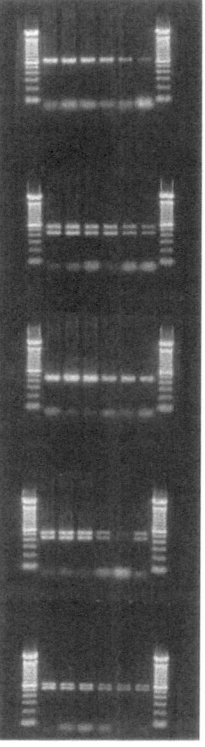

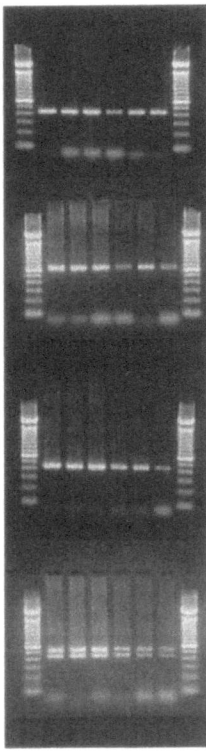

Figure 2. Comparison of the four DNA purification methods. Samples of the FTA bloodstain cards were purified using one of the four reagent systems: phenol/chloroform/isoamyl alcohol, poteinase K, Wizard genomic DNA reagents, or One-Step. DNA samples were amplified using the STR CSF1PO amplification system and analyzed on 2% agarose yield gels. Lanes 2-3 = One-Step, Lanes 4-5 = Phenol, Lanes 6-7 = Wizard, Lanes 8-9 = Proteinase K. Lanes 1 and 10 = Markers.

Figure 3. Comparison of amplification from FTA and S&S 903 blood stain cards. Whole blood samples from 9 individuals were spotted onto both FTA and S&S 903 blood stain cards. Following purification of the DNA with One-Step DNA reagent, the samples were amplified using the D1S80 amplification system. Following amplification, the samples were analyzed using 2% agarose yield gels. Lanes 1 & 8 = 100 Bp ladder; Lanes 2-4 = FTA; Lanes 5-7 = S&S903

4. The Rosys Workstation is an integral part of the FTA DNA system and can be programmed to perform not only DNA sample preparation, but PCR set-up in the 96-well plate format or standard reaction tube format.

5. The FTA DNA system is a safe, single reagent, automated procedure which begins with sample collection and finishes with high quality amplification products. This system is designed for high-throughput processing of DNA, and can provide hundreds of samples per day.

REFERENCES

1. Audrezet, M. P., Costes, B. (1993). Screening for Cystic Fibrosis in Dried Blood of Newborns. Mol. Cell Probes. 7:497-502

2. Cassol, S. (1991). Use of Dried Blood Spot Specimens in the Detection of Human Immunodeficiency Virus Type I by the Polymerase Chain Reaction. J. Clinical Microbiology. 29: 661-667

3. Raskin, S. (1992). Cystic Fibrosis Genotyping by Direct PCR Analysis of Guthrie Blood Spots. PCR Methods and Applications. 2: 154-156.

4. Nyambi, P., Fransen, K., De Beenhouwer, H., Ephantus, N., Temmerman, M., Ndinya-Achola, J., Piot, P., and van der Groen, G. (1994). Detection of Human Immunodeficiency Virus type 1 (HIV-1) in Heel Prick Blood on Filter Paper from Children Born to HIV-1-Seropositive Mothers. J. of Clin. Microbiol. Nov. p. 2858-2860.

5. Williams, P., Marino, M., Del Rio, S., Turner, K., Steighner, B., Burgoyne, L., and Turner, J. (1994). Evaluation of a Novel Matrix for the Analysis of DNA and its Application to Automated DNA sample processing. Proceedings from Fifth International Symposium on Human Identification, Promega Corp.

6. McCabe, E., and Haung, S. (1987). DNA Microextration From Dried Blood Spots in Filter Paper Blotters: Potenial Applications to Newborn Screening. Human Genetics 75: 213-216.

7. Carducci, C., Ellul, E., Antonozzii, I., and Pontecorvi, A. (1992). DNA Elution and Amplification by Polymerase Chain Reaction from Dried Blood Spots. Biotechniques 13:735-737.

8. Gregory, C., Myal, Y., and Shiu, R. (1995). Rapid Genotyping of Transgenic Mice Using Dried Blood Spots from Guthrie Cards for PCR Analysis. Biotechniques Vol. 18, No.5 759-760.

9. Harvey, M., King, T., Burghoff, R. (1995). Impregnated 903 Blood Collection Paper: A Tool for DNA Prepared From Dried Blood Spots for PCR Amplification. Presented at: American Association of Clinical Chemistry, 1995, Anehiem, CA.

STR TYPING WITHOUT DNA EXTRACTION USING AN INFRARED-BASED NON-RADIOACTIVE AUTOMATED DNA SEQUENCER

R.Roy, Ph.D.*, D.L. Steffens, Ph.D.**, B.O. Gartside**, G.Y. Jang, Ph.D.** and J.A. Brumbaugh, Ph.D.**

*Nebraska State Patrol, Lincoln, NE 68502 USA.
** LI-COR, inc., Lincoln, NE 69504 USA.

ABSTRACT: A LI-COR Model 4000 automated DNA sequencer using high sensitivity infrared (IR) fluorescence technology was used to detect STR allele patterns from bloodstains and simulated forensic samples using *Tth* polymerase. Two different amplification strategies were used for labeling. Multiplexing of three primer pairs in a single PCR amplification was accomplished using *Taq* polymerase. Typing of STR alleles was also achieved using a *GenePrint*™ STR System (Promega) for various forensic-like specimens. Genotyping of the O allele of the human ABO blood group locus as well as the gender differentiating amelogenin locus was also performed using both strategies. This system combines IR fluorescence chemistry and laser technology thus eliminating the need for radioactivity and the gel handling required with some methodologies. STR alleles are displayed as autoradiogram-like images during the run and can be computer analyzed.

MATERIALS AND METHODS: The procedure for collection, amplification and gel electrophoresis of samples is according to the protocol described by Roy et al (1995). Bloodstains were collected from volunteer donors on two types of sterilized fabrics: 100% cotton and a cotton + polyester mixture. Approximately 1 mm of bloodstained thread was placed in an autoclaved reaction tube and directly amplified using *Tth* polymerase and a high temperature incubation to extract DNA from blood cells. To validate the results from bloodstain analysis, STR alleles were also amplified using Chelex extracted DNA from bloodstains, saliva, hair roots, semen, vaginal fluid and other simulated forensic samples. Electrophoresis and detection were performed using a LI-COR Model 4000 Automated DNA Sequencer. DNA for multiplex reactions was purified using a Genomix blood DNA extraction kit from Washington Biotechnology (Bethesda, MD).

Two strategies for automated IR fluorescence detection of PCR products from polymorphic repeat regions were utilized: 1.) One of the PCR primers had a 19 base extension at its 5' end with the sequence 5'-CACGACGTTGTAAAACGAC-3'. This sequence is identical to an IR-labeled universal M13 Forward (-29) primer which is included in the amplification reaction. During PCR the tailed primer generates a complementary sequence to the M13 primer which is subsequently utilized for priming in the amplification reaction thereby generating IR-labeled PCR products. 2.) A limited quantity of an IR-labeled deoxynucleotide (dATP) was included in the amplification reaction. During DNA synthesis the polymerase occasionally incorporates a labeled molecule into the growing DNA chain thus producing a PCR product internally labeled with IR fluorophore.

STR loci analyzed included the following: ACTBP2, D2S436, D18S535, D20S470 & HUMTHO1. Primers for the amelogenin locus were derived from sequence described by Sullivan et al (1993) and synthesized by Genosys (The Woodlands, TX). For the internal labeling strategy, ameloginin amplification primers were also obtained from a *GenePrint*™ STR System (Promega Corporation; Madison, WI). Multiplex primers for CSF1PO, TPOX and THO1 loci were also obtained from *GenePrint*™ STR Multiplex Kit. Primers for the O allele of the ABO locus were obtained from Genosys using the sequence described by Crouse and Vincek (1995). Molecular weight markers primarily utilized consisted of one lane of a standard sequencing reaction.

CONCLUSIONS: STR loci were detected directly from dried bloodstained fabric using *Tth* polymerase without time consuming DNA extraction and purification. Multiplexing with either three tailed primers or the *GenePrint*™ Multiplex STR System with internal labeling using *Taq*

391

polymerase can be achieved in one reaction tube using extracted DNA. Automated determination of STR polymorphisms, gender and the O allele can be performed with this methodology. The actual raw data is visualized during gel electrophoresis and stored automatically into a database.

REFERENCES:
1. Crouse C, Vincek V (1995) Identification of ABO alleles on forensic-type specimens using rapid-ABO genotyping. Biotechniques 18: 478-483.
2. Roy R, Steffens DL, Gartside B, Jang GY, Brumbaugh JA (submitted for publication) Producing STR locus patterns from bloodstains and other forensic samples using an infrared fluorescent automated DNA sequencer. Journal of Forensic Sciences.
3. Sullivan KM, Armando M, Kimpton CP, Gill P (1993) A rapid and quantitative DNA sex test: fluorescence-based PCR analysis of X-Y homologous gene amelogenin. Biotechn 15: 636-639.

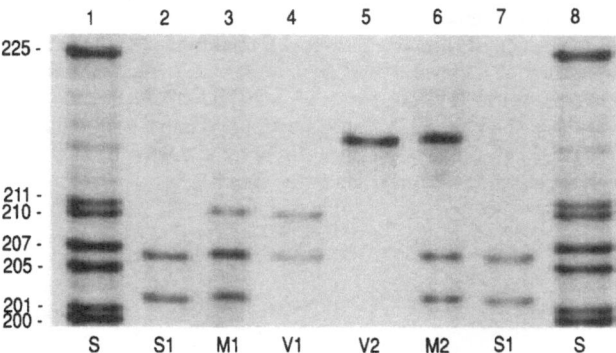

Figure 1. Allelic profiles for the HUMTHO1 locus from individual and mixed bloodstains directly amplified using *Tth* polymerase and tailed primer. Lanes 2 and 7 represent bloodstains from a suspect (S1) amplified from 100% cotton and cotton-polyester fabric, respectively. Lanes 4 and 5 represent bloodstains collected on 100% cotton from two victims (V1 and V2, respectively). Lane 3 (M1) represents a mixture of blood from S1 (bloodstains on 100% cotton) and V1. Lane 6 (M2) represents a mixture of blood from V2 and S1 (bloodstain on cotton-polyester fabric). Lanes 1 and 8 are molecular weight size standards (S) shown to the left of the image (in base pairs).

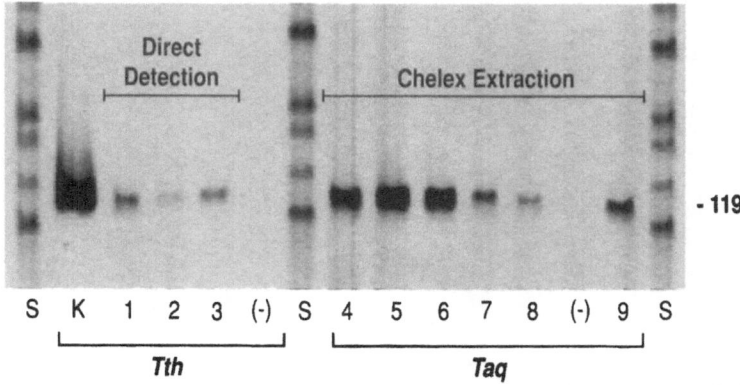

Figure 2. Amplification of O alleles (119 base pairs) from AO, BO and OO genotype individuals using tailed O primer and either *Tth* or *Taq* polymerase. K = K562 DNA (Promega). Lanes 1, 2 & 3 are direct detection using a high temperature incubation from bloodstained thread (100% cotton) from O, A & B phenotypic individuals, respectively. Lanes 4, 5 & 6 are Chelex extracted DNA from bloodstained thread (100% cotton) from three O individuals. Lanes 7 & 8 are Chelex extracted DNA from bloodstained cotton-polyester from A and B phenotypes, respectively. (-) = negative control. S = Molecular weight size standard.

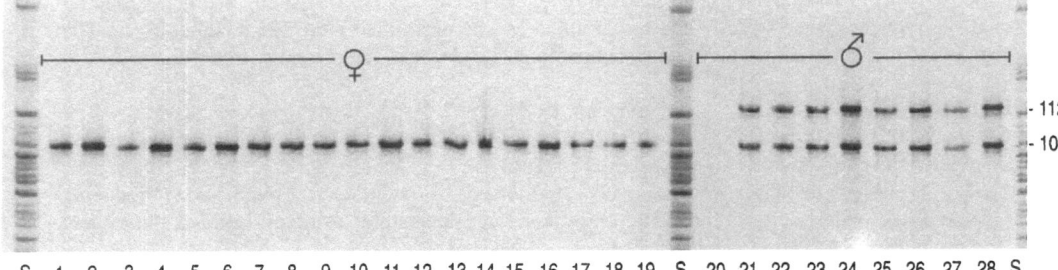

Figure 3. Amplification of extracted DNA from simulated forensic samples at the amelogenin locus using *Taq* polymerase and internal label. Blood (1), saliva (2), vaginal swab (3), vaginal wipe (4), hair (5), toe nail (6), earring (7), cigarette butt (8), toothbrush (9), head band (10), underarm (11), shed skin (12), earring (13), cigarette butt (14), rain soaked cigarette butt (15), vaginal swab (16&17), eyebrow (18) and saliva (19) samples from a female volunteer were analyzed. Negative control (20). Blood (21), semen-cloth (22), semen-paper (23), saliva (24), toe nail (25), toothbrush (26), cigarette butt (27) and hair (28) samples were from a male volunteer. S = Molecular weight size standard. Allele sizes are shown on the right of the figure.

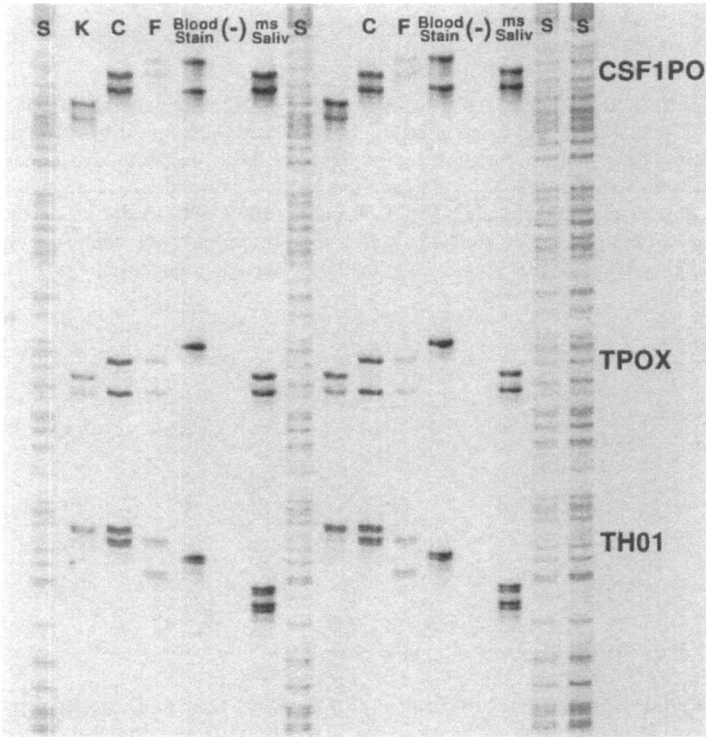

Figure 4. Detection of three polymorphic STR loci using purified DNA from a father (F) and child (C); and using Chelex extracted DNA from bloodstains and saliva using the *GenePrint*™ STR Multiplex System and internal label. K = K562, (-) = Negative Control, ms Saliv = saliva from an individual, S = Molecular weight size standard. STR loci are designated on the right of the image.

Evaluation of Hereditary Distance by Restriction Landmark Genomic Scanning (RLGS)

T. Sawaguchi, X. Wang, Y. Okazaki*, S. Nakamura,
O. Ohue, Y. Hayashizaki*, A. Sawaguchi

Dept. of Legal Medicine, Tokyo Women's Medical College, Tokyo JAPAN
* Genome Science Laboratory, Tsukuba Life Science Center, The Institute of
Physical and Chemical Research (RIKEN) Tsukuba JAPAN

The characteristics of RLGS

" Genome scanning" is defined as a high-speed survey for the simultaneous detection of signals from many loci throughout a genome by one process. By southern hybridization or polymerase chain reaction (PCR) only one locus can be detected in one process. By the fingerprint method or Alu-L1-PCR, some loci can be detected in one process but scanning is insufficient. To make up for this shortage in genome scanning, the restriction landmark genome scanning (RLGS) method has been developed. RLGS employs direct-end labeling of the genome digested with a restriction enzyme which high resolution two-dimensional electrophoresis is then carried out. In this method there is no hybridization procedure. After the first enzyme digestion (this will be used as a landmark), labeling is achieved. After the initial labeling, the second digestion is brought about by a second enzyme and then one-dimensional electrophoresis by agarose gel is carried out. After the one-dimensional electrophoresis, a third digestion is brought about by a third restriction enzyme and then two-dimensional electrophoresis by polyacrylamide gel is carried out. RLGS has the following advantages for genome scanning. (a) It has a speed-scanning ability. (b) The scanning field can be extended by the use of different kinds of landmarks in an additional series of electrophoreses. (c)This method can be applied to any organism. (d)The intensity of a spot reflects the copy number of the restriction landmark. Haploid and diploid genomic DNAs can be distinguished. (e)Using a methylation-sensitive enzyme, the methylated state of genomic DNA can be screened. (f)After finding spots of interest, the DNA fragments of those spots can be cloned from punched out gel. Figure 1 shows the principles and the entire procedure of the RLGS method.

Protocol

The Procedure of the RLGS method consists of 8 steps.
(i)Blocking: This is done to reduce the background generated by the incorporation of radioactivity in the nonspecifically damaged sites. The sample DNA was treated with 10 units of E. coli DNA polymerase I in the presence of 0.33mM dGTPaS, 0.33mM[α-^{32}P] dCTP and 0.33mM [α-^{32}P] dGTP.
(ii)Landmark cleavage by restriction enzyme A: This step is for cleavage of genomic DNA at the restriction landmarks. The blocked DNA is digested by 20 units of restriction enzyme A, whose site is used as a restriction landmark.
(iii)Labeling: The labeling method depends on the shape of the end of the restriction fragment. For a 5' protruding end, the reaction of [α-^{32}P] deoxy-nucleotide with E.coli DNA polymerase I is used. For a 3' protruding end or blunt end, the reaction of [α-^{32}P] dideoxy-nucleotide with deoxynucleotidyl terminal transferase is used.
(iv)Fragmentation of labeled DNA with restriction enzyme B: The samples were incubated with 20 units of restriction enzyme B, ddGTP, ddCTP and MgC1$_2$ at 37°C for 60 minutes.
(v)First fractionation by agarose gel electrophoresis: DNA restriction fragments were fractionated in one dimension by 1% agarose gel electrophoresis.

(vi)Fragmentation of labeled DNA with restriction enzyme C: A strip of the one-dimensional gel was treated with 1500 units of restriction enzyme C.

(vii)Second fractionation by polyacrylamide gel: The second fractionation was done in a two-dimensional 6% polyacrylamide gel electrophoresis after connection the agarose strip to the two-dimensional polyacrylamide gel.

(viii)Autoradiography: The final gel samples were dried and auto-radiographed.

Purpose

Polymorphism shows the diversity of form and characteristics within a species. Genetic polymorphisms are not often recognized visually. Polymorphism is the most important basis of variety in living organisms. The RLGS method is suitable for screening the physical state of genomic states at high speed. It has the best detection ability of all genome scanning methods. It can be effectively applied to the detection of DNA polymorphisms in mammals. In this report we have tried to evaluate the hereditary distance of the intersubspieces by the RLGS method.

Materials and Methods

Mice was examined for the calculation the DNA polymorphic rates as a means of evaluating the intraspieces hereditary distances: mice (B6, D2, M.spretus, M.m. domestics and M.m.molossinus). All tissues came from the liver and were immediately frozen in liquid nitrogen and genomic DNA extraction was performed.

The combination of three restriction enzymes are NotI, PvuII and PstI. The extracted DNA was treated using this combination of three restriction enzymes following the above-mentioned protocol of the RLGS method. After autoradiography, the polymorphic ratios were calculated by a comparison of two strains. The sum of the number of specific polymorphic spots and non-specific polymorphic spots of one strain was divided by the total number of countable polymorphic & non-polymorphic spots.

Results

The results are shown in Table 1 and Figure 1. In addition, The ratio of polymorphic spots between B6 and D2 was 13.4% and that between B6 and M.spretus was 50.9%. As you can see, the polymorphic rate between laboratory mouse B6 and wild mouse M. spretus was higher than that between laboratatory mice B6 and D2. Table 1 and Figure 1 show the same result of the intersubspieces. From this result, the polymorphic rate determined by the RLGS method seems to correlate with hereditary distance.

Reference

1. Hatada, I., Hayashizaki, Y. Hirotsune, S. et al: A Genomic Scanning Method of Higher Organisms Using restriction Sites as landmarks. Proc. natl. Acad. Sci. USA 88,9523-9527 (1991).

2. Hayashizaki, S.,Y., Hirotsune, S., Okazaki, Y. et al.: Restriction Landmark Genomic Scanning Method and Its Various Applications. Electrophoresis, 14, 251-258 (1993)

3. Hirotsune, S., Hatada, I., Komatsubara, H. et al.: New Approach for Detection of Amplification in Cancer DNA Using Restriction Landmark Genomic Scanning. Cancer Res. 52, 3642-3647 (1992).

4. Kawai, J., Hirotsune, S.,Hirose, K., et al.: Methylation profiles of genomic DNA of mouse developmental brain detected by restrction landmark genomic scanning (RLGS) Method. Nucl. Acid. Res. 21, 5604-5608 (1993).

5. Hayashizaki, Y., Shibata, H., Hirotsune, S. et al.: Identification of an imprinted U2af binding protein related sequence on mouse chromosome 11 using the RLGS

method. Nature Genetics. 6, 33-40 (1994).

6. Sawaguchi, T., Wang, X., Sawaguchi, A. et al.: Application of Restriction Landmark genomic Scanning (RLGS) to the detection of DNA polymorphism. DNA Polymorphism. 3, 79-83 (1995).
7. Hayashizaki, Y., Swaguchi, T., Sawaguchi, A. et al.: A new strategic plan for the detection of DNA polymorphisms: the Restriction Landmark Genomic Scanning (RLGS) method. DNA Polymorphism. 3, 10-15 (1995).

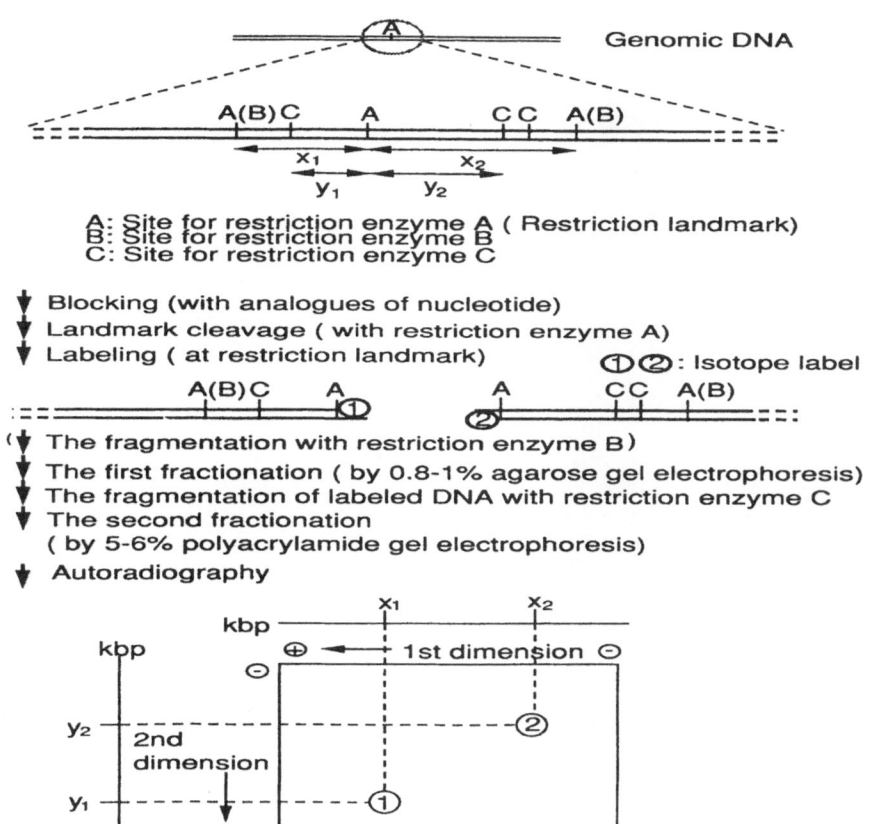

Figure1. Principle of RLGS method

Table 1. RLGS polymorphism among three Mus species

	M. m. domestics	M. m. molossinus	M. spretus
Mus musculus domestics (C3H/HeN)	-	33%	56%
Mus musculus molossinus	-	-	40%
Mus spretus	-	-	-

7 Conventional Markers

The PI System: Genetic Variation, Forensic Application and Clinical
Aspects

S. Weidinger

Medizinisch-Immunologische Laboratorien, Mittererstr. 3, D-80336 München,
Germany

INTRODUCTION

In the past two decades few polymorphic plasma proteins have attracted more
interest among scientists than the PI (protease inhibitor) system of alpha-
1-antitrypsin (α1AT). There are several reasons for this interest: (1) The
PI system was, from the beginning, associated with disease; (2) With the
development of high-resolution techniques, it was shown that the PI system
comprises a large number of codominant alleles, and (3) The findings of
linkage between the PI system and the Gm system of human IgG has contributed
to chromosome mapping.

On the basis of protein sequence homology, α1AT has been recognized as one
member of the large serine protease inhibitor (serpin) gene family (Hunt and
Dayhoff 1980). Although called antitrypsin, its prime role is an inhibitor
of neutrophil leucocyte elastase, and for this reason it is alternatively
called alpha-1-protease inhibitor. The PI locus has been mapped to chromosome 14q32.1, near the immunoglobulin heavy chain gene cluster (Rabin et al.
1986; Purrello et al. 1987). The α1AT gene is composed of seven exons
spanning 12.2 kb genomic DNA (Long et al. 1984). α1AT is a highly polymorphic
glycoprotein consisting of a single polypeptide chain of 394 amino acids
and a carbohydrate content of 12% (Carrell et al. 1982). The 52-kD protein
is synthesized primarily in hepatocytes. There are three carbohydrate
attachment sites at asparagine residues 46, 83 and 247, which result in
heterogeneous molecular species. For classification of PI phenotypes isoelectric focusing (IEF) is a widely used technique (Weidinger 1992).

GENETIC VARIATION

Alpha-1-antitrypsin shows a considerable amount of genetic variability. To
date, approximately 100 variants have been identified in the PI system by
either IEF of serum and/ or sequence analysis (Faber et al. 1994). The
variants can be conveniently categorized into four groups: normal, deficient,
null, and dysfunctional. Most of the PI alleles (including the M family) are
associated with normal concentrations of α1AT. PI M, which can be divided
into 10 subtypes (M1, M1M2, M2, M1M3, M2M3, M3, M1M4, M2M4, M3M4, and M4)
by high resolving IEF, is the most common phenotype in all populations
(frequency >90%). The nomenclature is very complex and is based on the
focusing position of the α1AT in IEF gels (Cox et al. 1980). The anodal
variants are designated from B to L, and variants cathodal to M are designated
from N to Z. In contrast to the normal alleles a number of deficiency alleles
(including null alleles and deficient M alleles) in the PI system is associated with reduced (or no detectable) serum α1AT levels. All rare alleles
are also named with the birthplace of the earliest known carrier. Figure 1
shows the band patterns of several normal and deficient PI phenotypes which
were obtained by IEF and immunoprinting.

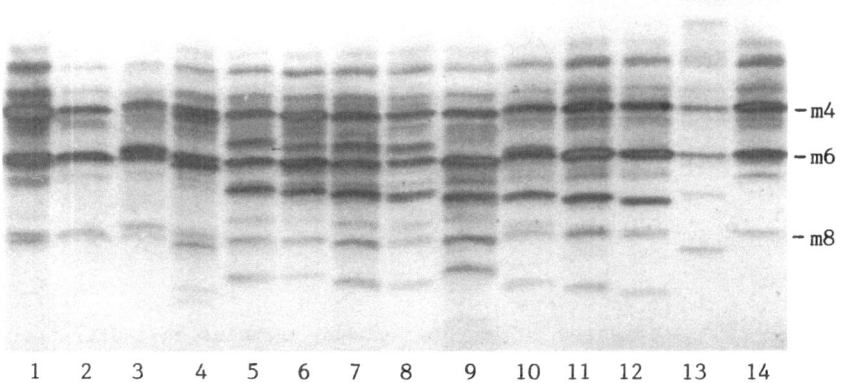

Figure 1. Banding patterns of several normal and deficient PI phenotypes obtained from sera by high-resolution IEF in a narrow pH gradient (pH range 4.2–4.9), followed by immunoprinting with a monospecific α1AT-antiserum. The isoprotein zones m4, m6, and m8 are indicated. Anode at the top. Lanes: (1) M1M2; (2) M3riedenburg-QOriedenburg; (3) M3-Lfrankfurt; (4) M2-Loffenbach; (5) M1-P; (6) M1-Pduarte; (7) M3-Psaint albans; (8) M1-Pdonauwoerth; (9) M3-Smunich; (10) M1-V; (11) M1-S; (12) M1-T; (13) M1-Z; (14) M1-Mpalermo.

Distribution of the PI alleles has now been determined in many populations (Table 1). The frequency of PI*M1 is the highest in all populations studied. M2 and M3 are the next most frequent. The additional subtype allele PI*M4 has been described in several ethnic groups, at a frequency of 0.01 to 0.05. The PI*S allele is rare or absent in black and oriental populations, highest in Spain and Portugal, next most frequent in other parts of Europe. PI*Z, which is the most common deficiency allele, seems to be absent in oriental and black populations.

Table 1. PI allele frequencies in selected populations

Population origin	No. tested	PI alleles M1	M2	M3	M4	S	Z	Other
Denmark	909	0.728	0.136	0.082	–	0.022	0.023	0.009
Netherlands	357	0.679	0.147	0.081	0.047	0.029	0.013	0.004
Germany	752	0.689	0.165	0.090	0.018	0.017	0.013	0.008
France	1030	0.667	0.143	0.101	–	0.063	0.018	0.008
Italy	965	0.661	0.162	0.107	–	0.024	0.041	0.005
Spain	340	0.596	0.156	0.112	0.013	0.112	0.007	0.004
U.S.(white)	904	0.724	0.137	0.095	–	0.023	0.014	0.007
U.S.(black)	549	0.981	–	–	–	0.015	0.004	–
Japan	746	0.785	0.153	0.062	–	–	–	–
China	1010	0.709	0.209	0.070	–	–	–	0.012

In addition to the extensive variation found in the protein by electrophoretic methods, further variation is found in the DNA sequence, as recognized by restriction enzymes, producing RFLP's (restriction fragment length polymorphism). Several genomic sequences have been obtained by using the probes 4.6 and 6.5. The allele frequencies for DNA polymorphisms are shown in Table 2.

Table 2. Allele frequencies for DNA polymorphisms

Probe	Restriction enzyme	Alleles (kb)	Allele frequency*			No. of haplotypes	PIC
-------	--------------------	--------------	+	−	0	------	-----
4.6	Sst I	1.8, 1.9	0.69	0.31	−	2	0.33
	Msp I	0.95, 0.98	0.47	0.53	−	2	0.38
	Ava II	0.9, 1.1	0.65	0.35	−	2	0.35
6.5	Mae III	2.3, 2.5	0.71	0.29	−		
	Mae III(3')	0.5, 0.7	0.65	0.35	−	4	0.33
	Ava II(5/7)	0.48, 0.68	0.22	0.78	−	4	0.44
	Ava II(1/4)(3')	0.72, 2.7	0.29	0.71	−		
	Taq I	1.4, 2.0	0.97	0.03	−		
	Taq I(3')	4.8, 6.7, 0	0.53	0.26	0.21	4	0.58
	Eco RI(3')	5.7, 8.6	0.23	0.77	−	2	0.29

*) + = Presence of restriction site; − = absence of site; 0 = no fragment.
PIC = Polymorphism information content.

The probe 4.6 includes the first exon of α1AT, and the probe 6.5 includes the coding region and some of the 3' flanking region (Kidd et al. 1983). Three polymorphisms have been described with probe 4.6, using the restriction enzymes Sst I, Msp I, and Ava II. Seven polymorphisms were detected with probe 6.5. Ava II detects polymorphisms both in the α1AT gene and the homologous sequence and was the first enzyme shown to produce a unique DNA haplotype for PI ZZ individuals (Cox et al. 1985).

FORENSIC APPLICATION

The considerable number of alleles, together with the highly reproducible techniques available for phenotyping and genotyping, make the PI system

Table 3. Comparison of highly polymorphic serum markers

System	Chromosomal assignment	Method	No. of alleles*	Silent alleles	Exclusion chance (%)
HP	16q	PAGIF	4 (> 20)	+	30.6
GC	4q	PAGIF/IP	3 (>120)	+	29.8
PI	14q	PAGIF	6 (> 90)	+	27.1
TF	3q	PAGIF	3 (> 30)	+	19.5
ORM1	9q	PAGIF/IP	3 (> 30)	+	21.0
AHSG	3q	PAGIF/IP	2 (> 30)	?	18.5
PLG	6q	AGIF/IF	2 (> 20)	+	19.8
F13B	1q	AGIF/IF	3 (> 20)	?	22.7

Abbreviations: HP = haptoglobin; GC = group-specific component; PI = protease inhibitor; TF = transferrin; ORM = orosomucoid; AHSG = alpha2-HS-glycoprotein; PLG = plasminogen; F13B = B subunit of coagulation factor XIII.
PAGIF = polyacrylamide gel isoelectric focusing; AGIF = agarose gel isoelectric focusing; IF = immunofixation; IP = immunoprinting.
*) No. of rare alleles in parenthesis.

valuable for forensic haemogenetics, especially paternity testing. In fact, a so-called classical exclusion constellation at the PI locus is considered to disprove paternity. The single exclusion chance in paternity cases is 27.1%, indicating that the protease inhibitor is a very powerful marker in forensic individualization and paternity testing. Table 3 shows a comparison of highly polymorphic serum markers in forensic haemogenetics. The theoretical exclusion probability of PI is similar to that of GC or vitamin D-binding protein (DBP), which is the highest polymorphic serum marker. Silent alleles were revealed for most of these proteins, and may lead to erroneous assumption of inverse homozygosity. Chromosomal assignment either from somatic cell hybrids or recombinant DNA has shown, with exceptance of TF and AHSG, that the structural genes of these markers are located on distinct chromosomes.

Only in cases of low producing alleles errors may arise in precise subtyping by IEF if there are heterozygous carriers with a highly deficient (null allele, deficient M allele) and one normal allele. Figure 2A presents PI phenotypes of a case of paternity in which an inverse homozygosity was found between the child (PI M1) and the alleged father (PI M3). The man could not

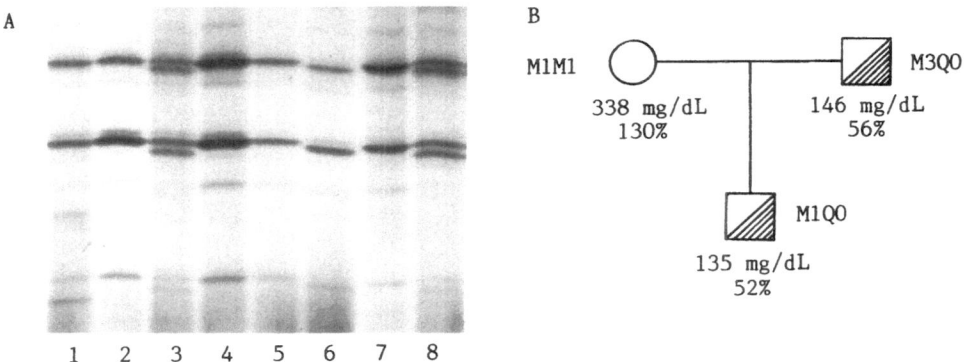

Figure 2. (A) Demonstration of PI M subtypes of mother, child, putative father and controls following high-resolution IEF of serum samples. Anode at the top. Lanes: 1= M1-Z; 2= M1M1; 3= M1M2; 4= M1M1 (mother); 5= M1QO (child); 6= M3QO (putative father); 7= M1M1; 8= M1M2. (B) Transmission of the PI*QO allele and α1AT serum levels.

be excluded as the father of this child in 26 other genetic systems. Biostatistical evaluation of the combined data yielded a paternity probability of W $\triangleq$ 99.99%. Because the band patterns of the two individuals were clearly reduced, it was assumed that they are PI M1QO and PI M3QO heterozygotes. This was consistent with their serum levels of 52% and 56% of normal, respectively (Figure 2B).

For characterization of the PI*QO allele direct sequencing of all exons after PCR amplification of genomic DNA was used (Faber et al. 1990). This method failed to reveal any molecular defect causing the PI QO phenotypes in these two individuals. DNA restriction analysis with two genomic probes of the α1AT gene revealed that the PI QO phenotype is caused by a major deletion of the gene (Poller et al. 1991). The newly deficiency allele has been preliminary named QOriedenburg. The frequency of the PI*QOriedenburg as well as other null alleles in the general population may be expected to be very low (0.001-0.0001).

CLINICAL ASPECTS

Alpha-1-antitrypsin deficiency is one of the most common inherited metabolic disorders. About 1 in 3000 of northern Europeans are homozygous for the PI Z mutation (Glu342 GAG → Lys AAG) (Cox 1989; Brantly et al. 1988). In comparison with some other disorders α1AT deficiency is only slightly less common than cystic fibrosis and it is more common than congenital adrenal hyperplasia (21-hydroxylase deficiency) and phenylketonuria (Table 4).

Table 4. Prevalence of inherited disorders

Disorder	Frequency
Cystic fibrosis	1/ 2 000
Alpha-1-antitrypsin deficiency	1/ 3 000
Congenital adrenal hyperplasia	1/ 7 000
Phenylketonuria	1/10 000
Sickle cell anemia	1/10 000
Cysteinuria	1/15 000
Galactosemia	1/40 000

Genetic deficiency of α1AT predisposes for the development of liver cirrhosis in early childhood (Sharp et al. 1969), and chronic degenerative lung disease in early adult life (Eriksson 1965). The most common sign of liver abnormality associated with α1AT deficiency is the "neonatal hepatitis syndrome". A deficiency should always be considered in a child with prolonged jaundice of unexplained origin, and PI typing should be an early diagnostic procedure. From 14 to 29% of infants with neonatal hepatitis have been found to possess PI ZZ (Moroz et al. 1976). Homozygote PI Z individuals have only about 15% of the normal α1AT level and a 20-30 fold increased risk of developing chronic obstructive pulmonary disease, specifically emphysema. In patients were shown that the basal lung regions are most severely affected. Although the majority of patients have emphysema, there are some symptoms of chronic bronchitis or bronchial asthma.

Longitudinal studies have demonstrated that PI ZZ individuals have reduced survival. The chance of being alive at the age of 50 is about 52%, compared with about 93% for the general population (Crystal et al. 1989). For those with a history of cigarette smoking, life expectancy is reduced by a further 10 years because of accelerated chronic degenerative lung disease. Heterozygotes of the type PI MZ are thought to have a moderately increased risk but only if they smoke. In addition to PI Z, there are a number of rare deficient PI M and PI null variants which are associated with diseases in the homozygous or compound heterozygous state.

REFERENCES

Brantly M, Nukiwa T, Crystal RG (1988) Molecular basis of alpha-1-antitrypsin deficiency. Am J Med 84 (6A): 13-31.
Carrell RW, Jeppsson J-O, Laurell C-B et al (1982) Structure and variation of human α1-antitrypsin. Nature 298: 329-34.
Cox DW (1989) α1-antitrypsin deficiency. In: Scriver C, Beaudet A, Sly W, Valle D, eds. The metabolic basis of inherited disease. 6th ed. New York: McGraw-Hill, pp 2409-37.
Cox DW, Johnson AM, Fagerhol MK (1980) Report of nomenclature meeting for α1-antitrypsin. Hum Genet 53: 429-33.

Cox DW, Woo SLC, Mansfield T (1985) DNA restriction fragments associated with alpha-1-antitrypsin indicate a single origin for deficiency allele PI Z. Nature 316: 79-81.

Crystal RG, Brantly ML, Hubbard RC et al (1989) The alpha-1-antitrypsin gene and its mutations. Chest 95: 196-208.

Eriksson S (1965) Studies in alpha-1-antitrypsin deficiency. Acta Med Scand Suppl 432: 1-85.

Faber J-P, Weidinger S, Olek K (1990) Sequence data of the rare deficient alpha-1-antitrypsin variant PI Zaugsburg. Am J Hum Genet 46: 1158-62.

Faber J-P, Poller W, Weidinger S et al (1994) Identification and DNA sequence analysis of 15 new α1-antitrypsin variants, including two PI*QO alleles and one deficient PI*M allele. Am J Hum Genet 55: 1113-21.

Hunt L, Dayhoff M (1980) A surprising new protein superfamily containing ovalbumin, antithrombin III, and alpha-1-proteinase inhibitor. Biochem Biophys Res Commun 95: 864-71.

Kidd VJ, Wallace RB, Itakura K, Woo SLC (1983) α1-antitrypsin deficiency detection by direct analysis of the mutation in the gene. Nature 304: 230-4.

Long GL, Chandra T, Woo SLC et al (1984) Complete sequence of the cDNA for human α1-antitrypsin and the gene for the S variant. Biochemistry 23: 4828-37.

Moroz SP, Cutz E, Cox DW, Sass-Kortsak A (1976) Liver disease associated with alpha-1-antitrypsin deficiency in childhood. J Pediatr 88: 19-25.

Poller W, Faber J-P, Weidinger S, Olek K (1991) DNA polymorphisms associated with a new α1-antitrypsin PI QO variant (PI QOriedenburg). Hum Genet 86: 522-4.

Purrello M, Alhadeff B, Whittington E et al (1987) Comparison of cytologic and genetic distances between long arm subtelomeric markers of human autosome 14 suggests uneven distribution of crossing-over. Cytogenet Cell Genet 44: 32-40.

Rabin M, Watson M, Kidd V et al (1986) Regional location of alpha-1-antichymotrypsin and alpha-1-antitrypsin genes on human chromosome 14. Somat Cell Mol Genet 12: 209-14.

Sharp HL, Bridges RA, Krivit W, Freier EF (1969) Cirrhosis associated with alpha-1-antitrypsin deficiency: A previously unrecognized inherited disorder. J Lab Clin Med 73: 934-9.

Weidinger S (1992) Reliable phenotyping of alpha-1-antitrypsin by hybrid isoelectric focusing in an ultranarrow immobilized pH gradient. Electrophoresis 13: 234-9.

A Parentage Testing Study Revealing a Possible Deletion at the PLG Locus

H. F. Polesky, M. Mount, S. Seim, L. Wiessner

Memorial Blood Centers of Minnesota, Minneapolis, Minnesota 55404, USA

INTRODUCTION

A routine paternity study of a black trio revealed reverse homozygosity (single indirect exclusion) between the alleged father and child in the PLG system. Additional testing revealed a second possible exclusion based on a single band in the RFLP system D6S132. Since both apparent exclusions are loci found on the same segment of Chromosome 6 (6q26-q27) it is unlikely that the discrepant results between father and child are evidence of non paternity.

METHODS

Standard methods were used to test for red cell antigens (ABO, RH, MNSs, Kell, Duffy, and Kidd), red cell enzymes (ESDi, ACP, and PGM1i), and serum proteins (Gci, BF, F13A, F13B, and PLG). Eight single locus DNA RFLP systems (D1S47, D2S44, D6S132, D7S104, D7S467, D12S11, D17S79, and D18S27) were tested using Pst1 for restrictions and colorometric detection with alkaline phosphatase labeled probes. For each DNA probe/enzyme combination, members of the trio were tested in the same batch and each included a mix of the alleged father and child as well as appropriate controls. A multi locus probe, DNF24, was also used to test this trio. Calculations of the paternity index was based on in house frequency tables for the majority of systems.

RESULTS

Initial testing showed only a possible exclusion in PLG (alleged father PLG 2, child PLG 1). Because of a high residual paternity index (26,362 if PLG assigned a value of 1 or 403 if a "PLG null" is assumed with a frequency of 0.0153, [Polesky 1987]) a family study was suggested. Testing of the parents (both PLG 1-2) and sister of the alleged father ruled out the possibility of a PLG null (see figure 1). Additional RFLP testing showed a second discrepancy in expected inheritance at the D6S132 locus using the probe/enzyme combination Sli1090/Pst1. The results (see figure 1) showed the child to have a single band (1.92 Kb) that matched with one of the maternal bands. The alleged father had two bands, 3.47 and 1.89. Although the 1.89 and 1.92 Kb bands are similar in size, the mix of child and alleged father showed three distinct bands (1.89, 1.92, 3.47). The paternity index based on the red cell antigens, red cell enzymes, serum proteins (except PLG), and seven single locus

RFLP systems (D6S132 not included) exceeded 2.7 billion.

DISCUSSION and CONCLUSION

The two loci that potentially exclude this alleged father are both assigned to the q26-q27 region of chromosome 6 [Ziegler,1991]. Since extensive testing of other genetic loci fail to exclude this man and testing of his family rules out the presence of a "PLG null", we have concluded that he is the father of the child in question. The finding of two apparent discrepancies at the same chromosomal region can best be explained by a deletion involving a single locus or two closely linked loci. This case illustrates the importance of comparing chromosomal locations for classic markers with the assignments of various DNA probes.

REFERENCES

Polesky HF, Souhrada JM (1987) A protocol for reporting single indirect exclusions. Advances in Forensic Haemogenetics 2: 600 - 602.

Ziegler A, Field LL, Sakaguchi AY (1991) Report of the committee on the genetic constitution of chromosome 6. Cytogenet Cell Genet 58: 295 - 336.

Fig 1.DW Family:PLG and D6S132 Results

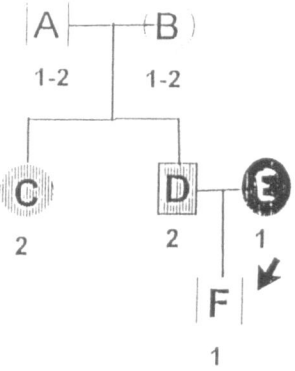

A: 3.47 / 4.13
B: 1.89 / 3.47
C: 1.89 / 3.47
D: 1.89 / 3.47
E: 1.92 / 2.73
F: 1.92

DETECTION OF THE ABO, GC, ACP and HLA-DQA1 POLYMORPHISMS AT THE DNA LEVEL USING PCR AND SSCP

J. Dissing and D. Christiansen

Department of Forensic Genetics, Institute of Forensic Medicine, University of Copenhagen, Frederik V's Vej 11, DK-2100 Copenhagen, Denmark.

INTRODUCTION

The formal genetics of the classical polymorphisms such as the ABO marker are well established via extensive World wide population studies, and gene frequencies are known for vast numbers of populations and subpopulation. The use of these polymorphisms as evidence in paternity testing and criminal case work has been accepted for decades by courts throughout the World. In step with the attainment of sequence information on the genes encoding classical markers it has become possible to design methods for genotyping based on DNA technology. We have developed methods for the detection of three of these markers, ABO, GC and ACP1, as well as for HLA-DQA1. The methods are based on PCR amplification of gene segments containing allele specific mutation sites followed by electrophoretic characterization of the separated DNA strands at non denaturing condition allowing the strands to attain sequence specific conformations (single strand conformation polymorphism, SSCP (Orita et al. 1989)).

MATERIALS AND METHODS

PCR amplification:
PCR reactions (50μl) were performed in 0.01M Tris pH 8.3, 50mM KCl, 1.5 - 2.5mM MgCl$_2$, 0.01% gelatine containing 2 U of TAQ polymerase (Perkin-Elmer Cetus), 0.2mM of each dNTP and 20 pmol of each primer using a Perkin-Elmer Cetus 480 thermocycler. A 404nt segment at the ACP1 locus was amplified using primers 10 and 16 as previously described (Lazaruk et al. 1993); a 186nt segment at the GC locus was amplified using primers flanking exon 11 (Witke et al. 1993, and Dissing et al. unpubl. results); a 198nt segment at the ABO locus was amplified using primers flanking positions 258 and 293 (Yamamoto and Hakomori, 1990; Yamamoto et al. 1990, and Dissing et al. unpubl. results); 239/242nt segments at the HLA DQα locus was amplified according to Saiki et al. (1989).

SSCP analysis:
SSCP analysis was performed using precast 20% polyacrylamide gels (PhastGels) and a semi automatic electrophoresis and staining system (PhastSystem, Pharmacia). Running conditions for ACP1/GC, ABO and DQα were 600Vh at 13°C, 400Vh at 14°C and 450Vh at 15°C, respectively. Silver staining was performed according to the recommendations of the manufacturer.

RESULTS AND DISCUSSION

GC and ACP1:
Codon 416 and 420 in exon 11 of the GC locus contain two mutational sites, and three combinations of base substitutions at these codons distinguish the GC*1F, *1S and *2 alleles (Reynolds and Sensabaugh, 1990; Witke et al. 1993). Primers flanking this region were used

for amplification of the GC locus. At the ACP1 locus a segment spanning two mutational sites in exon 3F and 3S, respectively, at which base differences distinguish the ACP1* A, *B and *C alleles was amplified (Lazaruk et al. 1993). Initially GC and ACP1 were analyzed separately and primer positions, PCR and electrophoretic conditions were optimized to obtain unequivocal genotypic SSCP patterns (results not shown). However, it was also possible to define conditions allowing multiplexing and SSCP analysis of these two markers in the same lane (Fig. 1).

ABO:

The ABO*O allele is characterized by a single-base deletion (nt 258) as detected in cDNA cloned from the corresponding glycosyltranferase gene (Yamamoto and Hakomori, 1990; Yamamoto et al. 1990). By analysis of a 250 nt segment spanning this site using denaturing gradient gel electrophoresis Johnson and Hopkinson (1992) detected four different O alleles, two B alleles and one A allele, which were assumed to be the result of combinations of different point mutations flanking nt 258. Using PCR and SSCP of a 198 nt segment spanning the same region we detected three O alleles, one A and one B allele in blood samples from 100 unrelated Danes (Fig. 2). The allele frequencies observed were: ABO*O1, 42%; *A, 27%; *O2, 19%; *B, 10%; *O3, 2%. Combined with the ability to detect heterozygosity with respect to the ABO*O alleles this greatly increases the informative value of the ABO polymorphism, thus the power of discrimination is increased from 62 to 86% and the theoretical rate of exclusion of non-fathers from 17 to 46%.

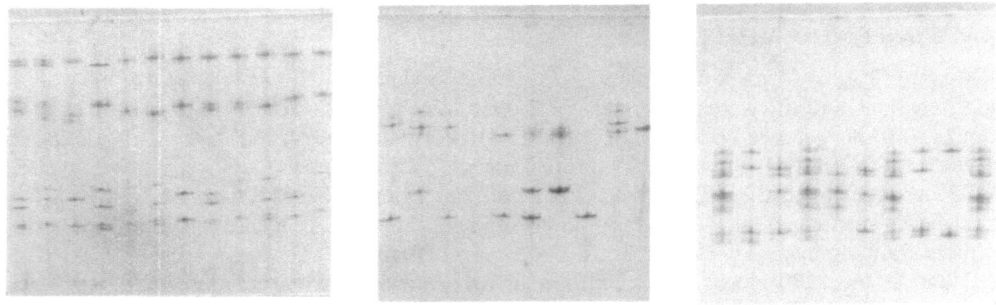

Fig. 1 (left). SSCP patterns of GC and ACP1 phenotypes using multiplexing and electrophoretic separation in 20% polyacrylamide gel for 600Vh at 13°C. GC (bottom) and ACP1 (top) phenotypes are from left to right (lanes 1-12): 1S,2/B,C; 1F,2/A,C; 1S/A,B; 1F,1S/C; 1F/B; 1F,1S/A; 2/B; 1S,2/A,B; 1F,2/A,B; 1F,1S/A; 1F/B.

Fig. 2 (middle). SSCP patterns of ABO phenotypes after electrophoretic separation in 20% polyacrylamide gel for 400Vh at 14°C. The phenotypes are from left to right (lanes 1-10): O1,O3; B,O2; B,O1; (the pattern in lane 4 does not reproduce well on the photograph); A,O1; O1,O2; O2; O1; A,B; A.

Fig. 3 (right). SSCP patterns of HLA-DQA1 phenotypes after electrophoretic separation in 20% polyacrylamide gel for 450Vh at 15°C. The patterns are from left to right (lanes 1-10): allelic ladder; 0101,0301; 0301,0501; allelic ladder; 0201,0501; 0301,0501; allelic ladder; 0102,0301; 0102; allelic ladder.

DQA1:

The HLA-DQA1 polymorphism is commonly detected by PCR and a reversed dot blot format as developed by Perkin-Elmer Cetus (Saiki et al. 1989). This method allows the detection of 6 alleles. Using a combination of PCR-RFLP and allele-specific amplification Cowland et al. (1995) were able to discriminate between 8 alleles, however, this procedure is rather laborious. Barros et al. (1994) have previously shown that DQA1 alleles are detectable using PCR and SSCP. We investigated this approach and conditions were determined for the unequivocal detection of 8 alleles (HLA-DQA1*0101, *0102, *0103, *0201, *0301, *0401, *0501, *0601) in a single electrophoretic run (Fig. 3).

CONCLUSIONS

Genotyping of classical genetic markers by PCR and SSCP is simple and fast and much less labour-intensive than classical phenotyping. The technique allows multiplexing. Except for the components of the PCR reaction the only other reagents needed are simple chemicals for silver staining. With the Pharmacia PhastSystem electrophoretic separation and staining can be accomplished in 2-3 hours. The cumulative power of discrimination of the GC/ACP1, ABO and DQA1 polymorphisms as described above is 99.93% and the theoretical chance of exclusion of non-fathers in paternity testing is 90%. Thus genotyping of "classical" structural loci by PCR and SSCP offers a valuable supplement to mutation prone VNTR and STR loci.

REFERENCES

Barros F, Munozbarus I, Lareu MV, Rodriguezcalvo MS, Carracedo A (1994) Double- and single-strand conformation polymorphism analysis of point mutations and short tandem repeats. Electrophoresis 15:566-571

Cowland JB, Madsen HO, Morling N (1995) HLA-DQA1 typing in Danes by two polymerase chain reaction (PCR) based methods. Forens Sci Int 73:1-13

Johnson PH, Hopkinson DA (1992) Detection of ABO blood group polymorphism by denaturing gradient electrophoresis. Hum Mol Genet 1:341-344

Lazaruk KDA, Dissing J, Sensabaugh GF (1993) Exon Structure at the Human Acp1 Locus Supports Alternative Splicing Model for f-Isozyme and s-Isozyme Generation. Biochem Biophys Res Commun 196:440-446

Orita M, Suzuki Y, Sekiya T, Hayashi K (1989) Rapid and sensitive detection of point mutations and DNA polymorphisms using the polymerase chain reaction. Genomics 5:874-879

Reynolds RL, Sensabaugh GF (1990) Use of the polymerase chain reaction for typing Gc variants. In: Polesky HF, Mayr WR (eds) Advances in Forensic Haemogenetics 3. Springer, Berlin: 158-161

Saiki RK, Walsh PS, Levenson CH, Erlich HA (1989) Genetic analysis of amplified DNA with immobilized sequence-specific oligonucleotide probes. Proc Natl Acad Sci USA 86:6230-6234

Witke WF, Gibbs PE, Zielinski R, Yang F, Bowman BH, Dugaiczyk A (1993) Complete structure of the human Gc gene: differences and similarities between members of the albumin gene family. Genomics 16:751-754

Yamamoto F-I, Clausen H, White T, Marken J, Hakomori S-I (1990) Molecular genetic basis of the histo-blood group ABO system. Nature 345:229-233

Yamamoto F-I, Hakomori S-I (1990) Sugar-nucleotide donor specificity of histo-blood group A and B transferases is based on amino acid substitutions. J Biol Chem 265:19259-19262

NOVEL POLYMORPHISMS IN THE CODING SEQUENCE OF THE COAGULATION FACTOR XIII A-SUBUNIT AND THEIR HAPLOTYPE DIVERSITY

Koichi Suzuki[1], Misa Iwata[1], Tatsushige Fukunaga[2], Goichi Ishimoto[2], Jürgen Henke[3], Lotte Henke[4], Maria Szekelyi[3], Shigenori Ito[1], Hiroko Tsuji[1], Akiyoshi Tamura[1]

[1]Department of Legal Medicine, Osaka Medical College, 2-7 Daigakumachi, Takatuski 569, Japan

INTRODUCTION

Genetic polymorphism of coagulation factor XIII A-subunit (F13A) is defined by four suballeles, F13A*1A, *1B, *2A, and *2B (Suzuki 1988). Some of the authors have recently determined nucleotide substitutions responsible for the allelic differences of the F13A protein by using the polymerase chain reaction (PCR) and direct sequencing, and have reported PCR-mediated typing procedure for the four alleles (Suzuki 1994). Further analysis of the coding sequences of the F13A gene has demonstrated several novel polymorphisms based on nucleotide substitutions in the coding sequences. Here, we present these nucleotide site polymorphisms and haplotypic combinations of them.

MATERIALS AND METHODS

Genomic DNA and/or plasma samples were obtained from 53 Finnish, 39 Russian, 16 German, and 50 Japanese individuals. Plasma samples were unfortunately unavailable from all of the Finnish individuals and some of the German individuals. Plasma samples were subjected to subtyping isoelectric focusing (IEF) (Suzuki 1988) and conventional IEF (Henke 1994). Genomic DNAs were PCR-amplified by using oligonucleotide primers (Suzuki 1994). Single strand conformational polymorphism (SSCP) was analyzed in mini-polyacrylamide gels. Single strands with altered mobilities were sequenced by the Sanger dideoxy method.

RESULTS AND DISCUSSION

The entire coding regions of each exon of the F13A gene were analyzed by SSCP after PCR amplification. Shifted band patterns were observed in three exons in addition to exons 12 and 14 where the nucleotide changes responsible for the differences between the four suballeles are located. Furthermore, a novel band was also detected for each of exons 12 and 14.

Direct sequence analysis showed nucleotide changes conferring each shifted band pattern. A novel band for exon 12 was based on an A to G transition at the third nucleotide of codon 567. Thus, three kinds of sequences occurred for exon 12 in the three Caucasian populations, corresponding to CTG·GAA, CCG·GAA, and CCG·GAG at positions 564 and 567. Interestingly, a novel band for exon 14 was found to correspond to GTT·CAG sequence at positions 650 and 651, where only two antithetic sequences, GTT·GAG (F13A*1A and *1B) and ATT·CAG (F13A*2A and *2B), were detected in a Japanese population. In addition, the GTT·CAG sequence was found to occur a little more frequently than the ATT·CAG sequence in the three Caucasian groups. Our previous prediction (Suzuki 1994) that the ATT·CAG mutated from the GTT·GAG via either of the GTT·CAG or the ATT·GAG was confirmed in this study.

Polymorphic nucleotide changes in exon 2, 5, 8, 12 and 14 were listed in Table 1. A G to T transversion in exon 2 and a A to T transversion in exon 5 result in amino acid changes without any detectable mobility shift in IEF. Nucleotide changes in exon 8 and 12 (codon 567) were found to be synonymous.

Next, we defined haplotypic combinations of the five polymorphic exons. For haplotype description, we gave numerical codes for each of allelic versions of the five exons as shown in Table 1. For instance, a single-heterozygotes such as 2/1-1/1-1/1-1/1-1/1 were able to be

[2]Department of Legal Medicine, Mie University School of Medicine, 2-174 Edobashi, Tsu 514, Japan
[3]Institut für Blutgruppenforschung, Hohenzollernring 57 Postfach 19 04 20, D-50501 Köln, Germany
[4]Institut für Blutgruppenforschung, Abtl. forensische Blutgruppenkunde und Molekulargenetik, Düsseldorf, Germany

unambiguously divided into the haplotypes, 21111 and 11111, and haplotypic combinations of some multiple-heterozygotes were also determined with the aid of pedigree data.

Table 1. Novel polymorphisms in the F13A coding sequences and nucleotide substitutions responsible for the allelic differences of the F13A protein.

exon	number of amino acid residue	codon	amino acid	corresponding alleles of protein	numerical code
2	34*	GTC	Val		1
		TTC	Leu		2
5	204	TAT	Phe		1
		TTT	Tyr		2
8	331	CCA	Pro		1
		CCC	Pro		2
12	564·567	CTG·GAA	Leu·Glu	A	2
		CCG·GAA	Pro·Glu	B	1
		CCG·GAG	Pro·Glu	B	3
14	650·651	GTT·GAG	Val·Glu	1	1
		GTT·CAG	Val·Gln	2	2
		ATT·CAG	Ile·Gln	2	3

*) Polymorphism at this site has been already reported in a Finnish population by Mikkola et al. (1994).

Of the predicted 72 haplotypic combinations, 18 haplotypes were delineated as shown in Table 2. When linkage disequilibrium between the five polymorphic exons was tested for the Finnish population, the frequencies of any two pairs were found not to deviate significantly from those

Table 2. Haplotypes of nucleotide polymorphisms in five exons.

sequence haplotype		Finn (n=58)		Russian (n=42)		German (n=28)		total (n=128)	
P1	11111	31	.5345	20	.4762	10	.3571	61	.4766
P2	21111	7	.1207	7	.1667	2	.0714	16	.1250
P3	12111	-	-	-	-	1	.0357	1	.0078
P4	11211	7	.1207	6	.1429	1	.0357	14	.1094
P5	11121	8	.1379	4	.0952	6	.2143	18	.1406
P6	11131	1	.0172	1	.0238	-	-	2	.0156
P7	11112	-	-	-	-	4	.1429	4	.0313
P8	11113	2	.0345	-	-	-	-	2	.0156
R1	21121	1	.0172	-	-	-	-	1	.0078
R2	11133	1	.0172	-	-	-	-	1	.0078
R3	21211	-	-	1	.0238	-	-	1	.0078
R4	11221	-	-	1	.0238	-	-	1	.0078
R5	11123	-	-	-	-	1	.0357	1	.0078
R6	11132	-	-	-	-	1	.0357	1	.0078
R7	21131	-	-	1	.0238	-	-	1	.0078
R8	21132	-	-	1	.0238	-	-	1	.0078
R9	11222	-	-	-	-	1	.0357	1	.0078
R10	21222	-	-	-	-	1	-	1	.0078

calculated under the assumption of random combinations of those exons. These findings led us to the idea that frequent recombinational events might equilibrate the combination of the exons of the F13A gene.

When assumed that the most frequent 11111 haplotype (P1) is the ancestral sequence, seven haplotypes (P2-P8) with a nucleotide change at a single site must result from the ancestor through a point mutation, and recombination between the seven haplotypes seem to lead to seven haplotypes (R1-R7) with polymorphic sites in two separate exons. The remaining three haplotypes (R8-R10) with polymorphic sites in more than two exons may also originate from recombination (Watt 1972; Strobeck and Morgan 1978) between the existing haplotypes.

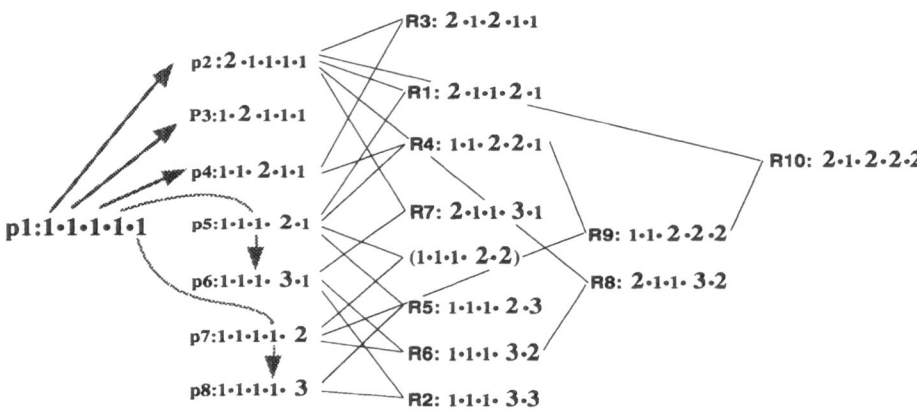

Figure 1. Hypothetic model for the generation of haplotypes. A pair of lines converging to the right indicate recombinations of any two of the existing haplotypes to produce novel haplotypes consisting of the existing polymorphic sites. A haplotype in parentheses is not defined in this study.

We detected the nucleotide site polymorphisms of the F13A gene in three Caucasian populations and only the substitution in exon 2 at a low frequency (1 in 50 individuals) in a Japanese population. Further investigations will be required for demonstrating occurrence of the site polymorphisms in other ethnic groups, especially in Negroid, and evidence of recombinational hot spots in the F13A gene region.

REFERENCES

Board PG (1979) Genetic polymorphism of the A subunit of human coagulation factor XIII. Am J Hum Genet 31:116-124

Henke J, Szekely M, Henke L (1994) On the occurrence of common and rare alleles in the coagulation FXIIIA system. Klin Lab 40:433-436

Mikkola H, Syrjälä M, Rasi V, Vahtera E, Hämäläinen E, Peltonen L, Palotie A (1994) Deficiency in the A-subunit of coagulation factor XIII: Two novel point mutations demonstrate different effects on transcript levels. Blood 84:517-525

Strobeck C and Morgan K (1978) The effect of intragenic recombination on the number of alleles in a finite population. Genetics 88:829-844

Suzuki K, Matsui K, Ito S, Fujita K, Matsumoto H (1988) Polymorphism of the A subunit of coagulation factor XIII: Evidence for subtypes of the FXIIIA*1 and FXIIIA*2 alleles. Am J Hum Genet 43:170-174

Suzuki K, Iwata M, Ito S, Matsui K, Uchida A, Mizoi Y (1994) Molecular basis for subtypic differences of the "a" subunit of coagulation factor XIII with description of the genesis of the subtypes. Hum Genet 94:129-135

Watt WB (1972) Intragenic recombination as a source of population genetic variability. Am Nat 106:737-753

NUCLEOTIDE CHANGES IN VARIOUS VARIANTS OF THE COAGULATION FACTOR XIII A-SUBUNIT

Koichi Suzuki, Jürgen Henke`, Misa Iwata, Lotte Henke``, Maria Szekelyi`, Shigenori Ito, Atsuko Uchida

Department of Legal Medicine, Osaka Medical College, 2-7 DaigakumachiTakatsuki 569, Japan
`Institut für Blutgruppenforschung, Hohenzollernring 57 Postfach 19 04 20, D-50501 Köln, Germany
``Institut für Blutgruppenforschung, Abtl. forensische Blutgruppenkunde und Molekulargenetik, Düsseldorf, Germany

INTRODUCTION

Blood coagulation factor XIIIa (F13A) is reported to be a polymorphic protein defined by two alleles (Board 1979), F13A*1 and *2, both of which are further classified into two suballeles (Suzuki 1988), F13A*1A, *1B, *2A, and *2B, by subtyping IEF. We have recently reported the molecular basis of the differences between the four suballeles (Suzuki 1994) and disclosed novel polymorphisms at five nucleotide sites in Caucasians (presented in this volume). These sites are located in codon 34 of exon 2, codon 204 of exon 5, codon 331 of exon 8, codon 567 of exon 12, and codon 651 of exon 14. These polymorphic sites including the protein allele-determining sites (codon 564 of exon 12 and codons 650-651 of exon 14) are segregated as sequence haplotypes.

This study presents molecular characterization of 16 rare F13A variant alleles and one silent allele sampled mainly from German and Japanese, together with the sequence polymorphisms underlying those variant alleles.

MATERIALS AND METHODS

Plasma and/or genomic DNA samples of various F13A variant alleles were derived from Buryat, Finnish, German, and Japanese individuals. The F13A genotype was determined for plasma samples by subtyping isoelectric focusing (IEF) (Suzuki 1988) and conventional IEF (Henke 1994). Each coding exon of the F13A genes was amplified by the polymerase chain reaction (PCR) (Suzuki 1994). Single strand conformational polymorphism (SSCP) was analyzed in mini-polyacrylamide gels followed by silver staining. PCR products showing mobility alterations in SSCP were subjected to sequencing by the Sanger dideoxy method.

RESULTS AND DISCUSSION

Because to the best of my knowledge at present there are no reference laboratories for identifying rare F13A alleles by comparing unknown samples with registered controls, we tentatively named the variant samples analyzed here according to the scheme presented by Dykes et al. (1988). The relative positions of the variants are presented in Fig. 1.

To detect mutations which cause changes in electrophoretic mobilities in IEF, the genomic DNAs from the individuals with F13A variant proteins were analyzed by PCR-SSCP. PCR products amplified from each of all the coding exons of variant alleles were indistinguishable from those amplified from the common four suballeles in agarose gel electrophoresis, indicating that no major alterations in length of coding regions were associated with the variants. PCR products were then subjected to SSCP electrophoresis.

Exons of which PCR products showed mobility shifts in SSCP analysis were then sequenced. The sequence changes of the variant alleles are listed in Table 1. For 16 variant alleles and one silent allele, we disclosed point mutations at 13 different sites in the coding exons, a deletion of a single codon, and a point mutation at a splice acceptor site, and at the same time, we determined their underlying sequence haplotypes. The amino acid changes inferred from those point mutations in the coding exons and from that single codon deletion seemed to be consistent with the mobility shifts of the corresponding variant proteins in subtyping IEF; but unfortunately we have had no chance to type the plasma sample of Fi.15 by IEF.

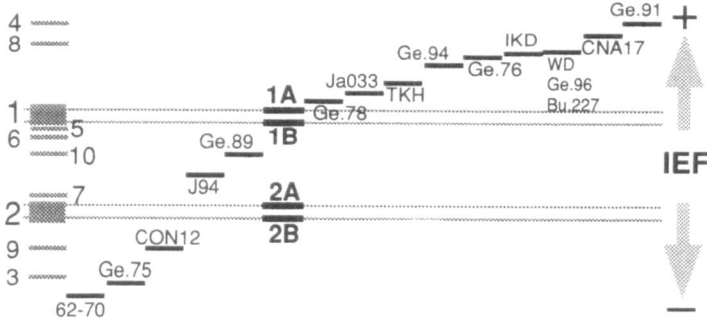

Fig.1 Relative positions of rare variant proteins on subtyping IEF. Genomic DNAs of CNA17, J94, CON12, 62-70 were unavailable and thus sequence changes of the variants were not delineated. Plasma of Ge.74, Ge.86, and Ge.79 were typed by conventional IEF and not depicted here. On the left lane are the relative positions of the two conventional alleles, *F13A*1* and **2*, and eight rare alleles presented by Dykes (1988).

Table 1. Nucleotide changes and sequence haplotypes in various variants.

sample code*	protein allele	exon involved	codon involved	nucleotide change (amino acid)	sequence haplotype exon				
					2	5	8	12	14
							codon		
					34	204	331	564 567	650 651
Ge.91	4	15	696	TGC CGG (Arg)→TGC TGG (Trp)	1	1	1	2	1
Ge.96 WD Bu.227	4	12	540	TTC CGG(Arg)→TTC CAG(Gln)	1	1	1	1	1
Ge.74	4	7	303	TAC CGG(Arg)→TAC CAG(Gln)	1	1	1	2	1
IKD	4	11	468	AAA CAA(Gln)→AAA GAA(Glu)	1	1	1	1	1
Ge.76	4	13	621	GCC AAG(Lys)→GGC GAG(Glu)	1	1	1	1	1
Ge.94	8	4	174	AGT CGA(Arg)→AGT CAA(Gln)	1or2	1	1	1	1
TKH	8	4	114	AAG GGA(Gly)→AAG GAA(Glu)	1	1	1	1	1
Ja.033	8	4	158	TTC CGC(Arg)→TTC TGC(Cys)	1	1	1	1	1
Ge.78	8	13	626	ACC GTG(Val)→ACC ATG(Met)	1	1	1	1	1
Ge.89	6or(5)	14	668	CTG GAT(Asp)→CTG GGT(Gly)	1	1	2	1	1
Ge.86	10or(6)	12	499	CTG ATG(Met)→CTG AAG(Lys)	2	1	1	1	1
Ge.79	7or(10)	12	509	ACA GAA(Glu)→ ACA ---	1	1	1	1	1
Ge.75	3or(9)	13	593	GGC GAG(Glu)→GGC AAG(Lys)	1or2	1	1or2	2	1
Fl.15	1B?	8	353	ATC TTC(Phe)→ATC TAC(Tyr)	1	1	1	1	1
Ge.84	Q0	intron V		···aataɡ TTT→···aataɡ TTT	1	1	1	1	1

*)Samples with the following headings, "Ge.", "Fi.", and "Bu." are German, Finn, and Buryat, respectively. WD, IKD, TKH, and Ja.033 are Japanese.

Ge.96, Bu.227, and WD, all typed as F13A*4, were found to share an identical nucleotide change on the same background of a sequence haplotype (11111) although they were of different ethnic origins. It is unknown now whether these three mutations occurred independently in the three groups or were due to historical interbreeding between them.

For a case in which a silent allele was transmitted from a mother (Ge.85:F13A 1) to her child (Ge.84:F13A 2), we have found a G to A transition at the splice acceptor site of intron V in both of them. An F13A deficiency resulting from the same mutation has been recently reported to be the resultant introduction of a premature stop codon due to frame shift that was caused by an alternative use of the first ApG dinucleotide downstream in exon 6 as a splice acceptor (Vreken 1995). Therefore, the homozygote of the silent allele must lead to the F13A deficiency.

The 14 different point mutations were shown to result from 11 transitions and 3 transversions. Seven (50%) of the mutations occurred in CpG dinucleotides. This high proportion is consistent with the relatively frequent occurrence of CpG dinucleotides in the coding region of the F13A gene, which has 60 (5.5%) CpG dinucleotides among 1098 dinucleotides as compared with 44 CpGs expected from an average G + C content (about 40%) in mammalian genomes. The high proportion of the mutations support the evidence that CpG dinucleotides act as a hot spot for mutation (Cooper and Youssoufian 1988).

All the mutants were further characterized for their haplotypic backgrounds by SSCP analysis of the sequence polymorphisms in exons 2, 5, 8, 12, and 14, 11 mutations (64.7%) occurring on the 11111 haplotype, 2 (11.8%) on the 11121 haplotype, 2 on the 21111 haplotype, 1 (5.9%) on the 11211 haplotype, and 1 on an undefined haplotype. This order of the frequencies agreed with that of the haplotype frequencies reported for Caucasian populations presented elsewhere in this volume.

In conclusion, much more polymorphisms can be latently harbored in the coding sequences of conventional marker genes than in their gene products, as shown in this study as well as in other genes. In addition to elucidating sequence differences between the alleles of the conventional markers, a full delineation of such hidden sites underlying common and rare alleles will serve as much more detailed characterization of human populations and also allow those rare alleles to be traced back to their founders. Thus, molecular analysis on the conventional marker genes will be required still in future.

REFERENCES

Board PG (1979) Genetic polymorphism of the A subunit of human coagulation factor XIII. Am J Hum Genet 31:116-124

Cooper DN, Youssoufian H (1988) The CpG dinucleotide and human genetic disease. Hum Genet 78:151-155

Dykes DD et al (1988) Incidence of rare variants among serum proteins and RBC enzymes in Us Whites and Blacks. In: Mayr WR (ed) Advances in Forensic Haemogenetics 2. Springer-Verlag, Berlin Heidelberg, p 125-131

Henke J et al (1994) On the occurrence of common and rare alleles in the coagulation FXIIIA system. Klin Lab 40:433-436

Suzuki K et al (1988) Polymorphism of the A subunit of coagulation factor XIII: Evidence for subtypes of the FXIIIA*1 and FXIIIA*2 alleles. Am J Hum Genet 43:170-174

Suzuki K et al (1994) Molecular basis for subtypic differences of the "a" subunit of coagulation factor XIII with description of the genesis of the subtypes. Hum Genet 94:129-135

Vreken P et al (1995) A point mutation in an invariant splice acceptor site results in a decreased mRNA level in a patient with severe coagulation factor XIII subunit A deficiency. Thromb Haemost 74:584-589

ABO GENOTYPING WITH PCR

Ulrike Schacker, Peter M. Schneider*, and Manuel Zapata

Lange Str. , 76530 Baden-Baden; *Institute of Legal Medicine, 55131 Mainz, Germany

Since Landsteiner discovered the bloodgroup antigens in 1902 more than 20 independent blood group systems have been identified by serological means. Altogether more than 250 different antigens are known to be present on human red cells. Their characterization has made rapid progress due to the developments in molecular biology. The application of DNA sequence analysis has allowed the identification of coding regions of the gene products. The molecular basis of ABO polymorphism has been known for about 30 years to be mediated via carbohydrate determinants and variant glycosyl transferases encoded by the ABO locus on the long arm of chromosome 9. Bloodgroup A individuals express an N-acetyl-D-galactosaminyl transferase and the B-encoded enzyme is a D-galactosyl transferase. AB individuals express both enzymes and 0 individuals exhibit none of the two enzymatic activities.

The molecular cloning of the ABO-specific mRNAs was carried out by Yamamoto et al. (1990). Sequence analysis revealed that the A gene differs from B by seven nucleotides which results in four amino acid substitutions. The 0 gene was found to be identical to the A coding sequence except for a single base deletion at nucleotide position 258 which leads to a frame shift mutation resulting in the synthesis of a functionally inactive transferase. In addition, it has recently been reported by Grunnet et al. (1994) that there is a second mutation in the gene also causing nonexpression and thus a second type of the 0 allele. In this allele, position 258 is not deleted, position 526 is identical to the B allel, and the actual mutation is located at position 802. In this position, the glycin has been replaced by an arginine possibly blocking the enzymatic activity. This allele has a frequency of 3.7 % in the population. The minor subtype of A, the A2 transferase, differs from A1 by a single base substitution at nucleotide 464, which can be distinguished by restriction analysis using Nae I (A_1) or Alu I (A_2).

Based on the sequence data a combination of PCR assays was developed. Single mutations can be detected either via allele-specific PCR (ASP) or restriction enzyme digestions of the PCR product. The differentiation of $A_{(1/2)}$ and B gene products was carried out with two allele-specific PCR assays. For the first PCR amplification a 407 bp fragment was chosen which contained the variable nucleotide positions responsible for A1,A2 and A,B differentiation. The nested PCR was carried out with the respective allele-specific primer for the $A_{(1/2)}$ and B loci.

Table 1: PCR primer sequences for ABO Genotyping

Primer	Sequence (5′ to 3′)
258-01-I	GAC ACC GTG GAA GGA TGT CCT C
258-01-II	CAA TGT CCA CAG TCA CTC GCC
523-I	TCC TGA AGC TGT TCC TGG AGA
523-II	AGT AGA AAT CGC CCT CGT CCT T
523-A	AGC TGT CAG TGC TGG AGG TGC
523-B	AGC TGT CAG TGC TGG AGG TGG

Table 2: PCR primer combinations for AB0 genotyping

Primer combination	Restriction analysis / size	AB0 allele
258-01-I + 258-01-II	Kpn I [+]: 171/28 bp	0_1
258-01-I + 258-01-II	Kpn I [-]: 200 bp	A, B
Nested PCR with 523-I + II:	407 bp	(use as template)
523-A + 523-II	266 bp	A_1 or A_2
523-B + 523-II	266 bp	B

Using these primers as well as the restriction enzyme Kpn I (Lee et al., 1992), the major blood groups A, B and 0 can be differentiated using the primers listed in Table 1 and combined in individual reactions as described in Table 2. The resulting PCR fragment lengths and patterns are shown schematically in Fig. 1. The smaller Kpn I fragments are clearly visible after polyacrylamide gel electrophoresis and silver staining. All A or B positive samples which show this additional smaller fragment after PCR and following restriction analysis are heterozygote null allele carriers. The ability of PCR analysis to identify AB0 genotypes should be useful for paternity testing and stain analysis.

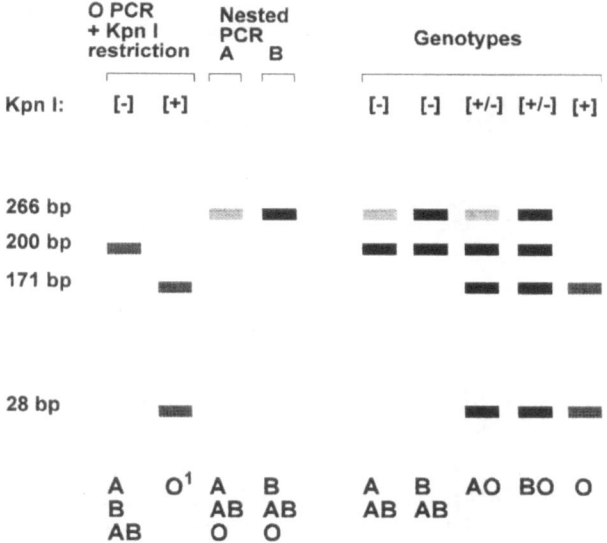

Fig. 1: PCR fragments and restriction fragments for AB0 genotyping. On the left, the individual PCR fragments from each amplification (as well as Kpn I digestion in case of the 200 bp fragment) are shown, and on the right the respective fragment combinations informative for the genotypes.

References

Grunnet N, Steffensen R, Bennett EP, Clausen H (1994) Evaluation of histo-blood group AB0 genotyping in a Danish population: frequency of a novel 0 allele defined as 0^2. Vox Sang 67:210-215

Lee JC, Chang JG (1992) AB0 genotyping by polymerase chain reaction. J Forensic Sci 37:1269-1275

Yamamoto F, Clausen H, White T, Marken J, Hakomori S (1990) Molecular genetic basis of the histo-blood group system. Nature 345:229-233

INDICATION FOR A SILENT ALLELE OF PROPERDIN FACTOR B POLYMORPHISM (BF*Q0) IN A PATERNITY CASE

Domenici R, Fornaciari S, Nardone M, Rocchi A, Spinetti I, Venturi M, Bargagna M

Department of Biomedicine, Section of Legal Medicine, University of Pisa, Italy

INTRODUCTION

The structural gene of factor B (BF), a component of the alternative complement pathway, is located in the class III region of the major histocompatibility complex (MHC) centromeric to the C2 gene and between the C4 and HLA B genes. Alpern *et al* (1972) first reported polymorphism of BF, by using immunofixation agarose gel electrophoresis: they identified two common (F and S) and two less common (F1 and S1 = S0.7) alleles, codominant at the same locus. Subsequently, a number of rare variants have been described and a nomenclature has been proposed (Geserick *et al* 1990). Further isoelectric focusing (IEF) studies revealed the occurrence of BF subtypes (Teng *et al* 1982; Geserick *et al* 1983) which could not be demonstrated by standard electrophoresis.

Until now, only a few families with an apparent silent allele of the factor B polymorphism (BF*Q0) have been published (Weidinger *et al* 1979; Sociu-Foca *et al* 1980; Tokunaga *et al* 1984; Bertrams *et al* 1985 and 1986; Weidinger *et al* 1989; Stanekova *et al* 1993). BF*Q0 allele frequency is estimated close to 0.001 (Polesky *et al* 1983). Recently, hypomorphic gene products of assumed BF*Q0 alleles were detected by means of advanced methods of IEF (Siemens *et al* 1992). In this paper we present further indication for a silent BF allele, in a case of disputed paternity.

MATERIALS AND METHODS

Blood samples were drawn from four apparently healthy individuals (mother [M], child [C] and two alleged fathers [AF1 and AF2, separate husband and current partner of M, respectively]) for paternity testing, after a private request.

The subjects were investigated - according to the protocol used in 1992 in our laboratory - in the following genetic systems: AB0, RH, MNS, HP, IGHG, IGK, GC, TF, PI, BF, ACP, PGM1, AK, ADA, GPT, GLO, ESD, DQA1, D1S80. BF typing was carried out by immunofixation with a monospecific BF antiserum (New Scientific Company) immediately after agarose gel electrophoresis, as described by Domenici *et al* (1986). Several electrophoretic runs were performed on the same blood samples, in order to confirm the results.

As new DNA polymorphisms were added to our protocol - after 1992 - also YNZ22, APOB, TH01, VWA and FES systems were determined on previously extracted and stored DNA.

RESULTS AND DISCUSSION

The first man [AF1] was excluded as the father of the child [C] in MNS, HP, PI and GLO systems. Only a single indirect exclusion in the BF polymorphism was found in the case of the second man [AF2]. AF2 was BF S, C was BF F (Fig. 1). Biostatistical evaluation of combined data (BF + other 18 systems) yielded, for AF2, a paternity probability of W = 96.73% (Fig. 2).

A request of new blood sample was rejected by mother and AF2, because the probability of paternity was "high enough" for them. So it was not possible to perform the second step of paternity analysis, including HLA system. Immunochemical and functional levels of factor B were not determined either.

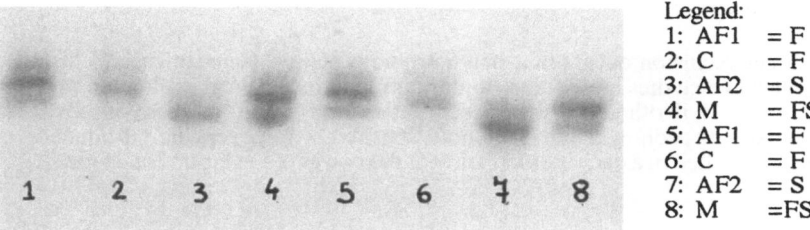

Legend:
1: AF1 = F
2: C   = F
3: AF2 = S
4: M   = FS
5: AF1 = F
6: C   = F
7: AF2 = S
8: M   =FS

Fig. 1: BF allotypes in the investigated family, after agarose gel electrophoresis and specific immuno-fixation.

After the study of five "new" DNA polymorphisms, the paternity of AF1 was excluded also in YNZ22, TH01 and VWA systems. On the other hand, the probability of paternity of AF2 raised to W = 99.995% (Fig 2). It is, therefore, very probable that he is the real father.

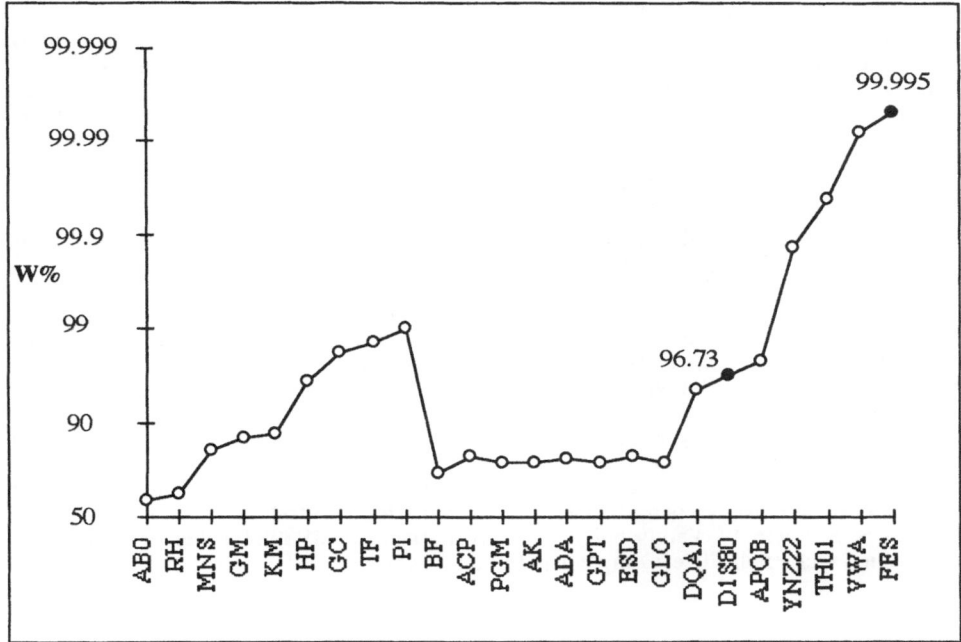

Fig. 2: Cumulative probability of paternity (W) of AF2 (logarithmic scale)

Our findings suggest that the inverse homozygosity between AF2 and C could be due to an (apparently) non-expressed BF allele.

Direct evidence on the nature of abnormal allele was not achieved. In this connection, quantitative analysis are believed to be useful, even if lowered plasma levels of factor B protein are not a reliable criterion, since factor B levels may vary considerably, due to its function as acute phase reactant (Bertrams *et al* 1985). Recently, the application of advanced methods of IEF for the determination of BF F subtypes showed that different hypomorphic BF products (BF QL = quantitatively low), with functional haemolytic activity, were expressed by assumed BF*Q0 alleles (Siemens *et al* 1992).

When a single indirect exclusion occurs in a polymorphic protein system, in case of disputed parentage, more extensive studies are needed: in our opinion biostatistical evaluation plays an important role, especially if other analyses (quantitative and functional essays, advanced determination methods) or pedigree studies are no practicable. Moreover, the introduction of DNA polymorphisms resulted in a decisive increasing of the power of the biostatistical tool.

REFERENCES

Alpern CA, Boenisch T, Watson L (1972) Genetic polimorfism in human glycine-rich beta-glycoprotein. J Exp Med 135:68-80

Bertrams J, Mauff G (1985) Another family with a silent allele of properdin factor B polymorphism (BF*Q0). Hum Genet 70:321-323

Bertrams J, Mauff G (1986) A silent allele of Properdin Factor B polymorphism (BF*Q0) in five family members. Adv Forens Haemogenet 1:93-96

Domenici R, Giari A, Bargagna M, Weidinger S (1986) Distribution of C3 and Bf allotypes in Tuscany (Italy). Hum Hered 36:330-332

Geserick G, Abbal M, Brenden M, Braun-Stilwell M, Mauff G, Siemens I (1990) Factor B (BF) nomenclature statement. Complement Inflamm 7: 255-260

Geserick G, Patzelt D, Schröder H, Nagai T (1983) Isoelectrofocusing in the study of the Bf system - existence of two common subtypes of the Bf*F allele. Vox Sang 44:178-182

Polesky HF, Souhrada JM, Dikes DD (1983) The frequency of "null" genes calculated from trios in disputed parentage cases. Proceedings in 10th Int Congr Soc Forens Haemogenet pp 161-166

Siemens I, Brenden M, Mauff G, Abbal M, Du Toit E, Bertrams J, Geserick G (1992) Apparently non-expressed alleles of factor B (BF) code for hypomorphic proteins. Immunogenetics 37:24-28

Sociu-Foca N, O'Neill G, Rubinstein P (1980) Evidence for the existence of possible Bf "null" allele. In: Teraski PI (ed) Histocompatibility testing 1980, UCLA TTL, Los Angeles, pp 935-936

Stanekova D, Niks M, Buc M, Starsia Z, Michalkova A (1993). Genetic polymorphism of factor B (Bf) and C3 component of complement in type 1 (insulin-dependent) diabetes mellitus: BF*QO allele observed in a diabetic child. Folia Biol (Praha) 93:117-123

Teng YS, Tan SG (1982) Subtyping of properdin factor B (Bf) by isoelectric focusing. Hum Hered 32:362-366

Tokunaga K, Omoto K, Yukiyama Y, Sakurai M, Saji H, Maruy E (1984) Further study on a BF silent allele. Hum Genet 67:449-451

Weidinger S, Schwarzfisher F, Cleve H (1979) Properdin Factor B polymorphism - An indication for the existence of a Bf°-allele. Z Rechtsmed 83: 259-164

Weidinger S, Schwerd W, Patutschnick W, Schwarzfisher F (1989) Further evidence for a properdin B factor null allele. Complement Inflamm 6:303

PRELIMINARY STUDIES ON THE POPULATION SUBSTRUCTURE FOR C1R PROTEIN IN CHINESE POPULATIONS

Qing Gou* Zemin Jin Yiping Hou Jin Wu Yunxiu Xu Meiyun Wu

Department of Forensic Biology, West China University of Medical Sciences,
Chengdu 610044, PR China
*Graduate Genetics Program, The George Washington University,
Washington DC 20052, USA

Introduction

Human complement subcomponent C1R is one of three distinct glycoproteins that constitute the macromolecular complex of the first complement component. It consists of two identical subunits with 170-180 kd molecular weight. Its normal concentration in human plasma is about 3-11 mg/dL. It plays an important role in activating the classical pathway of complement. The complete amino acid and nucleotide sequences of C1R have been determined (Journet and Tosi, 1986). The structural gene of C1R has been mapped on chromosome 12 (Leppert et al, 1987). The genetic polymorphism of C1R was originally described by Kamboh and Ferrell (1986). Two common alleles, C1R*1 and C1R*2, with some variants (C1R*3, C1R*4, C1R*5, C1R*6 and C1R*7) have been reported in several populations. The purposes of the present study are to investigate the polymorphism of C1R in 5 Chinese populations and to observe the genetic microdifferentiation of Chinese population by comparing allele distribution.

Materials and Methods

EDTA-blood samples were collected from 552 unrelated, healthy Chinese individuals living in 5 different geographic areas of China (fig.1). Plasma were separated within 12 h and store at -20°C until use.

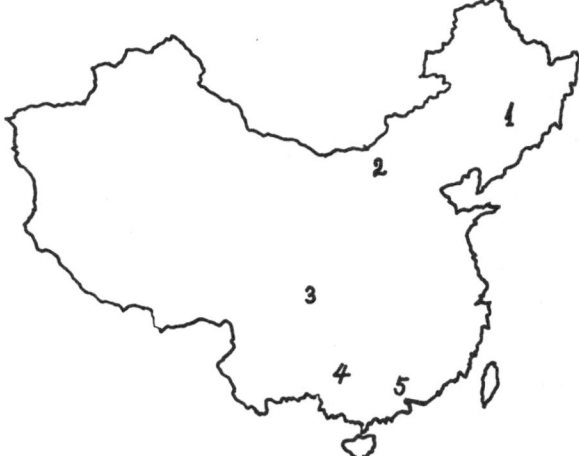

Fig.1. The geographic locations of five Chinese populations investigated.
1=Jilin 2=Inner Mongolia 3=Chengdu 4=Nanning 5=Guangzhou

Isoelectric focusing

Isoelectric focusing was carried out in 0.4mm thick 5%polyacrylamide gels containing 6mol/L urea and 2.5 (w/v) Pharmalyte pH4-6.5 (Pharmacia) as described by Kamboh. The electrode solutions were 0.1 mol/L sodium hydroxide for cathode and 0.1 mol/L phosphoric acid for anode. After 30 min prefocusing, native plasma were applied on the surface of gel near the anode. The electrofocusing was run for 5 hr at the maximum setting of 2000V with cooling temperature of 8^{0}C.

Immunoblotting

A nitrocellulose membrane (0.45um, China) was used for passive transfer of proteins. This membrane was incubated for 60 min in 3% BSA, followed by exposure to goat antihuman C1R antiserum (Atlantic, USA) at a 1:1000 dilution for 12 hr at 4^{0}C. After washing in PBS-Tween, the membrane was incubated for 4 hr in rabbit anti-goat IgG conjugated with peroxidase (Dako) at 1:500 dilution. The specific bands were developed by the solution of DAB.

Results and Discussion

Two common alleles, C1R*1 and C1R*2, were observed in all the studied Chinese populations. Some variants, C1R*5, C1R*6 and C1R*7 were encountered and designated according to the nomenclature recommended by Kamboh et al (1989).The distribution of C1R phenotypes and allele frequencies in 5 Chinese populations are presented in table 1 and table 2, respectively. The observed and expected values based upon Hardy-Weinberg equilibrium showed good agreement in all populations (table 2). For the purpose of studying the population substructure of C1R, two statistical analyses were conducted. Firstly, all comparisons of allele frequencies between these 5 groups were evaluated using a chi-test for significance and no significant differences were observed (P>0.05 for each pair). Secondly, a test for Hardy-Weinberg equilibrium was conducted when all the individuals studied were pooled together and no deviations from this equilibrium (x^2=10.7487, df=6, P>0.05) and no loss of heterozygotes were observed. All these data suggested that there was no population substructure for C1R in these 5 Chinese populations.

Table 1. Distributions of C1R phenotypes in 5 Chinese populations

Population	N	1-1	2-2	5-5	5-1	2-1	5-2	5-V	2-V	1-V	1-6	1-7
Jilin	105	28	7	4	20	35	5	2	1	1	1	1
Inner Mongolia	142	42	10	7	20	46	13	2	1	1	0	0
Chengdu	111	34	13	1	12	45	5	0	0	1	0	0
Nanning	93	26	15	0	5	39	6	0	0	2	0	0
Guangzhou	101	24	10	1	12	46	8	0	0	0	0	0
pooled	552	154	55	13	69	211	37	4	2	5	1	1

Table 2. C1R allele frequencies in 5 Chinese populations

Population	N	C1R allele frequencies				x^2	df	P
		C1R*1	C1R*2	C1R*5	C1R*Var§			
Jilin	105	0.5381	0.2619	0.1714	0.0286	4.78	6	>0.05
Inner Mongolia	142	0.5317	0.2817	0.1725	0.0141	6.93	6	>0.05
Chengdu	111	0.5676	0.3423	0.0856	0.0045	1.45	6	>0.05
Nanning	93	0.5269	0.4032	0.0591	0.0108	2.77	6	>0.05
Guangzhou	101	0.5248	0.3663	0.1089	-	2.83	3	>0.05
Pooled	552	0.5380	0.3261	0.1241	0.0118	10.75	6	>0.05

§: C1R*Var=C1R*V+C1R*6+C1R*7

There are two interesting features which make C1R a useful marker in population genetics and anthropological genetics studies. First, the allele distributions of C1R showed bimodal in Mongoloid populations, while it showed unimodal in Caucasoid and Negroid populations (table3). Second, the widespread distribution of C1R*5 among all Mongoloid populations and its low frequencies in Caucasoid populations suggested that it was a gene which characterizes the gene of Mongoloid populations.

Table 3. C1R allele frequencies in various populations

Population	N	C1R allele frequencies			
		C1R*1	C1R*2	C1R*5	C1R*Var
U.S. Whites	133	0.8910	0.1090	-	-
U.S. Blacks	109	0.8990	0.1010	-	-
Dogrib Indians	95	0.8320	-	0.1680	-
Aleuts	187	0.8930	0.0670	0.0400	-
Japanese	1000	0.4760	0.3260	0.1940	0.0080
Chinese	552	0.5380	0.3261	0.1241	0.0118

Acknowledgments

The authors are grateful to individuals who have helped us to collect samples. This project was accomplished under the grant from the National Natural Science Research Foundation of P.R.China and the grant from the Chinese Medical Board of New York.

Reference

1 Cooper NR (1985) Adv. Immunol 37:151-216.
2 Journet A, Tosi M (1986) Biochem J 240:783-787.
3 Leppert M, Ferrell RE, Kambol MI, Beasley J, P.O'Connell, Lathrop M, Lalouel JM, White R (1987) Cytogenet & Cell Genet 46:647.
4 Kamboh MI, Ferrell RE (1986) Am J Hum Genet 39:826-831.
5 Kamboh MI, Lyons LA, Ferrell RE (1989) Am J Hum Genet 44:148-153.
6 Kido A, Komatsu N, Kimura Y, Oya M (1991) Hum Hered 41(2):129-133.

A STUDY OF POLYMORPHISM OF ANTITHROMBIN III AT THE LEVEL OF BOTH PROTEIN AND DNA IN A CHINESE POPULATION

Qing Gou*   Yiping Hou   Youfang Zhang   Meiyun Wu

*Graduate Genetics Program, The George Washington University,
Washington DC 20052, USA
Department of Forensic Biology, West China University of Medical Sciences,
Chengdu 610044, PR China

Introduction

A systematical study of structure and genomic organization of antithrombin III (ATIII) (Lane and Caso, 1989) indicated that there are two polymorphisms: an intragenic polymorphism arising from a translationally silent A to G transition in condon 305, and a length polymorphism arising from the presence of 32 BP or 108 BP non-homologous sequences 345bp upstream from the translation intiation condon. Products of three ATIII codominant autosomal alleles have been revealed by IEF from Caucasoid and Negroid (Kambol and Ferrell, 1988). On the other hand, the fragment length polymorphism of ATIII has been studied by Southern blotting (Bock and Levitan, 1983) and by PCR (Seino, 1989) in Caucasian population.The purpose of this study is to reveal the genetic polymorphism of ATIII in a Chinese population at the level of both protein and DNA and to explore the relationship between these two kinds of polymorphisms.

Materials and Methods

EDTA-blood specimens were collected from 51 healthy unrelated Chinese individuals living in the Inner Mongolia antonomous Region of China. For family studies, the samples were collected from the members of two families residing in Chengdu, China.

Isoelectric focusing and immunoblotting for products of ATIII alleles
IEF was carried out in ultra-thin layer polyacrylamide gels containing 6M urea as described by Kambol and Ferrell (1988). An optimal pH gradient was obtained by mixing Pharmalyte of pH4.2-4.9 and of pH 4.5-5.4 at a ratio of 1:1. The power supply settings were 1500V, 5W, 6hr (gel dimension 120x80x0.4mm). Immunoblotting was achieved by diffusion blotting for 45 min onto nitrocellulose filter. The ATIII proteins on this filter were probed by rabbit anti-human ATIII serum . Horseradish-peroxidase-labeled goat anti-rabbit IgG was used as the second antibody and the DAB served as a detecting agent. The alleles for ATIII were named according to Kambol and Ferrell(1988).

Polymerase chain reaction for ATIII 5'locus

The oligonucleotides with sequences of 5'-CCACAGGTGAACATTGTGT-3' and 5'-GAGATAGTGTGATCTGAGGC-3' were used as the PCR primers. DNA was extracted using Chelex100 method. Reaction system of the PCR contained 2-100ng genomic DNA, 1xTaq buffer, 2 mM $MgCl_2$, $200uM$ each of dNTP, 40 pM each of primers and 1U Taq polymerase (Gibco BRL) in 25 ul. The reactions were subjected to 30 cycles consisting of 1min at 94^0C for denature, 1min at 54^0C for annealing and 4min at 71^0C for extension. The PCR products combined with the size marker of PBR322/HaeIII were electrophoresed on a

2.5% agarose gel containing ethidene bromide. The ATIII 5' alleles were identified relative to this marker and named according to Seino (1989).

Results

The IEF pattern of ATIII revealed in this study is similar to that reported by Kambol and Ferrell except that the ATIII*3 product was not encountered. Using the primers described above, two fragments (496 bp and 572 bp) were successfully amplified and named as ATIII5'*2 and ATIII5'*1 accordingly.

The pedigrees below show the distributions of ATIII genotypes at the level of both protein and DNA in two families. The codominant segregations of both ATIII alleles and ATIII5' alleles were observed, suggesting that their inheritance are in accordance with Mendelian law. Secondly, the ATIII5' polymorphism doesn't correlate with any specific one of the allelic IEF variations, implying that these two polymorphisms are independent.

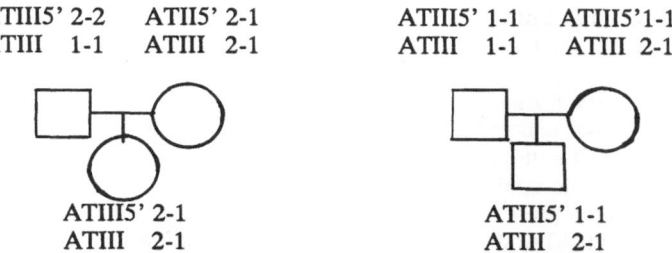

The distributions of genotypes and allele frequencies for ATIII and ATIII5' loci in Chinese population are given in table 1. The genotypes in each locus are in Hardy-Weinberg equilibrium. The PICs (Botstein et al, 1980) for ATIII5' locus and ATIII locus were 0.6018 and 0.0782, respectively. This indicated that the ATIII5' locus was more useful for genetic linkage analysis.

Table 1. Distributions of ATIII5' and ATIII genotypes in a Chinese population

Genotypes		No. observed	No. expected	Allele frequencies
ATIII5'	2-1	24	24.71	ATIII5'*1=0.4118
	1-1	9	8.65	ATIII5'*2=0.5882
	2-2	18	17.64	x^2=0.0419
				df=1
	total	51	51.00	P>0.05
ATIII	1-1	47	47.08	ATIII*1=0.9608
	2-1	4	3.83	ATIII*2=0.0391
	2-2	0	0.08	x^2=0.0877
				df=1
	total	51	51.00	P>0.05

The results of the estimation of pairwise haplotype frequencies and the linkage disequilibrium coefficient (Ott, 1985) between ATIII and ATIII5' are shown in table 2. The observed frequencies of both ATIII*1-ATIII5'*2 and ATIII*2-ATIII5'*1 were higher than those expected at linkage equilibrium, showing that these two haplotypes were preferred. However, the D linkage value was not significantly different from 0 (x^2=0.4178, P>0.05). So the linkage disequilibrium between ATIII and ATIII5' was not observed in this study.

Table 2. Estimation of haplotype frequencies for pairs of markers and D linkage value

No. of chromosomes examined	Haplotypes and their frequencies			
	ATIII1/ATIII5'1 (1)	ATIII1/ATIII5'2 (2)	ATIII2/ATIII5'1 (3)	ATIII2/ATIII5'2 (4)
102	0.3922	0.5686	0.0196	0.0196
D=(1)*(2)-(3)*(4)=-0.0034		x^2=0.4178	P>0.05	

Discussion

In the past, the polymorphisms of human plasma proteins were much concerned at the level of gene translation products. The main limitation of such studies is the low PIC. Therefore, both forensic biologists and geneticists are making great efforts to disclose the polymorphisms of genetic markers at DNA level. Among others, one of the advantages of such studies is that the polymorphisms arising from non-coding regions can be detected out. It can be imaged that studies of polymorphisms of both protein and DNA could provide some information about the relationship between genetic markers arising from these two level. In this study, we have successfully investigated the protein and DNA polymorphisms of ATIII. The results showed the polymorphisms of both ATIII described by Kambol and ATIII5' described by Seino can be detected from Chinese population. Furthermore, the family study and the association analysis revealed that ATIII5' amp-FLP and the ATIII IEF variants are independent, indicating that ATIII5' amp-FLP is not the primary factor in the determination of ATIII IEF variants.

It is interesting that the distributions of allele frequencies in these two systems are quite different, notwithstanding the same number of alleles in them. The polymorphic information contained in the exons of ATIII structural locus is much less than that in non-coding areas. This phenomenon is in accordance with the biological functions of exons and introns of a gene. In addition, it suggested that the mechanisms of polymorphism developments of exons and introns of a gene are quite different.

Acknowledgments

This work was accomplished under grant 39300072 from the National Natural Science Research Foundation of PR China, grant from the Ministry of Public Health of PR China and grant from the Chinese Medical Board of New York.

References

1 Lane DA & Case R (1989) Bailers Cline Haematol 2(4):961.
2 Kambol MI & Ferrell RE (1988) Ann Hum Genet 52:17-24.
3 Bock SC & Levitan DJ (1983) Nucl Acids Res 11:8569-8582.
4 Wu S, Seino S, Bell GI (1989) Nucl Acids Res 17(15):6433.
5 Botsein D, Raymond LW, Skolnick M (1980) Am J Hum Genet 32:314-331.
6 Ott J. Analysis of human genetic linkage (1985) The Johns Hopkins University Press, USA, pp147-152.

Genetic polymorphisms of Alpha-1-Antitrypsin and Group-Specific Component in Spanish Gypsy population.

Guisán A., López-Abadía I., Ruiz de la Cuesta J.M., Bandrés F.

*1 Escuela Med. Legal. Biología Forense. Fac. Med. UCM. 48040. Madrid.Spain.
*2 Fundación Laboral INI-SAS. Castelló 58. 28001. Madrid. Spain.

SERUM PROTEINS

Alpha-1-Antitrypsin (Pi) and Group-Specific Component (Gc).

POPULATION AND SAMPLE SIZE

Gypsies (Basque Country, Spain). N:165.

METHODS

Isoelectric focusing (IEF) in polyacrylamide gels: Allen y cols. (1974) for Pi and Hoste (1979) for Gc.

Interpretation of the results: direct staining (Coomassie Blue) for Pi and by precipitation for Gc.

RESULTS

The phenotypic distribution at all the loci was at Hardy-Weinberg equilibrium.

Observed genotypes for Pi (Table 1):

Gen.	Obs.	Gen.	Obs.	Gen.	Obs.	Gen.	Obs.
M1M1	105	M1S	18	M2M3	1	M2F	1
M1M2	18	M1F	3	M2S	3	M3M3	2
M1M3	6	M2M2	7	M2Z	1		

Observed genotypes for Gc (Table 2):

Gen.	Obs.	Gen.	Obs.	Gen.	Obs.
1S 1S	42	1S 2	54	1F 2	17
1S 1F	27	1F 1F	4	2 2	21

Allele frequencies for Pi (Table 3):

Allele	Frequency	Allele	Frequency	Allele	Frequency
M1	0.7727273	M3	0.0333333	Z	0.0030303
M2	0.1151515	S	0.0636364	F	0.0121212

Test P: $0.10 > p > 0.05$

Allele frequencies for Gc (Table 4):

Allele	Frequency	Allele	Frequency	Allele	Frequency
1S	0.5	1F	0.1575758	2	0.3424242

Test P: $p > 0.95$

COMMENTS

In this population, a high proportion of homozigosis stood out for the phenotype M1M1 (Pi). We also found a very high frequency for the allele F (Pi), the highest known among the frequencies studied up to the present time (1.2%).

This data may be used for paternity diagnosis and may contribute to studies regarding the gypsies in the world, as an ethnic group, since it is widely extended population, in all countries and in all continents.

REFERENCES

Allen RC, Harley RA, Talamo RC (1974). A new method for determination of alpha-1-antitrypsin phenotypes using isoelectric focusing on polyacrylamide gel slabs. Am J Clin Pathol 62:732-739.

Hoste B (1979). Group-specific component (Gc) and transferrin (Tf) subtypes ascertained by isoelectric focusing. A simple nonimmunological staining. Hum Genet 50:75-79.

Saha N y cols. (1990). The distribution of some serum protein and red cell enzyme polymorphisms in the Koch ethnic group of West Bengal, India. Jinrui Idengaku Zasshi 35:253-256.

Tills D, Kopec AC, Tills RE (1983). The distribution of the human blood groups and others polymorphisms. Suplement 1. Oxford University Press, Oxford.

Studies on Blood Genetic Markers in Some Mongoloid
Populations of Eastern Siberia

G.Ishimoto[1], K.Suzuki[2], H.Matsumoto[2],V.P.Wiebe[3] and V.Valentina[4]

1) Department of Legal Medicine, Mie University School of Medicine,Tsu, Japan 2) Department of Legal Medicine, Osaka Medical College,Osaka, Japan 3) Institute of Cytology and Genetics, Siberian Division of Russian Academy of Sciences, Novosibirsk, Russia 4) Department of Biology, Uladivostok Medical University, Uladivostok, Russia

To present new genetic information on northern peoples and to examine their relationship with Japanese, field-works were under-taken in summer in 1991 and 1993 to collect blood samples from indigenous populations of Mongoloid groupsin Eastern Siberia and the Primorsky region.

Materials

Buryat samples were provided from a hospital in Ulan-Ude. Evenki samples were collected at camp-sites and villages of Ust-Njukza, Ust-Urkema and Perbomaiskij near Tynda. Udeghe and Nanai samples were obtainedin villages of Agzu and Krasnii Yar.   Out of 687 samples only those whose parents were from a same ethnic group were chosen.

They were 180 for Buryats, 194 for Evenkis and 110 for Udeghes. The Nanai group is excluded in this report, because most were 'mixed'.

Results and Discussion

Table 1 presents allele frequencies for the 14 polymorphic systems invesitigated in the three Mongoloid populations in Russia.   Data for a Japanese population are also given as reference.

Compared with Japanese, the three indigenous populations showed much more polymorphic in ACP, HP and AHS systems, and far less poly-morphic in PGM, ESD and TF systems.

In addition, PLG*M5, responsible for producing an inactive form of plasminogen, was first detected except Japanese.   A considerably high incidence of GM*ST gene was again observed in the Buryat population. the C1R(subcomponent R of complement 1) system proved to be a useful marker for examining Mongoloid populations.

Table 1. Allele Frequencies for 14 Genetic Markers

	ABO			ACP		PGM				ESD		
	O	A	B	A	B	1A	1B	2A	2B	1	2	V
Buryat	0.518	0.194	0.267	0.325	0.675	0.750	0.065	0.172	0.013	0.769	0.231	-
Evenki	0.558	0.178	0.264	0.246	0.754	0.813	0.083	0.083	0.021	0.762	0.238	-
Udeghe	0.610	0.152	0.219	0.327	0.673	0.768	0.005	0.155	0.073	0.714	0.286	-
C(Jpn)	0.559	0.271	0.170	0.213	0.787	0.696	0.092	0.155	0.057	0.628	0.364	0.008

	HP		GC				TF			PI		
	1	2	1F	1S	2	V	1	2	V	1	2	3
Buryat	0.315	0.685	0.517	0.297	0.178	0.008	0.819	0.164	0.017	0.831	0.136	0.033
Evenki	0.406	0.594	0.598	0.299	0.103	-	0.866	0.121	0.013	0.732	0.196	0.071
Udeghe	0.358	0.642	0.636	0.091	0.273	-	0.918	0.073	0.009	0.854	0.141	0.005
C(Jpn)	0.263	0.737	0.472	0.247	0.253	0.028	0.747	0.239	0.014	0.740	0.210	0.050

	C1R				AHS			PLG			
	1	2	5	V	1	2	V	A	B	M5	V
Buryat	0.614	0.267	0.116	0.003	0.603	0.394	0.003	0.925	0.050	0.022	0.003
Evenki	0.353	0.235	0.412	-	0.613	0.382	0.005	0.987	0.013	-	-
Udeghe	0.432	0.259	0.305	0.005	0.536	0.459	0.005	0.991	0.009	-	-
C(Jpn)	0.456	0.338	0.196	0.010	0.732	0.268	-	0.953	0.010	0.015	0.022

	GM				BF				13A			
	ag	axg	ab³st	afb'b³	F	S	S07	FV	1A	1B	2A	2B
Buryat	0.444	0.132	0.281	0.143	0.222	0.744	0.031	0.003	0.225	0.556	0.008	0.208
Evenki	0.590	0.103	0.227	0.080	0.075	0.920	0.003	0.003	0.201	0.678	0.003	0.119
Udeghe	0.581	0.196	0.164	0.059	0.123	0.868	-	0.010	0.209	0.650	0.032	0.109
C(Jpn)	0.453	0.158	0.269	0.121	0.182	0.795	-	0.023	0.275	0.620	0.007	0.098

Nei' standard genetic distances for each pair of the populations in Table 1 were calculated (Table 2). Clustering was performed using the UPGMA method. Fig.1 is a dendrogram based on the above14 loci. The Buryat shows a great affinity with Japanese, whereas the rest of

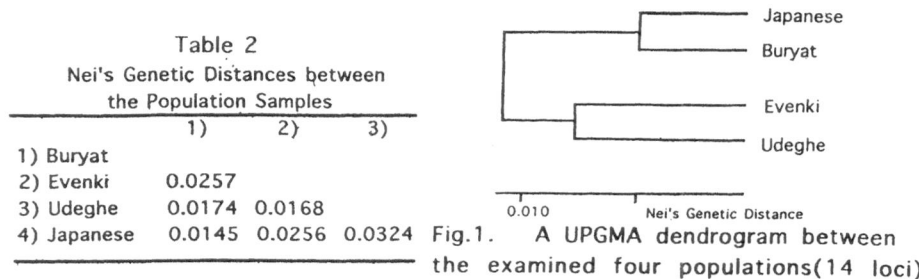

Table 2
Nei's Genetic Distances between
the Population Samples

	1)	2)	3)
1) Buryat			
2) Evenki	0.0257		
3) Udeghe	0.0174	0.0168	
4) Japanese	0.0145	0.0256	0.0324

Fig.1. A UPGMA dendrogram between the examined four populations(14 loci)

a same tungusic-speaking group forms another cluster.

Several Russian investigators have benn devoted to genetic studies of various isolated indigenous populations in Siberia, and have offered their results in literatures. Utilizing such data as well as those of neighboring countries, an additional "map" could be depicted. Fig. 2 is a dendrogram for 11 Mongoloid populations based on the 6 loci (ABO, HP, GC, TF, ACP and PGM- any not subtyped). It includes further 7 populations whose data source are indicated below.

There are two main clusters. One consists of populations of Arctic peoples in Northern Siberia. The other comprises the populations of the Altaic language family, which appear to be separated into two groups according to their language affiliation. The exception is of the Udeghe. A plausible explanation is probably due to Chinese effects to that ethnic group.

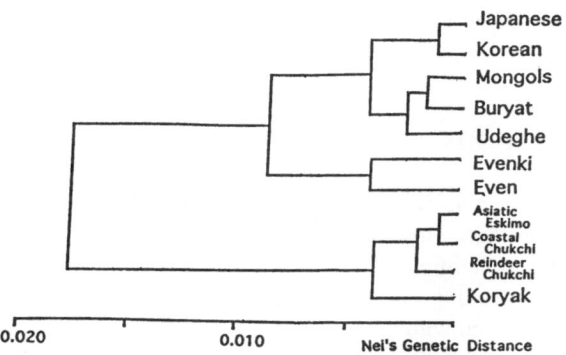

Fig.2. A UPGMA dendrogram between
eleven Mongoloid populations(6 loci)

Data source for furthrt 7 populations:
Asiatic Eskimo, Coastal Chukchi and Reindeer Chukchi: Solovenchuk LL,1984. Koryak: Solovenchuk LL et al.,1985 Even: Posukh OL et al. 1990 Mongols: Batsuur Zh et al.,1991 Korean: Ohkura K et al.,1989, Jiujin X et al.,1986, Matsumoto H et al.,1980, Goedde HW et al.,1984.

PI SUBTYPING IN DENTAL PULPS

Akira KIDO and Masakazu OYA

Department of Legal Medicine, Yamanashi Medical University, Yamanashi-ken 409-38, Japan

INTRODUCTION

Genetic polymorphism of human serum α_1-antitrypsin (PI) was first discovered by Fagerhol and Braend (1965) using acid starch gel electrophoresis. The common PI M type can be separated into six subtypes with three alleles, PI*M1, PI*M2 and PI*M3, by means of isoelectric focusing followed by direct protein staining with Coomassie Brilliant Blue (CBB) (Frants and Eriksson, 1976).

Recent introduction of the technique of immunoblotting has provided much better visualization of focused PI than the CBB staining method (Whitehouse et al., 1989). In the present study, PI subtyping was attempted from dental pulps using isoelectric focusing followed by immunoblotting.

MATERIALS AND METHODS

Teeth were collected from 43 patients who received treatment at the Dental Clinic of Yamanashi Medical University Hospital. Fifteen samples were examined immediately after extraction and the remaining 28 samples after storage at room temperature for various periods of week. Serum samples were also taken from the same 43 subjects as control. The tooth was crushed with a hammer, and the dental pulp was picked out from the pulp cavity. The pulp tissue weighing 10 to 20 mg was macerated in 30 μl distilled water and mashed with a glass rod. Eight μl of dental pulp lysates or serum samples were treated with 1 μl 0.1 M dithiothreitol for 30 min at room temperature and then with 1 μl 0.1 M iodoacetamide for 60 min at 4°C. Serum samples were diluted 1:20, but dental pulp samples were not diluted.

The amount of PI present in the dental pulp was quantitated using rocket immunoelectrophoresis (Laurell, 1966).

Isoelectric focusing was performed using a Bio-Phoresis Electrophoresis Cell (Bio-Rad) and a Model 3000 Xi Power Supply (Bio-Rad). Polyacrylamide gels (230 x 110 x 0.5 mm) were prepared with 20 ml acrylamide stock solution (5.25% acrylamide/0.25% N,N'-methylenebisacrylamide) containing 1 ml Pharmalyte pH 4.2-4.9 (Pharmacia), 0.3 ml 0.01% riboflavin, 2.5 g sucrose and 0.3 g N-(2-acetamide)-2-aminoethanesulfonic acid. The electrode paper strips were soaked with 1 M phosphoric acid for the anode and with 1 M sodium hydroxide for the cathode. After prefocusing at 1500 Vmax and 5 mAmax for 60 min, 10 μl of the samples was applied to the gel surface 2 cm from the cathode using 5 x 6 mm filter paper strips (Whatman No. 3). Electrofocusing was conducted at a constant voltage of 1500 V for 180 min. The sample applicators were removed after 60 min of focusing. During focusing the gel was cooled by circulating water at 4°C.

A sheet of nitrocellulose membrane (Bio–Rad) was placed on the gel surface and left for 60 min with 1 kg weight. Following blotting the membrane was rinsed in 20 mM Tris/500 mM sodium chloride buffer, pH 7.5, (TBS) for 10 min and immersed in TBS containing 3% gelatin for 30 min. After washing in TBS for 15 min, the membrane was incubated for 60 min in rabbit anti–human PI serum (DAKO) that was diluted 500–fold with TBS containing 0.05% Tween 20 (TTBS). Then the membrane was washed 3 times in TTBS for 30 min and incubated for 60 min in goat anti–rabbit IgG serum conjugated with alkaline phosphatase (Sigma) that was diluted 500–fold with TTBS. After 3 washes in TTBS for 30 min, the membrane was incubated in 50 ml of a staining solution (1.8 g sodium hydroxide and 3.7 g boric acid/1000 ml) containing 25 mg β–naphthyl phosphate, 25 mg Fast Blue BB salt and 60 mg magnesium sulfate for a few minutes.

RESULTS AND DISCUSSION

The amount of PI present in dental pulp lysates from 15 fresh tooth samples was determined by rocket immunoelectrophoresis. The values ranged from 0.29 to 1.90 mg/ml. The mean value was 0.82±0.11 mg/ml, which was about one third of the value in normal serum (2.42 mg/ml) (Blundell and Frazer, 1975).

Table 1 summarizes the results of PI subtyping in fresh teeth and in teeth stored at room temperature for various periods.

The PI patterns in fresh dental pulps were identified as clearly and intensely as those in serum samples, and the types observed in dental pulps agreed with those in the corresponding serum samples (Fig. 1). All the dental pulp samples examined were correctly subtyped after storage for up to 4 weeks. The pattern in dental pulps from teeth stored for 1 week at room temperature is shown in Fig. 2.

Table 1. Positive results of PI subtyping in dental pulps

Periods of storage	No. tested	Subtype			
		M1	M1M2	M2	M2M3
Fresh	15	9	5	1	
1 week	10	5	3	1	1
2 weeks	6	4	1		1
3 weeks	6	5	1		
4 weeks	6	4	2		

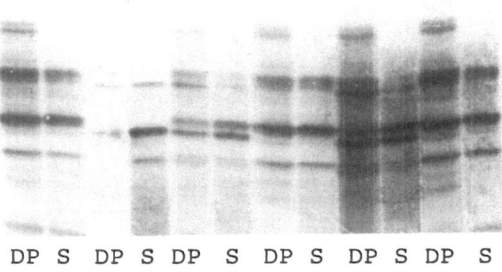

Fig. 1. Isoelectric focusing PI pattern in fresh dental pulps (DP) and the corresponding serum samples (S). 1: M1, 2: M2, 3: M1M2, 4: M1, 5: M1M2, 6: M1. The anode is at the top.

DP S DP S DP S DP S DP S DP S
1 1   2 2   3 3   4 4   5 5   6 6

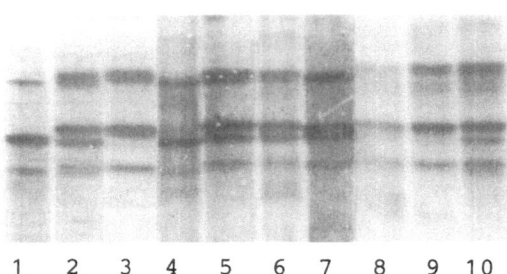

Fig. 2. Isoelectric focusing PI pattern in control sera (1–3) and dental pulps from teeth stored for 1 week at room temperature (4–10). 1: M2, 2: M1M2, 3: M1, 4: M2, 5: M1M2, 6: M1M2, 7: M2M3, 8: M1, 9: M1, 10: M1M2. The anode is at the top.

1   2   3   4   5   6   7   8   9   10

In conclusion, isoelectric focusing followed by immunoblotting permits reliable PI subtyping from teeth stored for up to 4 weeks and is therefore recommended to be used in medico–legal practice. The PI subtyping combined with the TF and GC typings is useful for personal identification of teeth, particularly in cases of mass disasters such as automobile accidents, aircraft crashes and explosions.

REFERENCES

Blundell G. and Frazer A. (1975) Alpha$_1$ antitrypsin phenotypes in Northern Ireland. *Ann. Hum. Genet.*, 38, 289–294.

Fagerhol M.K. and Braend M. (1965) Serum prealbumin: Polymorphism in man. *Science*, 149, 986–987.

Frants R.R. and Eriksson A.W. (1976) α_1–Antitrypsin: Common subtypes of Pi M. *Hum. Hered.*, 26, 435–440.

Laurell C.B. (1966) Quantitative estimation of proteins by electrophoresis in agarose gel containing antibodies. *Anal. Biochem.*, 15, 45–52.

Whitehouse D.B., Lovegrove J.U. and Hopkinson D.A. (1989) Variation in alpha–1–antitrypsin phenotypes associated with penicillamine therapy. *Clin. Chim. Acta*, 179, 109–116.

GC SUBTYPING IN SERUM AND SEMEN AFTER NEURAMINIDASE TREATMENT

Akira KIDO, Masakazu OYA and Masaaki HARA*

Department of Legal Medicine, Yamanashi Medical University, Yamanashi-ken 409-38, Japan
Department of Legal Medicine, Saitama Medical School, Saitama 350-04, Japan*

INTRODUCTION

Genetic polymorphism in the group-specific component (GC) of human serum was first described by Hirschfeld (1959) with two alleles, GC*1 and GC*2. Using isoelectric focusing, Constans and Viau (1977) demonstrated that GC 1 is resolved into GC 1F and GC 1S with a double-band pattern. Thus, six phenotypes are coded by three alleles, GC*1F, GC*1S and GC*2. Cleve and Patutshnick (1979) reported that the anodal bands of GC 1F and of GC 1S disappear after removal of sialic acid by neuraminidase treatment.

We have recently observed that in human semen the anodal bands of GC 1F and of GC 1S do not disappear by neuraminidase treatment. This paper describes GC subtyping in serum, semen and seminal stains using isoelectric focusing after treatment of the samples with neuraminidase.

MATERIALS AND METHODS

Blood and semen samples were obtained from 30 male volunteers with known phenotypes. Seminal stains were made on filter paper (Whatman No. 3) and stored at 4°C, room temperature and 37°C. Native serum samples were diluted 1:150 with distilled water. Serum samples were desialylated in 1/10 volume of 1 M potassium phosphate buffer (pH 7.0), containing 50 U/ml neuraminidase from *Clostridum perfringens* (Type V, Sigma), overnight at 4°C, followed by dilution of the mixture, 1:150, with distilled water. Native semen samples were diluted 1:10 with 6 M urea, containing 0.5% BSA. Semen samples were diluted 1:10 with 6 M urea, containing 0.5% BSA, and incubated in 1/10 volume of 50 U/ml neuraminidase. Seminal stains (5 x 5 mm) were extracted with 36 μl 6 M urea, containing 0.5% BSA, and incubated in 4 μl 50 U/ml neuraminidase overnight at 4°C.

Isoelectric focusing was performed using a Bio-Phoresis Electrophoresis Cell (Bio-Rad) and a Model 3000 Xi Power Supply (Bio-Rad). Polyacrylamide gels (230 x 110 x 0.5 mm) were prepared from 20 ml stock solution (5.25% acrylamide/0.25% N,N'-methylenebisacrylamid), containing 1 ml Pharmalyte pH 4.5-5.4 (Pharmasia), 0.3 ml 0.1% riboflavin and 2.5 g sucrose. The electrode paper strips were soaked with 1 M phosphoric acid for the anode and with 1 M sodium hydroxide for the cathode. Ten μl of the samples were applied to the gel surface 2 cm from the cathode using 5 x 6 mm filter paper (Whatman No. 3). Electrofocusing was conducted at a constant voltage of 2000 V for 240 min. The filter papers were removed after 60 min of focusing. During focusing the gel was cooled by circulating water at 4°C.

A sheet of nitrocellulose membrane (Bio–Rad) was placed on the gel surface and left for 60 min, applying a 1 kg weight. Following blotting the membrane was rinsed in 20 mM Tris/500 mM sodium chloride buffer, pH 7.5 (TBS), for 10 min and immersed in TBS containing 3% gelatin for 30 min. After washing in TBS for 15 min, the membrane was incubated for 60 min in goat anti–human GC serum (Atlantic Antibodies), diluted 500–fold with TBS containing 0.05% Tween 20 (TTBS). Next, the membrane was washed 3 times in TTBS for 30 min and incubated for 60 min in rabbit anti–goat IgG serum conjugated with alkaline phosphatase (Sigma) that was diluted 750–fold with TTBS. After 3 washes in TTBS for 30 min, the membrane was incubated in 50 ml staining solution (1.8 g sodium hydroxide and 3.7 g boric acid/1000 ml) containing 25 mg β–naphthyl phosphate, 25 mg Fast Blue BB salt and 60 mg magnesium sulfate for a few minutes.

RESULTS AND DISCUSSION

Figures 1 and 2 show the isoelectric focusing patterns of GC in samples of native serum, neuraminidase–treated serum, native semen and neuraminidase–treated semen from the same individuals. By neuraminidase treatment of the serum samples, the anodic bands of GC 1F and of GC 1S disappeared whereas the cathodic bands of GC 1F and of GC 1S and the GC 2 band remained unchanged. In semen samples, the GC 2 type exhibited 2 bands: the main GC 2 band and another fast band which focused at the position of

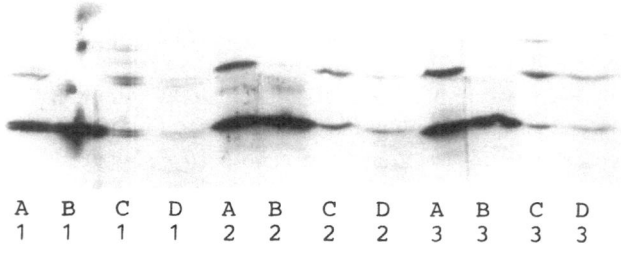

A	B	C	D	A	B	C	D	A	B	C	D
1	1	1	1	2	2	2	2	3	3	3	3

Fig. 1. A: native serum, B: neuraminidase–treated serum, C: native semen, D: neuraminidase–treated semen. 1: 1F1S, 2: 1F, 3: 1S. The anode is at the top.

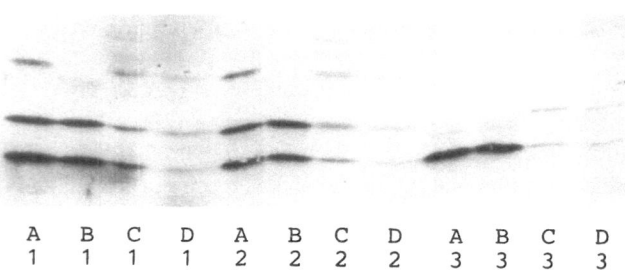

A	B	C	D	A	B	C	D	A	B	C	D
1	1	1	1	2	2	2	2	3	3	3	3

Fig. 2. A: native serum, B: neuraminidase–treated serum, C: native semen, D: neuraminidase–treated semen. 1: 2–1F, 2: 2–1S, 3: 2. The anode is at the top.

the cathodic band of GC 1F. The GC 2–1F type thus showed a three–band pattern, and the GC 2–1S type a four–band pattern. Moreover, some minor bands appeared towards the anode. When the semen samples were incubated with neuraminidase, these minor bands disappeared, but the double bands of GC 1F and of GC 1S as well as the above two GC 2 bands were not altered. It seems therefore that the seminal GC is devoid of sialic acid.

All the seminal stains examined were subtyped for GC at 4°C for periods of up to 10 weeks, at room temperature for periods of up to 8 weeks, and at 37°C for periods of up to 5 weeks. Figure 3 shows the isoelectric focusing pattern of GC in seminal stains stored for 1 week at room temperature. Our results for the determination limits are superior to those of Pötsch–Schneider and Klein (1988) who, using isoelectric focusing in an ultrathin immobilized pH gradient gel, demonstrated the GC patterns in seminal stains stored for 2 weeks at room temperature.

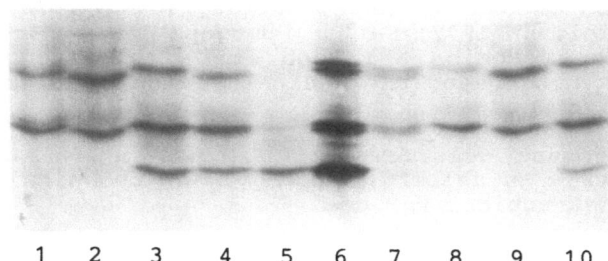

Fig. 3. 1: 1F, 2: 1S, 3: 2–1F, 4: 2–1S, 5: 2, 6: standard (mix of GC 1F1S and 2), 7: 1F1S, 8: 1F, 9: 1S, 10: 2–1F. The anode is at the top.

Isoelectric focusing and immunoblotting combined with neuraminidase digestion permit reliable GC subtyping from seminal stains stored for at least 5 weeks. The technique is simple and economical, and requires no specific equipment as compared with the immobilized isoelectric focusing method. The GC system provides a useful genetic marker for the forensic individualization of seminal stains.

REFERENCES

Cleve H. and Patutschnick W. (1979) Neuraminidase treatment reveals sialic acid differences in certain genetic variants of the Gc system (vitamin–D–binding protein). *Hum. Genet.*, 47, 193–198.

Constans J. and Viau M. (1977) Group–specific component: Evidence for two subtypes of the Gc[1] gene. *Science*, 198, 1070–1071.

Hirschfeld J. (1959) Immunoelectrophoretic demonstration of qualitative differences in human sera and their relation to the haptoglobin. *Acta Pathol. Micobiol. Scand.*, 47, 160–168.

Pötsch–Schneider L. and Klein H. (1988) Subtyping of group specific component (GC) in human semen, blood and vaginal fluids by isoelectric focusing in immobilized pH gradients. *Electrophoresis*, 9, 602–605.

SIMULTANEOUS FOCUSING OF PGM1 AND ACP PHENOTYPES USING
MINIATURIZED GELS AND 3-ELECTRODE TECHNIQUE

W. Kuchheuser, D. Krause

Institute for Forensic Medicine, University of Magdeburg
Leipziger Str. 44, D-39120 Magdeburg/FRG

Phosphoglucomutase (PGM1) and acid erythrocyte phosphatase (ACP) have been suitable erythrocyte enzyme markers in forensic paternity testing since their first description (Hopkinson, Spencer, Harris 1963; Spencer, Hopkinson, Harris, 1964). After the discovery of PGM_1-suballeles, IEF has been established as the method of choice (Bark, Harris, Firth 1976; Kühnl, Schmidtmann, Spielmann 1977; Sutton, Burgess 1978). In the present paper, we describe a method for simultaneous PGM1-subtyping and ACP-typing using ultrathin-layer gels and a reduced interelectrode distance.

We used ready-to-use precast gels SERVALYT[R] PRECOTES[R] PGM Kit (Cat. No. 42888; Serva, Heidelberg, FRG). For technical details see producers instructions for use.

Deviating from the usual procedure, the gels are horizontally divided by placing the cathode strip in the central position and the anode strips on the outer edges of the gel resulting in two gel halves with a common cathode and a distance of 5 cm to each anode.
Electrical parameters and running conditions have been adapted to the changed gel configuration: I= 10 mA, U= 2000 V, P= 10 W; 30 Vh (appr. 30 min.) prefocusing, up to 90 Vh (appr. 30 min.) focusing with samples, and up to 1200 Vh (appr. 1:30 h) focusing without samples. Cooling temperature is 8 °C.
Fresh or stored (-70 °C) stroma-free hemolysates are placed with 4 x 3 mm filter paper pieces (Desaga/FRG, No. 121231) 1 cm apart from the anodal strips.

After the focusing run, the gel is cut into two halves along the cathode strip. The detection steps take place for PGM1 and ACP in the upper, and the lower gel half, respectively. In this way, disturbancies caused by e. g. the considerable difference of the pH-optimum of the enzymes are avoided. The one half of the gel is covered with filter paper soaked in a solution of methylumbelliferylphosphate (solved in citrate buffer, pH 4.8), the other one with an agarose overlay (Sutton and Burgess 1978).
After 15 minutes at, 37 °C, the ACP-spots are visible under ultraviolet light. The PGM-spots appear as violet bands after about 30 minutes at 37 °C in a dark place.

The band configuration of the ACP phenotypes differs from that after conventional electrophoresis as described by other authors (Budowle 1984; Burdett and Whitehead 1977; Divall 1983; Dorrill and Sutton 1983). The A-band is located close to the focused hemoglobin near the cathode, whereas the B-band is

near to the anodal side, and the C-band more in the middle.
Fig. 1 shows the band configuration of both markers
schematically.
There is a marked difference between the PGM1 1A, 1B, 2B and
2A band concerning their position. Despite the reduced
resolving power using 5 cm interelectrode distance the
phenotypes of both markers are easy to differentiate without
any risk of mistyping. There is no need to use separators to
flatten the pH gradient (Gill and Sutton 1985).

The optimized method described here allows the typing of more
than 40 hemolysates per run for each marker or the double
number for one marker. The costs and the desired time are
reduced considerably.

After more than 1 year of use the three-electrode-technique
has turned out to be an economical and reliable procedure for
routine work. It is possible to use the 3-electrode-technique
for other markers, e. g. group specific component, transferrin
(Kuchheuser and Krause 1993), and coagulation factor 13B, too.

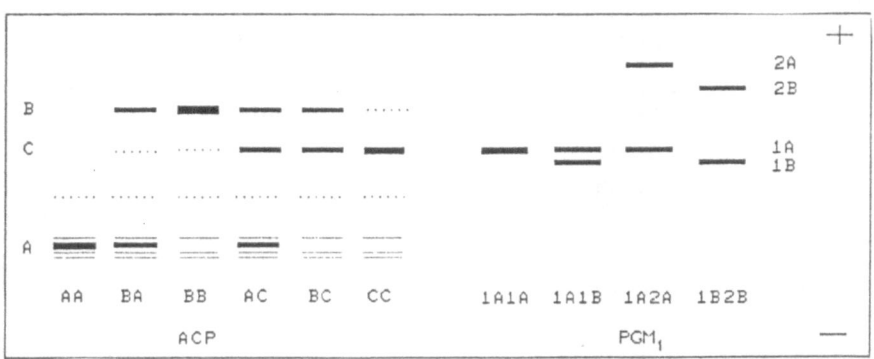

Fig 1: Schematic representation of ACP and PGM bands

References

Bark JE, Harris MJ, Firth MJ (1976) Typing of the common PGM1 variants using isoelectric focusing - a new interpretation of the PGM_1 system. Forens Sci Soc 16:115-120

Budowle B (1984) Rapid electrofocusing of erythrocyte acid phosphatase. Electrophoresis 5:254-255

Burdett PE, Whitehead PH (1977) The separation of the phenotypes of phosphoglucomutase, erythrocyte acid phosphatase, and some hemoglobin variants by isoelectric focusing. Analyt Biochem 77:419-428

Divall GB (1981) Studies on use of isoelectric focusing as a method of phenotyping erythrocyte acid phosphatase. For Sc Int 18:67-78

Dorrill MJ, Sutton JG (1983) Simultaneous isoelectric focusing of EAP and PGM_1 on 0.15 mm polyacrylamide gels. J For Sc Soc 23:131-134

Gill P, Sutton JG (1985) Enhanced resolution (PGM_1) by the addition of a separator to ultrathin isoelectric focusing gels. Electrophoresis 6:23-26

Hopkinson DA, Spencer N, Harris H (1963) Red cell acid phosphatase variants: A new human polymorphism. Nature (Lond) 199:969-971

Kuchheuser W, Krause D (1993) Possibilities for optimized representation of protein markers by isoelectric focusing. IAFS Düsseldorf, 22.-28.8.1993, 121

Kühnl P, Schmidtmann U, Spielmann W (1977) Evidence for two additional common allels at the PGM1 locus (Phosphoglucomutase-E.C.2.7.5.1). Hum Genet 35:219-223

Spencer N, Hopkinson DA, Harris H (1964) Phosphoglucomutase polymorphism in man. Nature 204:742-745

Sutton JG, Burgess R (1978) Genetic evidence for four common alleles at the phosphoglucomutase-1 locus (PGM_1) detectable by isoelectric focusing. Vox Sang 34:97-103

PLATELET & GRANULOCYTE ALLOANTIGEN TYPING USING SEQUENCE-SPECIFIC PRIMER (SSP) PCR AMPLIFICATION

C.Phillips, P. J. Lincoln, T. Annan, A. Waters*, J. Chapman* & M. Murphy*

Haematology Department, London Hospital Medical College
and *St. Bartholomews Hospital Medical College, London, U.K.

INTRODUCTION

A polymerase chain reaction (PCR) amplification technique has been investigated for the phenotyping of two medically important polymorphic loci: the platelet alloantigen marker HPA1 and the granulocyte alloantigen marker NA. HPA1 phenotyping is important in predicting the development of alloimmune thrombocytopenia (Metcalfe & Waters 1993). NA phenotyping similarly facilitates the prediction of allo- & autoimmune neutropenia (Stein *et al* 1994). Both systems have been previously phenotyped using serological techniques which require isolation of specific cell types from blood samples - a method which is particularly difficult with fetal or neonatal samples and requires reagents of limited availability. In this study, the usefulness of each locus in paternity analysis was assessed by studying false family trios constructed by using an unrelated individual as the putative father. Twenty five meioses in the form of the mother : child pairs in the above trios were analysed for mutations and mode of inheritance. A population database of 60 Caucasians was analysed for any deviation from Hardy Weinberg equilibrium.

MATERIALS & METHODS

Both HPA1 and NA are diallelic systems which allow the use of sequence specific primers in paired PCR reactions for each sample - one reaction in each pair containing the primer complimentary to one of the two alleles found in the system. Samples are subsequently scored for presence or absence of the appropriate PCR product using agarose electrophoresis.

The technique of sequence specific primer PCR relies on the principle that a single base mismatch between the 3' terminal base of the primer and the target sequence will block progress of the Taq1 polymerase, which, unlike other polymerases, is unable to repair single base mismatches efficiently. Thus, alleles differing by only one base can be distinguished, since a mismatch will result in very low levels of amplification compared to those produced when primer and target site match precisely.

In the case of HPA1, the two alleles differ at a single base in position 196 of intron 2 of the GPIIIa gene (allele 1a = T, allele 1b = C) (Newman *et al* 1989).

The NA locus has 3 distinct base substitutions which distinguish the 2 alleles, occurring within intron EC-1 of the FcRIII-1 gene; so primers exploiting the base mismatches at 2 of these sites can initiate amplification at different positions to give a product of a distinct size for each of the two alleles (Stein *et al* 1994).

Samples: Blood samples of mother : child pairs from paternity investigations performed at the LHMC were used. Samples from medical students were used as fathers to construct false family trios and as additional samples for the database. All samples were identified as Caucasian from photographs.

DNA Extraction: DNA was extracted using 5% chelating resin (Lareu *et al* 1994).

Primers: HPA $^{1A}/_{1B}$ 5' TCA GGT CAC AGC GAG GTG AGG CC$^A/_G$ 3'
         HPA common   5' CTG CAG GAG GTA GAG AGT CGC CAT AG 3'
         NA 1   5' CAG TGG TTT CAC AAT GTG AA 3'
         NA 2   5' CAA TGG TAC AGC GTG CTT 3'
         NA common   5' ATG GAC TTC TAG CTG CAC 3'

Amplification: HPA1 : 98°C x 1 min.   NA: 95°C x 1 min.
                  68°C x 1 min.   30 cycles   68°C x 2 mins.   26 cycles
                  72°C x 1 min.   72°C x 1 min.
                  (final extension - 5 mins)   (final extension - 5 mins)

       Both systems : 25µl PCR reaction volumes with 10µl DNA extract.
       All primers at 0.5µM and nucleotides at 200mM. 1.0U of Taq per amp.

Electrophoresis: 12µl of PCR sample was electrophoresed in 1.6% FMC Seakem LE®
               agarose stained with ethidium bromide. 8 volts / cm. x 30 mins.

RESULTS

Typical results for HPA1 and NA are shown in figures 1 and 2. Since low levels of amplification *can* occur when primer and target site mismatch, faint non-specific bands can be found with some samples. However there is relatively low levels of activity in comparison to bands produced when primer and target site match, so that the relative intensity of bands can be important in the interpretation of results. Both bands should be of equal intensity and when one band is relatively weak this cannot be considered to provide evidence for presence of the corresponding allele. With NA typing, non specific amplification products can result in additional bands but these would not be confused with the true NA products.

In order to provide an indication that the PCR reaction was working correctly, Human growth hormone (HGH) primers have been used by some workers as an internal DNA control for each PCR reaction : producing a monomorphic band of similar size (439 bp) to both HPA & NA bands. Our experience suggested difficulties in obtaining suitable concentrations of control primers in the reaction mix to avoid competition between HPA or NA primers and the HGH primers. In many respects, the primer bands, clearly discernable in figure 1, act as a control.

The results of the phenotyping of 60 unrelated Caucasians (medical students & mothers from the false family trios) and the analysis of 25 false family trios for each system are outlined in tables 1 & 2.

Both systems produced phenotypes in expected ratios, with no deviation from Hardy Weinberg equilibrium.

Each system gave clear indications of normal Mendelian inheritance between the mother and child in all the families studied.

The exclusion rates are similar to those predicted by the allele frequencies determined from the population survey in each system.

FIGURE 1. HPA typing (left to right : +/-, +/+, +/+, -/+, -/+ = 1a, weak 1a1b, 1a1b, 1b, 1b)

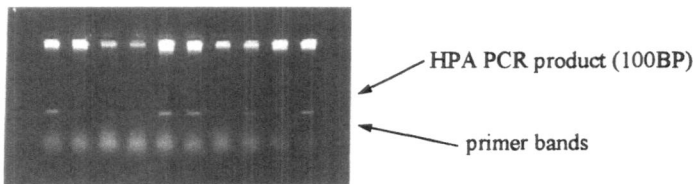

HPA PCR product (100BP)

primer bands

FIGURE 2. NA typing (left to right : +/+, +/+, +/+, +/-, -/+ = 2.1, 2.1, 2.1, 1, 2)

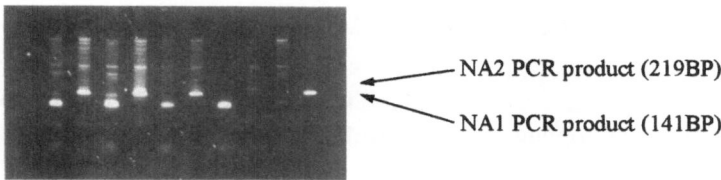

NA2 PCR product (219BP)

NA1 PCR product (141BP)

TABLE 1. HPA1 Analysis.

Phenotype	Obs. (%)	Expected	
1a	40 (66.7)	**40.05**	HPA 1a = **0.817**
1a1b	18 (30.0)	17.94	HPA 1b = **0.183**
1b	2 (3.3)	**2.01**	χ^2 = < **0.001 (not Significant)**

Observed No.of Exclusions : **3/25 (12%)**   Expected No. of Exclusions : **12.7%**

TABLE 2. NA Analysis

Phenotype	Obs (%)	Expected	
1	9 (15.0)	9.6	NA 1 = **0.4**
2.1	30 (50.0)	28.8	NA 2 = **0.6**
2	21 (35.0)	21.6	χ^2 = **0.104 (not significant)**

Observed No.of Exclusions : **4/25 (16%)**   Expected No. of Exclusions : **18.2%**

SUMMARY

It appears that SSP-PCR testing for the identification of the alleles in these two polymorphic systems provides a quick and simple method, where previous availability of reagents and adequacy of blood samples have made such typing difficult by other techniques.

The detection of the two polymorphisms described here and the further platelet and white cell polymorphic markers for which primers are becoming available, will provide a group of systems which could be used in problems of identification.

ACKNOWLEDGMENT

The authors would like to thank Dr. J. Bux, Giessen, GDR, Dr. M. Guttridge, NBTS, Cardiff and Dr. P. Metcalfe, NIBSC, Potters Bar, UK for the generous gifts of primers.

REFERENCES

Lareu MV, Phillips CP, Carracedo A, Lincoln PJ, Syndercombe Court DS & Thomson J *For. Sci. Int.* (1994) **66** 41-22.
Metcalfe P & Waters AH *Br. J. Haematol.* (1993) **85** 227-229.
Newman PJ, Derbes RS & Aster RH *J. Clin. Invest.* (1992) **83** 1778-1781
Stein EL, Bux J, Santoso S & Mueller-Eckhardt C *Br. J. Haematol.* (1994) **87** 428-430

Plasma protein markers in S.Tomé e Príncipe

M.F. Santos[1], A. Amorim[1], L. Manco[2] and M.J. Trovoada[2]

[1]Inst. Antropologia, Univ.Porto and IPATIMUP, 4050 Porto, Portugal
[2]Dept. Antropologia, Univ.Coimbra, 3000 Coimbra, Portugal

Systems and loci: BF (properdin factor B, 6p21.3)
GC (group specific component; 4q12-q13)
TF (transferrin, 3q21)

Population and sample sizes:
S.Tomé e Príncipe (Gulf of Guinea); BF: N=50; GC: N=77; TF: N=59

Methods:
Samples: chord blood plasmas from unrelated newborns.
Phenotyping: agarose gel electrophoresis (BF and TF types, essentially according to Hauptmann *et al.*, 1977) or isoelectric focusing (GC and TF subtypes, by the methods of Constans and Cleve, 1988 and Budowle, 1987, respectively, with minor modifications).

Results:

Observed phenotypes:

BF phenotypes	Obs.	GC phenotypes	Obs.	TF phenotypes	Obs.
F-F	16	1F-1F	43	C1-C1	41
F-Fv	1	1F-1S	10	C1-C2	13
F-S	19	1F-2	9	C1-D	4
Fv-Fv	1	1F-1C	4	C2-D	1
Fv-S	3	1S-1S	4		
S-S	9	1S-2	6		
S-Sv	1	2-2	1		
P=0.28		P=0.06		P=0.71	

Allele frequencies

BF Allele	Freq.	GC Allele	Freq.	TF Allele	Freq.
F	0.520	1F	0.708	C1	0.839
Fv	0.060	1S	0.156	C2	0.119
S	0.410	2	0.110	D	0.042
Sv	0.010	1C	0.026		

Comments:

Fv and Sv stand for fast and slow variants of BF; 1C stands for a variant cathodal to GC*1S.

Gene frequencies estimated in our sample were compared with those from West Africa (compiled by Parra *et al.*, 1995) and Cabo Verde Islands, another archipelago colonised by the Portuguese. For the three loci an intermediate situation was found, demonstrating that Caucasian influence in S.Tomé e Príncipe gene pool was much smaller than in Cabo Verde.

Particularly interesting are: (a) the absence of TF*C3 and relatively high frequencies of (b) GC*1C and (c) BF*Fv variants.

References

Constans J, Cleve H (1988) The group specific component / vitamin D binding protein (GC / DBP) system in the analysis of disputed paternities. Electrophoresis. 9: 349-403.

Budowle B (1987) Improved separation of the common transferrin variants in gels containing pH 5-7 Ampholines and HEPES. Electrophoresis. 8: 210-212.

Hauptmann G, Wertheimer E, Tongio MM, Mayer S (1977) Bf polymorphism: Another variant (S0.8). Hum. Hered. 36: 109-111.

Parra EJ, Teixeira Ribeiro JC, Caeiro JLB, Riveiro A (1995) Genetic structure of the population of Cabo Verde (West Africa): evidence of substantial European admixture. Am J Phys Anthrop. 97: 381-389.

Acknowledgements This work was partially supported by CNCDP (Comissão Nacional para as Comemorações dos Descobrimentos Portugueses, research contract nº 70).

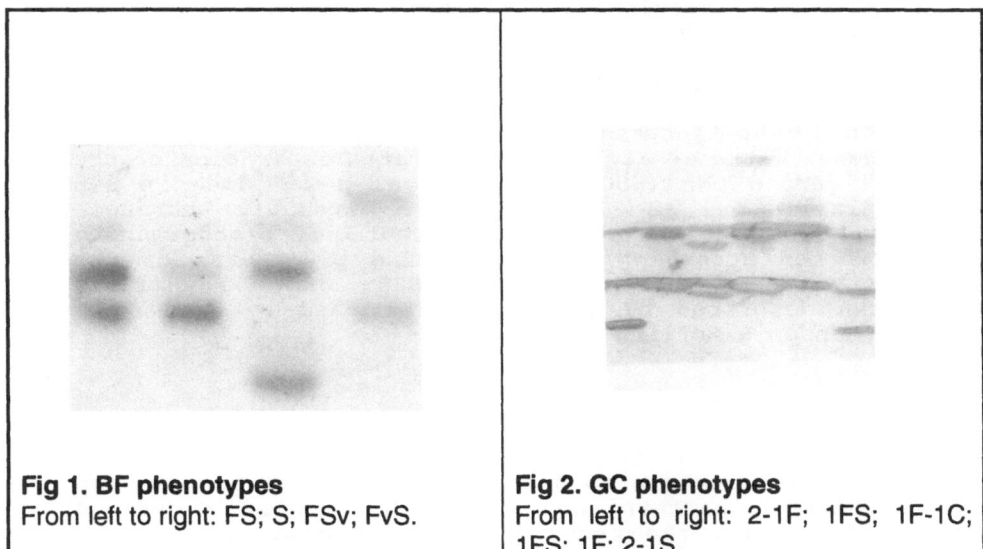

Fig 1. BF phenotypes
From left to right: FS; S; FSv; FvS.

Fig 2. GC phenotypes
From left to right: 2-1F; 1FS; 1F-1C; 1FS; 1F; 2-1S.

DETECTION OF A SILENT GC ALLELE IN A DANISH MOTHER AND CHILD

M.Thymann, H.E.Hansen and J.Dissing

Department of Forensic Genetics
Institute of Forensic Medicine, University of Copenhagen,
11 Frederik V´s Vej, DK-2100 Copenhagen, Denmark

INTRODUCTION

The Group-Specific Component (GC, vitamin-D binding protein, DBP) is a polymorphic plasmaprotein still used for paternity investigations in many laboratories (theoretical chance of exclusion 31%). In a Danish case of disputed paternity inverse homozygosity was observed in a mother and her child by isoelectric focusing. Extended investigations including conventional bloodtyping systems, RFLP- and AMP/FLP-examinations were carried out. PCR/SSCP analysis of a DNA fragment containing two mutation sites specific for the alleles GC 1F, GC 1S and GC 2 in exon 11 of the GC gene was also performed.

MATERIALS AND METHODS

Conventional GC typing was carried out by isoelectric focusing in polyacrylamide gel in a non-linear pH 4.5-5.5 gradient. Visualization was performed by immunoblotting and staining with indolylphosphate/nitrobluetetrazolium using rabbit anti-human GC as the first antibody and phosphatase conjugated swine anti-rabbit immunoglobulin as the second antibody. For GC typing by PCR/SSCP, amplification of exon 11 was performed by the use of 25- and 28-mer primers (Dissing unpublished result) designed from the known DNA sequence of the GC gene (Witke et al.) Electrophoretic separation of the single stranded DNA (SSCP, Orita et al.) was done in 20% polyacrylamide gel at 12°C using the automatic Pharmacia Phast System and silver staining. Conventional bloodgrouping was performed according to the routine procedures of the laboratory. The methods used for D1S80- and RFLP-analysis have been described by Thymann et al. and by Morling & Hansen; Hansen & Morling.

RESULTS AND DISCUSSION

The GC phenotypes of the mother (GC 2) and child (GC 1S) obtained by isoelectric focusing are shown in figure 1. The electrophoretic pattern gave no indication of decreased protein level and the results were confirmed by repeated examination of new samples. GC genotyping at the DNA level is possible due to the existence of allele specific base differences at codons 432 and 436 in exon 11 of the GC gene (Reynolds and Sensabaugh). Using PCR and SSCP a 186 bp-DNA fragment spanning this exon was analyzed. The GC type of the mother was detected as GC 1S,2 and that of the child as GC 1S (figure 2). The extended investigation comprised nine conventional bloodgrouping systems (ABO, MNS, RH, HP, PGM1, ACP1, GPT, ESD, GLO), seven VNTR single locus system D2S44 *YNH24*, D4S139 *pH30*, D5S43 *MS8*, D7S21 *MS31*, D7S22 *g3*, D12S11 *MS43a*, D16S309 *MS205*) and one AMPFLP system (D1S80 *MCT118*). The results obtained are given in table 1a and 1b. The calculated probability of maternity exeeded 10.000 to 1. The results of the SSCP analysis showed that the silent GC allele in the mother and child is not caused by a major deletion involving the entire GC gene since exon 11 appeared to be intact.

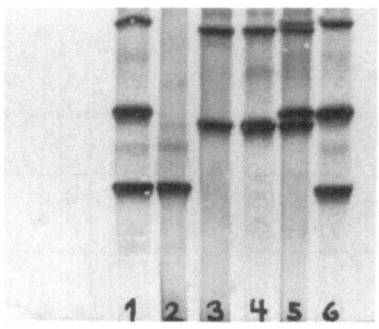

<u>Figure 1</u>
GC phenotypes of mother, child and several controls as obtained by IEF in polyacrylamide gel followed by immunoblotting. Anode at the top. (1) GC 1F,2; (2) mother GC 2; (3) child GC 1S; (4) GC 1S; (5) GC 1F,1S; (6) GC 1F,2.

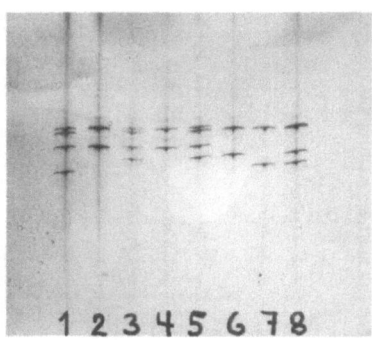

<u>Figure 2</u>
GC genotypes of mother, child and controls as obtained by PCR/SSCP analysis of a 186 bp DNA fragment of exon 11. (1) GC 1F,1S; (2) GC 1S; (3) mother GC 1S,2 (4) child GC 1S (5) GC 1S,2; (6) GC 2; (7) GC 1F; (8) GC 1F,2.

Table 1a. Results obtained by bloodgrouping of a Danish mother and child.

	GC	ABO	MN Ss	RH	HP	PGM1	ACP1	GPT	ESD	GLO
Mother	**2** IEF **1S**PCR **2**SSCP	0	M ss	cc D Ee	2FS	1F	A	1 2	1	1
Child	**1S**	0	M ss	cc D EE	1F 2FS	1F	A	2	1	1 2

Table 1b. Results obtained by DNA-analysis of a Danish mother and child.

	D1 S80	D2 S44	D4 S139	D5 S43	D7 S21	D7 S22	D12 S11	D16 S309
Mother	18	4.26 4.80	4.20 7.23	5.16 8.37	5.38 8.70	6.61 9.01	5.27 8.88	1.59 3.03
Child	18 31	3.28 4.76	7.24 8.13	2.80 5.19	5.36 5.48	7.07 9.07	8.77 10.00	2.78 3.01

CONCLUSION

Inverse homozygosity was observed in a Danish mother and child by GC phenotyping. Using isoelectric focusing the type of the mother was GC 2 and the type of the child GC 1S. GC genotyping was performed by PCR/SSCP analysis of exon 11 of the GC gene. The mother and child were typed as GC 1S,2 and 1S, respectively. After extended investigations the probability of maternity exeeded 10.000 to 1. The silent GC allele is not due to a major deletion of the entire GC gene since exon 11 appeared to be intact.

REFERENCES

Hansen H E and Morling N: Paternity testing with VNTR DNA systems. II.Evaluation of 271 cases of disputed paternity with the VNTR systems D2S44, D5S43, D7S21, D7S22, and D12S11. Int J Leg Med (1993) 105:197-202.
Morling N, and Hansen H E: Paternity testing with VNTR DNA systems. I.Matching criteria and population frequencies of the VNTR systems D2S44, D5S43, D7S21, D7S22, and D12S11 in Danes. Int J Leg Med (1993) 105:189-196.
Orita M, Suzuki Y, Sekiya T, and Hayashi K: Rapid and sensitive detection of point mutations and DNA polymorphisms using the polymerase chain reaction. Genomics (1989) 5:874-879.
Reynolds R L, and Sensabaugh G F: Use of the polymerase chain reaction for typing GC variants. Adv. Forensic Haemogenet (1990 3: 158-161
Thymann M, Nellemann L J, Masumba G, Irgens-Møller L, and Morling N: Analysis of the locus D1S80 by amplified fragment length polymorphism technique (AMP-FLP). Frequency distribution in Danes. Intra and inter laboratory reproducibility of the technique. Forensic Sci Internat (1993) 60:47-56.
Witke W F, Gibbs P E M, Zielinski R, Yang F, Bowman B H, and Dugaiczyk A: Complete structure of the GC gene: Differences and similarities between members of the Albumin gene family. Genomics (1993) 16: 751-754.

ABH-RELATED ANTIGENS PARTICIPATE IN THE SPERMATOGENESIS OF CATS AND RATS

I. Ushiyama*, M. Yamada**, A. Tanegashima*, A. Nishimura*, M. Kane*, Y. Yamamoto* and K. Nishi*

* Department of Legal Medicine, Shiga University of Medical Science, Ohtsu, Shiga 520-21, Japan
** Department of Human Life Science, Seibo-Jogakuin Women's College, Fushimi, Kyoto, Japan

The ABH antigens were expressed in the secretory cells of many mammals(1), including humans. Although the allelic cDNA of ABO blood group had been cloned and sequenced(2), no clear explanation of the biological significance of the ABH and related antigens has been proposed. In this study we examined the distribution of ABH related antigens in the urogenital organs from cats and rats in order to pro mote better understanding on the biological significance of the antigens, using monoclonal antibodies (MoAbs) against the ABH and related antigens, and lectins. The results obtained from the present study suggested that the ABH and related antigens may play certain roles in the processes of development of spermatogenic system. In view of forensic practice, the importance of species identification prior to ABO blood grouping from seminal, saliva and urinal stains are stressed on the basis of the present results.

Materials and Methods

Tissue specimens of salivary glands and male reproductive organs from rats and cats were used in this study. Tissues from animals were obtained from the Institute for Experimental Animals of Shiga University of Medical Science. The specimens were fixed in 10% formalin, embedded in paraffin and sectioned serially at 5μm. The staining procedures were described previously(3), using anti A, B, H, Le^a, Le^b, Le^x, and Le^y MoAbs and Erythrina cristagalli(ECA), Helix Pomatia (HPA) and Glycine max(SBA) lectins conjugated with horseradish peroxidase. Anti A and B MoAbs were purchased from Ortho Diagnosis Systems (Raritan, N.J. USA) and anti H and Le x MoAbs were from Dako (Santa Barbara, Ca., USA). Anti Lea and Le b MoAbs were obtained from Signet Laboratories (Cambridge, MA, USA) and anti Le^y was from Nihon Koutai (Gumma, Japan). Lectins was obtained from E.Y. Laboratories (San Mateo, Ca.,USA).

Results

a) antigen expression in cats

The ABO grouping of animal individuals examined in this study could be determined by the reactivity of anti A, B and/or H MoAbs with secretory cells of salivary gland. Although all individuals of cats examined were grouped into blood group A, they were classified into two subgroups according to the difference in the distribution of A and H antigens in the submandibular gland. In one group of cats, A antigen was expressed both in the mucous and duct cells of the glands but the H antigen was found only in the duct cells. In another group, the pattern of the expression of these antigens was reverse, i.e. H antigen was expressed both in mucous and duct cells while A antigen was expressed only in the duct cells. Although similar difference in staining pattern with anti H or A MoAbs were also recognized in the serous cells of von Ebner's glands and lingual glands in the tongues, no difference was observed in the reproductive organs. The reactivity by anti A, H,Le^x and Le^y MoAbs in the collecting tubules of kidney was also recognized.

In the seminiferous tubules of cats, ECA specific for Galß(1-4)-GlcNAc (4) stained the spermatogonium, spermatocytes, spermatids and tail of elongate spermatids. The acrosome granule and nuclear cap of spermatids were clearly stained by ECA. The reactivity of SBA specific for Gal(1-3 or 1-4) GlcNAc (4) was observed strongly in the nuclear cap and acrosome granule of the spermatids, and feebly in spermatocytes. Anti A, B, H, Le^a, Le^b, Le^x and Le^y MoAbs and HPA specific for GalNAc(4) showed no reactivity in the seminiferous tubules including the Sertoli cells. ECA showed striking staining of the epithelial cells(ECs) of the ductuli efferentes, however, the intensity is declining towards the corpus and cauda epididymis. SBA showed good reactivity with the stereocila on the free surface of ductuli efferentes and weak or feeble with the ECs of the ductus epididymidis. Anti A, H, Le^x and Le^y MoAbs stained the ECs of the ductuli efferentes and/or ampulla epididymidis, showing mosaic reactivity with the cells. Although anti A MoAb and HPA showed intense reactivity with the ECs, spermatozoa and secretory fluid in the lumen of the epididymis, anti H, Le^x and Le^y MoAbs showed no reactivity with the ECs in the corpus and cauda epididimidis. We could not examined the reactivity by MoAbs and lectins in the prostates and seminal vesicles of cats because no tissues of the organs could be obtained.

b) antigen expression in rats

The blood groups of rats were determined to be blood group B and AB. In blood group AB rats, anti A MoAb stained secretory cells of submandibular glands and anti H MoAb stained secretory cells and duct cells. Anti B, Le^a, Le^b and Le^y MoAbs stained the duct cells of the glands. Anti Le^x MoAb showed no reactivity in the salivary glands.

ECA and SBA clearly stained the nuclear cap of spermatocytes and elongate spermatids in the seminiferous tubules, while the tail of the spermatids was not stained by these lectins. Although the intense staining by these lectins was observed in the epithelial cells of the ductuli efferentes, and in the ECs in the ampulla epididymidis, the instensity was declining towards the corpus and cauda epididymidis.

MoAbs used in this study showed no reactivity in the seminiferous tubules including the Sertoli cells. However, HPA lectin specific for GalNAc and blood group A antigen showed intensive reactivity in the testis and epidydimidis. HPA stained the spermatocytes, spermatids and tail of spermatids in the seminiferous tubules and the ECs, secretory fluid and spermatozoa in lumen from the ampulla to cauda epididymidis obtained from all the rats examined. Anti A MoAb showed weak reactivity with the ECs of epididymidis from some rats and the B and H antigens were not detected in the epididymidis of rats. Anti Le^y MoAb clearly stained the ECs of prostates and anti Le^x weakly stained the ECs of the ductus deferens. Anti H, Le^a and Le^b MoAbs showed feeble or no reactivity with the ECs of the prostates of rats. ECA and SBA stains also the ECs of the prostate. The patterns of the reactivity in the prostate varied considerably according to the MoAbs and Lectins.

Discussion

We demonstrated previously (5) that the ABH and related antigens were expressed in the salivary glands, taste bud cells and kidneys of some mammals. The antigens were also expressed in the epididymidis and prostates from rats and/or cats in this study. However, the patterns of distribution of these antigens varied considerably between animals and organs. Although Le^a, Le^b ,Le^x and/or Le^y antigens were expressed in rats as well as human tissues, Le^a and Le^b antigens were not detected in the tissues of cats. Blood group ABH antigens in human tissues are mainly carried by either type 1 or type 2 carbohydrate chains (6). The Le a and Le b antigens are type 1 and Le x and Le y antigens are type 2 based antigens, respectively. The results obtained indicate that both the type 1 and 2 carbohydrate chains of the ABH antigens were secreted in the tissues of humans and rats whereas only type 2 chain antigens were expressed in tissues of cats. The distribution patterns of ABH antigens in the submandibular gland of cats and rats were different from those of humans. In cats, the A antigen was secreted only in duct cells from one group and both in the mucous and duct cells from another group. In group AB rats, the A antigen was secreted in the mucous cells and the B antigen was secreted in duct cells. In addition, non secretor types were not observed in rats and cats examined. These results indicate that the genetic control systems of the tissue specific expression of the blood group antigens in humans might be quite different from those of other mammalian species. On the other hand, based on the results obtained in this study, we must emphasize that the species identification prior to ABO blood grouping is indispensable because forensic materials such as the stains from saliva, urine and seminal fluid might be contaminated with the fluid from indoor pets.

Intratesticular spermatogenesis and the subsequent epididymal maturation of the sperm are hallmarked by substantial morphological and biochemical changes accompanied by important cell-surface modifications[7]. Pattern of carbohydrate expression changed dramatically during the process of spermatogenesis. It is well known that SBA and ECA lectins show the specificity to the precursor structure of H antigen [4]. The finding of ABH, related antigens and the precursor substance recognized by ECA and/or SBA in the reproductive organs of rats and cats may provide an important clue to the role of these antigens in the processes of spermatogenesis of these animals. It has been suggested that Le^x antigen plays a role in cell adhesion of the early mouse embryo, since the Le^x antigen appeared in the developing embryo at the compaction stage [8]. Nomura et al.[9] detected blood group B active glycosphingolipids in Xenopus laevis eggs and suggested that the B antigen plays a role in the cell-adhesion process of Xenopus embryonic cells.

Summary

The distribution of ABH and related antigens in reproductive organs of male rats and cats was examined using histochemical methods. Although the reactivity of MoAbs against ABH related antigens with the tissues were different and varied among the animal species, the antigens were expressed in the epithelial cells of reproductive organs from animals inhabiting around humans. The results obtained in this study and previous ones indicate that in view of forensic practice, the species identification prior to ABO blood grouping in the stain analysis are indispensable to avoid mistyping due to contaminated materials from indoor pets.

Pattern of the reactivity with MoAbs against ABH and related antigens and lectins changed dramatically during the process of spermatogenesis. In the seminiferous tubules, the reactivity of ECA and SBA with the precursor substance was intensively observed and the reactivity was declining towards the epididymidis, while the reactivity of anti A and/or HPA in the epidydimidis was increasing. The reactivity of anti H, Le^x and Le^y MoAbs was observed in the ductuli efferentes or ampulla epididymidis of cats. The ABH and related-antigens secreted in the reproductive organs might be involved in the processes of spermatogenesis and sperm maturation of rats and cats.

Acknowledgments

This work was supported in part by Grant-in-Aid (No. 07670488) from the Ministry of Education, Science and Culture, Japan.

References

(1). Nishi K., Fukunaga T., Yamamoto Y., Yamada M., Kane M., Ito N. and Kawahara S. Adv. Forens. Hemoge. (1992) 4. 407-409.

(2). Yamamoto F., Marken J., Tsuji T., White T., Clausen H., and Hakomori S-H., J Biol Chem (1990) 265, 1146-1151

(3). Nishi K., Fukunaga T., Yamamoto Y., Yamada M., Kane M., Tanegashima A., Rand S., and Brinkmann B., Int J Legal Med (1992) 105, 75-80

(4). Ito N., and Hirota T., Progr Histochem Cytochem (1992) 25, 1-85.

(5). Nishi k., Tanegashima A., Ushiyama I., Ymamoto Y., Nishimura A., ans Yamada Y ., Proceedings of the 5th Indo-pacific congress on Legal Med and Forens Sci. (6). Ito N., Nishi K., Nakajima M., Okamura Y., and Hirota T., J Histochem. Cytochem., (1990) 38 1331 - 1340.

(7) Koehler J K., Arch Andro (1981) 6, 197-217.

(8). Gooi H.C., Feizi T., Kapadia A., Knowles B. B., Solter D., and Evans M. J., Nature, (1981) 292, 156 - 158

(9). Nomura K., Nakajou N., Hidari K., Nomura H., Murata M., Suzuki M., Yamana K., and Hirabayashi Y., Biochem. J. (1995) 306 821-827.

Species Identification by Analysis of the Genes for ABO Blood Group.

Yamada M[1], Ushiyama I[2], Sato M[3], Ueyama H[3], Ohkubo I[3], Nishimura A[2] and Nishi K[2]

[1] Department of Human Life Science, Seibo Jogakuin Women's College, Fukakusa, Fushimi-ku, Kyoto 612, Japan, and
Departments of [2] Legal Medicine and [3] Medical Biochemistry,
Shiga University of Medical Science, Seta-Tsukinowacho, Otsu 520-21, Japan.

INTRODUCTION

The species identification is of a great importance in the forensic field. The immunological techniques have been utilized to distinguish human from other animal samples, such as blood stain, saliva or seminal fluid, however a keen method for identification of the origin of a sample has not been established. We have previously reported that ABH(O) blood group substances are detected in various species and that the lectin- and immuno-histochemistry can be available for species identification from tissue particles (Nishi 1992). It is considered that some animals possess the genes homologous to those for human ABO blood group. We have also reported the determination of ABO genotypes with DNAs extracted from fresh blood or formalin-fixed, paraffin-embedded tissues by PCR amplification and restriction enzymes digestion (Yamada 1994), depending on the polymorphism of the gene encoding blood group A-transferase. Here we describe that the DNA analysis of the genes for ABO blood group might be a tool of species identification.

MATERIALS AND METHODS

DNAs were prepared (Sambrook 1989) from the blood of human, Japanese monkeys, pigs, cats, rabbits, Chinese hamsters, rats (Wister and Fischer), mastomys and mice and from the liver of goldfishes.

Amplification with Taq DNA polymerase (Sambrook 1989) was performed with oligonucleotide primers 1) and 2), 3) and 4) (Lee 1992) and primers 5) and 6), those were designated as PCR-1+2, PCR-3+4 and PCR-5+6, respectively. Primers 1) and 2) were put across nucleotide 258 (a single base deletion site of the O allele) and primers 3) and 4) across nucleotide 700 (a single base substitution site in the A and B alleles) of cDNA at the human ABO gene locus (Yamamoto 1990). Primers 5) and 6) amplify the region includes three single base substitution sites, nucleotides 700, 793 and 800, in the human A and B alleles. Sequences of the primers used are as follows; 1) CACCGTGGAAGGATGTCCT C, 2) AATGTCCACAGTCACTCGCC, 3) TGGAGATCCTGACTCCGCTG, 4) GTAGAAATCGCCCTCGTCCT, 5) CTGGTGTGCGTGGAC and 6) ACCTCTTGCACCGACCC.

Amplified DNAs were electrophoresed on 6% polyacrylamide gels and the bands were visualized by ethidium bromide staining (Sambrook 1989).

The PCR products from human DNA, labelled with digoxigenin-dUTP by random primed, were used as probes. After electrophoresis, the DNAs were transferred on to Nylon membranes (Hybond N+, Amersham) followed by hybridization with the

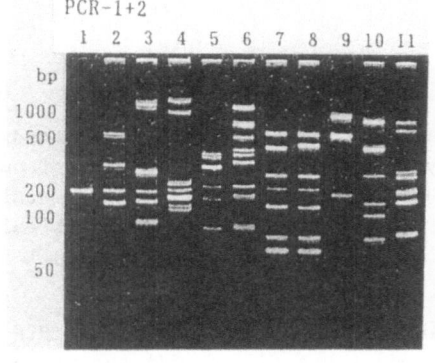

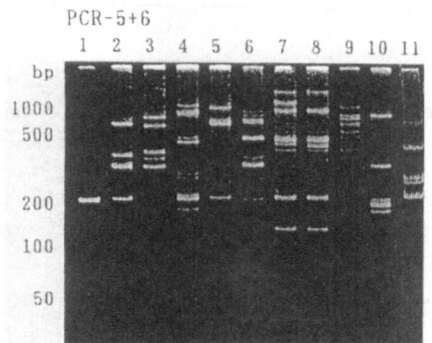

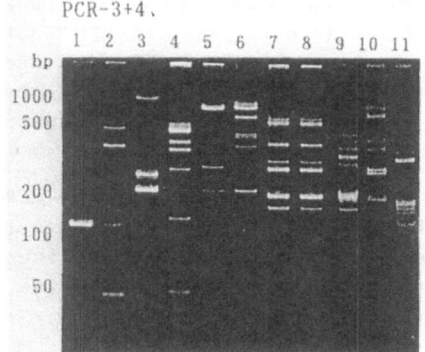

Figure 1. Electrophoretic Pattern of the PCR Product.

1; human, 2; Japanese monkey, 3; pig, 4; cat, 5; rabbit, 6; Chinese hamster,7; rat (Wistar), 8; rat (Fischer), 9; mastomys, 10; mouse and 11; goldfish.

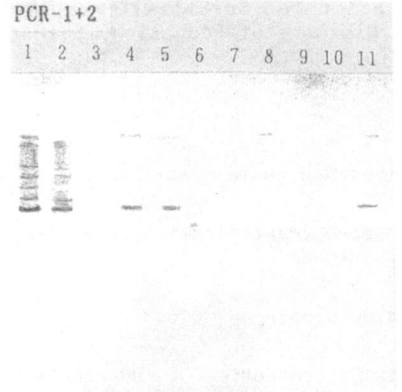

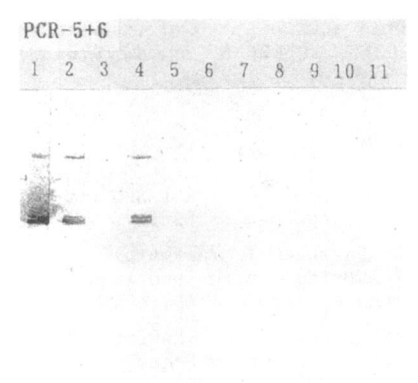

Figure 2. Hybridization Analysis.

Filters were washed in 0.1x SSC-0.1% SDS at 68 °C.

See the legend for Fig. 1.

corresponding probes. The filters were washed (Sambrook 1989) in 0.1x SSC-0.1% SDS at 68 °C or 2x SSC-0.1% SDS at 42 °C and the hybrids were detected by enzyme immunoassy (DNA Labelling & Detection Kit, Boehringer).

RESULTS AND DISCUSSION

Electrophoretic Analysis of The PCR Products (Fig. 1)

Every pair of primers presented a single band from human DNA and several bands from the other animals electrophoretically. The band patterns obtained from each species in PCR-1+2, PCR-3+4 and PCR-5+6 were distinct and no individual difference was observed (data not shown). Two strains of rat had identical electrophoretic patterns.

Hybridization Analysis (Fig. 2)

In Japanese monkey, cat, rabbit and goldfish, the amplified fragments in PCR-1+2 with the length as same as the human product hybridized with the probe, the human product, when washing at high stringency. After washed at lower stringency, the hybrids were observed in all the animals examined (data not shown). The PCR-3+4 fragments from mastomys and goldfish did not hybridize with the corresponding probe at both high and low washing stringencies (data not shown)and the PCR-5+6 fragments from Japanese monkey and cat showed hybridization.

Combination of the electrophoretic and hybridization analyses of the PCR products might be utilized for species identification. It is considered that the species identification followed by ABO typing might be desired when analyzing the stains of body fluids, such as saliva, semen and urine. Moreover, the sesults might explain the ABO substances detected in animals.

ACKNOWLEDGEMENTS

This work was supported in part by Grants-in-Aid for Scientific Research (#04670353, #05670387 and #07670488) from the Ministry of Education, Science and Culture of Japan.

REFERENCES

Lee JC-I, Chang J-G (1992) ABO genotyping by polymerase chain reaction. J Forens Sciences 37:1269-1275

Nishi K, Fukunaga T, Yamamoto Y, et al (1992) Species identification from tissue particles using lectin- and immuno-histochemical methods. Adv Forens Haemogenet4:407-409

Sambrook J, Fritsch EF, Maniatis T (1989) Molecular Cloning, 2nd edn. Cold Harbor Laboratory Press, New York

Yamada M, Yamamoto Y, Tanegashima A, et al (1994) Determination of ABO genotypes with DNA extracted from formalin-fixed, paraffin-embedded tissues. Int J Legal Med 106:285-287

Yamamoto F, Marken J, Tsuji T, et al (1990) Cloning and characterization of DNA complementary to human UDP-GalNAc:Fucα1$\rightarrow$2Galα1$\rightarrow$3GalNAc transferase (histo-blood group A transferase) mRNA. J Biol Chem 265:1146-1151

8 Population Genetics

Statistical Issues in DNA Profiling

B.S. Weir and J.S. Buckleton*

Program in Statistical Genetics, Department of Statistics
North Carolina State University, Raleigh NC 27695-8203, USA

INTRODUCTION

DNA profiles consist of pairs of variants, or alleles, at one or more genetic loci. If the profile from an evidentiary sample does not match that from a suspect in a crime, then the suspect is excluded from having contributed to the sample. When the two profiles do match, however, then the suspect is not excluded from being a contributor. In this case, it may be necessary to attach some numerical weight to the evidence of a match, and statistical issues arise.

As discussed by Evett and Buckleton in this volume, and as described fully by Aitken (1995), the appropriate weighting of evidence is by means of a likelihood ratio. If E is the evidence of matching DNA profiles, and C and $\bar{C}$ are alternative explanations for that evidence, then the relative merits of the two explanations can be compared by the ratio of the probabilities of the evidence under each:

$$L \;=\; \frac{\Pr(E|C)}{\Pr(E|\bar{C})}$$

A court can be told that the evidence is L times more likely under C than under $\bar{C}$.

It is often the case that the prosecution explanation C fully explains the evidence, in which case $\Pr(E|C) = 1$ and L becomes the reciprocal of the probability of E under the defense explanation $\bar{C}$. A major exception to this simplification is when the evidentiary sample gives a profile that must have come from more than one person but the crime was committed by one person. For single stains, however, it should be straightforward to determine the probability of the evidence under $\bar{C}$ from the principles of population genetics. Translating a theoretical probability into a numerical estimate on the basis of samples of profiles requires statistical methods.

SINGLE STAINS

Suppose the profile $A_i A_j$ is found for locus **A** from both an evidentiary sample and a suspect S. The circumstances of the crime imply that the sample was left by the perpetrator P, so that the evidence E can be written $S = A_i A_j, P = A_i A_j$. The two explanations are

$$
\begin{array}{lll}
\text{Prosecution} & C: & S = P \\
\text{Defense} & \bar{C}: & S \neq P
\end{array}
$$

The likelihood ratio is

$$
\begin{aligned}
L \;&=\; \frac{\Pr(S = A_i A_j, P = A_i A_j | S = P)}{\Pr(S = A_i A_j, P = A_i A_j | S \neq P)} \\[2mm]
&=\; \frac{\Pr(P = A_i A_j | S = A_i A_j, S = P)\,\Pr(S = A_i A_j | S = P)}{\Pr(P = A_i A_j | S = A_i A_j, S \neq P)\,\Pr(S = A_i A_j | S \neq P)} \\[2mm]
&=\; \frac{1}{\Pr(P = A_i A_j | S = A_i A_j, S \neq P)}
\end{aligned}
$$

* ESR:Forensic, Mt Albert Science Centre
Private Bag 92-021, Auckland, NEW ZEALAND

This last expression is from a "suspect-anchored" viewpoint, and requires knowledge of the probability with which an unknown person P has the profile when it is known that a different person S has that profile. It has been the assumption that this probability does not depend on S since $\bar{C}$ says that S and P are assumed to be different people. This assumption is obviously false if S and P are related, meaning that they share common recent ancestors, and it is also false when S and P are related in an evolutionary sense. The latter dependence is more of a factor when S and P belong to the same population, particularly if that population is small.

Suspect and Perpetrator Independent

Evidently the expression

$$L = \frac{1}{\Pr(P = A_i A_j)}$$

is a very special case, even though it is the one in general use. The probability refers to people in some population of "potential perpetrators" defined by the circumstances of the crime. Although genetic frequencies are determined by evolutionary forces, and will therefore differ between ethnic groups, it is unlikely that the circumstances of the crime will describe the ethnicity of the perpetrator with any precision. It is equally unlikely that the ethnicity of the suspect is the reason that person is considered to be in the potential perpetrator population, and this population is certainly not defined by the suspect's ethnicity.

The simplest means for attaching a numerical value to $P_{ij} = \Pr(P = A_i A_j)$ is to sample people and determine the proportion $\tilde{P}_{ij}$ of the sample with this genotype. Debate over the appropriate population to sample can be avoided by sampling the entire population or by presenting estimates from several different ethnic groups. In either case, the estimate can differ from the true value. If the sample was a random one of size n, then it is helpful to report an upper confidence limit with the estimate and this is

$$\tilde{P}_{ij} + 1.645\sqrt{\tilde{P}_{ij}(1 - \tilde{P}_{ij})/n}$$

for a 95% limit *providing* $\tilde{P}_{ij}$ is not too small. This is likely to be the case for conventional blood groups or STR loci with only a few alleles.

For VNTR loci or other systems with many alleles, genotype frequencies are too small to allow confidence limits to be given by the binomial/normal theory of the previous paragraph. Indeed, samples of a few hundred people may not even contain representatives of the genotype in question. This is the point at which independence of the two alleles A_i and A_j is assumed and the genotype frequency estimated as the product of sample allele frequencies

$$P_{ij} \,\hat{=}\, \begin{cases} \tilde{p}_i^2 & A_i = A_j \\ 2\tilde{p}_i\tilde{p}_j & A_i \neq A_j \end{cases}$$

Methods for testing for independence have recently been reviewed by Maiste and Weir (1995). The very conditions under which use of the product rule is needed are those which invalidate normal-theory confidence limits, so the expressions of Chakraborty et al. (1993) are to be avoided. Instead, numerical resampling procedures such as the bootstrap (Efron and Tibshirani 1993) can be used.

In practice, DNA profiles involve several loci. Each particular genotype is very rare and product-rule estimates, along with bootstrap confidence limits, are necessary.

Suspect and Perpetrator Dependent

Calculating the likelihood ratio when the suspect and perpetrator are close relatives can be complex, although methods are in place (Weir 1994). This situation will not be treated here. Methods for pairs of people in the same population are not yet fully developed. Conditional genotypic frequencies of the form $\Pr(A\,A\,|A\,A\,)$ or $\Pr(A\,A\,|A\,A\,)$ are required. Direct estimates of these quantities are under development but, as they refer to dependencies imposed by evolutionary forces, they cannot be estimated from a single population. The problem has been discussed extensively for the simpler case of pairs of allele frequencies $\Pr(A_i|A_i)$ in different individuals (e.g. Cockerham 1969).

It may be helpful to realize that

$$\Pr(A_i|A_i) = p_i + (1 - p_i)\theta$$

where θ is often written as F_{ST}. This parameter, quantifying the correlation of alleles between individuals within populations also gives the variance component between populations. It is logically impossible to estimate this quantity from a single population.

There is an analogous parameterization for frequencies such as $\Pr(A_iA_i|A_iA_i)$, although three-gene and four-gene analogs of θ are needed (Cockerham 1971, Weir 1994). The expressions given recently by Balding and Nichols (1994) are true only for populations at equilibrium under the evolutionary forces of drift and infinite-alleles mutation. The relevance of these expressions for actual human populations has not yet been explored fully.

MIXED STAINS

There is currently some debate over the interpretation of mixed stains, even though the appropriate methodology was laid out by Evett et al. (1991). For the present discussion, it will be assumed that there are no dependencies between any of the principals in a crime: suspects, victims or perpetrators. The simplest case is where an evidentiary sample contains four alleles A_i, A_j, A_k, A_l and circumstances of the crime imply this sample has DNA from the victim V and one perpetrator P. If the victim has profile A_iA_j and a suspect S has A_kA_l then the suspect is not excluded from having contributed to the sample. The prosecution explanation C_1 is that the sample has DNA from V and S, whereas the defense explanation $\bar{C}_1$ is that it has DNA from V and some unknown perpetrator P.

The likelihood ratio for C versus $\bar{C}_1$ is

$$L = \frac{\Pr(E|C_1)}{\Pr(E|\bar{C}_1)}$$

$$= \frac{\Pr(V = A_iA_j, S = A_kA_l, P = A_kA_l|S = P)}{\Pr(V = A_iA_j, S = A_kA_l, P = A_kA_l|S \neq P)}$$

$$= \frac{\Pr(S = A_kA_l, P = A_kA_l|S = P)}{\Pr(S = A_kA_l, P = A_kA_l|S \neq P)}$$

$$= \frac{1}{\Pr(P = A_kA_l)}$$

as in the single-stain case.

Another situation is where it is not known with certainty that the victim has contributed to the evidentiary sample, and the defense explanation $\bar{C}_2$ is that there are two unknown contributors $U1, U2$. Now the likelihood ratio is

$$L = \frac{\Pr(E|C_1)}{\Pr(E|\bar{C}_2)}$$

$$= \frac{\Pr(\text{evidence profile } A_iA_jA_kA_l|\text{contributors } S, V)}{\Pr(\text{evidence profile } A_iA_jA_kA_l|\text{contributors } U1, U2)}$$

$$= \frac{1}{\Pr(\text{evidence profile } A_iA_jA_kA_l|\text{contributors } U1, U2)}$$

The probability needed is that of finding the four distinct alleles A_i, A_j, A_k, A_l from two unknown people. Evidently these people must both be heterozygotes, but there are three possible heterozygote pairs: $A_iA_j \& A_kA_l$, $A_iA_k \& A_jA_l$ and $A_iA_l \& A_jA_k$. Under the assumption of allelic independence, therefore,

$$L = \frac{1}{24p_ip_jp_kp_l}$$

A third situation may have a prosecution explanation C_2 of S and some unknown person $U1$ being the contributors, and then the likelihood ratio for C_2 versus $\bar{C}_2$ is

$$L = \frac{\Pr(E|C_2)}{\Pr(E|\bar{C}_2)}$$

$$= \frac{\Pr(\text{evidence profile } A_iA_jA_kA_l|\text{contributors } S, U1)}{\Pr(\text{evidence profile } A_iA_jA_kA_l|\text{contributors } U1, U2)}$$

$$= \frac{\Pr(\text{profile } A_iA_j \text{ from } U1)}{\Pr(\text{profile } A_iA_jA_kA_l \text{ from } U1, U2)}$$

$$= \frac{2p_ip_j}{24p_ip_jp_kp_l}$$

$$= \frac{1}{12p_kp_l}$$

The interpretation of mixed stains must therefore take into account the alternative explanations being offered. The calculations all hinge on the probabilities with which mixed stain profiles are found among two (or more) people. There is no logic in considering the probability with which a single person has a genotype included in the mixture (NRC 1992), or in working with probabilities with which single people would be excluded from a compound profile.

The number of contributors to a mixed stain may be dictated by circumstances of the crime, but in other cases the number may not be known with certainty. This could be the case when a location associated with a crime has several blood stains, some of which reveal six alleles at a locus and some of which reveal four alleles. Were the latter stains left by two contributors, or were there actually three and some alleles were not detected? Some of these complexities are present in the following example.

EXAMPLE

In the case of People of the State of California v. Orenthal James Simpson (Los Angeles County Case BA097211), evidence was presented for blood stains on the center console of a Bronco automobile. Three RFLP profiles were determined by the California Department of Justice DNA Berkeley Laboratory, and the band lengths are shown in Table 1, along with band lengths for two of the principals in the case, defendant OS and victim RG. At D4S139 and D5S110, evidentiary sample bands a, b match those of OS and bands c, d match those of RG. At D2S44, bands a, b match those of OS and bands a, c match those of RG. None of the 11 bands match those of the third principal, victim NB.

The fragment frequencies shown in Table 1 are from four FBI databases: AA=African American, CA=Caucasian, SE=Southeast Hispanic, and SW=Southwest Hispanic. Frequencies are assigned by the fixed-bin method described by Budowle et al. (1991). Consistency of genotype frequencies in these databases with the assumption of independence has been demonstrated by Maiste and Weir (1995).

The evidentiary stain could not have come from one person, although it could have come from two contributors, and indeed can be explained if OS and RG were the contributors. Other stains in the Bronco, however, contain alleles at other loci that match those of victim NB. One stain, involving locus DQα, was claimed by the defense to require a contributor other than the three principals, so the court ordered that statistics be provided for three and four contributors.

Table 1 RFLP profiles for Bronco Center Console.

Locus	Allele	Fragment lengths			Frequency			
		Sample	OS	RG	AA	CA	SE	SW
D2S44	a	2931	2925	3017	.0316	.0859	.0983	.0387
	b	1874	1877		.0842	.0827	.0750	.0898
	c	1684		1689	.0926	.1073	.1050	.1109
D4S139	a	8899	8915		.0770	.0951	.1013	.1264
	b	3281	3301		.0525	.0311	.0241	.0189
	c	7203		7192	.1094	.1911	.1672	.1830
	d	5683		5733	.0837	.1077	.1061	.1472
D5S110	a	11356	11355		1.0000	1.0000	1.0000	1.0000
	b	4777	4778		.0581	.0391	.0385	.0515
	c	5717		5722	.0765	.0274	.0367	.0455
	d	3015		3022	.0765	.0910	.0927	.0758

An example of the kinds of calculations needed is shown in Table 2. This table shows the genotypes, in terms of allelic names, of two possible contributors. The corresponding frequencies, with those for one contributor being taken from the AA database, and the other from the CA database, are also shown. For loci D4S139 and D5S110 the calculations are straightforward, and just lay out all six possible pairs of heterozygotes. For locus D2S44, care is needed.

Table 2 Details of two-contributor calculations.

AA Type	CA Type	Frequency			AA Type	CA Type	Freq.
		D2S44				D4S139	
		$\phi = 0.0$	$\phi = 0.1$	$\phi = 0.5$	a b	c d	.000333
a a / a d	b c	.000018	.000130	.000579	a c	b d	.000113
a b	a c	.000098	.000098	.000098	a d	b c	.000153
a b	b c	.000094	.000094	.000094	b c	a d	.000235
a b	c c / c d	.000061	.000175	.000632	b d	a c	.000319
a c	a b	.000083	.000083	.000083	c d	a b	.000108
a c	b b / c d	.000040	.000137	.000524		D5S110	
a c	b c	.000104	.000104	.000104	a b	c d	.000579
b b / b d	a c	.000131	.000441	.001683	a c	b d	.001089
b c	a a / a d	.000115	.000383	.001455	a d	b c	.000328
b c	a b	.000222	.000222	.000222	b c	a d	.001618
b c	a c	.000287	.000287	.000287	b d	a c	.000487
c c / c d	a b	.000122	.000385	.001437	c d	a b	.000915

The forensic scientist reported a possible fourth allele d at D2S44 close in size to allele a, as would be consistent with the explanation that OS and RG were the contributors. If it is not certain that a fourth allele is seen, however, there is the possibility that the RFLP technology simply did not detect the fourth allele d implied by two contributors. For this reason, the evidentiary profile a, b, c contributors include both aa, bc and ad, bc genotype pairs, with the d in the second pair not being seen. This unseen allele is assigned a frequency ϕ, and the value $\phi = 0$ corresponds to the case when it is known the evidentiary profile contains only three alleles at the locus. Some estimates for unseen RFLP allele frequencies have been reported, and have not been greater than 0.05 (Chakraborty et al. 1994). An extremely conservative upper bound, not at all supported by any data, would be $\phi = 0.5$. Each of these three values of ϕ was used in Table 2.

Reciprocals of frequencies for all combinations of racial groups, and for 2, 3 or 4 contributors, are shown in Table 3. Note that there is no need to double frequencies (or halve reciprocals) for pairs of different racial groups as these are conditional frequencies. A reciprocal for the pair AA,CA is the same as for CA,AA and for (AA,CA or CA,AA).

Table 3 Reciprocals of frequencies with which unknown contributors would have the evidentiary profile. (D2S44 unseen band frequency $\phi = 0.1$).

		2 unknowns					4 unknowns	
	AA	AA	114,237,467	AA	AA	AA	AA	2,746,756,219
	AA	CA	62,197,505	AA	AA	AA	CA	1,228,857,678
	AA	SE	60,855,431	AA	AA	AA	SE	1,278,168,818
	AA	SW	68,058,586	AA	AA	AA	SW	1,287,152,804
	CA	CA	67,204,161	AA	AA	CA	CA	631,696,172
	CA	SE	66,357,214	AA	AA	CA	SE	661,957,388
	CA	SW	58,133,830	AA	AA	CA	SW	615,392,828
	SE	SE	68,882,220	AA	AA	SE	SE	698,478,400
	SE	SW	60,114,492	AA	AA	SE	SW	642,501,663
	SW	SW	74,741,492	AA	AA	SW	SW	646,894,041
				AA	CA	CA	CA	375,349,666
		3 unknowns		AA	CA	CA	SE	393,922,618
AA	AA	AA	199,297,316	AA	CA	CA	SW	346,965,288
AA	AA	CA	94,627,491	AA	CA	SE	SE	416,665,128
AA	AA	SE	96,111,383	AA	CA	SE	SW	365,353,456
AA	AA	SW	101,405,846	AA	CA	SW	SW	342,048,695
AA	CA	CA	58,701,786	AA	SE	SE	SE	443,988,463
AA	CA	SE	60,198,945	AA	SE	SE	SW	387,829,353
AA	CA	SW	55,377,118	AA	SE	SW	SW	360,009,506
AA	SE	SE	62,636,897	AA	SW	SW	SW	365,721,013
AA	SE	SW	56,784,217	CA	CA	CA	CA	269,572,101
AA	SW	SW	60,333,497	CA	CA	CA	SE	281,441,469
CA	CA	CA	49,958,156	CA	CA	CA	SW	238,546,758
CA	CA	SE	51,055,589	CA	CA	SE	SE	297,186,005
CA	CA	SW	43,324,748	CA	CA	SE	SW	252,291,022
CA	SE	SE	53,300,230	CA	CA	SW	SW	226,565,281
CA	SE	SW	45,246,827	CA	SE	SE	SE	317,154,522
CA	SW	SW	43,308,048	CA	SE	SE	SW	269,724,555
SE	SE	SE	56,752,747	CA	SE	SW	SW	242,188,143
SE	SE	SW	48,248,000	CA	SW	SW	SW	233,397,498
SE	SW	SW	45,998,948	SE	SE	SE	SE	341,890,383
SW	SW	SW	52,037,162	SE	SE	SE	SW	291,370,357
				SE	SE	SW	SW	261,840,024
				SE	SW	SW	SW	251,670,721
				SW	SW	SW	SW	266,668,092

Simply presenting the frequencies with which unknown contributors have (only) the evidentiary profile between them does not provide the full forensic implication of the match between that profile and the profiles of OS and RG. As discussed above, the weight to be attached to this match is obtained as the ratio of the frequencies under alternative pairs of explanations, as shown in Table 4. In each case the probability for explanation C is divided by the probability for explanation $\bar{C}$. For example, the evidence is between 58 and 114 million times more likely to have arisen if OS and RG were the contributors than if two unknown people were the contributors, and the frequency of unseen bands at D2S44 is 0.1. The range of values reflects all possible combinations of racial groups for the unknown people.

Table 4 Likelihood ratios for interpreting evidence.

Explanation C	Explanation $\bar{C}$	Likelihood ratio		
		$\phi = 0.0$	$\phi = 0.1$	$\phi = 0.5$
Two Contributors				
OS+RG	OS+U1	65,000–150,000	42,000–96,000	17,000–38,000
OS+RG	RG+U1	38,000–73,000	23,000–52,000	9,400–23,000
OS+RG	U1+U2	100,000,000–220,000,000	58,000,000–114,000,000	21,000,000–38,000,000
OS+U1	U1+U2	720–20,000	630–1,700	560–1,400
RG+U1	U1+U2	1,000–5,800	1,100–4,800	910–4,000
Three contributors				
OS+RG+U1	OS+U1+U2	2,000–5,000	1,200–2,800	480–1,000
OS+RG+U1	RG+U1+U2	1,200–3,600	740–2,400	290–1,000
OS+RG+U1	U1+U2+U3	1,000,000–4,600,000	490,000–1,700,000	100,000–320,000
OS+U1+U2	U1+U2+U3	400–1,100	290–800	150–410
RG+U1+U2	U1+U2+U3	650–2,100	410–1,300	190–670
Four contributors				
OS+RG+U1+U2	OS+U1+U2+U3	880–2,200	500–1,100	190–430
OS+RG+U1+U2	RG+U1+U2+U3	550–1,500	320–1,000	120–430
OS+RG+U1+U2	U1+U2+U3+U4	260,000–1,300,000	100,000–460,000	18,000–71,000
OS+U1+U2+U3	U1+U2+U3+U4	110–680	87–440	42–200
RG+U1+U2+U3	U1+U2+U3+U4	410–1,100	230–690	97–290

U1,U2,U3,U4 are distinct unknown people.

CONCLUSION

The statistical issues arising in DNA profiling are currently centering on ways in which to accommodate population structure and to interpret mixtures. There is no problem with either provided likelihood ratios and the principles of population genetics are used. The care with which forensic samples are collected and analyzed must be matched by care in statistical analysis, and in explaining these analyses to a court.

ACKNOWLEDGEMENTS

This work was supported in part by NIH grant GM45344, and by award 95-IJ-CX-0007 from the National Institute of Justice, Office of Justice Programs, U.S. Department of Justice. Points of view in this document are those of the authors and do not necessarily represent the official position of the U.S. Department of Justice. The cooperation of Mr. Gray Sims from the California Department of Justice is deeply appreciated.

464

REFERENCES

Aitken CGG (1995) Statistics and the Evaluation of Evidence for Forensic Scientists. Wiley, New York.

Balding DJ, Nichols RA (1993) DNA profile match probability calculation: how to allow for population stratification, relatedness, database selection and single bands. Foren Sci Int 64:125–140.

Budowle B, Giusti AM, Waye JS, Baechtel FS, Fourney RM, Adams DE, Presley LA, Deadman HA, Monson KL (1991) Fixed-bin analysis for statistical evaluation of continuous distributions of allelic data from VNTR loci, for use in forensic comparisons. Am J Hum Genet 48:841-855.

Chakraborty R, Zhong Y, Jin L, Budowle B (1994) Nondetectability of restriction fragments and independence of DNA fragment sizes within and between loci in RFLP typing of DNA. Am J Hum Genet 55:391–401.

Chakraborty R, Srinivasan MR, Daiger SP (1993) Evaluation of standard error and confidence interval of estimated multilocus genotype probabilities, and their implications in DNA forensics. Am J Hum Genet 52:60-70

Cockerham CC, (1969) Variance of gene frequencies. Evolution 23:72-84

Cockerham CC (1971) Higher order probability functions of identity of alleles by descent. Genetics 69:235–246.

Efron B, Tibshirani RJ (1993) An Introduction to the Bootstrap. Chapman and Hall, New York.

Evett IW, Buffery C, Wilott G, Stoney D (1991) A guide to interpreting single locus profiles of DNA mixtures in forensic cases. J Foren Sci Soc 31:41–47

Maiste PJ, Weir BS (1995) Comparison of tests for independence in the FBI RFLP databases. Genetica 96:125-138.

NRC (National Research Council) (1992) DNA Technology in Forensic Science. National Academy Press, Washington, DC

Weir BS (1994) Effects of inbreeding on forensic calculations. Ann Rev Genet 28:597–621.

POPULATION GENETICS OF D1S80, HUMVWFA31/A AND HUMF13A1 FROM PORTUGAL AND GOA(INDIA)

H. Geada[1,2], R. Espinheira[1], T. Ribeiro[1] and L. Reys[1,2]

Institute of Legal Medicine, Lisbon[1]
Department of Legal Medicine, Faculty of Medicine, Lisbon[2],
Portugal

INTRODUCTION

Analysis of variable number of tandem repeats (VNTR) loci is widely used for individualization in forensic testing. VNTR locus D1S80 is successfully amplified by PCR. STR loci HUMVWFA31/A and HUMF13A1 are also two informative PCR based identification systems. The aim of this paper is to provide information about estimate allele frequencies for the three loci in **Portuguese and Goa (India) populations**, due to the Portuguese presence in Goa during four centuries.

MATERIAL AND METHODS

Unrelated Portuguese blood samples from paternity cases were studied for population analysis:D1S80-187 samples, HUMVWFA31/A-114 samples and HUMF13A1- 108 samples. These samples mainly from the South of Portugal, include Continental as well as Madeira and Açores Islands. Goa blood samples were obtained from unrelated persons from Portuguese origin living in Goa: D1S80-120 samples, HUMVWFA31/A-102 samples and HUMF13A1-95 samples.

DNA was extracted from blood by **Chelex method. D1S80 amplification** was carried out under the following conditions: 95°C 60sec, 65°C 60sec, 70°C 8min, 30 cycles (1). **HUMVWFA31/A and HUMF13A1 amplifications** were performed according to the EDNAP protocol(2), with slight modifications, using 0.5 uM of each primer in a 50 ul reaction volume, of which one primer was labelled with fluorescein. Amplification conditions: 94°C 45sec, 52°C 60sec, 72°C 60sec, 30 cycles.

D1S80 and the two STR systems were simultaneously analysed on an Automatic Laser Fluorescent (A.L.F.) **DNA sequencer** in a 4% hydrolink gel. Allelic ladders were used as external standards and three internal size markers (114bp, 402bp, 821bp) were added into each lane (3).

RESULTS AND DISCUSSION

In the Portuguese Population, we have obtained 27 alleles for **D1S80** locus, ranging from 15-48 number of repeats and in Goa Population 19 alleles, ranging from 14-36. The allele frequency differences in both populations are the allele 14, 16 and 19 presence and a higher 31 allele frequency in Goa Population (Table1, Fig.1).

TABLE 1. D1S80 allele frequencies in Portuguese and Goa populations

Allele	Port	Goa	Allele	Port	Goa	Allele	Port	Goa
14	-	0.0042	22	0.0321	0.0471	30	0.0107	0.0083
15	0.0027	0.0042	23	0.0107	0.0083	31	0.0267	0.1083
16	-	0.0167	24	0.3449	0.3167	32	0.0027	-
17	0.0027	0.0042	25	0.0401	0.0333	33	0.0027	-
18	0.2593	0.3208	26	0.0133	0.0083	34	0.0054	-
19	-	0.0208	27	0.0160	0.0125	35	-	0.0083
20	0.0160	-	28	0.0668	0.0417	36	0.0080	0.0042
21	0.0348	0.0125	29	0.0695	0.0250	37-48	0.0349	-

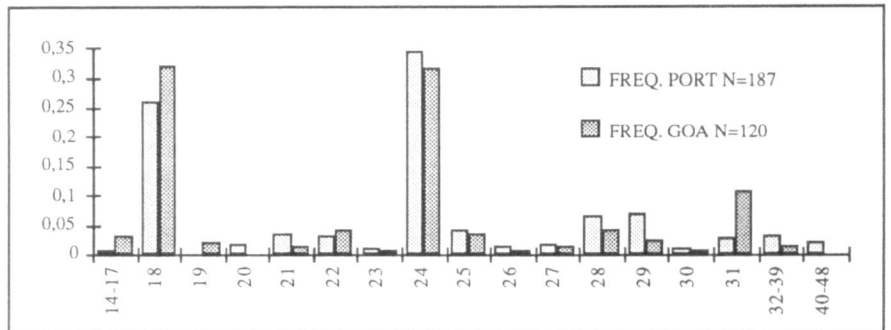

Fig.1. D1S80 allele frequency distribution in Portuguese and Goa Populations

For **HUMVWFA31/A**, Portuguese and Goa Populations are in good agreement withHWE(Port-X^2=6.766,d.f.=10,0.70<p<0.80;Goa- X^2=13.41, d.f.=10, 0.20<p<0.30), showing frequency differencies in alleles 14 and 19. **HUMF13A1** is also in good agreement for HWE (Port X^2=11.99,d.f.=10,20<p<0.30; Goa X^2=6.039,d.f.=10,0.80<p<0.90), with higher frequencies in alleles 14 to 17 and mainly in allele 3.2 in Goa Population (Table2,Fig.2).

TABLE 2. HUMVWFA31/A and HUMF13A1 allele frequencies in Portuguese and Goa Populations

HumVWFA31/A			HumF13A1		
Allele	Port	Goa	Allele	Port	Goa
12	0.0044	-	3.2	0.0741	0.1947
13	-	0.0098	4	0.0417	0.0474
14	0.0746	0.1373	5	0.2222	0.3368
15	0.1272	0.0833	6	0.2870	0.1684
16	0.2149	0.2255	7	0.3056	0.1895
17	0.2632	0.3088	8	0.0185	0.0053
18	0.1667	0.1471	9	0.0370	-
19	0.1140	0.0539			
20	0.0263	0.0343	14	-	0.0158
21	0.0087	-	15	0.0093	0.0263
			16	0.0046	0.0105
			17	-	0.0053

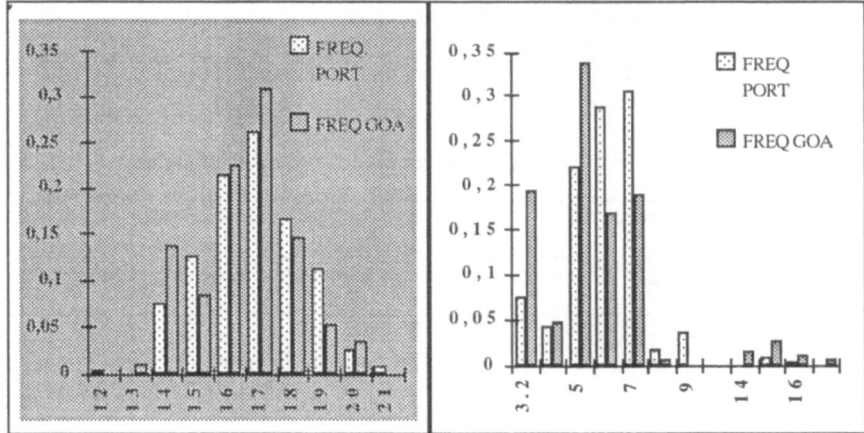

Fig.2. HumVWFA31/A(right) and HumF13A1(left) allele frequency distribution in Portuguese and Goa Populations

In conclusion, Goa population database has been established for theVNTR locus D1S80 and two STR loci HumVWFA31/A and HumF13A1, and although from Portuguese origin, it is in agreement with other Indian populations studied.

Acknowledgements: To Dr. Joaquim Santana da Silva for Goa samples

REFERENCES

1. Barros F et al. (1992) Detection of polymorphisms of human DNA after polymerase chain reaction by miniaturized SDS-PAGE, Forensic Sci Int , 55:27-36.
2. Kimpton C et al. (1995) Report on the second EDNAP collaborative STR exercise, Forensic Sci Int, 71:137-152.
3. Lango A et al. (1993) Simultaneous analysis of STR and VNTR polymorphisms, Advances in Forensic Haemogenetics 5, 109-111.

GENETIC SUBSTRUCTURE AT THE STR LOCI HUMTH01 AND HUMVWA IN HAN POPULATIONS, CHINA

Yiping Hou   Hubert Walter*
Institute of Forensic Medicine, West China University of Medical Sciences
610044 Chengdu, Sichuan, PR China
*Department of Human Biology, University of Bremen
D-28334 Bremen, Germany

Systems and loci: HUMTH01 (11p15-p15.5) and HUMVWA (12p12-pter)
Populations and sample size: Han populations living in 3 different geographic areas in China, Guangzhou(S China) N: 101, Chengdu(SW China) N:121 and Changchun(N China) N: 92.

Methods:
Primers for HUMTH01 and HUMVWA (Kimpton et al 1993).
PCR amplification conditions: Hou et al (1994a).
Electrophoresic methods: native polyacrylamide gels with discontinuous buffer system and silver stain (Hou et al 1994a).Typing for HUMTH01 and HUMVWA was performed by comparison with sequenced allele ladders according to the published ISFH guidelines(1994)

Results:
Table 1. Distribution of HUMTH01 genotypes in three Han populations of China

	Observed				Observed		
Genotype	Guangzhou	Chengdu	Changchun	Genotype	Guangzhou	Chengdu	Changchun
6-6	5	2	-	7-10	-	2	1
6-7	2	9	3	8-9	9	7	5
6-8	-	1	1	8-9.3	-	-	2
6-9	12	15	7	8-10	1	2	-
6-9.3	4	-	-	9-9	23	26	29
6-10	2	3	-	9-9.3	3	4	3
7-7	7	7	5	9-10	3	5	3
7-8	2	2	4	9.3-9.3	1	-	-
7-9	26	32	26	9.3-10	-	1	-
7-9.3	1	3	3				

Table 2. Distribution of allele frequencies for HUMTH01

	Frequency				Frequency		
Allele	Guangzhou	Chengdu	Changchun	Allele	Guangzhou	Chengdu	Changchun
6	0.149	0.132	0.060	9	0.490	0.475	0.554
7	0.223	0.256	0.255	9.3	0.049	0.033	0.044
8	0.059	0.050	0.065	10	0.030	0.054	0.022

Test for Hardy-Weinberg Equilibrium (Hou et al 1994b): each population P>0.05

Table 3. Distribution of HUMVWA genotypes in three Han populations of China

	Observed				Observed		
Genotype	Guangzhou	Chengdu	Changchun	Genotype	Guangzhou	Chengdu	Changchun
13-18	-	1	-	16-16	1	1	3
14-14	5	6	5	16-17	6	11	14
14-15	5	2	4	16-18	10	8	5
14-16	8	11	9	16-19	3	4	3
14-17	15	18	9	16-20	1	1	-
14-18	11	7	6	17-17	6	12	3
14-19	3	5	4	17-18	8	13	7
14-20	1	1	-	17-19	5	6	1
15-15	1	-	-	17-20	2	1	2
15-16	-	1	4	18-18	2	4	2
15-17	1	-	4	18-19	7	7	4
15-18	-	-	1	19-19	-	1	1
15-19	-	-	1				

Table 4. Distribution of allele frequencies for HUMVWA

	Frequency				Frequency		
Allele	Guangzhou	Chengdu	Changchun	Allele	Guangzhou	Chengdu	Changchun
13	-	0.004	-	17	0.243	0.302	0.234
14	0.262	0.232	0.228	18	0.198	0.182	0.147
15	0.040	0.012	0.076	19	0.089	0.099	0.081
16	0.148	0.157	0.223	20	0.020	0.012	0.011

Test for Hardy-Weinberg Equilibrium(Hou et al 1994b): each population P>0.05

Comments:
In order to assess the genetic substructure in Chinese populations and analyse human evolution on the basis of DNA sequences, three populations of the Chinese Han nationality from northern and southern as well as from southwestern China, respectively, were directly sampled. The distributions of genotype and allele frequencies at two STR loci HUMTH01 and HUMVWA in these population samples are shown in tables 1-4. The most common allele at the HUMTH01 locus in the Chinese Han population is allele 9, while at the HUMVWA locus the most frequently observed alleles are 14 and 17. No evidence of deviation from Hardy-Weinberg equilibrium was observed in these population samples using the modified statistical approach (Hou et al 1994b). In search of the relationship between the Chinese Han nationality and major racial groups, a phylogenetic tree of 11 populations was constructed on the basis of allele frequencies at the loci HUMTH01 and HUMVWA (figure 1). As shown in figure 1, at the level of a genetic distance of 0.136, the 11 populations were clustered in three major groups, corresponding to Mongoloids, Negroids and Caucasoids. At the level of a genetic distance of 0.023, the Chinese Han nationality was divided into two subgroups, north and south. The comparison of the data showed that the distribution of the frequency of allele 6 at HUMTH01 locus between northern Han and southern Han was significantly different (Changchun:Guangzhou, x^2=7.36, df=2, P<0.05. Changchun: Chengdu, x^2=6.15, df=2,

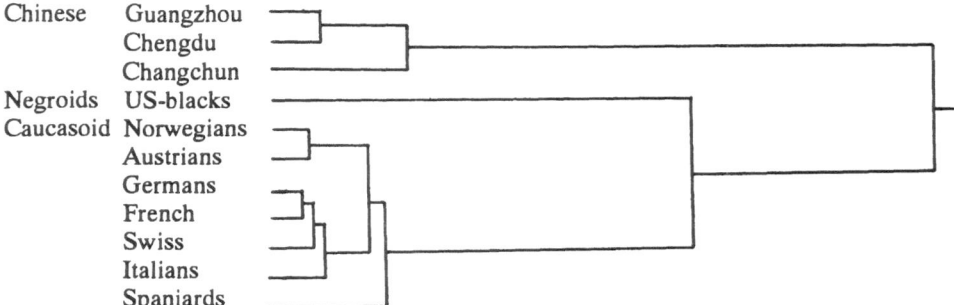

Fig 1. Phylogenetic tree of 11 populations

P<0.05), but when x^2 and P values were calculated using a 2-way R*C contingency table, there were no statistical difference in the distributions of allele frequencies for the loci HUMTH01 and HUMVWA within the Chinese Han population samples. In contrast, the ethnic distributions of allele frequencies for the two loci between the compared populations were always significantly different. The implication of these results is that the greatest genetic differences of allele frequencies for the loci HUMTH01 and HUMVWA appear between major racial groups and that there is some substructure in the Chinese Han population at HUMTH01 locus, but the statistical effect of such subdivision on the match probability may be minor. More effort should be put into further clarification of allele frequency distribution for various Chinese nationalities in order to evaluate the necessity to include a ceiling principle approach for forensic application of the two STR loci.

Acknowlegment
This research was supported by a grant from the Alexander von Humboldt Foundation, Germany.

References
1. Kimpton CP, Gill P, Walton A, Urquhart A, Millican ES, Adams M (1993) PCR Methods and Applications 1993;3:13-22.
2. Hou Y, Gill P, Staak M, Schmitt C, Prinz M (1994) In: Bär W, Fiori A, Rossi U (eds) Advances in Forensic Haemogenetics 5. Springer-Verlag, Berlin Heidelberg New York, 508-510.
3. Hou Y, Prinz M, Staak M (1994) In: Bär W, Fiori A, Rossi U (eds) Advances in Forensic Haemogenetics 5. Springer-Verlag, Berlin Heidelberg New York, 511-514.
4. DNA recommendations (1994) Int J Leg Med 107:159-160.
5. Edwards A, Hammond HA, Jin L, Caskey CT, Chakraborty R(1992) Genomics 12:241-253
6. Dupuy BM, Berg ES, Olaisen B (1994) In: Bär W, Fiori A, Rossi U (eds) Advances in Forensic Haemogenetics 5. Springer-Verlag, Berlin Heidelberg New York, 539-541.
7. Klintschar M, Kubat M (1995) Int J Leg Med 107:329-330.
8. Hochmeister MN, Jung JM, Budowle B, Borer UV, Dirnhofer R (1994) Int J Leg Med 107:34-36.
9. Pascal O, Levayer T, Aubert D, Peneau A, Markey P, Moisan JP (1994) In: Bär W, Fiori A, Rossi U (eds) Advances in Forensic Haemogenetics 5. Springer-Verlag, Berlin Heidelberg New York, 542-544.
10. Pestoni C, Lareu MV, Rodriguez MS, Munoz I, Barros F, Carracedo A (1995) Int J Leg Med 107:283-290.
11. Buscemi L, Tagliabracci A, Cucurachi N, Mencarelli R, Porro D, Giorgetti R, Ferrara SD (1994) In: Bär W, Fiori A, Rossi U (eds) Advances in Forensic Haemogenetics 5. Springer-Verlag, Berlin Heidelberg New York, 475-477.

COLLABORATIVE STUDY ON THE POLYMORPHISM OF THE D1S80 LOCUS IN THE ITALIAN POPULATION.

G. Graziosi, Editor.

Department of Biology, University of Trieste, 34127 Trieste, Italy

Contributors. M.Alù, Medicina Legale, Modena; A.Asmundo, Medicina Legale, Messina; E.Carnevali, Medicina Legale, Perugia; N.Cerri, Medicina Legale, Brescia; P.Cortivo, Medicina Legale, Padova; N.Cucurachi, Medicina Legale, Parma; E.d'Aloia, Medicina Legale, U.C.S.C., Roma; F.De Ferrari, Medicina Legale, Brescia; F.De Stefano, Medicina Legale, Genova; C.Di Nunno, Medicina Legale, Bari; R.Domenici, Dip. Biomedicina Sperimentale, Pisa; P.Fattorini, Medicina Legale, Trieste; F.Florian, Dip. Biologia, Trieste; G.Pappalardo, Medicina Legale, Bologna; G.Pasqui, Medicina Legale, Camerino; G.Peloso, Medicina Legale, Pavia; S.Pelotti, Medicina Legale, Bologna; P.F. Pignatti, Dip. Biologia e Genetica, Verona; B.Porfirio, Dip. Fisiopatologia Clinica, Firenze; C.Previderè, Medicina Legale, Pavia; U.Ricci, Dip. di Genetica Umana, Firenze; D.Scimmi, Medicina Legale, Perugia; G.Sciacca, Medicina Legale, Catania; F.Suadoni, Medicina Legale, Perugia; A.Tagliabracci, Medicina Legale, Ancona; E.Trabetti, Dip. Biologia e Genetica, Verona; M.Venturi, Medicina Legale, Ferrara.

Summary.

Twenty Italian laboratories were involved in a collaborative study on the polymorphism of the locus D1S80. A total of 1720 blood samples of unrelated people collected in 19 Italian towns were analysed. The allelic frequencies reported by the participant laboratories were statistically homogeneous with the exception of one laboratory. More than 33 different alleles were found, ranging from 14 to over 41 repeats. Four interalleles were found and five alleles were larger than 41 repeats. A total of 146 genotypes was found. Phenotypic classes with expected frequency >4 were tested for Hardy-Weinberg equilibrium: the observed frequencies of the 51 classes did not differ significantly from the expected frequencies. No mutant allele was detected in 465 mother-child pairs.

Introduction.

Since the first appearance on the forensic scene of the use of DNA polymorphism analysis for personal identification and paternity testing there has been concern on a number of issues such as the reproducibility of the results, population differences and population stratification. In line with the recommendation of the EDNAP, the Italian Group of Forensic Haematologists (G.E.F.I.) launched a series of collaborative studies to standardise the techniques and to collect population data all over Italy. One of these studies concerned the polymorphic locus D1S80. This locus shows a large number of alleles and the collaborative study allowed the collection of a relatively large sample of the Italian population for the establishment of a reference data bank of allelic and genotypic frequencies.

Materials and methods.

Each participant laboratory was invited to collect and analyse a minimum of 50 blood samples obtained from residents in the corresponding region. The main characteristics of the common protocol adopted were: primers as reported by Kasai et al (1990), reference allelic ladder (T14-T40) and amplification conditions as for the commercial kit Cetus D1S80, allele separation and gel staining as reported by Budowle et al (1991). Some laboratories run the electrophoresis on agarose gels. Each participant was given a reference DNA with alleles widely separate to control possible preferential amplification and two bloodstains as a blind control.

Results.

Twenty laboratories took part in the collaborative exercise and a total of 1720 blood samples of unrelated people of 19 towns were analysed (Genova, Pavia, Brescia, Verona, Padova, Trieste, Parma, Modena, Ferrara, Bologna, Firenze, Pisa, Ancona, Camerino, Terni, Roma, Bari, Messina and Catania). The number of samples analysed by each laboratory ranged from 34 to 380. All laboratories correctly characterised the reference DNA and the two blind samples, although 4 laboratories gave no answer for the bloodstains.

Table 1.
Simplified allelic frequencies

Alleles	Obser.	%
14-18	680	20.97
19-21.5	166	5.12
22-23.5	231	7.13
24-24.5	1,227	37.85
25-26	201	6.20
27-29	422	13.02
30-42	315	9.72
Total	3,242	100

The allelic frequencies for each laboratory were computed and an homogeneity test among laboratories was performed. Because of the high number of alleles, the allelic frequencies were grouped into 7 allelic classes (see Table 1) to have the lowest expected frequency >4. The homogeneity test showed a highly significant variation among laboratories (X^2 =391.87 df=120 p<0.01). The pairwise comparison between laboratories showed that the majority of the variation was introduced by Laboratory 9 as reported in Table 2. This was probably due to laboratory 9 which changed the allelic ladder during the analyses and moreover included, (for a specific purpose of the laboratory), a population sample with 4 autochthonous grandparents. To avoid a possible bias, the data of this laboratory were excluded from further analyses. The remaining significant heterogeneity was scattered between laboratories and the allelic groups as would be expected for such a large comparison with large sample variation.

Table 2.
Pairwise comparisons between laboratories: X^2 test of the simplified allelic frequencies.

Lab.	1	2	3	4	5	6	7	8	9	10	11	12	13	14	15	16	17	18	19	20
1	0																			
2	6.18	0																		
3	8.92	8.95	0																	
4	7.19	6.15	8.32	0																
5	6.71	3.75	10.3	5.55	0															
6	2.66	6.52	6.21	4.69	5.26	0														
7	**17.3**	11.6	**19.1**	7.26	10.4	3.49	0													
8	2.11	9.52	11.3	5.07	6.52	3.01	12.3	0												
9	**87.2**	**73.6**	**75.7**	**78.7**	**92.1**	**74.5**	**46.4**	**78.0**	0											
10	**14.7**	11.8	**17.9**	11.7	10.0	**13.8**	10.5	13.7	**59.9**	0										
11	9.95	**14.0**	6.67	10.4	9.17	6.40	**16.6**	8.37	**67.7**	11.2	0									
12	2.17	11.0	6.07	10.5	**13.4**	2.99	**21.3**	4.03	**87.6**	**19.1**	6.72	0								
13	4.16	6.33	8.35	1.48	3.87	3.49	12.0	3.07	**97.6**	**14.7**	8.75	7.28	0							
14	7.36	5.13	11.8	5.63	3.55	4.39	4.80	6.34	**48.0**	3.33	7.41	9.35	6.49	0						
15	9.58	8.49	8.98	3.42	9.65	7.46	**13.6**	7.42	**96.8**	6.56	5.78	9.96	5.27	4.85	0					
16	**13.1**	**13.1**	**18.7**	9.80	**12.7**	5.72	4.94	9.33	**82.3**	**14.3**	**16.5**	**15.4**	**13.9**	1.59	**18.4**	0				
17	10.0	6.81	9.55	2.03	5.37	7.41	9.72	7.84	**96.2**	**17.5**	**13.4**	**14.4**	2.71	9.10	8.80	**18.5**	0			
18	7.62	5.47	**15.6**	5.62	3.29	7.01	9.42	7.93	**45.1**	5.72	10.5	11.5	8.57	3.15	9.80	5.80	11.5	0		
19	8.97	6.95	**14.3**	5.44	6.08	6.42	3.37	7.77	**34.9**	7.62	11.0	12.3	6.78	4.73	7.92	4.51	7.20	6.77	0	
20	5.23	4.73	5.09	1.62	3.88	3.04	7.90	4.41	**69.1**	11.1	7.61	7.43	0.79	5.82	4.46	9.33	1.02	8.35	6.41	0

Bold values show a significant difference (p<0.05).

A total of 33 different alleles were observed (Table 3), ranging from 14 to over 41 repeats, notably four of these alleles dropped in between the rungs of the allelic ladder and they were provisionally designated with an interallelic value. Five alleles were larger than 41 repeats and they were all grouped in the 42 repeat class. The most frequent alleles were the 18 (20.4%) and the 24 (37,8%). As reported in other sudies, no 39 repeat allele was found: presumably this allele is either missing or very rare.

Of the 561 possible phenotypes only 146 were observed (Table 4). The most frequent phenotypes were: 18/24 (15.2%) and 24/24 (14.1%). The phenotypic classes with expected frequency >4 were tested for Hardy-Weinberg equilibrium: the 51 classes did not differ significantly from the expected frequencies (X^2=42.04, d.f.=31, P>0.05).

A total of 465 mother-child pairs was analysed to assess the mutation rate. No mutant allele was detected.

Discussion.

No new allele of the D1S80 genetic system was reported, in fact the interalles listed here were previously described by Schwartz et al (1994). Notably the allelic frequencies reported by the 19 participant laboratories were relatively homogeneous, suggesting a relative uniformity in the Italian population. Nevertheless we cannot exclude that there may be small allelic frequency variations in different regions. In fact there were wide differences in the number of samples and it is possible that more data could disclose small but statistically significant variations.

The allelic frequencies reported here are also very similar to those reported for other European populations (Advances in Forensic Haemogenetics, Vol.5; Skowasch et al, 1992) and for the American Caucasian population (Budowle et al, 1991). On one hand, this result confirms the D1S80 Caucasian population structure and, on the other, validates the results reported by the participant laboratories.

In conclusion, the success of the collaborative exercise allowed the establishment of a reference D1S80 data bank for the Italian population and proved that a reasonable standardisation of methods can be achieved.

Table 3.
Allelic frequencies

Allele	Obs.	%
14	2	0.06
15	2	0.06
16	9	0.28
17	5	0.15
18	662	20.42
19	12	0.37
20	68	2.10
21	86	2.65
22	181	5.58
22.5	1	0.03
23	48	1.48
23.5	1	0.03
24	1226	37.82
24.5	1	0.03
25	137	4.23
26	64	1.97
27	42	1.30
28	172	5.31
29	208	6.42
30	49	1.51
31	154	4.75
31.5	1	0.03
32	29	0.89
33	9	0.28
34	13	0.40
35	4	0.12
36	15	0.46
37	20	0.62
38	7	0.22
39	0	0.00
40	8	0.25
41	1	0.03
> 41	5	0.15
Total	3,242	100

References.

Budowle B, Chakraborty R, Giusti AM, Eisemberg AJ, Allen RC (1991) Analysis of the VNTR Locus D1S80 by PCR Followed by High-Resolution PAGE. Am J Hum Genet 48:137-144.

Kasai K, Nakamura Y, White R (1990) Amplification of Variable Number of Tandem Repeats (VNTR) Locus (pMCT118) by the Polymerase Chain Reaction (PCR) and its application to Forensic Science, J. Forensic Sci 35:1196-1200.

Schwartz DWM, Jungl EM, Krenek OR, Mayr WR. Phenotype and allele frequencies of 4 VNTR-AMPFLP's in an Austrian population sample. In: Advances in Forensic Haemogenetics 5 (Eds. W Bär, A Fiori & U Rossi) Springer-Verlag Berlin Heidelberg (1994) pp 578-580.

Skowasch K, Wiegand P, Brinkmann B (1992) pMCT118 (D1S80): a new allelic ladder and an improved electrophoretic separation lead to the demonstration of 28 alleles. Int J Leg Med 105:165-168.

Table 4.
Genotypic frequencies.

Alleles Lower	Upper	%	Obs.	Expcted	X² test
14	29	0.12	2	0.13	
15	18	0.06	1	0.41	
15	22	0.06	1	0.11	
16	16	0.06	1	0.01	
16	18	0.06	1	1.84	
16	20	0.06	1	0.19	
16	22	0.06	1	0.50	
16	24	0.12	2	3.40	
16	29	0.12	2	0.58	
17	22	0.06	1	0.28	
17	23	0.06	1	0.07	
17	24	0.12	2	1.89	
17	29	0.06	1	0.32	
18	18	5.18	84	67.59	3.98
18	20	0.86	14	13.89	0.00
18	21	1.17	19	17.56	0.12
18	22	1.97	32	36.96	0.67
18	22.5	0.06	1	0.20	
18	23	0.37	6	9.80	1.47
18	23.5	0.06	1	0.20	
18	24	15.18	246	250.3	0.08
18	25	1.79	29	27.97	0.04
18	26	0.62	10	13.07	0.72
18	27	0.37	6	8.58	0.77
18	28	1.85	30	35.12	0.75
18	29	2.53	41	42.47	0.05
18	30	0.56	9	10.01	0.10
18	31	1.67	27	31.45	0.63
18	32	0.43	7	5.92	0.20
18	33	0.12	2	1.84	
18	34	0.06	1	2.65	
18	35	0.12	2	0.82	
18	36	0.12	2	3.06	
18	37	0.25	4	4.08	0.00
18	40	0.06	1	1.63	
18	>41	0.06	1	1.02	
19	21	0.06	1	0.32	
19	24	0.37	6	4.54	0.47
19	25	0.06	1	0.51	
19	26	0.06	1	0.24	
19	27	0.06	1	0.16	
19	28	0.06	1	0.64	
19	29	0.06	1	0.77	
20	20	0.12	2	0.71	
20	22	0.25	4	3.80	
20	24	1.67	27	25.71	0.06
20	25	0.06	1	2.87	
20	26	0.19	3	1.34	
20	28	0.37	6	3.61	
20	29	0.25	4	4.36	0.03
20	31	0.12	2	3.23	
20	37	0.06	1	0.42	
20	40	0.06	1	0.17	
21	21	0.31	5	1.14	
21	22	0.19	3	4.80	0.68
21	23	0.19	3	1.27	
21	24	1.85	30	32.52	0.20
21	25	0.25	4	3.63	
21	26	0.06	1	1.70	
21	28	0.19	3	4.56	0.54
21	29	0.25	4	5.52	0.42
21	31	0.43	7	4.09	2.08
21	32	0.06	1	0.77	
22	22	0.56	9	5.05	3.08
22	23	0.12	2	2.68	
22	24	4.87	79	68.45	1.63
22	25	0.31	5	7.65	0.92
22	26	0.31	5	3.57	
22	27	0.25	4	2.34	
22	28	0.56	9	9.60	0.04
22	29	0.37	6	11.61	2.71
22	31	0.37	6	8.60	0.78
22	32	0.06	1	1.62	

Alleles Lower	Upper	%	Obs.	Expected	X² test
22	33	0.06	1	0.50	
22	34	0.12	2	0.73	
22	41	0.06	1	0.06	
23	24	1.11	18	18.15	0.00
23	25	0.19	3	2.03	
23	28	0.19	3	2.55	
23	29	0.19	3	3.08	
23	30	0.12	2	0.73	
23	31	0.19	3	2.28	
23	34	0.12	2	0.19	
23	37	0.06	1	0.30	
23	38	0.06	1	0.10	
24	24	14.07	228	231.8	0.06
24	25	2.96	48	51.81	0.28
24	26	1.67	27	24.20	0.32
24	27	1.05	17	15.88	0.08
24	28	4.07	66	65.04	0.01
24	29	5.12	83	78.66	0.24
24	30	1.36	22	18.53	0.65
24	31	3.39	55	58.24	0.18
24	32	0.74	12	10.97	0.10
24	33	0.31	5	3.40	
24	34	0.12	2	4.92	1.73
24	35	0.12	2	1.51	
24	36	0.62	10	5.67	3.30
24	37	0.43	7	7.56	0.04
24	40	0.25	4	3.03	
24	>41	0.06	1	1.89	
25	25	0.37	6	2.89	
25	26	0.06	1	2.70	
25	27	0.12	2	1.77	
25	28	0.31	5	7.27	0.71
25	29	0.62	10	8.79	0.17
25	30	0.19	3	2.07	
25	31	0.49	8	6.51	0.34
25	32	0.12	2	1.23	
25	36	0.12	2	0.63	
25	37	0.12	2	0.85	
26	26	0.06	1	0.63	
26	28	0.37	6	3.40	
26	29	0.19	3	4.11	0.30
26	30	0.12	2	0.97	
26	31	0.12	2	3.04	
26	37	0.06	1	0.39	
27	28	0.19	3	2.23	
27	29	0.12	2	2.69	
27	30	0.06	1	0.63	
27	31	0.25	4	2.00	
27	32	0.06	1	0.38	
27	38	0.06	1	0.09	
28	28	0.56	9	4.56	4.32
28	29	0.31	5	11.04	3.30
28	30	0.19	3	2.60	
28	31	0.43	7	8.17	0.17
28	32	0.06	1	1.54	
28	33	0.06	1	0.48	
28	37	0.12	2	1.06	
28	38	0.06	1	0.37	
28	>41	0.06	1	0.27	
29	29	0.56	9	6.67	0.81
29	30	0.25	4	3.14	
29	31	0.86	14	9.88	1.72
29	34	0.25	4	0.83	
29	36	0.06	1	0.96	
30	38	0.06	1	0.45	
30	32	0.19	3	0.44	
31	31	0.43	7	3.66	
31	32	0.06	1	1.38	
31	34	0.12	2	0.62	
32	32	0.12	2	0.13	
32	37	0.06	1	0.18	
38	38	0.12	2	0.01	
40	40	0.06	1	0.01	
	Total	100	1621	1621	42.04

DNA-FINGERPRINTING IN BALEARIC POPULATION

Albalá I.; Picornell A.; Castro J.A.; Ramón M.M.

Lab. de Genètica. Dept. Biologia Fonamental i Ciències de la Salut.

Universitat de les Illes Balears. Palma de Mallorca 07071 (Spain)

INTRODUCTION:

The genetic structure of the Balearic Islands populations has been studied by means of the blood group polymorphism, serum proteins and erythrocyte enzymes and mtDNA polymorphisms (Picornell 1992; Massanet 1995). The global results revealed that the Balearic populations have a genetic differentiation with respect to those of the Iberian peninsula and the circunmediterranean ones. In Majorca Island we find an autochthonous group, the Chuetas, which are descendents of the persecuted Sephardic Jews in the last "autos de-fe" of the Inquisition. They remained isolated from the Christian Balearic population until the middle of this century in spite of their official conversion to Christianity (15th century). Although many other schemes remain to be addresed we focus in the present work our attention on the minisatellite regions, in order to know better the genetics of the Balearic populations. We use a probe based on a tandem-repeat of the core sequence which can detect many highly variable loci simultaneously and can provide an individual specific DNA "fingerprint" of general use in human genetic analysis (Jeffreys et al., 1985)

MATERIALS AND METHODS:

The sample was composed of 80 unrelated individuals, 36 of them were autochthonous of Majorca island, 21 from the Chueta population and 23 from the Iberian Peninsula resident in Majorca. The DNA was extracted, digested to completion with Hinf I, and 10 µg samples electrophoresed in a 0.7% agarose gel, during 48 hours DNA was transferred by blotting to a Hybond-N membrane (Amersham), and southern blot hybridized with alkaline phosphatase labelled probe 33.15. The number of bands shared and unshared was estimated, and the similarity index, S (Lynch M., 1990) was employed to compare the diversity of the populations.

RESULTS AND DISCUSION:

A multilocus probe, like 33.15, binds to alleles at a high (but unknow) number of loci. The resulting profiles consist of a series of bands, whose number and position will be different from one individual to another, according to the distint electrophoretic mobilities of the DNA fragments (Donnelly P., 1995). We have determined the number of bands (with a size >5kb) for each individual to calculate the mean number of bands and the band-sharing for each population.

POPULATION	CHUETA	MAJORCA	IBERIAN P.
Nº OF INDIVIDUALS	21	36	23
MEAN Nº OF BANDS	11.38±3.47	11.6±2.30	14.3±2.20
MEAN Nº OF SHARED BANDS	1.56±1.28	1.18±0.95	1.06±0.84
MEAN BAND-SHARING FR. (S)	0.15±0.009	0.11±0.03	0.07±0.012

Jeffreys et al. (1991b), using the multilocus probes 33.6 and 33.15, reported around 17 bands on average in the scored region (>3.5kb) for each profile and probe, with a range from 5 to 35 bands. Our scored region was lower (only bands >5kb). For this reason the number of bands we found were also lower than Jeffreys' results and different in each population: Chueta population showed 11 bands on average, with a range from 7 to 19; in Majorcan samples we scored 11.6 bands, with a range from 7 to 18 bands; and the population of the Iberian peninsula showed 4.3 bands, with a range from 10 to 21 bands. As can be seen, the average number of bands is higher in the Peninsula than in Majorca and Chueta population, which have similar values (slightly higher in Majorca). This indicating a major degree of heterozigosity in the sample of the Iberian Peninsula.

The average of band-sharing frequency (S) is 0.15 in Chuetas, 0.11 in Majorca population and 0.07 in Iberian peninsula. Jeffreys et al. 1991b, in a study of Caucasian population found an index of 0.14, but, as we have indicated, this study was made with a larger region. Moreover, this value depends of the different scored regions, for example values of 0.248, 0.201 and 0.068 were found for the regions 4-6 kb, 6-9kb and 9-23 kb and 0.14 was only an average. We can see that the major value of band-sharing frequency belongs to the region of 4-6 Kb that we have not scored. The band-sharing frequency estimated by Jeffreys did not show significant changes among the different ethnic groups, although a study involving a highly inbred small community from Gaza strip, where the consanguineos marriages are a cultural norm, indicated that the band-sharing coefficient among unrelated individuals significantly increased (Bellamy et al., submitted; Jeffreys et al. 1991a). Now we can say that the Chueta population has a high value of band-sharing and showing, therefore, a higher level of consanguinity than the other populations sampled. This study would confirm the information about the existence of a high level of consanguinity detected in Chuetas by other markers.

REFERENCES:
Donelly P. (1995). Genetica **96**: 55-67.
Jeffreys A.J. et al. (1991a). Pp 1-18 in T. Burke, G. Dolf, A.J. Jeffreys, and R. Wolf eds. DNA fingerprinting: Approaches and applications. Birkhauser, Basel.
Jeffreys A.J.; Turner M.; Debenham P. (1991b). Am. J. Hum. Genet. **48**, 824-840.
Jeffreys A.J.; Wilson V.; Thein S.L. (1985). Nature, **314**, 67-73.
Lynch M. (1990). Mol. Biol. Evol. **7** (5), 478-484.
Massanet M.F. (1995). Tesis de licenciatura. University of Balearic Islands.
Picornell A. (1992). Ph D. Thesis. University of Balearic Islands.

HLA DQA1 AND D1S80 IN THE POPULATION OF VALENCIA (SPAIN)

M. Aler, M.V. Lareu (1), F. Verdú, C. Pestoni (1) and M.S. Gisbert
U.D. Medicina Legal. Universidad de Valencia. Spain
(1) Instituto de Medicina Legal. Santiago de Compostela. Spain

System and locus: HLA DQA1 (6p21.3)

Population and sample size: 107 unreleated people from the district of Valencia (Eastern Spain).

Methods:
Primers: GH26 and GH27 (Lareu et al. 1993).
PCR amplification conditions (Lareu et al. 1993).
Method of detection: Dot-blot with AmpliType HLA DQA1 (Perkin-Elmer)

Results:

Observed genotypes

Gen.	Obs.	Gen.	Obs.	Gen.	Obs.	Gen.	Obs.
0101-0101	2	0101-0501	13	0103-0201	3	0301-0301	3
0101-0102	4	0102-0102	1	0103-0501	7	0301-0501	11
0101-0103	3	0102-0103	3	0201-0201	3	0501-0501	9
0101-0201	9	0102-0201	7	0201-0301	5		
0101-0301	6	0102-0301	5	0201-0501	13		

Allele frequencies

Allele	Frequency	Allele	Frequency	Allele	Frequency
0101	0.1822	0103	0.0748	0301	0.1542
0102	0.0981	0201	0.2009	0501	0.2897

χ^2: 16.345 (d.f. 16); p:0.450

Comments: Significant differences with other SW European populations (i.e. P<0.01 with the population of Galicia). h: 0.8072, DP: 0.9335, CE: 0.6074.

References:
Lareu MV, Muñoz I, Pestoni C, Rodriguez MS, Vide C, Carracedo A (1993) The distribution of HLA DQA1 and D1S80 (pMCT118) alleles and genotypes in the population of Galicia and Central Portugal. Int J Leg Med 106:124-128.

System and locus: pMCT 118 (D1S80)

Population and sample size: 115 unreleated people from the district of Valencia (Eastern Spain).

Methods:
Primers: Kasai et al. (1990).
PCR amplification conditions (Lareu et al. 1993).
Method of detection: Miniaturized polyacrylamide gels (Phast-Gels 8-25, Pharmacia) followed by silver-staining.

Results:

Observed genotypes

Gen.	Obs.	Gen.	Obs.	Gen.	Obs.	Gen.	Obs.
16-29	1	18-31	2	23-27	1	24-33	1
17-18	1	19-24	1	23-29	1	24-35	1
18-18	9	20-24	3	23-31	1	24-36	1
18-20	1	20-28	1	24-24	17	25-27	1
18-21	1	21-22	1	24-25	3	26-30	1
18-22	2	21-24	1	24-26	4	26-31	1
18-24	15	21-25	1	24-27	4	28-29	1
18-25	2	22-24	2	24-28	2	29-29	1
18-26	1	22-29	1	24-29	5	29-31	1
18-28	2	22-30	1	24-30	1	31-31	1
18-29	4	23-23	1	24-31	7		
18-30	1	23-24	2	24-32	2		

Allele frequencies

Allele	Frequency	Allele	Frequency	Allele	Frequency	Allele	Frequency
16	0.0043	21	0.0174	26	0.0304	31	0.0609
17	0.0043	22	0.0304	27	0.0261	32	0.0087
18	0.2174	23	0.0304	28	0.0261	33	0.0043
19	0.0043	24	0.3870	29	0.0696	35	0.0043
20	0.0217	25	0.0304	30	0.0174	36	0.0043

Exact test p= 0.104

Comments: No significant differences with other SW European populations
h:0.7915, DP:0.9116, CE: 0.6208

References:

-Kasai K, Nakamura Y, White R (1990) Amplification of variable number of tandem repeats (VNTR) locus (pMCT118) by PCR and its aplication of Forensic Science. J Forensic Sci 35: 1196-1200.

-Lareu MV, Muñoz I, Pestoni C, Rodriguez MS, Vide C, Carracedo A (1993) The distribution of HLA DQA1 and D1S80 (pMCT118) alleles and genotypes in the population of Galicia and Central Portugal. Int J Leg Med 106:124-128.

GENE FREQUENCIES OF HUMAN POPULATIONS ALONG PYRENEAN CHAIN

Aluja, MªP. (1); Nogués, RMª; Sevin, A.(2); Larrouy, G. (3)

(1) U. Antropologia. Fac. Ciències. UAB 08193. Spain
(2) C.R.P.G. du C.N.R.S. Hopital Purpan. Toulouse. France
(3) Lab. Parasitol. et Ecol. Humaine. Univ. Paul Sabatier. Toulouse. France.

INTRODUCTION

The Pyrenees are an important range of mountains which have been a significant geographical barrier for the expansion of living species and, have more concretely played a great role in the establishment and differentiation of human cultures and populations.

Clines E-W are classically described for some blood group frequencies (ABO, for example) along the Pyrenees, and these clines extend from the Basque pole (wich represents an isolation area) to the Mediterranean zone wich constitutes an area of cultural and populational crossbreeding.

In spite of this, the existence of complex orographie with many N-S pointed valleys, surrounded by high peaks around 3,000 m., enhance the interest to establish if the isolation of valleys could vary or interrupt the regularity of cline. In fact, the isonimic studies show that the Pyrenean valleys reveal noteworthy individuality.

This short paper provides a brief discussion to establish the relationship between the different frequencies of blood markers and the variations of Pyrenaic geography.

MATERIALS AND METHOD

We have closely studied the hemotypology, internal mobility, migrations and isonimy of some characteristic valleys -La Cerdanya, Val d´Aran and Andorra- (1,2,3,4). Considering the genetic results we obtained, together with other Pyrenean populational data (5,6,7,8,9), we have drawn a genetic map which can show both the general cline of the mountain range and the peculiarities of its valleys.

The present analysis has been carried out for five groups (ABO, Rh, Fy, Kell, MN) on both sides of the Pyrenees. We have considered the 16 populations which have been reported for these markers (Fig. 1).

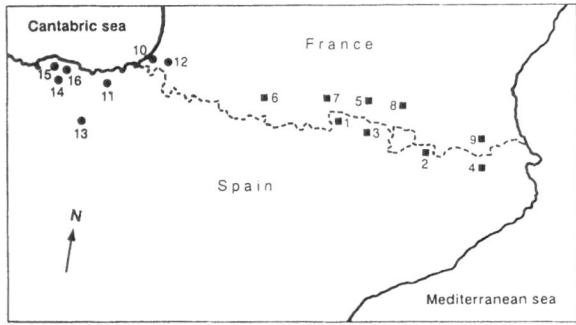

1: Val d'Aran
2: La Cerdanya
3: Pallars Sobirà
4: Garrotxa/Ripoll.
5: Bassin du Salat
6: Bigorre
7: Comminges
8: Pays de Foix
9: Eastern Pyrenees
10: French Basques
11: Spanish Basques
12: Macaya
13: Araba
14: Bizkaia
15: Arratia
16: Bizkaia

Fig.1: Geographical situation of Pyrenean populations considered.

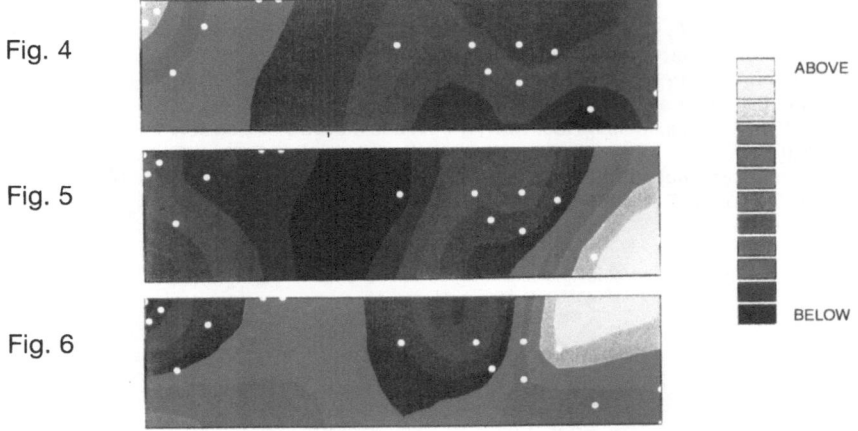

ABOVE	2.40
2.00 -	2.40
1.60 -	2.00
1.20 -	1.60
0.80 -	1.20
0.40 -	0.80
- -	0.40
-0.40 -	.
-0.80 -	-0.40
-1.20 -	-0.80
-1.60 -	-1.20
BELOW	-1.60

Fig. 2

ABOVE	3.15
2.70 -	3.15
2.25 -	2.70
1.80 -	2.25
1.35 -	1.80
0.90 -	1.35
0.45 -	0.90
0.00 -	0.45
-0.45 -	0.00
-0.90 -	-0.45
-1.35 -	-0.90
BELOW	-1.35

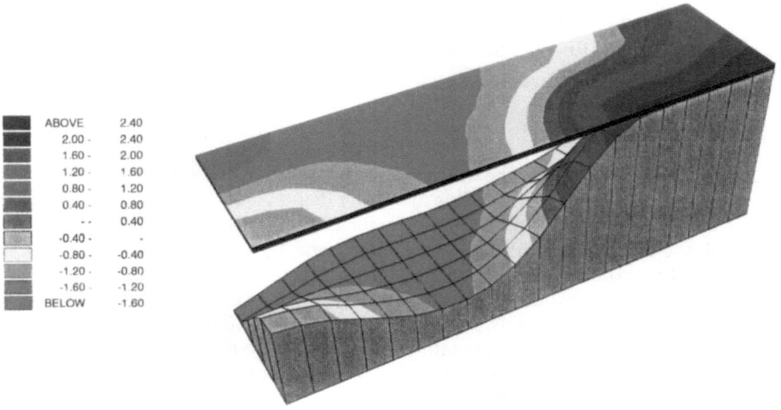

Fig. 3

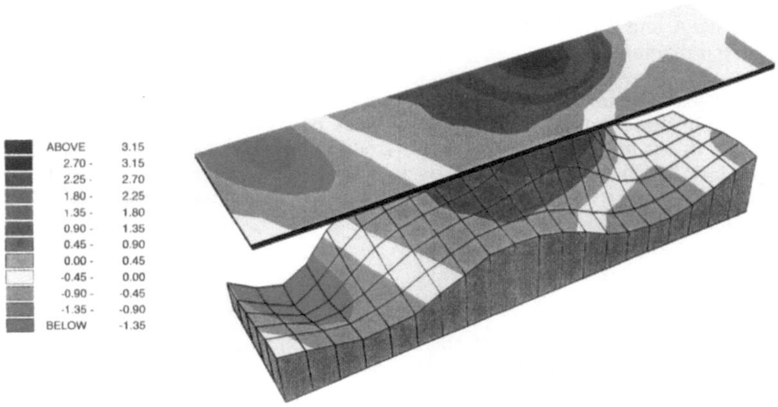

Fig. 2 and Fig. 3: Three-dimensional colour diagram of axes 1 and 2 of Principal Componen Analysis.

Fig. 4

Fig. 5

Fig. 6

ABOVE

BELOW

Fig. 4, Fig. 5 and Fig. 6: Rh(d), ABO (p) and Fy^a gene frequencies on geographical map.

We have analised many genetical markers but in this study we only consider 5 blood groups (ABO, Rh, Fy, MN and Kell) in 16 autochthonous populations on both slopes of Pyrenees whose genetical results are published. So we have always worked on definite date avoiding extrapolations.

RESULTS AND DISCUSSION

Fig. 2 is a three dimensional colour diagram of axe 1 for the PCA on all the considered blood groups. The cline E-W is clearly visible along the diagonal of the above rectangle. Fig. 3, shows the axe 2 of the PCA. In this graphic more influenced by Fy^a, the cline no longer appears. Considering the graphics wich correspond to each system one by one, we can apreciate some interesting peculiarities. For example, the allelic frequency of d on the geographical map (Fig. 4) also shows a clear cline from the Basque to Mediterranean populations, whereas the frequency of ABOp (Fig. 5) does not show it, but reveals a minimal value near the Central Pyrenees. The frequency of Fy^a (Fig. 6), on the other hand, also presents some characteristics like the isopleth (line of equal value) between Barèges and Comminges, and the Basque populations. This could be a reminiscence of an ancient Basque occupation since up to the VIth. century Basque was spoken in the area. Similar conclusions can be inferred from the PCA analysis of allelic frequencies for the locus A, the locus B and both A and B of the HLA system, and also from the analysis of genetic distances for the considered markers.

From the expounded data it can be deduced that although for the ABO system exists a clear continuity in the distribution of the frequencies between the North and the South slopes of the Pyrenees, this is not so clear for the Duffy and Rhesus Systems. These partially show clines N-S (and no E-W like in the case of ABO) as can be deduced from Fig. 4 and Fig. 6. We could consider that the E-W clines are reflection of the Neolithic migrations, while the N-S clines reveal the Indoeuropean population movements.

REFERENCES

1 ALUJA MªP: Estudi de diversos polimorfismes bioquímics a la comarca de La Cerdanya. Bellaterra, Universitat Autònoma de Barcelona, 1987.
2 ALUJA MªP, ERCILLA G, FONT A: HLA gene and haplotipe frequencies in a Spanish East Pyrenean population. Humanbiol. Budapest., 1989;19:129-135
3 NOGUES RMª, ALUJA MªP, MALGOSA A, MAS J: Variability of the Rh system in a Central Pyrenean population (Aran Valley). Gene Geography, 1992;6:97-108
4 ALUJA MªP, NOGUES RMª, MALGOSA A: Situation hémotypologique des populations de deux valles Pyrénéennes: quelques repères sur leurs origines. Rivista di Antropologia,1992; v. LXX:81-89.
5 MOURANT AE, KOPEC A, DOMANIEWSKA-SOBZAK K: The Distribution of the Human Blood Groups and Other Polymorphismes. Oxford University Press, 1976.
6 MORENO P, MORAL P, PANADERO AM: Sistemas de grupos sanguíneos ABO, Lewis, Rh, K, Duffy y P, en el Pallars Subirà. Trab. Antropol., 1986;20: 333-350.
7 MORENO P, MORAL P: Sistemas MNSs, Duffy y P en una muestra de población de Gerona. Trab. Antropol., 1986;20: 49-57.
8 ITURRIOZ R: Polimorfismos eritrocitarios de la población autóctona vizcaína y población mixta, Munibe, 1984;36:105-117.

Multiplex PCR and Automated Fluorescence Detection of Four Tetrameric STRs in a Western Austrian Population

E. Ambach[*], W. Parson[*], H. Niederstätter[*], B. Budowle[**]

* Institute for Forensic Medicine, University of Innsbruck, Muellerstraße 44, 6020 Innsbruck, Austria, Europe
** FSRTC, FBI Academy, Quantico, VA 22135, USA

Introduction

Short Tandem Repeats (STR) loci, also known as microsatellites, consist of repetitive sequences, generally 2 to 6 nucleotides in lenght. Because of their highly polymorphic nature, STR loci offer high discrimination amongst individuals which can be valuable in forensic matters. The fact that STRs are amplifiable by the Polymerase Chain Reaction (PCR) from small quantities of DNA (about 1 ng or less) and even substantially degraded DNA samples, makes the use of STRs desirable for genetic characterization in a number of forensic cases.
In the study, four STR loci (HUMTH01, HUMvWA31/A, HUMFES/FPS, HUMF13A1) were amplified and typed simultaneously to generate a database of a Western Austrian population.

Material and Methods

Blood was obtained from 382 unrelated individuals living in Western Austria. DNA was isolated from blood samples following digestion in Proteinase K (Boehringer Mannheim) and extraction by phenol/chloroform.
1–3 ng DNA were amplified by multiplex PCR in a total volume of 25 µl consisting of 1x PCR Buffer I, 1.7 mM $MgCl_2$, 250 µM each dNTP and 2 units AmpliTaq®–Polymerase (all Perkin Elmer). Oligonucleotide primer were synthesized commercially and labeled with fluorescent dye markers, either 6–FAM (6–carboxyfluorescein) or HEX (6–carboxy–2′,4′,7′,4, 7–Hexachlorofluorescein) coupled with an aminohexyl linker (Applied Biosystems, Weiterstadt, Germany).
PCR Amplification was carried out on a 9600 GeneAmp PCR Thermocycler (Perkin Elmer): 28 cycles at 94 °C for 45 sec, 54 °C for 45 sec and 72 °C for 90 sec, and a final incubation at 72 °C for 10 min. Prior to PCR all samples were incubated at 95°C for 5 min and hot–started with a deluted Taq–start mix.

Primer

TC11/f	(11p15–15.5)	5′–GTGATTCCCATTGGCCTGTTCCTC–3′
TC11/r		5′–6–FAM–GTGGGCTGAAAAGCTCCCGATTAT–3′
VWA/f	(12p12–pter)	5′–HEX–CCCTAGTGGATGATAAGAATAATCAGTATG–′3′
VWA/r		5′–GGACAGATGATAAATACATAGGATGGATGG–3′
FES/f	(15q25–qter)	5′–GGGATTTCCCTATGGATTGG–3′
FES/r		5′–6–FAM–GCGAAAGAATGAGACTACAT–3′
F13A1/f	(6p24–25)	5′–GAGGTTGCACTCCAGCCTTT–3′
F13A1/r		5′–HEX–ATGCCATGCAGATTAGAAA–3′

1 µl aliquots of the amplification products were combined with 1.2 fmol internal lane standard GeneScan–350 Tamra (Perkin Elmer), prepared by *PstI* digestion of plasmid DNA, subsequently digested by *BstU I* to yield DNA fragments containing a single TAMRA dye to ensure single peaks for unambigious standard calculation. Prior to loading on a denaturating polyacrylamid sequencing gel (6%T, 5%C; 8.3M urea; 1xTBE) the samples were denaturated at 90 °C for 2 min.

Gels were electrophoresed on an 373A Strech DNA Sequencer (ABI) for 5 hours at constant power (30 W), using filterwheel B. Analysis was performed with 672 GeneScan software (ABI) using the local southern method for fragment size estimation.

Statistical analysis

The frequency of each allele for each locus was calculated from the numbers of each genotype in the sample set. Unbiased estimates of expected heterozygosity were computed as described by Edwards, et al. (4). Possible divergence from Hardy–Weinberg expectations (HWE) was determined by calculating the unbiased estimate of the expected homozygote/heterozygote frequencies (3,9,10), the likelyhood ratio test (2,4,11), and the exact test (5).

The precision of band size estimation by the GeneScan 672 software for each allele at a distinct locus was calculated according to Kimpton et al (8). Polymorphic information content (PIC) was calculated using the formula of Botstein et al (1). An interclass correlation criterion (7) was used for detecting disequilibrium between loci.

Results and Discussion

We typed four tetrameric Strs in a multiplex reaction optimizing amplification parameters in order to yield a maximum signal–to–noise ratio. Firstly, we put a 2 min cooling ramp between denaturation and annealing step to get clear peaks with a weak background, which was rather time–consuming. This procedure also resulted in a preferential amplification of systems with higher Tm–values (i.e. HUMTH01, VWA). As we dropped the ramp, denaturation was exceeded up to 90 sec which led to a well–balanced result.

The distribution of observed allele frequencies for the four loci in a population sample of 382 unrelated individuals living in Western Austria are shown in Table 1.

Table 1: Allele frequencies (N=382).

Allele	HUMTH01	VWA	F13A1	FES
3.2			0.086	
4			0.045	
5			0.190	
6	0.229		0.285	
7	0.157		0.346	
8	0.122		0.003	0.004
9	0.152			
9.3	0.331			
10	0.009			0.298
11			0.005	0.450
12			0.003	0.200
13			0.003	0.046
14		0.102	0.005	0.001
15		0.124	0.020	
16		0.206	0.008	
17		0.246	0.003	
18		0.213		
19		0.090		
20		0.016		
21		0.003		
% precision[a]	99,93	99,88	99,92	99,94
SD	0,02	0,11	0,04	0,04
range[b]	0,41–0,85	0,62–0,98	0,01–1,1	0,06–0,99
PIC	0,74	0,79	0,71	0,61

a) across gels
b) fragment size estimated by the GeneScan 672 software for a given allele across gels

The genotype frequency distributions for HUMTH01, VWA and FES do not deviate from HWE based on the homozygosity test, likelyhood ratio test, and the exact test (Table 2). The F13A1 locus does depart from Hardy–Weinberg expectations.

The chi–square test for total homozygotes and heterozygotes does not detect departures from expectations for F13A1 (p=0,347). This is misleading and demonstrates the limited power of the particular test. The number of 5–5, 6–6, and 7–7 observed F13A1 homozygotes in our sample population was 22, 19, and 43, respectively. However, the expected number of homozygotes is 13.8, 31, and 45.7, respectively. Obviously, only the 7–7 observed and expected number of homozygotes are similar. The 5–5 and 6–6 homozygote situation tends to cancel one another.

The more powerful tests, such as the exact test, readily detect the departure (p=0,002). The apparent departure should not raise substantial concern for the use of the F13A1 locus and the product rule in human identity testing. The counting method (i.e., the frequency of an observed genotype) could be used for estimating an F13A1 type.

However, one should not confuse statistical significance with practical or *forensic significance*. When comparing the frequency of the F13A1 alleles in Western Austrians with other studies, such as that described by Hammond, et al. (6) for United States Caucasians, there is very little difference. For example, the frequencies of F13A1 alleles 3.2, 4, 5, 6, and 7 in West Austrians is 0.086, 0.045, 0.190, 0.285, and 0.346, respectively, and in United States Caucasians the frequencies are 0.083, 0.020, 0.192, 0.345, and 0.325, respectively. Under the assumption of independence using either database would yield similar estimates of the frequency of F13A1 types. The data suggest that it might be considered more appropriate to assume independence at the F13A1 locus in the Western Austrian sample population to obtain a valid estimate of the rarity of F13A1 types.

An analysis was performed to determine whether or not there were any detectable associations between any pair–wise comparisons of the four STR loci. An inter–class correlation test analysis demonstrated that there were no departures from expectation (Table 3).

Table 2:Tests for independence on STR loci.

	HUMTH01	VWA	F13A1	FES
Obs. Homozygosity	23.3%	16.8%	22.5%	34.6%
Exp. Homozygosity[a]	22.4%	18.2%	24.6%	33.3%
Homozygosity Test[b]	0.665	0.478	0.347	0.607
LikelyhoodRatio Test[b]	0.268	0.972	0.003	0.153
Exact Test[b]	0.459	0.956	0.002	0.218

Table 3: Test for independence between loci

Loci	Probability
HUMTH01/VWA	0.585
HUMTH01/F13A1	0.476
HUMTH01/FES	0.677
VWA/F13A1	0.974
VWA/FES	0.262
F13A1/FES	0.867

a) Expected homozygosity is an unbiased estimate.
b) These values are probability values.

References

1. Botstein, D., White, R.L., Skolnick, M., Davis, R.W. (1980) **Am.J.Hum.Genet.** 32:314–331.
2. Chakraborty R, Fornage M, Guegue R, et al. (1991) in: Burke T, Dolf G, Jeffreys AJ, Wolff R, (ed) DNA Fingerprinting: Approaches and Applications. Berlin: Birkhauser Verlag, 127–143.
3. Chakraborty, R., Smouse, P.E., Neel, J.V. (1988) **Hum.Genet.** 43:709–725.
4. Edwards, A., Hammond, H.A., Jin, L., Caskey, T., Chakraborty, R. (1992) **Genomics** 12:241–253.
5. Guo, S.W., Thompson, E.A. (1992) **Biometrics** 48:361–372.
6. Hammond, H.A., Jin, L., Zhong, Y., Caskey, C.T., Chakraborty, R. (1994) Am.J.Hum.Genet. 55:175–189.
7. Karlin, S., Cameron, E.C., Williams, P.T. (1981) **Proc.Natl.Acad.Sci USA** 78:2664–2668.
8. Kimpton C.P., G.P., Walton A. (1993) **Cold Spring Harbour Laboratory Press** 3:13–22.
9. Nei, M. (1978) **Genetics** 89:583–590.
10. Nei, M., Roychoudhury, A.K. (1974) **Genetics** 76:379–390.
11. Weir, B.S. (1992) **Genetics** 130:873–887.

Population and formal genetics of the STRs
TPO, TH01 and VWFA31/A in North Portugal

A. Amorim, L. Gusmão and M. J. Prata

Inst. Antropologia, Univ.Porto and IPATIMUP, 4050 Porto, Portugal

Systems and loci

TPO, repeat (AATG), intron 10 of thyroid peroxidase gene (2p23-pter)
TH01, repeat (TCAT), intron 1of tyrosine hydroxylase gene (11p15.5-p15)
VWFA31/A, repeat (TCTR), intron 40 of von Willebrand factor gene (12p12-pter).

Population and sample sizes:

North Portugal. TPO: N=273; TH01: N=197; VWFA31/A: N=255

Methods:

Samples: blood or buccal swabs from unrelated individuals and mother/child pairs; DNA extraction: method of Lareu *et al.* (1994); electrophoresis according to Luis and Caeiro (1995); silver staining: Budowle *et al.*(1992); genotyping was performed by side-by-side comparison with an allelic ladder made up from previously typed samples.

TPO: primers (Anker *et al.*, 1992); amplification conditions: 5 min at 93°; 94°: 1 min; 63°: 0.5 min; 72°: 1.5 min; 27-35 cycles

TH01: primers (Gill *et al.*, 1994); amplification conditions: 5 min at 93°; 94°: 1 min; 54°: 1 min; 72°: 1 min; 27-35 cycles

VWFA31/A: primers (Kimpton *et al.*, 1992); amplification conditions: the same as for TH01.

Results:

Allele frequencies

TPO		TH01		VWFA31/A	
Allele	**Freq.**	**Allele**	**Freq.**	**Allele**	**Freq.**
6	0.005	6	0.193	12	0.002
7	0.004	7	0.191	13	0.002
8	0.511	8	0.140	14	0.121
9	0.084	9	0.201	15	0.110
10	0.060	9.3	0.256	16	0.214
11	0.291	10	0.019	17	0.300
12	0.042			18	0.176
13	0.002			19	0.061
				20	0.012
				21	0.002

Observed genotypes

TPO Genotypes	Obs.	TH01 Genotypes	Obs.	VWFA31/A Genotypes	Obs.
6-8	1	6-6	8	12-17	1
6-9	1	6-7	13	13-16	1
6-11	1	6-8	13	14-14	4
7-8	2	6-9	17	14-15	6
8-8	73	6-9.3	19	14-16	9
8-9	17	6-10	2	14-17	25
8-10	17	7-7	11	14-18	10
8-11	83	7-8	8	14-19	3
8-12	12	7-9	16	14-20	1
8-13	1	7-9.3	19	15-15	4
9-9	2	7-10	1	15-16	19
9-10	3	8-8	5	15-17	12
9-11	17	8-9	11	15-18	6
9-12	4	8-9.3	15	15-19	3
10-10	1	8-10	1	15-20	2
10-11	10	9-9	9	16-16	11
10-12	1	9-9.3	19	16-17	35
11-11	21	9-10	2	16-18	15
11-12	6	9.3-9.3	16	16-19	6
		9.3-10	2	16-20	2
				17-17	14
				17-18	37
				17-19	14
				17-21	1
				18-18	9
				18-19	4
				19-20	1

| P=0.9 | P=0.9 | P=0.7 |

Comments:

Mother-child pairs analyses (nr. of pairs: 159, 121 and 160 for each system, respectively) show no exclusions and no deviations to mendelian rules.

In TPO system two new alleles (7 and 13) were found, and frequencies estimated in this sample are similar to those reported up to now for Caucasians.

For TH01, allele 9 is more frequent than in other Caucasians, allele 9.3 being correspondingly rarer.

Concerning VWFA31/A, a new allele (12) with 130 bp was found; gene frequencies are similar to those described in other Caucasian populations.

References

Anker R, Steinbrueck T, Donis-Keller H (1992) Tetranucleotide repeat polymorphism at the human thyroid peroxidase (hTPO) locus. Hum Mol Genet 1: 137

Budowle B, Chakraborty R, Giusti AM, Eisenberg AJ, Allen RC (1991) Analysis of the VNTR locus D1S80 by the PCR followed by high-resolution PAGE. Am J Hum Genet 48: 137-144

Gill P, Kimpton C, D'Aloja E, Andersen JF, Bar W, Brinkmann B, Holgersson S, Johnson V, Kloosterman AD, Lareu MV, Nellemann L, Pfitzinger H, Phillips CP, Scmitter H, Schneider PM, Stenersen M (1994) Report of the European DNA profiling group (EDNAP)- twoards standardisation of short tandem repeat (STR) loci. Forensic Sci Int 65: 51-59

Kimpton C, Walton A, Gill P (1992) A further tetranucleotide repeat polymorphism in the vWF gene. Hum Mol Genet 1: 287

Lareu MV, Phillips CP, Carracedo A, Lincoln PJ, Court DS, Thomson JA (1994) Investigation of the STR locus HUMTH01 using PCR and two electrophoresis formats: UK and Galician Caucasian population surveys and usefulness in paternity investigations. Forensic Sci Int 66: 41-52

Luis JR, Caeiro B (1995) Application of two STRs (VWF and hTPO) to human population profiling. A survey in Galicia. Human Biology (in press)

Acknowledgements: This work was partially supported by JNICT (Junta Nacional de Investigação Científica e Tecnológica, BD/2849/93-ID and PBIC/C/CEN/1174/92) and CNCDP (Comissão Nacional para as Comemorações dos Descobrimentos Portugueses, research contract nº 70).

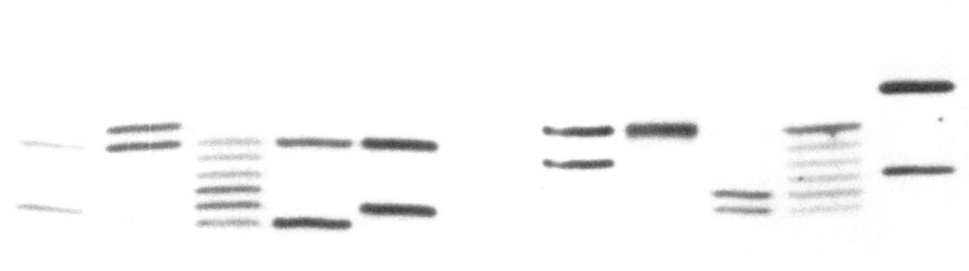

Fig 1. TPO genotypes
From left to right: lane 1: 8-12; lane 2: 7-8; lane 3: ladder; lane 4: 8-13; lane 5: 8-12;

Fig 2. VWFA31/A genotypes
From left to right: lane 1: 14-16; lane 2: 14-14; lane 3: 18-19; lane 4: ladder; lane 5: 12-17;

POPULATION GENETICS OF THREE STRs: TH01, CSF1PO AND TPOX IN SOUTHERN SPAIN

ANDRES MI, PRIETO V, FLORES IC, SANZ P.

National Institute of Toxicology. Seville. Spain.

Human systems under study

TH01: Tyrosine hydroxylase gene (11p15.5); AATG repeat; alleles 5, 6, 7, 8, 9, 9.3, 10, 11.
CSF1PO: c-fms protooncogene for CSF-1 receptor gene (5q33.3-34); AGAT repeat; alleles 8, 9, 10, 11, 12, 13, 14.
TPOX: Thyroid peroxidase gene (2p13); AATG repeat; alleles 8, 9, 10, 11, 12.

Population and sample size: Andalusian (Southern Spain) N:150.

Methods:

Blood samples from casework and staff. Extraction: Chelating Agent (Sigma).
Amplifications: simultaneous amplification using the Gene Print STR multiplex from Promega.
Typing: 6% denaturing gel electrophoresis followed by silver staining according to Promega protocols (1994).

Results

Table 1 TH01 observed genotypes

Gen.	N	Freq.	Gen.	N	Freq.	Gen	N	Freq.
6-6	3	0.0203	7-7	8	0.0541	8-9	7	0.0473
6-7	8	0.0541	7-8	8	0.0541	8-9.3	11	0.0743
6-8	9	0.0608	7-9	6	0.0405	9-9	7	0.0473
6-9	13	0.0878	7-9.3	13	0.0878	9-9.3	13	0.0878
6-9.3	16	0.1081	7-10*	4	0.0270	9-10*	1	0.0068
6-10*	3	0.0203	8-8*	6	0.0405	9.3-9.3	12	0.0811

$X^2 = 8.1088$ df$=7$ p$=0.3231$ % Heterozygosity$= 75.68$ * pooled classes
Discrimination Power$= 0.9312$ Average Power of exclusion$= 54.71$ %

Table 2 TPOX observed genotypes

Gen.	N	Freq.	Gen.	N	Freq.	Gen	N	Freq.
6-9*	1	0.0067	8-12†	4	0.0268	10-10‡	1	0.0067
8-8*	32	0.2148	9-9†	2	0.0134	10-11	2	0.0134
8-9	14	0.0940	9-10†	2	0.0134	11-11	18	0.1208
8-10	13	0.0872	9-11‡	3	0.0201	11-12	5	0.0336
8-11	51	0.3423	9-12‡	1	0.0067			

$X^2 = 7.5555$ df=3 p=0.0561 % Heterozygosity= 64.43 *,†,‡ different pooled classes
Discrimination Power= 0.8027 Average Power of exclusion= 38.13 %

Table 3 CSF1PO observed genotypes

Gen.	N	Freq.	Gen.	N	Freq.	Gen	N	Freq.
8-9*	2	0.0136	10-10	8	0.0544	11-13	10	0.0680
8-10*	1	0.0068	10-11	22	0.1497	11-14‡	1	0.0068
8-11*	1	0.0068	10-12	24	0.1633	12-12‡	19	0.1293
9-10*	2	0.0136	10-13	2	0.0136	12-13	8	0.0544
9-11*	3	0.0204	10-14†	1	0.0068	12-14○	2	0.0136
9-12*	1	0.0068	11-11†	15	0.1020	12-15○	1	0.0068
9-14*	1	0.0068	11-12	21	0.1429	13-14○	2	0.0136

$X^2 = 7.2439$ df=3 p=0.0645 % Heterozygosity=71.43 *,†,‡,○ different pooled classes
Discrimination Power= 0.8912 Average Power of exclusion= 48.05 %

Table 4 TH01 allele frequencies

Allel.	N	Freq.	Allel.	N	Freq.	Allel.	N	Freq.
5	0	0.0000	8	47	0.1588	10	8	0.0270
6	55	0.1858	9	54	0.1824	11	0	0.0000
7	55	0.1858	9.3	77	0.2601			

Table 5 TPOX allele frequencies

Allel.	N	Freq.	Allel.	N	Freq.	Allel.	N	Freq.
6	1	0.0034	9	25	0.0839	12	10	0.0336
7	0	0.0000	10	19	0.0638	13	0	0.0000
8	146	0.4899	11	97	0.3255			

Table 6 CSF1PO allele frequencies

Allel.	N	Freq.	Allel.	N	Freq.	Allel.	N	Freq.
7	0	0.0000	10	68	0.2313	13	22	0.0748
8	4	0.0136	11	88	0.2993	14	7	0.0238
9	9	0.0306	12	95	0.3231	15	1	0.0034

Comparison with other caucasian populations:

TH01 genotype frequencies were compared with two Spanish published data (Philipe, 1994; Lorente, 1994) using a Rx C contingency table X^2 test for homogeneity. The allele distributions were similar (p=0.8 and p=0.3 respectively). Up to date, enough genotype frequency data were not available for TPOX and CSF1PO in other Spanish caucasian populations.

Examples from casework

1.- PATERNITY CASE: After the implementation of STRs an old conflicting paternity case was reconsidered. The two alleged fathers were brothers of the mother. Paternity could not be solved at the time of the study: RFLPs could not be applied because blood samples, inadequately conserved, were deteriorated on arrival at the laboratory, DNA was highly degraded and no more blood samples could be obtained. Only DQA1 and D1S80 were added to the set of conventional genetic markers. No exclusions were found due to a high degree of consanguinity within the family group for several generations. The probabilities of paternity were 98.62% for alleged father 1 and 94.26% for alleged father 2. With the investigation of STRs (TH01, CSF1PO and TPOX) the probability of paternity for alleged father 1 increased to 99.89% and one exclusion was detected for alleged father 2 in TH01 (two additional exclusions were found when investigating other STR loci).

2.- SEXUAL ASSAULT: Samples: Victim and suspect blood samples, vaginal swab, blood stain on the suspect's underpants. Pubic hair obtained from pubic combing of the victim. The following results were obtained:

	DQA1	D1S80	CSF1PO	TPOX	TH01
Victim	1.3,2	T24T29	10-12	8-11	6-7
Suspect	2,3	T20T28	11-13	8-11	6-9
Spermatozoa	2,3	ND	11-13	8-11	6-9
Blood Stain	1.3,2(3)	T24T29 (T20T28)	10-12	8-11	6-7(9)
Pubic hair	2,3	ND	11-13	8-11	6-9

ND= not detected   ( )= weak signal

References

- Lorente JA, Lorente M, Budowle B, Wilson MR, Villanueva E (1994) Analysis of the HumTH01 Allele Frequencies in the Spanish Population. JFSCAS 39(5): 1270-1274

- Philips CP, Laren MV, Lincoln PJ, Carracedo A, Thomson JA (1994) In: Bär W, Fiori A, Rossi U (eds) Advances in Forensic Haemogenetics 5. Springer Verlag, Berlin

- Puers C, Lins AM, Sprecher CJ, Brinkmann B, Schumm JW (1993) Analysis of polymorphic STR loci using well characterized Allelic ladders. Fourth International Symposium on human identification, Promega

- Promega (1994) Gene Print STR Systems. Technical Manual

FREQUENCY MULTIVARIATE ANALYSIS OF LDLR, GYPA, HBGG, D7S8 AND GC IN 12 DIFFERENT POPULATIONS.

E. Arroyo, C. Asperilla, L. Prieto, M. Herrera, J. M. Ruiz de la Cuesta.

Departamento de Toxicología y Legislación Sanitaria. Escuela de Medicina Legal. Facultad de Medicina. Universidad Complutense de Madrid. 28040-Madrid. Spain.

INTRODUCTION

The object of this work is to establish comparisons among those populations studied for LDLR, GYPA, HBGG, D7S8 and GC loci, all of them contained in the "Amplitype PCR PM Amplification and Typing Kit". As far as we know, just twelve populations have been studied for the whole set of markers. Other authors have carried out comparisons among different populations tested for the same set of loci, but none have established a multivariate relation among the series. In this paper, a twofold multivariate analysis was tried: first, a Dendrogram Analysis (DA) and then a Principal Component Analysis (PCA).

MATERIAL AND METHODS

First of all, a matrix was constructed with the gene frequencies cited in the literature plus a sample studied in the Forensic Biology Laboratory of the Legal Medicine School of the Complutense University (207 apparently health non related individuals living in Madrid , Spain).
The set of samples obtained can not be considered a worldwide distribution of frequencies, since it is a mainly caucasian set of samples. However, other racial groups could also be included. The gene frequency matrix was analyzed with the SPSS/PC+ package for microcomputers. A genetic distance matrix was obtained from the gene frequencies matrix and then, a dendrogram was constructed with the former matrix. To calculate the genetic distances between populations a cosine transformation, similar to that proposed by Cavalli-Sforza and Edwards (1967), was used. The UPGMA algorithm was used to construct the dendrogram. Then, to extract the Principal Components (PC), Kaiser-Meyer-Olkin measure of sampling adequacy to the PC model was used and PC's were extracted and plotted. Both multivariate analyses allow to evaluate graphically the genetic proximity of the populations considered.

RESULTS AND DISCUSSION

In the figure 1 a UPGMA dendrogram for the eleven series can be seen. Caucasian samples appear together in the same cluster and at a very short distance: Swiss and Bavarian populations and two series of U.S. caucasians are clustered together with a sample of Hispanics from the south-east of the U.S.A. Spanish series (Galicia and Madrid), plus a sample of American caucasians, are also grouped together and very close to the former caucasian cluster. The other Hispanic samples remain

```
                        Rescaled Distance Cluster Combine

     C A S E   List of 0        5        10       15       20       25
     Label     Ref.   +---------+---------+---------+---------+---------+

  Hisp-SE-USA    2     -+
  Swiss          3     -¦
  Cauc-USA(2)    2     -+-+
  Bavarians      4     -+ +-----+
  Cauc-USA(1)    5     -+ ¦     ¦
  Madrid         6     -+-+     +--------------+
  Galicia        7     -+       ¦              ¦
  Hispanics-USA  5     --------+              +-----------------------+
  Hisp-SW-USA    2     ---+     ¦              ¦                       ¦
  Chinese        8     -------------------+---+                       ¦
  Blacks-USA(1)  5     -------------------------------------------+---+
  Blacks-USA(2)  2     -+
```

Figure 1. Dendrogram using Average Linkage (Between Groups). UPGMA.

(2) Budowle et al., 1992. (3) Hochmeister MN et al., 1994. (4) Hausmann R et al., 1995. (5) Perkin Elmer. Manufacturer's protocol, 1994. (6) Herrera M., 1995, (7) Pestoni C. , 1995. (8) Huang and Budowle, 1995.

together and, finally, mongoloid and negroid populations - Chinese plus the two U.S. black samples - cluster separately of the caucasian and Hispanic groups. Black samples are at a very short distance between each other and far away from the rest of populations. In conclusion, the DA reflects very well a three major racial groups model.

In the case of PC analysis, the gene frequency matrix was evaluated for Kaiser-Meyer-Olkin statistic (0.47105). The result showed a not very good sampling adequacy. However, the initial set of variables could be reduced to three PC's, the first of them explaining 47.4% of the total variance of the data, the second 35.3% and the third 13.5%. The three PC's explain the 96.3% of the total variance of the data.

In the figure 2, a plot of the two first PC's (82.8% of the total variance) can be seen. The

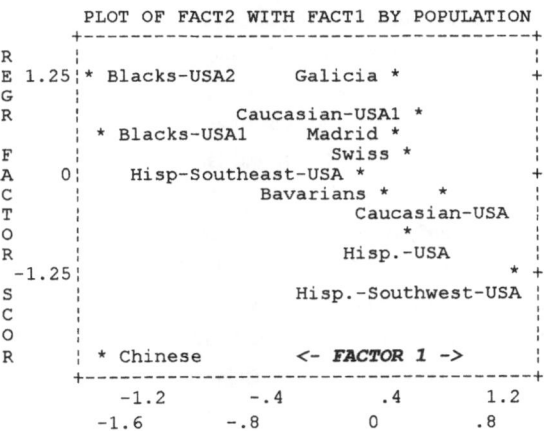

```
                PLOT OF FACT2 WITH FACT1 BY POPULATION
        +-----------------------------------------+
   R    ¦                                         ¦
   E  1.25¦* Blacks-USA2       Galicia *          +
   G    ¦                                         ¦
   R    ¦          Caucasian-USA1 *               ¦
        ¦    * Blacks-USA1      Madrid *          ¦
   F    ¦                       Swiss *           ¦
   A   0¦       Hisp-Southeast-USA *              +
   C    ¦                    Bavarians *     *    ¦
   T    ¦                       Caucasian-USA     ¦
   O    ¦                            *            ¦
   R    ¦                       Hisp.-USA         ¦
    -1.25¦                                   * +
   S    ¦                       Hisp.-Southwest-USA ¦
   C    ¦                                         ¦
   O    ¦                                         ¦
   R    ¦ * Chinese          <- FACTOR 1 ->       ¦
        +-----------------------------------------+
            -1.2      -.4        .4       1.2
          -1.6      -.8        0        .8
```

Figure 2. Plot of the two first Principal Components (82.8% of the total variance).

results meets quite well the conclusions of the DA: a group of caucasoid populations are very close to each other. Two Hispanic samples plot at the same distance of the caucasian group, and U.S. black samples appear separate of the other populations, the Chinese sample being the most separate of the set. Some subjetive interpretations of the PC plot can be avoided with the help of the DA which shows clearly the grouping of the series based on the genetic distance matrix. Finally, we can list the three following conclusions:

- A twofold multivariate approach can resolve some subjetivity, mainly in the case of PC plotting.

- The combination of DA and PCA seems to support a three major racial groups model for the populations considered in the study.

- The "Amplitype PCR PM Amplification and Typing Kit" is a usefull tool for genetic comparison of populations.

However, it would be better to carry out more studies in order to check the adequacy of the markers contained in the kit for population genetics studies.

REFERENCES

Budowle B, Lindsey JA, DeCou JA, Koos BW, Giusti AM, Comey CT (1995) Validation and population studies of thhe loci LDLR, GYPA, HBGG, D7S8 and GC (PM loci) and HLA-DQ alpha using a multiplex amplification and typing procedure. J. Forensic Sci. 40(1): 45.

Cavalli-Sforza LL, Edwards AWF (1967) Phylogenetics analysis: models and estimation procedures. Am. J. Hum. Genet. 19: 233-257.

Hausmann R, HAntschel M, Loetterle J (1995) Frequencies of the 5 PCR-based genetic markers LDLR, GYPA, HBGG, D7S8 and GC in a North Bavarian population. Int. J. Legal Med. 107(4): 227.

Herrera M (1995) Estudio del "Amplitype Polymarker PCR Amplification and Typing Kit". Doctoral Thesis. Universidad Complutense de Madrid.

Hochmeister MN, Budowle B, Borer UV, Dirnhofer R (1994) Swiss population data on the loci HLA-DQA1, LDLR, GYPA, HBGG, D7S8, GC and D1S80. Forensic Sci. Int. 67: 175-184.

Huang NE, Budowle B (1995) Chinese population data on the PCR-based loci HLA-DQ Alpha, Low-Density-Lipoprotein Receptor, Glycophorin A, Hemoglobin γ^G, D7S8, and Group-Specific Component. Hum. Hered. 45: 34-40.

Pestoni C, Muñoz JL, Rodríguez-Calvo MS, Bellas A, García Rivero A, Lareu MV, Barros F, Carracedo A (1995) Actas VII Jornadas Soc. Esp. Med. Legal y Forense. Lérida 4-6 Mayo. p. 473-481.

Perkin Elmer Corp., USA (1994). Amplitype PCR PM Amplifying and Typing Kit Manual. Part. No. N808-0057. p. 3.

WORLDWIDE DISTRIBUTION OF D1S80 POLYMORPHISM. COMPARISON OF GENETIC DISTANCES AND CLUSTER ANALYSIS

C. Asperilla, E. Arroyo, L. Prieto, J. M. Ruiz de la Cuesta

Departamento de Toxicología y Legislación Sanitaria. Facultad de Medicina. Universidad Complutense de Madrid. 28040 - Madrid. Spain.

INTRODUCTION

Some studies have tried to compare the homogeneity of D1S80 frequencies in populations of various origins. However, as far as we know, only conventional approaches with a small set of populations have been tested.

In this study we compare through a multivariate analysis a set of 48 populations which comprise of wide sample of the populations of the world.

MATERIALS AND METHODS

A data matrix was constructed with as many populations as possible and then proceed with the statistical package SPSS/PC+ for microcomputers.

The genetic disimilarity matrix (distance matrix) was calculated according to cosine transformation. This algorithm is similar to that of Cavalli-Sforza and Edwards (1967). The distance matrix was clustered with the UPGMA algorithm to obtain the final dendrogram.

RESULTS AND DISCUSSION

Several main clusters can be observed within the dendrogram (See dendrogram below). A big cluster comprising most of the caucasian populations plus a sample of US-Hispanics can be clearly differentiated from the rest. Another caucasian cluster contains two samples of US-caucasians plus portuguese and Galician samples. The oriental samples have clustered together and appear well apart from the caucasians cluster and a small cluster, which comprises all the populations of black african background, is situated at some distance from the former clusters.

Between caucasian and oriental clusters, a small group of Hispanic and caucasian populations (Russians, Finns and Indians) can be noticed.

However, some populations can not clearly classified within any of these clusters. A sample of papuans from New Guinea highlands clusters in intermediate positions between the former caucasian-Hispanic and oriental groups. Also, Pehuenche indians from central Chile remains between oriental populations and a set of heterogeneous populations from Birmania (Kachari) and Polynesia. The sample of Zoró indians from Brazil is separated from the rest of the clusters, probably due to some kind of genetic isolation.

```
Dendrogram using Average Linkage (Between Groups). UPGMA.

                              Rescaled Distance Cluster Combine

A S E          List of   0        5        10       15       20       25
Label       References   +--------+--------+--------+--------+--------+

Danes               26   -+
Caucasian-USA        5   -¦
Caucasian-USA       10   -¦
Swiss               12   -¦
Germans-NW          24   -¦
Germans-Münster     21   -¦
Austrians           14   -¦
Madrid-1             2   -¦
Madrid-2             6   -¦
Dutch               15   -¦
Germans-1            9   -+-+
Germans-2           23   -¦ ¦
Caucasian-USA       20   -¦ ¦
Caucasian-USA       17   -¦ ¦
Barcelona            3   -¦ ¦
Hisp-SE-USA          5   -+ ¦
Caucasian-USA       22   -+ ¦
Caucasian-USA        4   -¦ ¦
Galicia             16   -¦ ¦
Coimbra             16   -+-+
Brazil-whites       11   -¦ ¦
Slavonians          19   -+ +-+
Russians             7   -+ ¦ ¦
Indians              8   -¦ ¦ ¦
Finns               22   -+-+ ¦
Hispanics-USA       20   -¦ ¦ +------+
Mexican-USA         17   -¦ ¦ ¦      ¦
Hispanics-USA       10   -+ ¦ ¦      ¦
Hisp-SW-USA          5   ---+ ¦      ¦
New Guinea           9   -----+    +---+
Japan-2             18   ---+      ¦   ¦
Orientals            5   -+ ¦      ¦   ¦
Japan-1             25   ---+      ¦ +---+
Chinese              8   -- +------+ ¦   ¦
Malaysians           8   ---+        ¦   ¦
Chinese             13   ---+        ¦ +---+
Pehuenche In.        9   -------------+ ¦   ¦
Samoa-USA            9   -----------+   ¦   ¦
Western Samoa        9   ---+       +---+   ¦
Kachari              9   ----------+  +---+ ¦
Brazil-Xavant       11   -------+     ¦     ¦     +---------------------+
Dogrib Indians      11   -------------+     ¦     ¦                     ¦
African-USA         17   -----+             ¦     ¦                     ¦
African-USA          5   -+   ¦             ¦     ¦                     ¦
African-USA         20   ---------+         ¦     ¦                     ¦
Brazil-blacks       11   -----+   +-------------+ ¦                     ¦
African-USA         10   ---------+             ¦                       ¦
Brazil-Zoró         11   -----------------------------------------------+
```

In conclusion, a three major racial group model - caucasian, negroid and mongoloid - seems to be elucidated from the dendrogram, despite south-east asian and polynesian samples cluster separately. In general, the results show quite clearly that D1S80 genetic system is variable worldwide and a useful tool to diferentiate populations.

REFERENCES

1.- Cavalli-Sforza LL, Edwards AWF (1967) Phylogenetic analysis: models and estimation procedures. Am. J. Hum. Genet. 19: 233-257.

2.- Alonso A, Martín P, Albarran C, Sancho M (1993) Amplified fragment length polymorphism analysis of the VNTR locus D1S80 in central Spain. Int. J. Legal Med. 105: 311-314.

3.- Asperilla C, Herrera M, Prieto L, Giménez D, Arroyo E, Ruiz de la Cuesta JM (1995) Amplified fragment length polymorphism frequencies of the D1S80 locus in Northern east Spain. Int. J. Legal Med. (In press).

4.- Budowle B, Chakraborty R, Giusti AW, Eisenberg AJ, Allen RC (1991) Analysis of the VNTR locus D1S80 by PCR followed by high-resolution PAGE. Am. J. Hum. Genet. 48: 137-144.

5.- Budowle B, Baechtel FS, Smerick JB, Presley KW, Giusti AM, Parsons G, Alevy MC, Chakraborty R (1995) D1S80 population data in African Americans, Caucasians, Southeastern Hispanics, Southwestern Hispanics, and Orientals. J. Forensic Sci. 40: 38-44.

6.- Cabrero C, Díez A, Valverde E, Carracedo A, Alemany J (1995) Allele frequency distribution of four PCR-amplified loci in the Spanish population. Forensic Sci. Int. 71(2): 153-164.

7.- Chistiakov DA, Gavrilov DK, Ovchinnikov IV, Nosikov VV (1993) The use of PCR techniques for the VNTR allele distribution analysis of 120 unrelated russian individuals living in Moscow. Mol. Biol. (Mosk.) 27(6): 1304-1314.

8.- Chuah SY , Tan WF, YAp KH, Tai HE, Chow ST (1994) Analysis of the D1S80 locus by amplified fragment length polymorphism technique in the Chinese, Malays and Indians in Singapore. Forensic Sci. Int. 68(3): 169-180.

9.- Deka R, DeCroo S, Jin L, MacGarvey ST, Rothhammer F, Ferrel RE, Chakraborty R (1994) Population genetic characteristics of the D1S80 locus in seven human populations. Hum. Hered. 94: 252-258.

10.- Eisenberg M, Maha G (1991) AMPFLP Analysis in Parentage testing. In: Promega Corporation (Eds.). Proceedings from the Second International Symposium on Human Identification. Madison, USA. pp. 129-154.

11.- Heidrich E, Hutz MH, Salzano FM, Coimbra CEA, Santos RV (1995) D1S80 locus variability in three Brazilian Ethnic groups. Human Biol. 67: 311-319.

12.- Hochmeister MN, Budowle B, Borer UV, Dirnhofer R (1994) Swiss population data on the loci HLA-DQα, LDLR, GYPA, HBGG, D7S8, Gc and D1S80. Forensic Sci. Int. 67: 175-184.

13.- Huang NE, Chakraborty R, Budowle B (1994) D1S80 allele frequencies in a Chinese population. Int. J. Leg. Med. 107: 118-120.

14.- Klintschar M, Kubat M, Ebersold A (1995) The distribution of D1S80 (pMCT118) alleles in an Asutrian population sample - Description of two new alleles. Int. J. Legal Med. 107: 225-226.

15.- Kloosterman AD, Budowle B, Daselaar P (1993) PCR-amplification and detection of the human D1S80 VNTR locus. Int. J. Legal Med. 105: 257-264.

16.- Lareu MV, Muñoz I, Pestoni C, Rodriguez MS Vide C, Carracedo A (1993) The distribution of HLA DQA1 and D1S80 (pMNT118) alleles and genotypes in the populations of Galicia and Central Portugal. Int. J. Legal Med. 106: 124-128.

17.- Latorra D, Stern CM, Shanfield MS (1994) Characterization of Human AFLP systems Apolipoprotein B, Phenylalanine Hydroxylase, and D1S80. PCR methods and applications 3: 351-358.

18.- Nagai A, Yamada S, Bunnai Y, Ohya I (1994) Analysis of the VNTR locus D1S80 in a Japanese population. Int. J. Leg. Med. 106: 268-270.

19.- Nosikov VV, Chistyakov DA, Gavrilov DK, Ovchinnnikov IV, Chelnokova MV (1992) Analysis of PCR-based VNTR polymorphism within an East Slavonic population. European Soc. Human Genetics 24th Annual Meeting Helsigor, Denmark.

20.- Perkin Elmer (1994). Amplitype PCR PM Amplifying and Typing Kit Manual. Part. No. N808-0057. p. 3.

21.- Rand S (Personal Communication).

22.- Sajantila A , Budowle B, Ström M, Johnsson, Lukka M, Peltonen L, Ehnholm C (1992) PCR Amplification of Alleles at the D1S80 locus: Comparison of a Finnish and a North American Caucasian population sample, and forensic casework evaluation. Am. J. Hum. Genet. 50: 816-825.

23.- Schnee-Griese J, Bläss G, Herrmann S, Schneider HR, Föster R, Bässler G, Pflug W (1993) Frequency distribution of D1S80 allleles in the German population. Forensic Sci. Int. 59: 131-136.

24.- Skowasch K, Wiegand P, Brinkmann B (1992) pMCT118 (D1S80): a new allelic ladder and an improved electrophoretic separation lead to the demonstration of 28 alleles. Int. J. Legal Med. 105: 165-168.

25.- Sugiyama E, Honda K, Katsuyama Y, Uchiyyama S, Tsuchikane A, Ota M, Fukushima H (1993) Allele frequency distribution of the D1S80 (pMCT118) locus polymorphism in the Japanese population by the polymerase chain reaction. Int. J. Legal Med. 106: 111-114.

26.- Thymann M, Nellemann LJ, Masumba G, Irgens-Moller L, Morling N (1993) Analysis of the locus D1S80 by amplified fragment length polymorphism technique (AMP-FLP). Frequency distribution in Danes. Intra and inter laboratory reproducibility of the technique. Forensic Sci. Int. 60(1-2): 47-56.

Allele frequency distributions of three STR-loci in a population from Northern Germany

C. Augustin, M. Sanchez-Hanke and K. Püschel
Institute of Legal Medicine, 22529 Hamburg, Germany

Systems and loci: HUMVWA (12p12-12pter)
                               HUMFES/FPS (15q25-25qter)
                               HUMF13B (1q31-q32.1)

Population and sample size: Northern Germany,
                                        N = 307 (VWA), 387 (FES), 289 (F13B)

Methods: Primers: HUMVWA (Kimpton et al. 1992)
                               HUMFES/FPS (Polymeropoulos et al. 1991)
                               HUMF13B (Nishimura and Murray 1992)

PCR amplification conditions: Möller et al. 1994

Electrophoretic methods: non denaturing polyacrylamide gel electrophoresis (6% T, 1.5% C (HUMFES/FPS) or 6% T, 4.5% C (HUMVWA and HUMF13B), 0.5 mm), 60 mM formate (pH 9.0), 20 cm separation distance, running conditions: 600 V, 25 mA, 10 W until the bromophenolblue front reaches the anode, visualzation by silver staining according to Budowle et al. 1991.

Allele designation: according to the repeat number. Alleles 10a and 11a of HUMFES/FPS are designated according to Möller et al. 1994.

Results:

Observed genotypes of HUMVWA

Gen.	Obs.	Gen.	Obs.	Gen.	Obs.	Gen.	Obs.
14/14	7	15/16	9	16/19	9	18/19	17
14/15	6	15/17	26	16/20	2	18/20	2
14/16	8	15/18	16	17/17	31	19/19	3
14/17	10	15/19	5	17/18	32	19/20	3
14/18	14	16/16	11	17/19	12		
14/19	5	16/17	33	17/20	1		
14/20	1	16/18	31	18/18	13		

Allele frequencies of HUMVWA

Allele	Frequency	Allele	Frequency	Allele	Frequency
13	-	16	0.186	19	0.093
14	0.094	17	0.287	20	0.015
15	0.101	18	0.225	21	-

P-value (exact test):	0.063 +/- 0.007
Observed Heterozygosity:	0.788
Allelic diversity:	0.806 +/- 0.044
Discrimination power:	0.93
Mean exclusion chance:	0.62

Exact-test: Guo and Thompson 1992, Allelic diversity: Nei 1978, Discrimination power: Jones 1972, Mean exclusion chance: Krüger et al. 1968

Genotype frequencies of HUMFES/FPS

Gen.	Obs.	Gen.	Obs.	Gen.	Obs.	Gen.	Obs.
8/10a	2	10a/10a	4	10/10	2	11a/12	7
8/10	1	10a/10	62	10/11a	1	11/11	68
8/11a	1	10a/11a	38	10/11	27	11/12	74
8/11	10	10a/11	4	10/12	10	11/13	13
8/12	4	10a/12	2	10/13	2	12/12	17
9/12	1	10a/13	1	11a/11	9	12/13	5

Allele frequencies of HUMFES/FPS

Allele	Frequency	Allele	Frequency	Allele	Frequency
8	0.023	10	0.066	12	0.224
9	0.001	11a	0.028	13	0.031
10a	0.199	11	0.428		-

P-value (Exact test):	0.951 +/- 0.0059
Observed Heterozygosity:	0.726
Allelic diversity:	0.722 +/- 0.045
Discrimination power:	0.88
Mean exclusion chance:	0.49

Genotype frequencies of HUMF13B

Gen.	Obs.	Gen.	Obs.	Gen.	Obs.	Gen.	Obs.
6/6	2	7/8	2	8/9	26	9/10	54
6/8	15	7/9	1	8/10	54	9/12	1
6/9	11	7/10	4	8/11	1	10/10	50
6/10	28	8/8	19	9/9	20	10/11	1

Allele frequencies of HUMF13B

Allele	Frequency	Allele	Frequency	Allele	Frequency
6	0.100	9	0.230	12	0.002
7	0.012	10	0.417		
8	0.235	11	0.004		

P-value (Exact test): 0.872 +/- 0.009
Observed Heterozygosity: 0.685
Allelic diversity: 0.709 +/- 0.052
Discrimination power: 0.87
Mean exclusion chance: 0.46

References

1. Budowle B, Chakraborty R, Giusti AM, Eisenber AJ, Allen RC (1991) Analysis of the variable number of tandem repeats locus D1S80 by the polymerase chain reaction followed by high resolution polyacrylamide gel electrophoresis. Am J Hum Genet 48:137-144
2. Guo SW, Thompson EA (1992) Performing the exact test of Hardy-Weinberg proportion for multiple alleles. Biometrics 48:361-372
2. Jones DA (1972) Blood samples: Probabilities of discriminations. J Forensic Sci Soc 12:355-359
3. Kimpton CP, Walton A, Gill P (1992) A further tetranucleotide repeat polymorphism in the vWF gene. Hum Mol Gen 1:28
4. Krüger J, Fuhrmann W, Lichte KH, Steffens C (1968) Zur Verwendung der sauren Erythro-cytenphosphatase bei der Vaterschaftsbegutachtung. Dtsch Z Gerichtl Med 64:127-146
5. Möller A, Meyer E, Brinkmann B (1994) Different types of structural variation in STRs: Hum-FES/FPS, HumVWA und HumD21S11. Int J Leg Med 106:319-323
6. Nei M (1978) Estimation of average heterozygosity and genetic distance from a small number of individuals. Genetics 89:583-590
7. Nishimura DY, Murray JC (1992) A tetranucleotide repeat for the F13B locus. Nucleic Acids Res 20:1167
8. Polymeropoulos MH, Rath DS, Xiao H, Merril RM (1991) Tetranucleotide repeat polymorphism at the human c-fes/fps proto-oncogene (FES). Nucleic Acids Res 19:4018

ALLELE FREQUENCY DISTRIBUTION OF THREE STRs LOCI: HUMARA, HUMPLA2 AND VS17T IN THE SPANISH POPULATION

C. Cabrero, A. Díez, E. Valverde and J. Alemany
Depart. Biología Molecular, PharmaGen, Madrid, SPAIN

INTRODUCTION

The use of short tandem repeat loci for population genetic studies, genetic analysis of inherited diseases and individual identification purposes requires the stablishment of databases for each reference population. Some groups have reported a number of STR´s loci amenable to Polymerase Chain Reaction (PCR) analysis, as Edwards et al. (HUMTH01, HUMARA), Polymeropoulos et al. (HUMPLA2A), Kimpton (vWF) or Sharma (D21S11 or VS17T).

In the present study we have analysed the variability at three STRs loci (HUMARA, HUMPLA2A and VS17T), in a representative sample of the Spanish population.

METHODS

SAMPLES: Blood samples were obtained from 180 volunteer donnors belonging to the Spanish population. DNA was extracted following the perchlorate protocol. The geographical distribution of the donors is similar to that given in Valverde et al.

PCR REAGENTS: All amplifications were performed in a final volume of 50 μl in a Perkin Elmer thermocycler. Each reaction contained 2-200 ng of genomic DNA, 10 mM Tris-HCl (pH 8.3), 50 mM KCl, 1,5 mM $MgCl_2$ and 1.25 U AmpliTaq Polymerase. One of each pair of primers was end-labelled with ^{32}P-γ-ATP.

PRIMER SEQUENCES:
HUMPLA2A:

> 5´CTAGGTTGTAAGCTCCATGA3´
> 5´TTGAGCACTTACTCTGTGCC3´

VS17T:

> 5´GTGAGTCAATTCCCCAAG3´
> 5´GTTGTATTAGTCAATGTTCTCC3´

HUMARA:

> 5´GCTGTGAAGGTTGCTGTTCCTCAT3´
> 5´TCCAGAATCTGTTCCAGAGCGTGC3´

CYCLE TEMPERATURES: 95 °C (1 min), 54 °C (1 min) and 72 °C (1 min), 28 cycles. Prior to the first cycle the DNA was denatured at 95 °C for 10 min, and after the last cycle an additional extension at 72 °C for 10 min was performed.

RESULTS

Figures 1, 2 and 3 represent the allele frequency distribution of 180 unrelated Spanish individuals for the VS17T, HUMPLA2A and HUMARA loci respectively, and the table gives some statistical parameters.

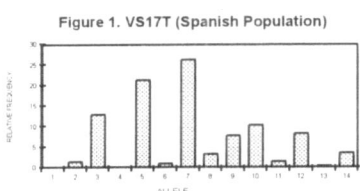

Figure 1. VS17T (Spanish Population)

	Heterozygosity	Chance of exclusion
HUMARA	0.744	0.506
HUMPLA2	0.743	0.504
VS17T	0.859	0.714

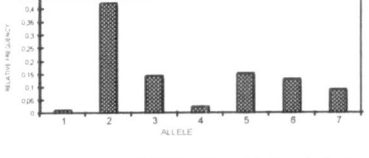

Figure 2. HUMPLA2A (Spanish Population)

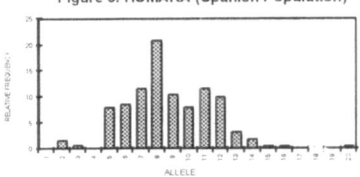

Figure 3. HUMARA (Spanish Population)

REFERENCES

1.- Edwards, A. et al. (1992). Genomics 12, 241-253

2.- Polymeropoulos, M.H. et al. (1991). Nucl. Acids Res .19, 195

3.- Kimpton, C. et al. (1992). Hum. Mol. Genet. 1, 287

4.- Kimpton, C.P. et al. (1993). PCR Methods and Applications 3, 13-22.

5.- Valverde, E. et al. Advances in Forensic Haemogenetics, Vol. 4, Springer-Verlag, Berlin, 1992, pp. 187-189.

6.- Díez, A. et al. Sangre, 37, (1992) 275-278.

7.- Valverde, E. et al. Int. J Leg. Med., 105 (1993) 251-256

Determination of the Allele and Genotype Frequencies of Loci HLA-DQA1, LDLR, GYPA, HBGG, D7S8 and GC in Bogota-Colombia.

M.I. Castillo, M. Paredes, C. Peñuela, I. Bustos, M. Jimenez and A. Galindo.

Laboratorio de DNA, Instituto Nacional de Medicina Legal y Ciencias Forenses, Carrera 13 No. 7-46 Bogotá - Colombia

The analysis of the allele and genotype frequencies for the reference population is necessary for studies of forensic identification. In Colombia, this work began with the determination of the allele and genotype frequencies of the loci HLA-DQA1, LDLR, GYPA, HBGG, D7S8 and GC of the whole blood samples obtained from 151 volunteer donors of blood banks, randomly selected and unrelated, who live in Bogotá.

DNA was extracted using the Chelex procedure. The Amplitype™ HLA DQA1 and Amplitype™ Polymarker PCR Amplification and Typing kits were used to detect the alleles in each system. In this sample 18 of the 21 possible HLA-DQA1 genotypes were observed. The 1.2,2, 1.3,1.3 and 1.3,2 were not represented. The allele and genotype frequencies of HLA-DQA1, HBGG, LDLR, GYPA, D7S8 and GC are shown below. (Tables 1,2,3,4,5 and 6)

Results:

Table 1. HLA-DQA1 Observed genotypes

Gen.	Obs.	Gen	Obs.	Gen.	Obs.	Gen.	Obs.
1.1, 1.1	3	1.1, 4	20	1.3, 3	3	3, 3	13
1.1, 1.2	4	1.2, 1.2	3	1.3, 4	7	3, 4	26
1.1, 1.3	3	1.2, 1.3	2	2, 2	4	4, 4	7
1.1, 2	3	1.2, 3	10	2, 3	6		
1.1, 3	14	1.2, 4	15	2, 4	8		

X^2 , 23.2426; P, 0.0826; d.f., 15

n = 151

Table 2. HLA-DQA1 Allele frequencies

Allele	Frequency	Allele	Frequency	Allele	Frequency
1.1	0.1656	1.3	0.0497	3	0.2815
1.2	0.1225	2	0.0828	4	0.2980

Table 3. LDRL, GYPA and D7S8 Observed genotypes

System	Gen.	Obs.	System	Gen.	Obs.	System	Gen.	Obs.
LDLR	AA	58	GYPA	AA	76	D7S8	AA	59
	AB	68		AB	51		AB	70
	BB	25		BB	24		BB	22

GYPA: X^2, 8.2411; P<0.005; d.f., 1
n =151

Table 4. HBGG and GC observed genotypes

System	Gen.	Obs.	System	Gen.	Obs.
HBGG	AA	31	GC	AA	10
	AB	59		AB	15
	AC	5		AC	36
	BB	51		BB	7
	BC	5		BC	35
	CC	0		CC	48

n = 151

Table 5. LDRL, GYPA, D7S8 Allele frequencies

System	Allele	Freq.	System	Allele	Freq.	System	Allele	Freq.
LDLR	A	0.6093	GYPA	A	0.6722	D7S8	A	0.6225
	B	0.3907		B	0.3278		B	0.3775

Table 6.   HBGG and GC Allele frequencies

System	Allele	Freq.	System	Allele	Freq.
HBGG	A	0.4172	GC	A	0.2351
	B	0.5497		B	0.2119
	C	0.0331		C	0.5530

The distribution of alleles in our sample is similar to those reported for US hispanic populations. (AmpliType™ User Guide; Fildes1990,).

The observed genotype frequencies for HLA-DQA1, LDLR, D7S8, HBGG and GC systems indicate that the studied population is in Hardy Weinberg equilibrium with each one of them. The only system that is not in H-W equilibrium is GYPA.

References:

Fildes N, Reynolds R. (unpublished data, Roche Molecular Systems, Inc.).

Perkin-Elmer, AmpliType User Guide, Version 2

ALLELE DISTRIBUTION OF THE AMPLITYPE PM COAMPLIFICATION SYSTEM IN A POPULATION OF NORTHERN ITALY

N.Cerri, R.Mignola and F. De Ferrari

Institute of Forensic Medicine - University of Brescia - Spedali Civili - P.le Ospedale 1, I - 25100 Brescia

INTRODUCTION

Forensic application of any genetic marker requires a study to carry out a data base of the relevant population for a correct use of the analysis results. According to this guideline the allele distribution of 5 different PCR polymorphisms (LDLR, GYPA, HBGG, D7S8 and GC) were investigated.
LDLR, the Low Density Lipoprotein Receptor, is a two codominant allele (A and B) system that is placed on Cr. 19. His PCR product give band at 214 bp.
GYPA, Glycophorin A, is a system with two alleles (A and B) but additional low frequency alleles are identified in the African American population. It is placed on CR. 4 and his PCR product is setting at 190 bp.
HBGG, the Hemoglobin G Gammaglobin, with a PCR product of 172 bp, is a three (A, B and C) system placed on Cr. 11.
D7S8, a locus of Cr. 7, shows two alleles (A and B) at 151 bp.
Finally GC, the Group Specific Component (GC) is composed by three different alleles (A, B and C) corrisponding to the IEF: 2, 1F and 1S, located on Cr. 4, and are visible at 138 bp.

MATHERIAL AND METHODS

For genotype frequency determination DNA was extracted from whole blood (drawn in EDTA tubes) from 100 unrelated individuals living in Brescia area (Northern Italy)
DNA extraction and purification was carried out by standard protocols using Phenol/ Chloform reagents. The samples (100 microlitres total volume) have been amplified by using Amplitype PM Kit by Perkin Elmer following the manufacturer's recommended protocol. Amplification was carried out with DNA Thermal Cycler - Perkin Elmer ; the amplified fragments were controlled in a 2% agarose gel electrophoresis in TBE 1X and the allele resolution was performed with the reverse Dot Blot technique.

RESULTS AND DISCUSSION

The observed genotypes , the expecrted and the allele frequencies of the systems are shown in Table 1 (LDLR, GYPA and D7S8) and Table 2 (HBGG and GC). The results of the statistical analysis demonstate no deviation from Hardy Weinberg expectation.
In LDLR system the most frequent allele is B, while, either in GYPA or in D7S8 is A.
About the two systems with three alleles we note that in HBGG the most frequent allele is A followed by B and C, while in GC, C is followed by A and B.
Oue allele distribution is similar to other Caucasian population except for HBGG system where the data obtained are different from Swiss population.

TABLE 1

Genotypes	Observed	Expected	X	Allele Frequencies
LDLR				
AA	16	15.61	0.0097	A = 0.395
AB	37	37.60	0.0044	
BB	47	47.79	0.0130	B = 0.605
Total	100	100	0.0271	0.7<p<0.9
GYPA				
AA	34	30.25	0.4649	A = 0.550
AB	24	20.25	0.6945	
BB	42	49.50	1.1363	B = 0.450
Total	100	100	2.2957	0.1< p<0.2
D7S8				
AA	44	42.90	0.0282	A = 0.655
AB	13	11.90	0.1017	
BB	43	45.20	0.1071	B = 0.345
Total	100	100	0.2370	0.5<p<0.7

TABLE 2

Genotypes	Observed	Expected	X	Allele Frequencies
HBGG				
AA	20	25.50	1.1863	A = 0.505
AB	60	48.99	2.4698	
BB	18	23.50	1.2955	B = 0.485
AC	1	1.01	0.0001	
BC	1	0.97	0.0000	C = 0.010
CC	-	0.01	0.0100	
Total	100	100	4.9616	0.1<p<0.2
GC				
AA	7	8.12	0.1545	A = 0.285
AB	7	10.83	1.3545	
BB	3	3.61	0.1030	B = 0.190
AC	36	29.93	1.2310	
BC	25	19.95	1.2783	C = 0.525
CC	22	27.56	1.2616	
Total	100	100	5.2429	0.1<p<0.2

REFERENCES

1) Yamamoto T., Davis C.G., Brown M.S., Schneider W.J., Casey M.L., Goldestein J.L. and Russel D.W. 1984. The human LDL Receptor: A cysteine- rich protein with multiple Alu sequences in its mRNA. Cell 39: 27-38

2) Siebert P.D. and Fukuda M. Molecolar cloning of a human glycophorin B cDNA: nucleotide sequence and genomic relationship to glycophorin A. Proceedings of the National Academy of Sciences, USA 84: 6735- 6739

3) Slightom J.L., Blechl A.E. and Smithies O. 1980. Human fetal Gy-and Ay- globin genes: complete nucleotide sequences suggest that DNA can be exchanged between these duplicated genes. Cell 21: 627-638

4) Yang F., Brune J.L., Naylor S.L., Apples R.L. and Naberhaus K.H. 1985. Human group-specific component (Gc) is a member of the albumin family.
Proceedings of the National Academy of Sciences, USA 82: 7994-7998

5) Hochmeister M.N., Budowle B., Borer U.V. and Dirnhofer R. 1994. Swiss population data on the loci HLA-DQalpha, LDLR, GYPA, HBGG, D7S8, Gc and D1S80. For. Sci.Int. 67: 175-184

6) Garcia O., Martin P., Albarran C. and Alonso A. 1995. Allele frequencies of HLA-DQalpha, LDLR, GYPA, HBGG, D7S8 and GC in the resident population of the Basque Country. XVI Congress of the International Academy of Legal Medicine and Social Medicine Strasbourg, France 31/5 2/6 1995. Personal Communication

ALLELE DISTRIBUTION OF THE AMPLITYPE PM COAMPLIFICATION SYSTEM IN A POPULATION OF NORTHERN ITALY

N.Cerri, R.Mignola and F. De Ferrari

Institute of Forensic Medicine - University of Brescia - Spedali Civili - P.le Ospedale 1, I - 25100 Brescia

Systems and Locus:

LDLR	Cr. 19	214 bp
GYPA	Cr. 4	190 bp
HBGG	Cr. 11	172 bp
D7S8	Cr. 7	151 bp
GC	Cr. 4	138 bp

Population and sample size: 100 unrelated individuals living in Brescia area (Northern Italy)

Methods:

- DNA extraction: Phenol/ Chloform

- Amplification by using Amplitype PM Kit by Perkin Elmer

- Allele resolution: reverse Dot Blot technique.

Results:

LDLR
- A = 0.95
- B = 0.605

GYPA
- A = 0.55
- B = 0.45

D7S8
- A = 0.655
- B = 0.345

HBGG
- A = 0.505
- B = 0.485
- C = 0.010

GC
- A = 0.285
- B = 0.190
- C = 0.525

Comments:

Our allele distribution is similar to other Caucasian population except for HBGG system where the data obtained are different from Swiss population.

CHARACTERIZATION OF YNZ 22 LOCUS FOR FORENSIC PURPOSES .
ALLELE AND GENOTYPES FREQUENCIES IN A NORTHERN ITALIAN POPULATION .

N.Cerri, S.Pivetti and F. De Ferrari.

Institute of Forensic Medicine - University of Brescia - Spedali Civili - P.le Ospedale, 1 - Brescia (Italy)

INTRODUCTION

PCR amplification discriminates several polymorphic VNTR regions also in forensic situations, where limited amounts of DNA are available .
One of the most highly polymorphic region is YNZ 22 (HGM locus D17S30)(1). This genomic locus contains 70 base pair sequence tandemly repeated a variable number of times.
The allele frequencies distribution of this VNTR system was investigated in order to create an own database for pratical applications in paternity testing and identification of stains.

MATERIALS AND METHODS

100 samples of unrelated subjects living in Brescia (Northern Italy) were considered . DNA was extracted from EDTA blood using proteinase K, phenol-chloroform isoamylalcohol and ethanol precipitation. DNA concentration was extimated by agarose minigel (0,8%) electrophoresis .
PCR amplification was performed according to the following conditions :

Denaturation   95°C   3 min.
Annealing   55°C   1 min.
Extention   72°C   1 min.

The amplification products were separated in agarose electrophoresis gel (2%).
The bands were visualized by ethidium bromide staining at the concentration of 1 mg/ml .
The fenotypes were identified by comparision with 123 BRL ladder.

RESULTS AND DISCUSSION

Table 1 shows the calculated allele frequencies while the Table 2 reports the observed genotypes and their frequencies.
A total of 22 different genotypes corresponding to 9 alleles, were found for YNZ 22 in 100 blood samples examined. The most frequent genotypes were the homozygotes 2 and 4, followed by the heterozygotes 3-4 and 2-4.
This distribution is different from that found in previous studies on Italian groups (Central Italy) (2-5). In fact, with regard to the allele frequencies, we observed that the frequencies of the allele 2 exceeded the allele 4 frequency.(Figure 1)
We propose to continue compiling a more complete and wide database to have a better and more precise valuation of these results, with special regard to the great number of homozygotes 2. This could depend on real higher value of the frequency or a selective amplification of the low WM allele.

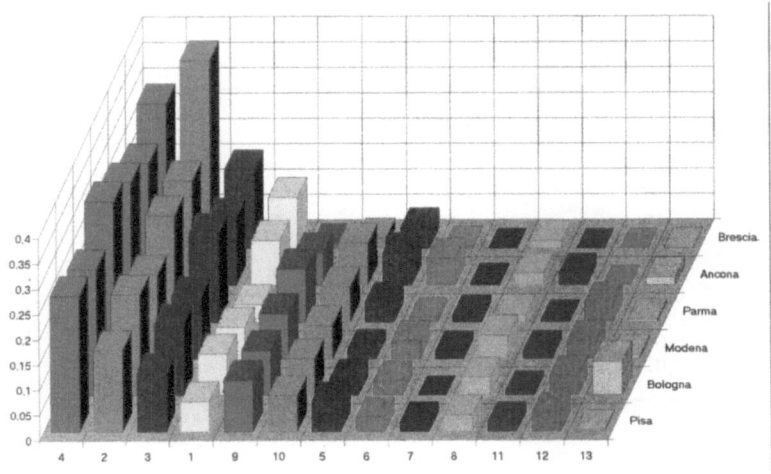

Figure 1: Distribution of YNZ22 alleles in Italy

REFERENCES

(1) G.T.Horn,B. Richards , K.W.Klinger (1989) Amplification of a highly polymorphic VNTR segment by the polymerase chain reaction.Nucleic Acid Res.17:2140

(2) L.Buscemi, N.Cucurachi, R.Mencarelli, B.Sisti, A.Tagliabracci, S.D.Ferrara (1994) PCR typing of the locus D17S30 (YNZ 22 VNTR) in an Italian sample. Int J Leg Med 106:200-204

(3) M.Alu', F.De Fazio (1994) Study of the YNZ 22 locus polymorphism in the district of Modena (Italy). XVI th Congress of the International Academy of Legal Medicine . Strasburg, France 31 May-2 June 1994

(4) S.Pelotti, P.Degli Esposti, V.Mantovani, E.Collina, G.Pappalardo (1994) Study of D17S5 (YNZ22) locus polymorphism in an Italian population sample.XVI th Congress of the International Academy of Legal Medicine. Strasburg, France 31May-2June 1994

(5) R.Domenici.Personal communication (1995).

TABLE 1

ALLELE FREQUENCIES		OBSERVED
YNZ 22 1	0,1	20
YNZ 22 2	0,37	74
YNZ 22 3	0,155	31
YNZ 22 4	0,285	57
YNZ 22 5	0,04	8
YNZ 22 6	0,005	1
YNZ 22 8	0,015	3
YNZ 22 9	0,01	2
YNZ 22 10	0,02	4

TABLE 2

GENOTYPE	OBSERVED	FREQUENCY	EXPECTED
1-1	3	0.03	1.0
1-2	4	0.04	7.4
1-3	2	0.02	3.1
1-4	7	0.07	5.7
1-5	1	0.01	0.8
2-2	27	0.27	13.69
2-3	7	0.07	11.47
2-4	8	0.08	21.09
2-9	1	0.01	0.74
3-3	5	0.05	2.4025
3-4	11	0.11	8.835
3-5	1	0.01	1.24
4-4	14	0.14	8.1225
4-5	1	0,01	2.28
4-8	1	0.01	0.855
4-10	1	0.01	1.14
5-5	1	0.01	0.16
5-6	1	0.01	0.04
5-8	1	0.01	0.12
5-10	1	0.01	0.16
8-9	1	0.01	0.03
10-10	1	0.01	0.04

CHARACTERIZATION OF YNZ 22 LOCUS FOR FORENSIC PURPOSES.
ALLELE AND GENOTYPES FREQUENCIES IN A NORTHERN ITALIAN POPULATION.

N.Cerri, S.Pivetti and F. De Ferrari.

Institute of Forensic Medicine - University of Brescia - Spedali Civili - P.le Ospedale, 1 - Brescia (Italy)

System and locus: YNZ 22 (HGM D17S30)

Population and sample size: Brescia (Northern Italy). 100 unrelated blood donors

Methods: - DNA extracted from EDTA blood using proteinase K, phenol-chloroform
· isoamylalcohol and ethanol precipitation.
- PCR amplification : Denaturation 95°C 3 min., Annealing 55°C 1 min.,
Extention 72°C 1 min.
- Electrophoretic method: agarose gel (2%) at 80 V. with ethidium bromide
- The fenotypes were identified by comparision with 123 BRL ladder.

Results:

ALLELE FREQUENCIES		OBSERVED
YNZ 22 1	0,1	20
YNZ 22 2	0,37	74
YNZ 22 3	0,155	31
YNZ 22 4	0,285	57
YNZ 22 5	0,04	8
YNZ 22 6	0,005	1
YNZ 22 8	0,015	3
YNZ 22 9	0,01	2
YNZ 22 10	0,02	4

Comments:

The allele distribution is different from that found in other Italian population. We propose to continue compiling a more complete and wide database to have a better and more precise valuation of these results, with special regard to the great number of homozygotes 2. This could depend on real higher value of the frequency or a selective amplification of the low WM allele.

D1S80 POPULATION DATA IN NORTH-EAST OF SPAIN

M.Crespillo, J.A.Luque, R.M.Fernández, P.García, E.Ramírez and J.L.Valverde.

Sección de Biología. Instituto Nacional de Toxicología. Ministerio de Justicia e Interior. Merced 1. 08002 Barcelona, Spain.

System and locus: D1S80

Population and sample: Catalonia (N.E. of Spain). N=183.

Methods:

Primers and PCR conditions: D1S80 Forensic DNA Amplification Reagent Set (Perkin Elmer) in a Linus DualCycler thermocycler.

Electrophoretic method: vertical electrophoresis on 0.75 mm thick native polyacrylamide gels (GeneAmp Detection Gel, Perkin Elmer) and silver staining [1]. The electrophoresis ran for one hour at a constant voltage of 500 V. To size the PCR products, a 27-allelic ladder supplied by the manufacturer was used. ISFH recommendations were followed [2,3].

To estimate Hardy-Weimberg equilibrium, the chi square test was made pooling alleles into five groups.

Table 1. Observed genotypes

Gen.	Obs.	Gen.	Obs.	Gen.	Obs.	Gen.	Obs.	Gen.	Obs.
16 -31	1	18 -29	2	21 -29	2	24 -27	4	26 -31	1
17 -24	1	18 -31	1	21 -31	1	24 -28	8	27 -28	1
18 -18	9	18 -32	2	22 -23	1	24 -29	2	27 -31	1
18 -19	4	18 -40	1	22 -24	12	24 -30	1	28 -31	2
18 -20	2	19 -24	1	22 -25	1	24 -31	10	28 -37	1
18 -21	3	20 -20	1	22 -26	1	24 -32	1	29 -29	1
18 -22	6	20 -24	2	22 -31	1	25 -25	2	29 -31	3
18 -23	2	20 -25	1	23 -24	1	25 -30	1	29 -35	1
18 -24	28	20 -34	2	24 -24	18	25 -31	1	29 -37	1
18 -25	6	20 -36	1	24 -25	7	26 -28	1	30 -31	1
18 -26	1	21 -24	6	24 -26	2	26 -29	1	31 -31	1
18 -28	7								

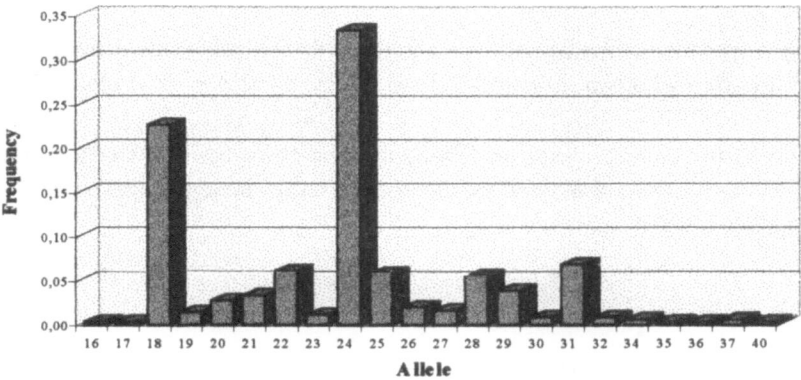

Figure 1. Distribution of D1S80 alleles in north-east of Spain

Table 2. Allele frequencies.

Allele	Frequency	Allele	Frequency	Allele	Frequency
16	0.00273	24	0.33333	31	0.06831
17	0.00273	25	0.05738	32	0.00820
18	0.22678	26	0.01913	34	0.00546
19	0.01366	27	0.01639	35	0.00273
20	0.02732	28	0.05464	36	0.00273
21	0.03279	29	0.03825	37	0.00546
22	0.06011	30	0.00820	40	0.00273
23	0.01093				

Table 3. Evaluation

	Pooled alleles				
Group	I	II	III	IV	V
Alleles	14-18	19-23	24	25-28	29-40
Chi^2=15.57; d.f.=10; P=0.11					

Observed heterozygosity	0.825
Allelic diversity (h ±s.e.) [4]	0.821 ±0.028
Power of exclusion (PE) [5]	0.664
Power of discrimination (PD) [6]	0.949

Comments:

The D1S80 genotype frequencies do not deviate from Hardy-Weimberg expectations, and show a bimodal distribution with two main peaks at the 18 and 24 alleles, as in others Caucasian populations.

In our study twenty-two different alleles and fifty-six different genotypes were identified, showing that the D1S80 locus is highly polymorphic and therefore the D1S80 locus provides a useful system for forensic applications and paternity testing.

References:

1. Bassam B, Caetano-Anolles G and Gresshof PM (1991) Fast and sensitive silver staining of DNA in polyacrylamide gels. Anal Biochem 196:80-83

2. DNA Commission of the ISFH (1992) Second DNA recommendations - 1991 report concerning recommendations of the DNA commission of the International Society for Forensic Haemogenetics relating to the use of DNA polymorphisms. Int J Leg Med 104:361-364

3. DNA Commission of the ISHF (1992) DNA recommendation - 1992 report concerning recommendations of the DNA Commission of the International Society for Forensic Haemogenetics relating to the use of PCR-based polymorphisms. Int J Leg Med 105: 63-64

4. Nei M, Roychoudhury AK (1974) Sampling variances of heterozygosity and genetic distance. Genetics 76:379-390

5. Garber RA, Morris JW (1983) General equations for the average power of exclusion for genetic systems of n codominants alleles in one-parent and no-parent cases of disputed parentage. In: Walker RH (ed) Inclusion probabilities in parentage testing. American Association of Blood Banks, Arlinton, pp 277-280

6. Jones DA (1972) Blood samples: probability of discrimination. J Forensic Sci Soc 12:355-359

POPULATION STUDY FOR THE HLA-DQA1, LDLR, GYPA, HBGG, D7S8 AND GC LOCI IN NORTH-EAST OF SPAIN

M.Crespillo, J.A.Luque, P.García, E.Ramírez, R.M.Fernández and J.L.Valverde

Sección de Biología. Instituto Nacional de Toxicología. Ministerio de Justicia e Interior. Merced 1. 08002 Barcelona, Spain.

System and locus: PM loci: low density protein receptor (LDLR)
glycophorin A (GYPA)
hemoglobin G gammaglobin (HBGG)
D7S8
group specific component (GC)
HLA-DQA1 locus

Population and sample: Catalonia (N.E. of Spain)
N: 146 (PM loci), 195 (HLA-DQA1)

Results:

Primers and PCR amplification conditions: Amplitype® PM and the HLA-DQα PCR Amplification and Typing kit (Perkin-Elmer) in a Linus DualCycler thermocycler. All samples for the HLA-DQA1 locus were single amplified.

Characterization of the alleles: by hybridization to filter strips carrying immobilised allele specific oligonucleotide DNA probes (reverse dot-blot) using the strips and recommendations of the manufacturer.

Results:

Table 1. Allele frequencies

Locus	Allele	Frequency	Allele	Frequency	Allele	Frequency
LDLR	A	0.48288	B	0.51712		
GYPA	A	0.51027	B	0.48973		
HBGG	A	0.46233	B	0.51712	C	0.02055
D7S8	A	0.55137	B	0.44863		
GC	A	0.33219	B	0.16096	C	0.50685
HLA-DQA1	1.1	0.16154	1.2	0.13846	1.3	0.05897
	2	0.20000	3	0.12051	4	0.32051

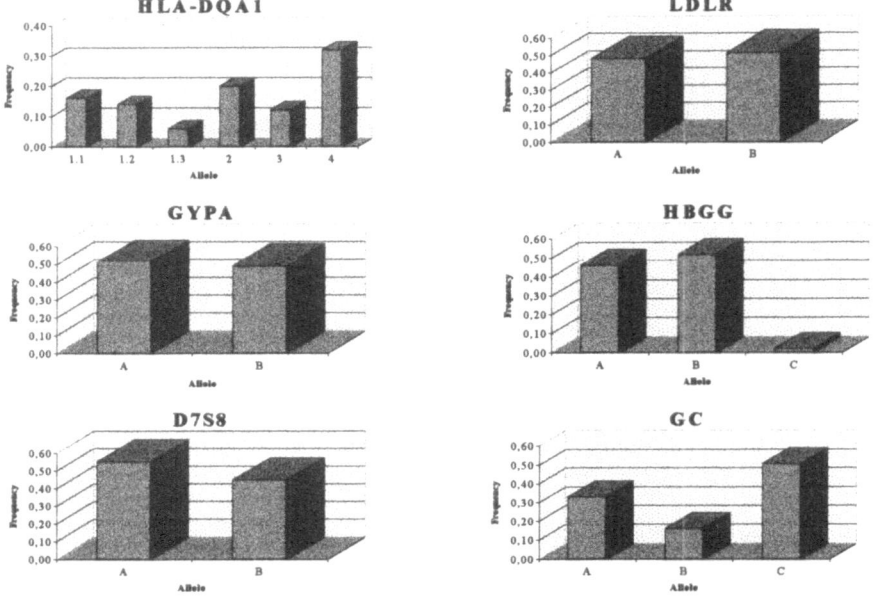

Figure 1. Distribution of HLA-DQA1 and PM loci alleles in North-East of Spain

Table 2. Observed genotypes

	Gen.	Obs.	Gen.	Obs.	Gen.	Obs.
LDLR	A-A	38	A-B	65	B-B	43
GYPA	A-A	39	A-B	71	B-B	36
HBGG	A-A	28	A-B	75	A-C	4
	B-B	37	B-C	2		
D7S8	A-A	49	A-B	63	B-B	34
GC	A-A	18	A-B	12	A-C	49
	B-B	5	B-C	25	C-C	37
HLA-DQA1	1.1-1.1	6	1.1-1.2	7	1.1-1.3	4
	1.1-2	16	1.1-3	6	1.1-4	18
	1.2-1.2	5	1.2-1.3	2	1.2-2	13
	1.2-3	7	1.2-4	15	1.3-1.3	1
	1.3-2	3	1.3-3	2	1.3-4	10
	2-2	8	2-3	8	2-4	22
	3-3	5	3-4	14	4-4	23

Table 3. Evaluation

Locus	Power of discrimination PD [1]	Power of exclusion PE [2]	Allelic diversity h (±s.e.) [3]	P value Chi square test
HLA-DQA1	0.929	0.599	0.796±0.029	0.91
LDLR	0.625	0.187	0.501±0.041	0.19
GYPA	0.625	0.187	0.502±0.041	0.74
HBGG	0.653	0.213	0.520±0.041	0.61
D7S8	0.622	0.186	0.496±0.041	0.12
GC	0.770	0.322	0.609±0.040	0.68
Combined	0.9997	0.885		

Comments:
The distribution of phenotypes is in agreement with Hardy-Weimberg expectations for the six loci. The Amplitype® PM and the HLA-DQα PCR Amplification and Typing kit provide two important advantages: they can be used as a fast and high sensitive screening of the samples; on the other hand, we need less template DNA to type six loci at a time with a high combined power of discrimination.
We use in routinely forensic casework this multiplex system.

References:

1. Jones DA (1972) Blood samples: probability of discrimination. J Forensic Sci Soc 12:355-359
2. Garber RA, Morris JW (1983) General equations for the average power of exclusion for genetic systems of n codominants alleles in one-parent and no-parent cases of disputed parentage. In: Walker RH (ed) Inclusion probabilities in parentage testing. American Association of Blood Banks, Arlinton, pp 277-280
3. Nei M, Roychoudhury AK (1974) Sampling variances of heterozygosity and genetic distance. Genetics 76:379-390

ALLELE FREQUENCIES OF FOUR STRs (HUMTH01, HUMVWFA31, HUMF13A01, HUMFESFPS) IN NORTH-EAST OF SPAIN

M.Crespillo, J.A.Luque, E.Ramírez, P.García, R.M.Fernández and J.L.Valverde.

Sección de Biología. Instituto Nacional de Toxicología. Ministerio de Justicia e Interior. Merced 1. 08002 Barcelona, Spain.

System and locus: HUMTH01 (11p15.5)
HUMVWFA31 (12p12-pter)
HUMF13A01 (6p24-25)
HUMFESFPS (15q25-qter)

Population and sample: Catalonia (N.E. of Spain)
N: 116 (TH01), 120 (VWF), 118 (FESFPS), 117 (F13)

Methods:
Primers and PCR amplification conditions: GenePrint STR system (Promega) in a Linus DualCycler thermocycler.
Electrophoretic method: vertical electrophoresis on 0.75 mm thick 4% denaturing polyacrylamide gels (19:1 acrylamide:bisacrylamide, 7M urea, 24 cm length) and silver staining [1]. The electrophoresis ran for 1h (45 min for VWF) at a constant voltage of 1000V with a fixed temperature of 51°C.
Alleles were assigned by means of ladders supplied by Promega. ISFH recommendations were followed [2,3,4].

Results:

Table 1. Allele frequencies.

HUMTH01		HUMVWFA31		HUMFESFPS		HUMF13A01	
Allele	Frequency	Allele	Frequency	Allele	Frequency	Allele	Frequency
5	0.00431	14	0.12500	8	0.02119	4	0.11111
6	0.16379	15	0.12083	9	0.00424	5	0.21368
7	0.13362	16	0.17500	10	0.25847	6	0.25214
8	0.15948	17	0.25833	11	0.47881	7	0.39316
9	0.25431	18	0.21667	12	0.19492	8	0.00427
9.3	0.28448	19	0.09167	13	0.03814	9	0.00427
		20	0.01250	14	0.00424	14	0.01709
						15	0.00427

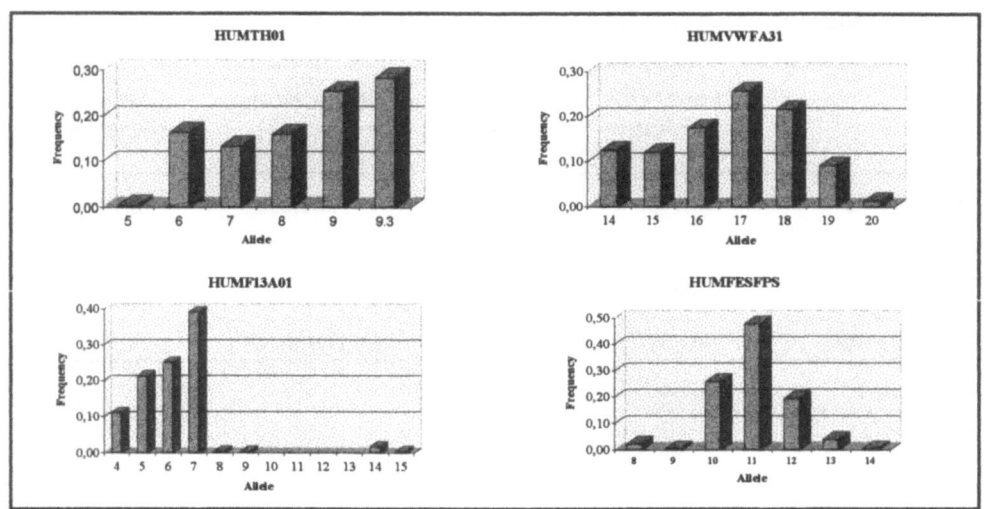

Figure 1. Allele frequency distribution of four STR's in north-east of Spain

Table 2. Observed genotypes

HUMTH01

Gen.	5-9	6-6	6-7	6-8	6-9	6-9.3	7-7	7-8	7-9	7-9.3	8-8
Obs.	1	1	6	6	12	12	1	8	5	10	3

Gen.	8-9	8-9.3	9-9	9-9.3	9.3-9.3
Obs.	10	7	7	17	10

HUMVWFA31

Gen.	14-14	14-15	14-16	14-17	14-18	14-19	15-16	15-17	15-18	15-19	15-20
Obs.	2	4	4	8	7	3	3	11	7	2	2

Gen.	16-16	16-17	16-18	16-19	17-17	17-18	17-19	17-20	18-18	18-19
Obs.	4	11	11	5	9	10	3	1	4	9

HUMFESFPS

Gen.	8-10	8-11	8-12	8-13	9-11	10-10	10-11	10-12	10-13	11-11	11-12
Obs.	2	1	1	1	1	6	30	15	2	25	26

Gen.	11-13	12-12	12-13	12-14
Obs.	5	1	1	1

HUMF13A01

Gen.	4-4	4-5	4-6	4-7	5-5	5-6	5-7	5-8	6-6	6-7	6-14
Obs.	2	6	7	9	6	13	18	1	8	20	3

Gen.	7-7	7-9	7-14	7-15
Obs.	21	1	1	1

Table 3. Evaluation.

LOCUS	Power of discrimination PD [5]	Power of exclusion PE [6]	Allelic diversity h (±s.e.) [7]	P value Chi square test
HUMTH01	0.919	0.574	0.788±0.038	0.70
HUMVWFA31	0.941	0.635	0.820±0.035	0.55
HUMFESFPS	0.833	0.409	0.667±0.043	0.25
HUMF13A01	0.877	0.483	0.727±0.041	0.29
Combined	0.999	0.952		

Comments:

For all STRs loci the Hardy-Weimberg equilibrium was tested by Chi square test, and no significant deviations were found (table 3).
These STR systems show a high power of discrimination (combined power of exclusion of 0.9999) and probability of exclusion (cumulated probability of exclusion of 0.95). The use of these four STRs provides an important tool in forensic and paternity testing. Now we use them in routinely forensic casework.

References:

1. Bassam B, Caetano-Anolles G and Gresshof PM (1991) Fast and sensitive silver staining of DNA in polyacrylamide gels. Anal Biochem 196:80-83
2. DNA Commission of the ISFH (1992) Second DNA recommendations - 1991 report concerning recommendations of the DNA commission of the International Society for Forensic Haemogenetics relating to the use of DNA polymorphisms. Int J Leg Med 104:361-364
3. DNA Commission of the ISHF (1992) DNA recommendation - 1992 report concerning recommendations of the DNA Commission of the International Society for Forensic Haemogenetics relating to the use of PCR-based polymorphisms. Int J Leg Med 105: 63-64
4. DNA Commission of the ISFH (1995) DNA recommendations - 1994 report concerning further recommendations of the DNA Commission of the ISFH regarding PCR-based polymorphisms in STR (short tandem repeat) systems. ISFH newsletter March 1995: Annex 2
5. Jones DA (1972) Blood samples: probability of discrimination. J Forensic Sci Soc 12:355-359
6. Garber RA, Morris JW (1983) General equations for the average power of exclusion for genetic systems of n codominants alleles in one-parent and no-parent cases of disputed parentage. In: Walker RH (ed) Inclusion probabilities in parentage testing. American Association of Blood Banks, Arlinton, pp 277-280
7. Nei M, Roychoudhury AK (1974) Sampling variances of heterozygosity and genetic distance. Genetics 76:379-390

GERMAN DATA ON THE LOCI LOW-DENSITY-LIPOPROTEIN RECEPTOR, GLYCOPHORIN A, HEMOGLOBIN γ^G, D7S8, GROUP-SPECIFIC COMPONENT AND HLA-DQα

Huckenbeck W[a], Scheil H-G[b], Cremer U[c], Makuch D[d], Eiermann TH[e], Kuntze K[a], Bonte W[a]

[a] Institute of Forensic Medicine, Heinrich-Heine-University Düsseldorf
[b] Institute of Human Genetics and Anthropology, Heinrich-Heine-University Düsseldorf
[c] Institute of Forensic Medicine, RWTH Aachen
[d] Institute of Forensic Medicine, University of Saarland
[e] Institute of Transfusion Medicine, University of Ulm

Summary

This paper reports on the allele and genotype frequencies for six polymerase chain reaction-based loci. The loci Low-Density-Lipoprotein Receptor, Glycophorin A, Hemoglobin γ^G, D7S8 and Group-Specific Component have been typed in samples from Düsseldorf (n=371), Aachen (n=107) and Saarland (n=100) (Germany). The HLA-DQα system was examined in a sample from Düsseldorf (n=579), Aachen (n=107) and Ulm (n=168). Typing was carried out by using the AmpliType® PM PCR amplification and typing kit and the HLA-DQα Forensic DNA Amplification and Typing Kit (AmpliType™, Perkin Elmer Cetus). The loci were tested for possible divergences from Hardy-Weinberg expectations (HWE). The gene frequencies found can be used in forensic analyses and paternity tests.

Materials and Methods

DNA extraction was performed from German Caucasians. For amplification and visualization the AmpliType® PM and the HLA-DQα PCR amplification and typing kits were used. Preparation of the samples, hybridization and visualization have been previously described (Perkin Elmer). Gene frequencies have been calculated by gene counting, the power of exclusion was calculated according to Krüger et al 1968.

Results and Discussion

AmpliType® PM Kit: The distributions of observed and expected genotypes are shown in table 1. No deviations from the Hardy-Weinberg equilibrium were found. In the case of Glycophorin A (Aachen and Saarland) no χ^2-test was practicable because of df = 0, but comparison of observed and expected values results in good agreement.

The gene frequencies found in our three samples are shown in table 2 together with the data of 3 other German samples.

The AVACH values for the Düsseldorf sample [pooled German data (2166 genomes) in Italics] are LDLR (18.62 %; *18.50 %*), GYPA (18.62 %; *18.62 %*), HBGG (19.79 %; *19.87 %*), D7S8 (18.08 % ; *18.24 %*) and GC (29.39 %; *30.06 %*) which result in a AVACH value of (69.27 %; *69.61 %*) for the five loci together.

AmpliType® HLA-DQα Kit: The distributions of observed and expected genotypes are shown in table 3. The Ulm sample is not with the Hardy-Weinberg equilibrium. Because we could exclude possible mistakes (foreigners eg) we think that this fact is caused by the size of the sample. The AVACH value for the Düsseldorf sample is 59.78%, for the Aachen sample 53.05 %. The pooled German data result in an AVACH value of 60.02 %.

For all six systems the AVACH value (pooled data) is 87.90 %.

	Düsseldorf observed n	%	expected n	%	Aachen observed n	%	expected n	%	Saarland observed n	%	expected n	%
Low-Density-Lipoprotein Receptor (LDLR)												
A	80	21.56	75.17	20.26	24	22.43	23.36	21.83	23	23	20.70	20.70
B	117	31.54	112.17	30.24	31	28.97	30.36	28.38	32	32	29.70	29.70
AB	174	46.90	183.65	49.50	52	48.60	53.27	49.79	45	45	49.60	49.60
Σ	371	100.00	370.99	100,00	107	100.00	106.99	100,00	100	100.00	100.00	100.00
	$\chi^2=1.03$ df=1 30>p>50				$\chi^2=0.06$ df=1 80>p>90				$\chi^2=0.86$ df=1 30>p>50			
Glycophorin A (GYPA)												
A	110	29.65	112.72	30.38	34	31.78	31.44	29.38	29	29	28.09	28.09
B	72	19.41	74.72	20.14	25	23.36	22.44	20.97	23	23	22.09	22.09
AB	189	50.94	183.55	49.48	48	44.86	53.12	49.64	48	48	49.82	49.82
Σ	371	100.00	370.99	100.00	107	100.00	107.00	99.99	100	100.00	100.00	100.00
	$\chi^2=0.33$ df=1 50>p>70				$\chi^2=0.99$ df=1 30>p>50				$\chi^2=0.13$ df=1 70>p>80			
Hemoglobin γ^G (HBGG)												
A	95	25.61	93.75	25.27	22	20.56	21.09	19.71	26	26	27.04	27.04
B	92	24.80	88.79	23.93	34	31.78	31.98	29.89	20	20	21.16	21.16
C	0	0.00	0.02	0.01	0	0.00	0.01	0.01	1	1	0.04	0.04
AB	178	47.98	182.47	49.18	49	45.79	51.93	48.54	51	51	47.84	47.84
AC	5	1.35	3.02	0.81	2	1.87	0.88	0.82	1	1	2.08	2.08
BC	1	0.27	2.94	0.79	0	0.00	1.09	1.02	1	1	1.84	1.84
Σ	371	100.01	370.99	99.99	107	100.00	106.98	99.99	100	100.00	100.00	100.00
	$\chi^2=0.24$ df=1 50>p>70				df=0				df=0			
D7S8												
A	145	39.08	140.14	37.77	38	35.51	35.35	33.04	32	32	35.40	35.40
B	60	16.17	55.11	14.85	22	20.56	19.35	18.08	13	13	16.40	16.40
AB	166	44.74	175.76	47.37	47	43.93	52.30	48.88	55	55	48.20	48.20
Σ	371	99.99	371.01	99.99	107	100.00	107.00	100.00	100	100.00	100.00	100.00
	$\chi^2=1.14$ df=1 20>p>30				$\chi^2=1.10$ df=1 20>p>30				$\chi^2=1.99$ df=1 10>p>20			
Group-Specific Component (GC)												
A	30	8.09	24.58	6.63	7	6.54	8.41	7.86	8	8	10.56	10.56
B	7	1.89	7.86	2.12	5	4.67	1.58	1.48	2	2	2.72	2.72
C	141	38.01	132.24	35.64	39	36.45	38.28	35.78	21	21	26.01	26.01
AB	32	8.63	27.81	7.50	6	5.61	7.29	6.81	9	9	10.73	10.73
AC	99	26.68	114.02	30.73	40	37.38	35.89	33.54	40	40	33.15	33.15
BC	62	16.71	64.50	17.38	10	9.35	15.55	14.53	20	20	16.83	16.83
Σ	371	100.01	371.01	100.00	107	100.00	107.00	100.00	100	100.00	100.00	100.00
	$\chi^2=4.58$ df=3 20>p>30				$\chi^2=3.21$ df=2 20>p>30				$\chi^2=4.07$ df=2 10>p>20			

Table 1 Polymarker kit: frequency distribution of observed and expected genotypes in the samples from Düsseldorf (n=371), Aachen (n=107) and Saarland (n=100).

Population		Germany Düsseldorf	Germany Saarland	Germany Aachen	Germany Mainz	Germany N.Bavaria	Germany Hannover	*Germany*
Genomes		742	200	214	310	300	400	*2166*
References		this study	this study	this study	Schneider et al	Hausmann et al	Rothämel et al	
Locus	Alleles							
LDLR	A	0.4501	0.4550	0.4673	0.4480	0.3770	0.3825	*0.4293*
	B	0.5499	0.5450	0.5327	0.5520	0.6230	0.6175	*0.5707*
GYPA	A	0.5512	0.5300	0.5421	0.5290	0.5870	0.5500	*0.5499*
	B	0.4488	0.4700	0.4579	0.4710	0.4130	0.4500	*0.4501*
HBGG	A	0.5027	0.5200	0.4439	0.5190	0.5000	0.5500	*0.5092*
	B	0.4892	0.4600	0.5467	0.4740	0.4830	0.4500	*0.4819*
	C	0.0081	0.0200	0.0093	0.0060	0.0170	0.0000	*0.0088*
D7S8	A	0.6146	0.5950	0.5748	0.5900	0.6000	0.5950	*0.5997*
	B	0.3854	0.4050	0.4252	0.4100	0.4000	0.4050	*0.4003*
GC	A	0.2574	0.3250	0.2804	0.3230	0.2930	0.3050	*0.2890*
	B	0.1456	0.1650	0.1215	0.1130	0.1570	0.1425	*0.1414*
	C	0.5970	0.5100	0.5981	0.5650	0.5500	0.5525	*0.5698*

Table 2 Polymarker kit: gene frequencies in German samples

	Düsseldorf				Aachen				Ulm			
	observed		expected		observed		expected		observed		expected	
	n	%	n	&	n	%	n	%	n	%	n	%
1.1-1.1	13	2.25	11.76	2.03	1q	0.94	1.70	1.59	2	1.19	2.50	1.49
1.1-1.2	36	6.22	36.77	6.35	3	2.80	5.81	5.43	5	2.98	9.27	5.52
1.1-1.3	8	1.38	8.27	1.43	0	0.00	0.38	0.35	3	1.79	3.54	2.11
1.1-2	24	4.15	20.94	3.62	8	7.48	3.66	3.42	16	9.52	6.46	3.85
1.1-3	29	5.01	24.93	4.31	4	3.74	2.90	2.71	3	1.79	4.03	2.40
1.1-4	42	7.25	50.59	8.74	10	9.35	10.85	10.14	10	5.95	12.69	7.55
1.2-1.2	31	5.35	28.74	4.96	6	5.61	4.94	4.62	9	5.36	8.60	5.12
1.2-1.3	9	1.55	12.93	2.23	1	0.94	0.64	0.60	6	3.57	6.56	3.91
1.2-2	30	5.18	32.74	5.65	5	4.67	6.23	5.83	11	6.55	11.99	7.41
1.2-3	42	7.25	38.98	6.73	5	4.67	4.95	4.62	6	3.57	7.46	4.44
1.2-4	79	13.64	79.10	13.66	20	18.69	18.49	17.28	30	17.86	23.52	14.00
1.3-1.3	0	0.00	1.45	0.25	0	0.00	0.02	0.02	3	1.79	1.25	0.74
1.3-2	9	1.55	7.36	1.27	0	0.00	0.41	0.38	3	1.79	4.57	2.72
1.3-3	10	1.73	8.77	1.51	0	0.00	0.32	0.30	1	0.60	2.85	1.70
1.3-4	22	3.80	17.79	3.07	2	1.87	1.20	1.13	10	5.95	8.97	5.34
2-2	11	1.90	9.32	1.61	1	0.94	1.97	1.84	2	1.19	4.18	2.49
2-3	20	3.45	22.20	3.83	1	0.94	3.12	2.91	7	4.17	5.20	3.10
2-4	42	7.25	45.06	7.78	13	12.15	11.65	10.89	12	7.14	16.40	9.76
3-3	12	2.07	13.22	2.28	1	0.94	1.24	1.15	1	0.60	1.62	0.96
3-4	50	8.64	53.65	9.27	11	10.28	9.25	8.64	14	8.33	10.21	6.08
4-4	60	10.36	54.43	9.40	15	14.02	17.28	16.15	14	8.33	16.10	9.59
Σ	579	99.98	579.00	99.98	107	100.03	107.01	100.00	168	100.02	167.97	100.01

$\chi^2=7.39$ df=14 90 > p > 95 $\chi^2=6.25$ df= 5 20 > p > 30 $\chi^2=25.65$ df=11 0.1 > p > 1

Table 3   HLA-DQα:Observed and expected genotype frequencies in Düsseldorf, Aachen and Ulm (this study)

	Alleles		1.1	1.2	1.3	2	3	4
	Population	Ref.	Genomes					
1	Germany Düsseldorf	this study	1158	0.1425	0.2228	0.0501	0.1269	0.1511	0.3066
2	Germany Wuppertal	Huckenbeck et al	298	0.1409	0.2315	0.0772	0.0906	0.1678	0.2920
	Germany Aachen	this study	214	0.1262	0.2150	0.0140	0.1355	0.1075	0.4019
	Germany Ulm	this study	336	0.1220	0.2262	0.0863	0.1577	0.0982	0.3095
3	Germany Mainz	Schneider et al	318	0.154	0.230	0.069	0.104	0.135	0.308
4	Germany Southwest	Reinhold et al	604	0.140	0.210	0.093	0.136	0.112	0.308
5	Germany Munich	Weichhold et al	426	0.106	0.185	0.080	0.134	0.160	0.336
	Germany		*3018*	*0.1368*	*0.2160*	*0.0650*	*0.1244*	*0.1414*	*0.3165*

Table 4   HLA-DQα system: gene frequencies in Germany; *Germany*: pooled data without Ulm

References

HAUSMANN R, HANTSCHEL M, LÖTTERLE J, 1995: Frequencies of the 5 PCR-based genetic markers LDLR, GYPA, HBGG, D7S8 and GC in a North Bavarian population. - Int. J. Leg. Med. 107, 227-228; HUCKENBECK W, ZENS V, SCHEIL H-G, 1994: HLA-DQα-System: Allelfrequenzen und Genotypenverteilung in den Großräumen Düsseldorf und Wuppertal. Rechtsmedizin 4: 107-109; REINHOLD J, ARNOLD J, 1994: PCR based analysis of HLA-DQα, D1S80 and Apo B loci in paternity testing. In BÄR W, FIORI A, ROSSI U (eds) Advances in Forensic Haemogenetics 5. Springer Verlag, Berlin-Heidelberg-New York. pp 229-231; SCHNEIDER PM, VEIT A, RITTNER C, 1991: PCR-typing of the human HLA-DQα locus: population genetics and application in forensic casework. In BERGHAUS G, BRINKMANN B, RITTNER C, STAAK M (eds.) DNA-technology and its forensic application. Springer, Berlin-Heidelberg. pp: 85-91; SCHNEIDER PM, LUMMER J, RITTNER G, RITTNER C, 1995: Populationsgenetik und forensische Anwendung der PCR-typisierten Genorte LDL-Rezeptor, Glycophorin A, Hämoglobin γG, D7S8 und gruppenspezifische Komponente. (In preparation);; WEICHHOLD GM, KEIL W, EULITZ A, BAYER B, 1994: HLA-DQα PCR system: frequencies of a South Bavarian population and family data. In BÄR W, FIORI A, ROSSI U (eds) Advances in Forensic Haemogenetics 5. Springer Verlag, Berlin-Heidelberg-New York. pp 599-601; ROTHÄMEL T, TRÖGER HD, 1994: Multiplex-PCR der Loci LDLR, GYPA, HBGG, D7S8 und GC: spurenkundliche Anwendbarkeit, Sensitivität, Linearität bri Misch-DNA und Populationsgenetik. Zbl. Rechtsmed.42, p 494;

ALLELE FREQUENCIES OF VWA, FESFPS, FXIIIA1 AND D21S11 IN AN ITALIAN POPULATION SAMPLE

M. Dobosz, M.Pescarmona, A. Moscetti, A. Caglià, E. D'Aloja, L. Grimaldi and V.L.Pascali*

Immunohematology laboratory, Istituto Medicina Legale, Università Cattolica, Largo F.Vito,1, 00168 Roma, Italy; (*) Istituto Medicina Legale, Università di Verona

Systems and loci: D21S11; FXIIA1 (6p25-p25); FESFPS (15q25qter); vWA (12p12-12pter)

Population: Central and Southern Italy

Method: primers and PCR according to the relevant articles cited below; electrophoresis on ALF DNA sequencer

Results:

D21S11 observed genotypes and allele frequencies (N: 135)

Gen.	Obs.	Gen.	Obs.	Gen.	Obs.	Gen.	Obs.
29-29	4	28-31	2	29-34.2	1	31-32.2	1
30-30	7	28-32	1	30-30.2	1	31-33.2	7
31-31	11	28-32.2	1	30-31	12	31-34.2	2
32-32	2	28-33.2	3	30-32	5	32-32.2	1
32.2-32.2	1	28-36	1	30-32.2	7	32-33.2	1
33.2-33.2	4	29-30	6	30-33.2	7	32.2-33.2	1
26-30	1	29-31	10	30-34.2	3	32.2-34.2	3
26-31	2	29-32	4	30.2-32.2	1	33.2-34.2	1
28-29	2	29-32.2	5	30.2-34.2	1		
28-30	2	29-33.2	7	31-32	4		

Allele	Frequency	Allele	Frequency	Allele	Frequency
26	0.0111	30,2	0.0111	33.2	0.1296
28	0.0444	31	0.2296	34.2	0.0407
29	0.1593	32	0.0741	36	0.0037
30	0.2148	32.2	0.0815		

rXIIIA1 observed genotypes and allele frequencies (N: 221)

Gen.	Obs.	Gen.	Obs.	Gen.	Obs.	Gen.	Obs.
3-3	1	3-17	1	5-7	37	6-16	1
5-5	15	4-5	6	5-8	3	7-8	2
6-6	19	4-6	7	5-12	1	7-11	1
7-7	15	4-7	8	5-15	1	7-13	2
3-4	1	4-8	3	5-16	4	7-14	1
3-5	9	4-9	1	6-7	38	7-15	1
3-6	11	4-15	1	6-8	1		
3-7	10	5-6	19	6-15	1		

Allele	Frequency	Allele	Frequency	Allele	Frequency
3.2	0.0769	8	0.0204	14	0.0023
4	0.0611	9	0.0023	15	0.0090
5	0.2489	11	0.0023	16	0.0113
6	0.2624	12	0.0023	17	0.0023
7	0.2941	13	0.0045		

FESFPS observed genotypes and allele frequencies (N: 258)

Gen.	Obs.	Gen.	Obs.	Gen.	Obs.	Gen.	Obs.
10-10	17	8-10	2	10-11	53	11-13	8
11-11	41	8-11	1	10-12	35	11-14	1
12-12	23	8-12	2	10-13	10	12-13	6
13-13	1	9-11	1	11-12	54	13-14	3

Allele	Frequency	Allele	Frequency	Allele	Frequency
8	0.0097	11	0.3876	14	0.0078
9	0.0019	12	0.2771		
10	0.2597	13	0.0562		

vWA observed genotypes and allele frequencies (N: 374)

Gen.	Obs.	Gen.	Obs.	Gen.	Obs.	Gen.	Obs.
14-14	4	13-17	2	15-16	22	16-20	5
15-15	5	14-15	2	15-17	22	17-18	40
16-16	14	14-16	14	15-18	24	17-19	9
17-17	32	14-17	21	15-19	6	17-20	2
18-18	13	14-18	18	16-17	52	18-19	15
19-19	1	14-19	6	16-18	26	18-20	3
13-16	1	14-20	1	16-19	12	19-20	2

Allele	Frequency	Allele	Frequency	Allele	Frequency
13	0.0040	16	0.2139	19	0.0695
14	0.0936	17	0.2834	20	0.0174
15	0.1150	18	0.2032		

References:

Polymeropoulos, M.H., Rath, D.S., Xiao, H., and Merrill, C.R. (1992a) (FES). *Nucleic Acids Res.* **19**: 4018.

Polymeropoulos, M.H., Rath, D.S., Xiao, H., and Merrill, C.R. (1992b). (F13A1). *Nucleic Acids Res.* **19**: 4306.

Kimpton, C., Walton, A., and Gill, P. (1992) (vWA) . *Hum. Mol. Genet.* **1**: 287.

Sharma V., Litt M. (1992) (D21S11) *Hum. Molec.Genet.* **1**: 67.

STR Analysis - HUMTH01 and HUMFES/FPS for Forensic application

R. Espinheira, H. Geada, T. Ribeiro, L. Reys

Institute of Legal Medecine and Medical Faculty of Lisbon

The tetrameric short tandem repeat loci HUMTH01 and HUMFES/FPS were studied.

Population and sample size: Portugal (South) N: 124

Methods: Amplification was performed according to EDNAP protocol (Kimpton et al.)
Electrophoretic methods: 6% polyacrilamide denaturing gel electrophoresis (Lango et al.). The gels were run for 120min. at 800V on the ALF DNA Sequencer. Typing was performed by comparison with allelic ladders.

Results:

HUMTH01 Allele Frequencies

Allele	Frequency	Allele	Frequency	Allele	Frequency
3	0.0040	7	0.1532	9.3	0.2742
5	0.0040	8	0.1452	10	0.0081
6	0.1935	9	0.2097	11	0.0081

$X^2 = 9.6092$ df = 10 $0.30 < p < 0.50$ CE = 0.5820 HI = 0.79

HUMFES/FPS Allele Frequencies

Allele	Frequency	Allele	Frequency	Allele	Frequency
8	0.0161	11	0.3952	14	0.0040
9	0.0040	12	0.2460		
10	0.2823	13	0.0524		

$X^2 = 8.7928$ df = 10 $0.50 < p < 0.70$ CE = 0.441 HI = 0.70

Comments:

Eigth alleles for HUMTH01 (154-178 bp) and seven for HUMFES/FPS (213-238 bp) were observed.
A HUMTH01 smaller allele (145.7 bp) was found and designated as 3 n° of repeats.
The two markers were in genetic equilibrium according to Hardy-Weinberg. HUMTH01 and HUMFES/FPS loci have a similar allele distribution to other already published Caucasian population groups.

References:

Walsh P. et al.	Biotechniques	10: 506-513 (1991)
Lango A. et al.	Adv.For.Haemogent.	5: 109-111 (1993)
Kimpton C. et al.	For.Sci.Int.	71: 137-152 (1995)

PROFILING A NORTH-EAST ITALIAN POPULATION BY FOUR HIGHLY POLYMORPHIC DNA PROBES

P. Fattorini*, F. Florian§, S. Tafuro§, F. Cossutta*, B.M. Altamura* and G. Graziosi§

*Istituto di Medicina Legale e delle Assicurazioni dell'Universita' di Trieste, Trieste (Italy)
§Dipartimento di Biologia dell'Universita' di Trieste, via Giorgieri 5, 34100, Trieste (Italy)

INTRODUCTION

After the forensic validation of the SBA (Southern Blot Analysis), the use of SLPs (single locus probes) has been used in the forensic laboratory for personal identification and paternity testing since the end of the 1980s. Even if expensive and time consuming, the SBA remains the most informative approach in some circumstances, for example in those paternity cases where either the alleged father is unavailable or the paternity index achieved by PCR-based polymorphisms is too low to prove paternity. In this work the allele frequenciy distributions at four highly polymorphic loci (D1S7, D7S21, D12S11 and D7S22) are described in a population living in the Trieste and Gorizia areas (North-East Italy).

MATERIALS AND METHODS

Profiling the samples High molecular weight DNA was purified from Na_2EDTA blood samples from randomly selected donors living in North-East Italy following standard procedure. About 2 μg of each DNA was fully digested with Hinf I and the samples were then electrophoresed according to the following conditions: 20 cm 0.7 % agarose gel in 1xTBE buffer (134 mM Tris, 75mM H_3B0_3, 2.5 mM Na_2EDTA) at 40 V until all fragments <2 Kb had run off the gel. Southern blot, hybridisation and washing were carried out following established conditions; the purified fragments of the clones λMS1 (locus D1S7), λMS31 (locus D7S21), λMS43 (locus D12S22) and pλg3 (locus D7S22) were P^{32} labelled and used as probes (Wong, 1987). All the samples showing only one fragment were redigested and run through a 20 cm 0.85 % agarose until the 0.5 Kb marker was at 3 cm from the end of the gel. This procedure was introduced both to avoid bands running off the gels and to obtain a good resolution of the low molecular weight fragments. The samples showing only one band even after the second electrophoresis were run again through a 25 cm 0.6 % agarose gel until the 3 Kb marker was at the end of the gel. This last precaution was taken to show the possible coalescence of the bands (or pseudohomozygosity condition). The DNA of the cell line K562 was used as a reference standard.

Sizing the DNA fragments The films were scored independently by two operators and the migration of the DNA fragments was measured by a ruler following conventional methods (Gill, 1991; Pascali, 1992). The P^{32} 1Kb ladder was used as reference molecular weight marker. The fragment size was determined by he method of Elder and Southern (1987).

Creating the database For each locus studied, two databases were created. The first contains the observed genotypes and the molecular weight of the alleles expressed in bp. In order to estimate the allele frequency distributions, a second database was created and the fixed bin method was adopted (Bubowle, 1991) with bins of 0,1 Kb.

Testing for Hardy-Weinberg Equilibrium The number of expected homozygotes (EH) at each locus was calculated by $EH= X_1^2+ X_2^2+ X_3^2+ ...+ X_n^2$ where X_1 is the frequency of the alleles at bin 1, X_2 is the frequency of the alleles at bin 2, etc (Weir and Hill, 1993).

Comparison between the expected and observed values was carried out by χ^2 test when the expected frequencies were more than four.

RESULTS

The mobility of the fragments of the standard DNA K562 differed by less than +/- 2.5 % on different gels and therefore the molecular weight of the alleles detected in this study should fall in this range. The final results are summarised in Tab. 1. The allele frequency distributions at loci studied are shown in the Figures. These data refer to the results after the third cycle of electrophoresis and the number of "single band profiles" after each cycle of electrophoresis is reported in Table 2. However, no divergences from H-W equilibrium were observed at loci D7S21 and D7S22 while a low discrepancy was shown at locus D12S11 (Table 2).

DISCUSSION

The data reported here do not differ from those of others reports on the Caucasian populations as far as heterozygosity and allele frequencies are concerned. This fact is even more relevant if we take in account that the population studied is composed of a majority of Italians, a minority of Slovenians and minor contributions by Croats, Serbs, Greeks, Germans and Hungarians. These ethnic groups moved to the region centuries ago and, apparently, as reported both by historical studies and blood group analyses, did not give rise to apparent population stratification. However, in the first years after the second World War, about 300.000 Italians moved from Istria and Dalmatia to our area and not less than 50-60.000 refugees settled in the Trieste area (more then 25 % of the inhabitants of Trieste). Therefore they would be expected to have contributed to modify the genetic structure to some degree. Nevertheless, our results, as well as those reported for the locus D2S44 (Fattorini, 1991), do not show stratification or subpopulation phenomena and suggest genetic homogeneity between our local population and other Caucasian populations. However, no deviation from H-W equilibrium could be demonstrated with the exception at the locus D12S11 but the reasons for this apparent excess of homozygosity have been pointed out (Devlin, 1990; Weir and Hill, 1993).

REFERENCES
Budowle B., Giusti AM, Waye JS, Beachtel FS, Fourney RM, Adams DE, Presley LA, Deadman MA, Monson KL (1991) Fixed bin analysis for statistical evaluation of continuous distributions of allelic data from VNTR loci for use in forensic comparisons. Am J Hum Genet 12:841-855
Devlin B, Risch N, Roeder K (1990) No excess of homozygosity at loci used for DNA fingerprinting. Science 249:1416-1420
Elder JK, Southern JM (1987) Computer-aided analysis of one dimensional restriction fragment gel. In: Bishop MJ and Rawlings CJ (eds) Nucleic acid and protein sequence analysis- a practical approach. IRL, Oxford, pag. 165-172
Fattorini P, Callegaro AP, Florian F, Fabbro D, Frisan T, Altamura BM, Graziosi G (1991) Analysis of allele frequencies of two polymorphic loci in a north-east italian population. In: Berghaus G, Brinkmann B, Rittner C, Staak M (eds) DNA-technology and its forensic application. Springer-Verlag, Berlin- Heidelberg, pp. 134-140
Gill P, Evett S, Woodroffe S, Lygo LE, Millican E, Webster M (1991) Databases, quality control and interpretation of DNA profiling in the Home Office Forensic Science Service. Electrophoresis 12:204-209
Pascali VL, Moscetti A, Dobosz M, Pescamora M, D'Aloja E (1992) Error in sizing bands of hypervariable profiles on autoradiograms: are they Gaussian? Electrophoresis 13:341-345
Wong Z, Wilson V, Patel T, Povey S, Jeffreys AJ (1987) Characterization of a panel of highly variable minisatellites cloned from human DNA. Ann.Hum.Genet. 51:269-288
Weir BS and Hill WG (1993) Population genetics of DNA profiles. J.Forensic Sci.Soc 33(4):218-225

ACKNOWLEDGEMENTS
We thank Prof. A.J. Jeffreys (University of Leicester, U.K.) and P. Debenham (Cellmark Diagnostics) for providing us with the minisatellite probes. We thank also Dr. S. Rand (University of Münster) for his helpful suggestions in preparing this manuscript.

Table 1. n: number of blood samples tested; Ht: heterozygosity; Kb: allele range.

locus	n	Ht	Kb
D1S7	332	0,9879	0,4-27
D7S21	340	0,9529	2,5-20
D12S11	339	0,9471	1,7-13
D7S22	332	0,9518	1,3-17

Table 2. Number of "single band profiles" observed after the 1st, the 2nd and 3rd cycle of electrophoresis (frequency in brackets). The results of the χ^2 test are reported in the last column; *: not carried out.

locus	1st	2nd	3rd	χ^2
D1S7	35 (0,105)	6 (0,018)	4 (0,012)	*
D7S21	19 (0,056)	19 (0,056)	16 (0,047)	3,239 (p>0,05)
D12S11	25 (0,073)	24 (0,071)	18 (0,053)	5,950 (p>0,05)
D7S22	96 (0,289)	17 (0,051)	16 (0,048)	0,201 (p>0,05)

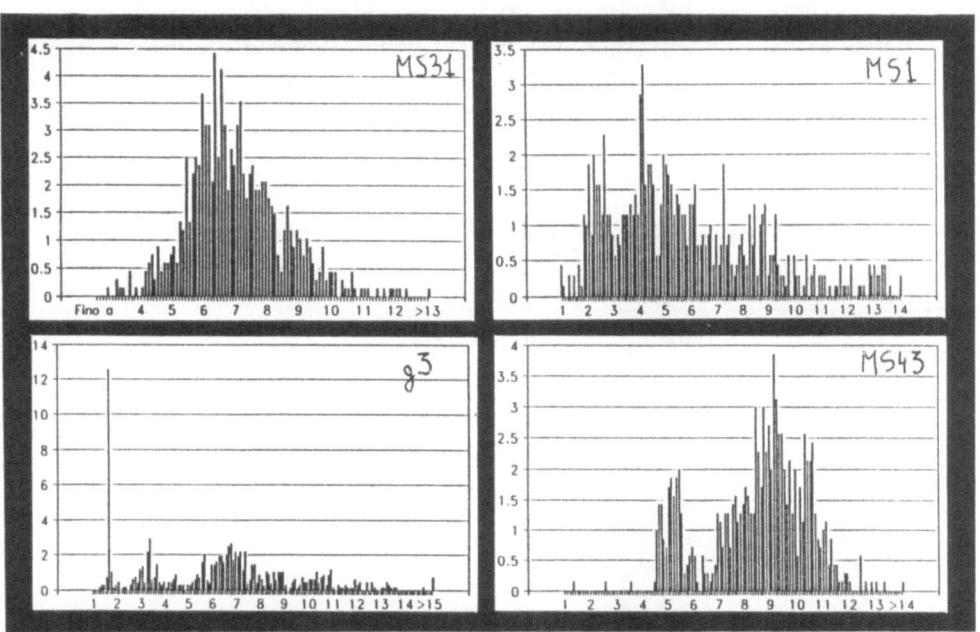

Allele frequencies of HLA-DQα, LDLR, GYPA, HBGG, D7S8 and GC in the resident and autochthonous populations of the Basque Country

O. García[1], P. Martín[2], B. Budowle[3], C. Albarrán[2], A. Alonso[2]

[1] Laboratorio UTAP, C/ María Díaz de Haro, 3-2ª Planta, 48013 Bilbao

[2] Sección de Biología, Instituto Nacional de Toxicología, Madrid

[3] FSRTC, FBI Academy, Quantico, Virginia 22135, USA

Systems and loci: HLA-DQα (6p21.3)
LDLR (19p13.1→p13.3)
GYPA (4q28→q31)
HBGG (11q)
D7S8 (7cen→q22)
GC (4q11→q13)

Populations and sample size: Basque Country resident population N = 208
Basque Country autochthonous population N = 206

Methods

DNA was extracted by the chelex method. The amplification by PCR and the typing by reverse dot-blot methodology using ASO probes were performed according to the AmpliType HLA DQα and AmpliType PM PCR Amplification and Typing kit protocol provided by the manufacturer (Perkin-Elmer Cetus). All samples carrying the allele 4 in the HLA-DQα system were digested using 2 restriction enzymes (Rsa I and Fok I) [1]. The digested fragments were separated by vertical discontinuous polyacrylamide gel electrophoresis using the Tris-chloride/Tris-glycine buffer system [2] and detected by silver stain.

Results

Observed allele frequency distribution for HLA-DQα locus

Allele	Autochthonous	Residents
1.1	0.190	0.156
1.2	0.180	0.184
1.3	0.101	0.087
2	0.204	0.158
3	0.108	0.153
4.1	0.180	0.238
4.2	0.034	0.021
4.3	0.002	0.002

HWE test for independence on HLA-DQα locus

	Autochthonous	Residents
Obs. Homozygosity	20.7 %	19.8 %
Exp. Homozygosity[a] [3]	16.4 %	16.9 %
Homozygosity test[b] [4-6]	0.095	0.265
Likelihood ratio test[b] [3,7-8]	0.224	0.839
Exact test[b] [9]	0.205	0.900

[a] Expected homozygosity is an unbiased estimate
[b] These values are probability values

Observed allele frequency distribution for PM loci

Allele	Autochtonous	Residents
LDLR*A	0.524	0.438
LDLR*B	0.476	0.562
GYPA*A	0.541	0.514
GYPA*B	0.459	0.486
HBGG*A	0.524	0.534
HBGG*B	0.476	0.459
HBGG*C	0.000	0.007
D7S8*A	0.515	0.575
D7S8*B	0.485	0.425
GC*A	0.330	0.339
GC*B	0.104	0.096
GC*C	0.566	0.565

HWE test for independence on PM loci in a Basque Country autochthonous sample population

	LDLR	GYPA	HBGG	D7S8	GC
Obs. Homozygosity	47.6 %	51.9 %	55.3 %	46.6 %	38.4 %
Exp. Homozygosity[a]	50.0 %	50.2 %	50.0 %	49.9 %	43.8 %
Homozygosity test[b]	0.487	0.621	0.125	0.341	0.113
Likelihood ratio test[b]	0.471	0.663	0.147	0.364	0.033*
Exact test[b]	0.570	0.663	0.116	0.429	0.035*

[a] Expected homozygosity is an unbiased estimate
[b] These values are probability values

HWE test for independence on PM loci in a Basque Country resident sample population

	LDLR	GYPA	HBGG	D7S8	GC
Obs. Homozygosity	54.8 %	46.2 %	61.1 %	48.6 %	47.1 %
Exp. Homozygosity[a]	50.7 %	49.9 %	49.4 %	51.0 %	44.2 %
Homozygosity test[b]	0.232	0.277	0.001*	0.482	0.396
Likelihood ratio test[b]	0.253	0.277	0.003*	0.476	0.095
Exact test[b]	0.253	0.337	0.003*	0.476	0.054

[a] Expected homozygosity is an unbiased estimate
[b] These values are probability values

Discussion

The genotype frequency distributions for most of the loci do not deviate from HWE based on the homozygosity test, likelihood ratio test and the exact test. Those loci that depart from HWE are marked with an asterisk. It should be noted that even for the highly significant departure from HWE for HBGG in the resident population, there would still be little impact for forensic identity purposes. The differences between observed and expected genotype frequencies in this case would not substantially alter the estimated rarity of a DNA profile and thus would not result in bias to an accused individual. An interclass correlation test analysis [10] demonstrated that there is little evidence for correlation between the alleles at any pairs of loci (data not shown).

In conclusion, a Basque Country population database has been established for six PCR-based polymorphic loci. The data can be used for deriving estimates of multiple locus profile frequencies for identity testing purposes using the product rule under the assumption of independence.

References

[1]   Ju, L.Y.; Gu, X.F.; Larger, E.; Krishnamoorthy, R.; Charrom, D. Electrophoresis 12: 270-273 (1991).

[2]   Alonso, A.; Martín, P.; Albarrán, C.; Sancho, M. Int. J. Leg. Med. 105: 311-314 (1.993).

[3]   Edwards, A.; Hammond, H.; Jin, L.; Caskey, C.T., Chakraborty, R. Genomics, 12: 241-253 (1992).

[4]   Chakraborty, R.; Smouse, P.E.; Neel, J.V. Am. J. Hum. Genet. 43: 709-725 (1988).

[5]   Nei, M.; Roychoudhury, A.K. Genetics 76: 379-390 (1974).

[6]   Nei, M. Genetics 89: 583-590 (1978).

[7]   Chakraborty, R.; Fornage, M.; Guegue, R.; Boerwinkle, E. In: DNA fingerprinting: Approaches and applications (Burke, T.; Dolf, G.; Jeffreys, A.J.; Wolff, R. -eds-) Birkhauser Verlag, Berlin, pp. 127-143 (1991).

[8]   Weir, B.S. Genetics, 130: 873-887 (1992).

[9]   Guo, S.W.; Thompson, E.A. Biometrics 48: 361-372 (1992).

[10] Karlin, S.; Cameron, E.C.; Williams, P.T. Proc. Natl. Acad. Sci. USA 78: 2664-2668 (1.981).

STUDY OF HUMACTBP2 STR POLYMORPHISM, PERFORMED BY PCR AND AUTOMATED LASER FLUORESCENCE (ALF) SEQUENCER IN A POPULATION SAMPLE OF CATALONIA

M. Gené, E. Huguet, M. Luna, P. Moreno, M.V. Lareu, A. Carracedo

Forensic Genetics Laboratory. School of Medicine. University of Barcelona. 28028 BARCELONA. Spain.

System and Locus: HUMACTBP2 (also named SE33). Located in the 5' flanking region of the human beta-actin related pseudogene H-beta-Ac-psi-2 (Moos 1983) on chromosome 5 (Warne 1991) or 6 (Polymeropoulos 1992). $(AAAG)_n$ tandem repeat.

Population and sample sizes: Catalonia (NE Spain). Western ·Mediterranean caucasoid population. N:154

Methods: Standard PCR amplifications were accomplished with fluorescein labelled primers described by Polymeropoulos (1992). Electrophoretic methods: 6% polyacrylamide denaturing gel electrophoresis. The gels were run for 4h. at 1450 V, 38 mA, 45W, 50°C and laser power at 3 mW on the ALF DNA Sequencer. Cocktail allelic ladder of sequenced known alleles and nomenclature proposed by Möller (1994) were used.

Results: Table 1. Observed ACTBP2 genotypes in a sample population of Catalonia

	7-1	13-2	13	14	15	16	17	18	19	20	21-2	21	22-4	22-2	22	23	24	25	26	27	28	29	30	31	32	33-1	33	34-2	34	36	42
7-1			1																												
13-2				1																											
13			1	1																		1					1				
14					1		1	1		2						1	1				2	1	1	1					1		
15				1	1		2		1							1	2		1		1	1									
16						3	3	1	2										1	2	2		1		1		1				
17							1	2		2		1		1	1	3	2	1			3	1	1	1							
18							1	5	3			1		1	1	1		1			3	1	2	2	1						
19								1	3								2	2			1	1					1		1		
20																1		1	1	2		1									
21-2												1								1											
21									1		1								1		1		1						1		1
22-4									1			1				2	1		1	1											
22-2																			1												
22																	1		1												
23																															
24																					1										
25																					1		1		1						
26																			1	2	1		1				1				
27																				2	2		1	1							
28																					1	1									
29																							3						1	1	
30																															
31																															
32																															
33-1																															
33																															
34-2																															
34																															
36																															
42																															

Table 2. Allele frequencies

	Allele		Frequency		Allele		Frequency
1.-	07-1	=	0.0032	17.-	24	=	0.0260
2.-	13-2	=	0.0032	18.-	25	=	0.0195
3.-	13	=	0.0162	19.-	26	=	0.0519
4.-	14	=	0.0454	20.-	27	=	0.0584
5.-	15	=	0.0422	21.-	28	=	0.0519
6.-	16	=	0.0747	22.-	29	=	0.0649
7.-	17	=	0.0844	23.-	30	=	0.0390
8.-	18	=	0.0974	24.-	31	=	0.0227
9.-	19	=	0.0682	25.-	32	=	0.0130
10.-	20	=	0.0552	26.-	33-1	=	0.0097
11.-	21-2	=	0.0130	27.-	33	=	0.0065
12.-	21	=	0.0260	28.-	34-2	=	0.0065
13.-	22-4	=	0.0357	29.-	34	=	0.0065
14.-	22-2	=	0.0130	30.-	35	=	0.0032
15.-	22	=	0.0260	31.-	42	=	0.0032
16.-	23	=	0.0130				

Table 3. Forensic diagnosis suitability results.

	HUMACTBP2
Heterozygosity Index (HI)	93.50
Power discrimination (PD)	0.99
Chance Exclusion (CE)	0.89
Essen-Möller mean value (EM)	8.94

Comments: HUMACTBP2 has a polemic length and sequence polymorphism [4] because a high number of alleles have been described, some of which may vary by as little as 1 base, moreover its AT-rich sequence may have anomalous migration rates in different electrophoretic systems. Nevertheless as it is one of the most powerful PCR markers, we describe the experience in our laboratory. A high degree of variability observed in a population sample of Catalonia, could makes it an extremely useful marker in forensic genetics diagnosis. In general, HUMACTBP2 is an interesting polymorphism that needs standardization of the experimental conditions, in order to obtain allele identification that is reproducible in all forensic laboratories. In this sense, the use of sequenced allelic ladder is very important.

References

Möller A, Brinkmann B (1994) Locus ACTBP2 (SE33). Sequencing data reveal considerable polymorphism. Int J Leg Med 106:262-267
Moos M, Gallwitz D (1983) Structure of two human beta-actin-related processed genes one of which is located next to a simple repetitive sequence. EMBO J. 2:757-761
Polymeropoulos MH, Rath DS, Xiao H, Merril CR (1992) Nucleic Acids Res 20:1432
Warne D, Watkins C, Bodfish P, Nyberg K, Spurr NK (1991) Nucleic Acids Res 19:6980

AYMARA AND QUECHUA AMERINDIAN POPULATIONS CHARACTERIZED BY HUMTH01 AND HUMVWA STR POLYMORPHISMS

M. Gené, E. Huguet, P. Moreno, M. Fuentes, J. Corbella, J. Mezquita

Forensic Genetics Laboratory. School of Medicine. University of Barcelona. 28028 BARCELONA. Spain

Systems and Loci: HUMTH01 (TC11, 11p15.5), HUMvWA (12p12-12pter).

Populations and sample sizes: Quechuas and Aymaras are two ancient precolumbian ethnic groups in South-America. Quechua samples (n= 68) were collected in Dalence (Oruro. Bolivia), and Aymara samples (n=80) in Pacajes and Murillo provinces (La Paz. Bolivia). DNA samples were obtained from single hairs.

Methods: Standard PCR amplifications were accomplished with fluorescein labelled primers. HUMTH01 primers (Edwards 1992) HUMVWA primers (Kimpton 1992). Electrophoretic methods: 6% polyacrylamide denaturing gel electrophoresis. The gels were run for 4h. at 1450 V, 38 mA, 45W, 50°C and laser power at 3 mW on the ALF DNA Sequencer. The allelic ladders used were composed by a cocktail of samples with alleles of known size from each polymorphism.

Results:

Table 1. Observed genotypes in a Aymara population sample.

HUMTH01		HUMVWA31	
6/6	3	14/15	1
6/7	21	14/16	2
6/9	2	15/16	4
6/9.3	5	15/17	3
7/7	36	15/20	1
7/9	1	16/16	8
7/9.3	11	16/17	17
9.3/9.3	1	16/18	3
		16/19	3
		17/17	9
		17/18	1
		17/19	2

Chi^2= 4.42		Chi^2= 18.74
df= 6		df= 21
0.750 > p > 0.500		0.650 > p > 0.600

Table 2. Observed genotypes in a Quechua population sample.

HUMTHO1		HUMVWA31	
6/6	1	15/16	1
6/7	15	15/17	1
6/9.3	3	15/18	1
7/7	26	16/16	3
7/9.3	6	16/17	17
9.3/9.3	7	16/18	5
		16/19	3
		17/17	16
		17/18	10
		17/19	4
		18/18	3
		18/19	2
$Chi^2=$	4.61	$Chi^2=$	2.59
df=	3	df=	10
$0.250 > p > 0.100$		$0.995 > p > 0.975$	

Table 3. Allele frequencies in a Aymara sample population.

	HUMTHO1 n= 80				HUMVWA31 n= 54		
Allele	Freq.	bp.[a]		Allele	Freq.	bp.[a]	
6	0.2125	184		14	0.0277	138	
7	0.6562	188		15	0.0833	142	
8	0			16	0.4166	146	
9	0.1875	196		17	0.3796	150	
9.3	0.1125	199		18	0.0370	154	
10	0			19	0.0463	158	
11	0			20	0.0092	162	

(a) Fragment sizes determined automatically using Fragment Manager v.1.1 software Pharmacia

Table 4. Allele frequencies in a Quechua sample population.

	HUMTHO1 n= 68			HUMVWA31 n= 66	
Allele	Freq.	bp.[a]	Allele	Freq.	bp.[a]
6	0.1470	184	14	0	
7	0.6103	188	15	0.0227	142
8	0		16	0.2424	146
9	0		17	0.4848	150
9.3	0.2426	199	18	0.1818	154
10	0		19	0.0681	158
11	0		20	0	

(a) Fragment sizes determined automatically using Fragment Manager v.1.1 software Pharmacia

Table 5. Forensic diagnosis suitability results.

	Aymara HUMTHO1	Aymara HUMVWA31	Quechua HUMTHO1	Quechua HUMVWA31
HI.	50	68.52	50	66.66
PD.	0.70	0.83	0.73	0.84
CE.	0.27	0.42	0.29	0.42
EM	9.78	9.65	9.79	9.68

Comments: The allelic frequencies, compared to other populations, show a high degree of variation between amerindians and caucasoids.

Acknowledgments: The authors are very grateful to the Aymara and Quechua populations for their contribution.

References

Edwards A, Hammond HA, Jin L, Caskey CT, Chakraborty R (1992) Genetic variation at five trimeric and tetrameric tandem repeat loci in four human population groups. Genomics 12:241-253

Kimpton C, Walton A, Gill P (1992) A further tetranuceotide repeat polymorphism in the VWF gene. Hum Mol Genet 1:287

SUITABILITY OF THE HUMTH01, HUMCD4, AND HUMVWA STR POLYMORPHISMS FOR LEGAL MEDICINE INVESTIGATIONS IN THE POPULATION OF CATALONIA (NORTH-EAST SPAIN)

M. Gené, E. Huguet, P. Moreno, C. Sánchez, J. Corbella, J. Mezquita

Forensic Genetics Laboratory. School of Medicine. University of Barcelona. 28028 BARCELONA. Spain.

Systems and loci: HUMTH01 (11p15.5), HUMCD4 (12p), HUMvWA (12p12-12pter)

Population and sample sizes: Catalonia (NE Spain). European Western Mediterranean population. HUMTC11 n=161. HUMCD4 n=117. HUMVWA n=122

Methods: Standard PCR amplifications were accomplished with fluorescein labelled primers. HUMTH01 primers (Edwards A 1992), HUMCD4 primers (Edwards MC 1991), HUMVWA primers (Kimpton 1992). Electrophoretic methods: 6% polyacrylamide denaturing gel electrophoresis. The gels were run for 4h. at 1450 V, 38 mA, 45W, 50°C and laser power at 3 mW on the ALF DNA Sequencer. The allelic ladders used were composed by a cocktail of samples with alleles of known size from each polymorphism.

Results:

Table 1. Observed genotypes.

HUMTH01		HUMCD4		HUMVWA31	
6/6	10	1/1	14	14/15	2
6/7	10	1/2	21	14/16	6
6/8	10	1/6	15	14/17	10
6/9	13	1/7	6	14/18	3
6/9.3	22	1/8	3	14/19	3
6/10	3	2/2	14	15/15	1
7/7	2	2/4	1	15/16	11
7/8	11	2/6	15	15/17	5
7/9	17	2/7	5	15/18	2
7/9.3	10	2/8	2	15/19	4
8/8	4	6/6	15	15/20	1
8/9	5	6/7	4	16/16	7
8/9.3	8	6/8	2	16/17	13
8/R1	1	16/18	8		
9/9	6	16/19	3		
9/9.3	16	17/17	10		
9/11	1	17/18	12		
9/R2	1	17/19	7		
9.3/9.3	11	18/18	9		
		18/19	5		

$Chi^2=36.25$	$Chi^2= 11.86$	$Chi^2= 27.35$
df= 36	df= 15	df= 21
$0.500> p > 0.450$	$0.790 > p > 0.789$	$0.250 > p > 0.100$

Table 2. Allele frequencies.

HUMTHO1 n=161			HUMCD4 n=117			HUMVWA31 n=122		
Allele	Freq.	bp.[a]	Allele[b]	Freq.	bp.[a]	Allele	Freq.	bp.[a]
6	0.2422	184	1	0.3119	86	14	0.0983	138
7	0.1614	188	2	0.3076	91	15	0.1106	142
8	0.1335	192	3	0		16	0.2254	146
9	0.2018	196	4	0.0042	101	17	0.2746	150
9.3	0.2422	199	5	0		18	0.1967	154
10	0.003	200	6	0.2820	112	19	0.0902	158
11	0.003	203	7	0.0641	117	20	0.0041	162
R1	0.003	209	8	0.0299	123			
R2	0.009	215						

(a) Fragment sizes determined automatically using Fragment Manager v.1.1 software Pharmacia
(b) Smallest allele in the HUMCD4 cocktail was therefore arbitrarily designated as "1" and the others were enumerated consecutively towards the cathode.

Table 3. Forensic diagnosis suitability results.

	HUMTHO1	HUMCD4	HUMVWA31
Heterozygosity Index (HI)	79.50	63.25	77.87
Power discrimination (PD)	0.93	0.87	0.93
Chance Exclusion (CE)	0.59	0.47	0.61
Essen-Möller mean value (EM)	9.55	9.65	9.53

Comments: The high degree of variability of each PCR polymorphism makes these markers very useful in forensic genetics diagnosis.

References

Edwards A, Hammond HA, Jin L, Caskey CT, and Chakraborty R (1992) Genetic variation at five trimeric and tetrameric tandem repeat loci in four human population groups. Genomics, 12: 241-253
Edwards MC, Clemens PR, Tristan M, Pizzuti A, Gibbs RA (1991) Pentanucleotide repeat length polymorphism at the human CD4 locus. Nucleic Acids Res, 19, 17: 4791
Kimpton C, Walton A, Gill P (1992) A further tetranuceotide repeat polymorphism in the VWF gene. Hum Mol Genet, 1: 287

Population and formal genetics of the STR system MBP - locus B - in North Portugal

L. Gusmão, M.J. Prata, A. Amorim

Inst. Antropologia, Univ. Porto and IPATIMUP, 4050 Porto, Portugal

System and locus: MBPB, myelin basic protein, locus B (18q22-qter)

Population and sample size: North Portugal; N=109

Methods

Samples: blood or buccal swabs from unrelated individuals and mother/child pairs.

DNA extraction: method of Lareu *et al.* (1994)

Primers: Polymeropoulos *et al.* (1992)

Amplification conditions: 5 min at 93°; 94°: 1 min; 62°: 0.5 min; 72°: 1 min; 27-35 cycles.

Electrophoresis: according to Luis and Caeiro (1995); silver staining: Budowle *et al.* (1992). Genotyping was performed by side-by-side comparison with an allelic ladder made up from previously typed samples.

Results:

Observed Genotypes

Genotypes	Obs.	Genotypes	Obs.	Genotypes	Obs.
7-7	17	7-13	1	10-11	6
7-9	4	9-9	1	10-12	3
7-10	11	9-10	1	11-11	15
7-11	21	9-11	3	11-12	15
7-12	6	10-10	2	12-12	3

P=0.5

Allele frequencies

Allele	Freq.	Allele	Freq.	Allele	Freq.
7	0.353	10	0.115	12	0.138
9	0.045	11	0.344	13	0.005

Comments:

Observed genotype distribution does not deviate significantly from Hardy-Weinberg expectations. The difference between observed (0.65) and expected (0.72) heterozygosities are also non-significant (χ^2= 2.7, 1df, P=0.10).

Estimated allele frequencies in our sample are similar to those reported for Germany (Möller *et al.* 1994).

In 59 mother-child pairs analysed, an exclusion (mother 7-7/child 11-11) was observed. This finding is in accordance with the results presented by Möller *et al.* (1994), demonstrating that this system must be used with care for forensic purposes.

References

Budowle B, Chakraborty R, Giusti AM, Eisenberg AJ, Allen RC (1991) Analysis of the VNTR locus D1S80 by the PCR followed by high-resolution PAGE. Am J Hum Genet 48: 137-144

Lareu MV, Phillips CP, Carracedo A, Lincoln PJ, Court DS, Thomson JA (1994) Investigation of the STR locus HUMTH01 using PCR and two electrophoresis formats: UK and Galician Caucasian population surveys and usefulness in paternity investigations. Forensic Sci Int 66: 41-52

Luis JR, Caeiro B (1995) Application of two STRs (VWF and hTPO) to human population profiling. A survey in Galicia. Human Biology (in press)

Möller A, Wiegand P, Grüschow C, Seuchter SA, Baur MP, Brinkmann B (1994) Population data and forensic efficiency values for the STR systems HumVWA, HumMBP and HumFABP. Int J Legal Med 106: 183-189

Polymeropoulos MH, Xiao H, Merril CR (1992) Tetranucleotide repeat polymorphism at the human myelin basic protein gene (MBP). Hum Mol Genet 1: 658

Acknowledgements: This work was partially supported by JNICT (Junta Nacional de Investigação Científica e Tecnológica, BD/2849/93-ID and PBIC/C/CEN/1174/92) and CNCDP (Comissão Nacional para as Comemorações dos Descobrimentos Portugueses, research contract nº 70).

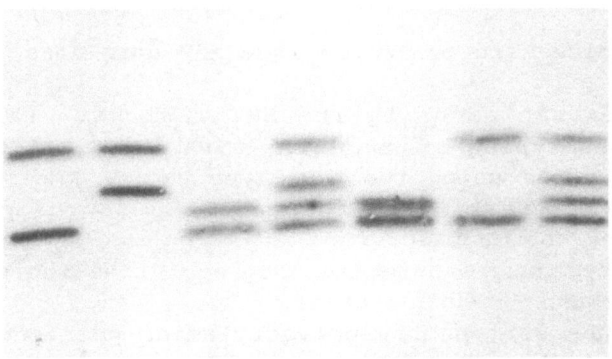

MBP-B genotypes after polyacrylamide electrophoresis of the amplified fragments. From left to right: lane 1: 7-11; lane 2: 7-9; lane 3: 10-11; lane 4: ladder; lane 5: 10-11; lane 6: 7-11; lane 7: ladder.

Allele Frequency Distribution of Five Loci (LDLR, GYPA, HBGG, D7S8 and GC) in a Japanese Population

M. Hara, A. Kido*, K. Saito, A. Takada, K. Yabe, T. Murai and H. Watanabe

Department of Legal Medicine, Saitama Medical School, Saitama-ken, Japan
Department of Legal Medicine, Yamanashi Medical University, Yamanashi-ken, Japan*

Introduction

Recently, a kit for the simultaneous genotyping of low density lipoprotein receptor (LDLR)[1], glycophorin A (GYPA)[2], hemoglobin G gammaglobin (HBGG)[3], D7S8 [4] and group specific component (GC)[5] has been commercially available which is based on the techniques of PCR amplification and reverse dot blot hybridization. With this new kit we have determined the distribution of genotypes and allele frequencies of the above five loci in a Japanese population. Moreover, we have investigated the relationship between MN blood types and GYPA genotypes and the relationship between serum GC subtypes and GC genotypes.

Materials and Methods

Blood samples were collected from 257 unrelated Japanese individuals.

DNA was extracted using the SMI TEST kit (Sumitomo Kinzoku). Genotyping of the LDLR, GYPA, HBGG, D7S8 and GC loci was performed using the AmpliType PM PCR Amplification and Typing kit (Perkin Elmer) according to the protocol recommended by the manufacturer.

MN blood types were determined by agglutination with the use of anti-M and -N sera (Ortho).

Serum GC was subtyped by polyacrylamide gel isoelectric focusing followed by immunoblotting [6].

Results and Discussion

The distributions of genotypes and allele frequencies of the five loci LDLR, GYPA, HBGG, D7S8 and GC are shown in Tables 1 and 2. The population data at each locus fitted the Hardy-Weinberg law. The cumulative probability of paternity exclusion for the 5 loci was calculated at 0.690. The cumulative discrimination power for the 5 loci was as high as 0.992.

Table 1. Distribution of genotypes of LDLR, GYPA, HBGG, D7S8 and GC in 257 unrelated Japanese

Genotype	LDLR	GYPA	HBGG	D7S8	GC
AA	0.027	0.335	0.144	0.377	0.066
AB	0.237	0.494	0.455	0.486	0.237
BB	0.735	0.171	0.401	0.136	0.257
AC			0.000		0.121
BC			0.000		0.253
CC			0.000		0.066

Table 2. Distribution of allele frequencies of LDLR, GYPA, HBGG, D7S8 and GC in 257 unrelated Japanese

Allele	LDLR	GYPA	HBGG	D7S8	GC
A	0.146	0.582	0.372	0.621	0.245
B	0.854	0.418	0.628	0.379	0.502
C			0.000		0.253

Table 3 shows the relationship between MN blood types and GYPA genotypes in 257 Japanese. A complete correspondence of M = GYPA A and N = GYPA B was confirmed.

Table 3. Relationship between MN blood types and GYPA genotypes in 257 unrelated Japanese

MN blood type	GYPA genotype		
	AA	AB	BB
M	86	0	0
MN	0	127	0
N	0	0	44
Total	86	127	44

Table 4 shows the relationship between serum GC subtypes and GC genotypes in 200 Japanese. 187 out of 200 individuals were common subtypes and a correspondence of GC*2 = GC A, GC*1F = GC B and GC*1S = GC C was observed. However, the remaining 13 individuals were variant types; GC 2-1A2 and GC 2-1A9 were GC AB, GC 1F-1A2 and GC 1A3-1A9 were GC

BB, GC 1S-1A2 was GC BC. Thus, GC*1A2, GC*1A3 and GC*1A9 corresponded to GC B as GC*1F did.

Table 4. Relationship between serum GC subtypes and GC genotypes in 200 unrelated Japanese

Serum GC subtype	GC genotype					
	AA	AB	AC	BB	BC	CC
2	13	0	0	0	0	0
2-1F	0	43	0	0	0	0
2-1S	0	0	27	0	0	0
1F	0	0	0	46	0	0
1F1S	0	0	0	0	47	0
1S	0	0	0	0	0	11
2-1A2	0	3	0	0	0	0
2-1A9	0	1	0	0	0	0
1F-1A2	0	0	0	4	0	0
1A3-1A9	0	0	0	1	0	0
1S-1A2	0	0	0	0	4	0
Total	13	47	27	51	51	11

The AmpliType PM PCR kit system permits combined genotyping of LDLR, GYPA, HBGG, D7S8 and GC on a single dot blot strip. The technique is simple, rapid and therefore recommendable to be routinely used for individual identification as well as paternity testing. Because of the frequent occurrence of various GC variants, however, the GC genotyping by the present kit cannot be substituted for the serum GC subtyping.

References

1 Yamamoto T, Davis CG, Brown MS, Schneider WJ, Casey ML, Goldstein JL, Russell DW (1984) Cell, **39**, 27-38.
2 Siebert PD, Fukuda M (1987) Proc Natl Acad Sci USA, **84**, 6735-6739.
3 Slightom JL, Blechl AE, Smithies O (1980) Cell, **21**, 627-638.
4 Horn GT, Richards B, Merrill JJ, Klinger KW (1990) Clin Chem, **36**, 1614-1619.
5 Yang F, Brune JL, Naylor SL, Cupples RL, Naberhaus KH, Bowman BH (1985) Proc Natl Acad Sci USA, **82**, 7994-7998
6 Kido A, Kimura Y, Oya M (1995) Electrophoresis, **16**, 1024-1026.

FREQUENCY DATA ON THE LOCI LDLR, GYPA, HBGG, D7S8 AND GC IN A POPULATION RESIDENT IN MADRID (SPAIN).

M. Herrera, C. Asperilla, M. A. Aumente, L. Prieto, E. Arroyo, J. M. Ruiz de la Cuesta.

Departamento de Toxicología y Legislación Sanitaria. Escuela de Medicina Legal. Facultad de Medicina. Universidad Complutense de Madrid. 28040 - Madrid. Spain.

System and loci: LDLR, GYPA, HBGG, D7S8 AND GC.

Population and sample size: Madrid (Central Spain). N: 207.

Methods: Standard procedure according to Amplitype PCR PM Amplification and Typing Kit Manual. (Perkin Elmer, USA). The comparison between expected and observed genotypes resulted in Hardy-Weinberg equilibrium through a common chi-square test.

Results:

Observed genotypes		
LDLR	AA	48
	AB	89
	BB	70
GYPA	AA	50
	AB	114
	BB	43
HBGG	AA	53
	AB	104
	AC	2
	BB	47
	BC	1
	CC	0
D7S8	AA	55
	AB	106
	BB	46
GC	AA	19
	AB	19
	AC	75
	BB	6
	BC	33
	CC	55

Allele frequencies.

Alleles->	A	B	C
LDLR	.4468	.5531	-
GYPA	.5169	.4830	-
HBGG	.5120	.4806	.0072
D7S8	.5217	.4782	-
Gc	.3188	.1545	.5265

Hardy-Weinberg equilibrium:

System	d.f.	X^2	p
LDLR	1	3.514	0.1>p>0.05
GYPA	1	2.184	0.2>p>0.1
HBGG	3	0.375	0.95>p>0.9
D7S8	1	0.141	0.75>p>0.7
Gc	3	1.069	0.8>p>0.75

Statistical parameters of medico-legal interest:

Discrimination Power (DP), Chance of Exclusion (CE) and Heterozygosity Index (H) were included separately for each marker and combinned in the case of the two first parameters. The DP was calculated following the method of Fisher (1951).

System	DP	CE	H
LDLR	.6471	.1860	0.4299
GYPA	.5952	.1873	0.5507
HBGG	.6304	.1965	0.5169
D7S8	.6178	.1872	0.5120
Gc	.7550	.3157	0.6135
COMB.	.9950	.7044	-

Comments:

The calculated values for DP, CE and H are similar to those obtained in other caucasoid population studies (Hochmeister et al., 1994; Perkin Elmer, PM kit Manual).

References:

Fisher RA (1951) Standard calculations for evaluating a blood group system. Heredity 5: 95-102.

Hochmeister MN, Budowle B, Borer UV, Dimhofer R. (1994) Swiss population data on the loci HLA-DQA1, LDLR, GYPA, HBGG, D7S8, GC and D1S80. Forensic Sci. Int. 67: 175-184.

Perkin Elmer Corp., USA (1994) Amplitype PM PCR Amplification and Typing Kit Manual. Part. No. N808-0057. p. 3.

GERMAN DATA ON THE PCR BASED LOCI HUMVWA31, HUMTH01, HUMFES/FPS, HUMF13B AND D1S80

Huckenbeck W[a], Scheil H-G[b], West S[c], Demir K[a], Kanja J[a], Kaiser A[a], Hees V[c], Meyer W[c], Scholten D[a], Stancu V[a], Bronczek M[d], BonteW[a]

[a] Institute of Forensic Medicine, Heinrich-Heine-University Düsseldorf
[b] Institute of Human Genetics and Anthropology, Heinrich-Heine-Universität Düsseldorf
[c] Landeskriminalamt of Northrhine Westphalia, Düsseldorf
[d] Court of Langenfeld

Summary

To create a preliminary data base for the PCR based loci HUMVWA31, HUMTH01, HUMFES/FPS, HUMF13B AND D1S80 population data from Germany were collected and additional population studies have been carried out on ethnic Germans living in Northrhine Westphalia. With exception of the D1S80 system no deviations from the Hardy-Weinberg-equilibrium have been detected. The German samples have been pooled by calculating the weighted arithmetical means to be useful as preliminary data base for forensic purposes.

Material and Methods

DNA was isolated from ethnic Germans living in Northrhine Westphalia. Isolation was carried out using a commercially available kit (Qiagen, Germany). The samples were typed according to Kimpton et al, 1994. AVACH values have been calculated according to Krüger et al, 1968.

Results and Discussion

The German gene frequencies for the loci HUMVWA31, HUMTH01, HUMFES/FPS, HUMF13B and D1S80 are presented in table 1 - table 5. For the Northrhine Westphalian samples no deviations from the Hardy-Weinberg-equilibrium were found: HUMVWA31 (χ^2 = 8.17, df = 10, 50 > p > 70); HUMTH01 (χ^2=15.64, df=9, 5 > p > 10); HUMFES/FPS (χ^2=5.09,df=4, 20>p>30).

The German AVACH values (samples pooled by calculating weighted arithmetical means) are HUMVW31 (0.6163), HUMTH01 (0.5645), HUMFES/FPS (0.4136), HUMF13B (0.4328) and D1S80 (0.6425).

Locus HUMVWA31

Population	n	Ref.	12	13	14	15	16	17	18	19	20	21
Düsseldorf	608	(1)	0.0000	0.0049	0.0477	0.1118	0.2385	0.2714	0.2105	0.1020	0.0115	0.0016
NRW	488		0.0020	0.0000	0.1086	0.0963	0.1947	0.3053	0.2111	0.0738	0.0082	0.0000
Münster	642	(2)	0.0000	0.0047	0.1100	0.0980	0.2100	0.2700	0.2100	0.0770	0.0170	0.0016
Germany	*1738*		*0.0006*	*0.0035*	*0.0878*	*0.1024*	*0.2157*	*0.2804*	*0.2105*	*0.0848*	*0.0126*	*0.0012*

Table 1   HUMVWA31A system: allele frequencies in Germany; *Germany* pooled by calculating the weighted arithmetical means of the allele frequencies; n = number of examined genomes; Ref. = references: (1) Huckenbeck et al 1996[a], (2) Möller et al. 1994.

Locus HUMTH01

Population	n	Ref.	5	6	7	8	9	9.3/10	11
Düsseldorf	604	(1)	0.0166	0.1722	0.1705	0.1291	0.1639	0.3377	0.0099
NRW	546		0.0092	0.2234	0.1429	0.1044	0.1648	0.3553	0.0000
Münster	220	(2)	0.0020	0.2310	0.1630	0.1120	0.1920	0.2890	0.0100
North Germany	536	(3)	0.0000	0.2180	0.1600	0.1030	0.1720	0.3470	0.0000
Germany	*1906*		*0.0081*	*0.2065*	*0.1588*	*0.1127*	*0.1697*	*0.3397*	*0.0043*

Table 2   HumTH01 system: allele frequencies in Germany; *Germany* calculated by weighted arithmetical means (n=numbers of genomes; Ref=references: (1) Huckenbeck et al 1996[b], (2) Wiegand et al 1993, (3) Berschick et al 1994).

Locus HUMF13B

Population	n	Ref.	6	7	8	9	10	11
Düsseldorf	602	(1)	0.0648	0.0017	0.2691	0.2342	0.4302	0.0000
Münster	524	(2)	0.0878	0.0030	0.2443	0.2557	0.4084	0.0038
Germany	*1126*		*0.0755*	*0.0023*	*0.2576*	*0.2442*	*0.4201*	*0.0018*

Table 3   HumF13B system: allele frequencies in Germany; *Germany* calculated by weighted arithmetical means (n=number of genomes; Ref=references: (1) Huckenbeck et al 1996[c], (2) Serac 1995

Locus HUMFES/FPS

Population	n	Ref.	8	9	10	11	12	13	14
Düsseldorf	600	(1)	0.0033	0.0033	0.2850	0.4667	0.2033	0.0383	0.0000
NorthrhineWestphalia	446		0.0157	0.0000	0.2960	0.3991	0.2242	0.0628	0.0022
Münster	266	(2)	0.0075	0.0075	0.2854	0.4624	0.1842	0.0526	0.0052
Germany	*1312*		*0.0084*	*0.0030*	*0.2888*	*0.4428*	*0.2065*	*0.0495*	*0.0018*

Table 4   HumFES/FPS system: allele frequencies in Germany; *Germany* calculated by weighted arithmetical means (n=genomes; Ref= references:(1) Huckenbeck et al 1996[d] (2) according to Serac (1994).

Locus D1S80

Alleles			14	15	16	17	18	19	20	21	22	23	24	25	26
Population	Ref.	n													
Germany Düsseldorf	(1)	756			0.003	0.005	0.253	0.013	0.024	0.029	0.033	0.017	0.343	0.046	0.012
Germany Bonn	(2)	308			0.003		0.279	0.006	0.042	0.026	0.032	0.010	0.341	0.039	0.010
Germany Northwest	(3)	436			0.002	0.009	0.245	0.002	0.037	0.018	0.035	0.021	0.378	0.052	0.007
Germany	(4)	500			0.006		0.198	0.002	0.028	0.032	0.050	0.018	0.346	0.044	0.030
Germany		*2000*			*0.004*	*0.004*	*0.242*	*0.007*	*0.031*	*0.027*	*0.038*	*0.017*	*0.351*	*0.046*	*0.015*

Alleles			27	28	29	30	31	32	33	34	35	36	37	38	39	40+
Population	Ref.	n														
Germany Düsseldorf	(1)	756	0.005	0.042	0.081	0.012	0.057	0.007	0.005	0.005		0.001	0.007			
Germany Bonn	(2)	308	0.020	0.020	0.055	0.003	0.087	0.010	0.010			0.006				
Germany Northwest	(3)	436	0.007	0.060	0.039	0.007	0.048		0.002	0.009		0.002	0.009		0.002	0.002
Germany	(4)	500	0.006	0.060	0.058	0.010	0.058	0.012	0.004	0.008		0.010	0.016			0.004
Germany		*2000*	*0.008*	*0.047*	*0.062*	*0.009*	*0.060*	*0.007*	*0.005*	*0.006*		*0.004*	*0.009*		*0.004*	*0.001*

Table 5   D1S80 system: allele frequencies in Germany; *Germany* pooled by calculating the weighted arithmetical mean (n=genomes; Ref.=references; allele 40 (includes alleles >40), all numbers of alleles include anodal and cathodal variants; (1) Huckenbeck et al 1996°, (2) Huber & Holtz 1994, (3) Skowasch et al. 1992, (4) Schnee-Griese et al. 1993.

References

Berschick, P., Henke, L., Henke, J., 1994: Analysis of the short tandem repeat polymorphism TC 11 (HUMTH01): allele frequencies and family studies. - Adv. Forens. Haemogent. 5, 469-471; **Huber, P., Holtz, J.**, 1994: Anwendbarkeit der Polymerase Kettenreaktion am D1S80 (pMCT 118) Locus in der forensischen DNA-Analytik. - Arch. f. Kriminol. 194 (1,2), 47-54.: **Huckenbeck, W., Demir, K., Scheil, H.-G., Alt, K.W., Bonte, W.**, 1996: German data on the HUMVWA31 locus. - Anthrop Anz 54/1 (in press); **Huckenbeck, W., Scheil, H.-G., West, S., Kanja, J.,Bonte, W.**, 1996: Northrhine Westphalian data on the locus HumTH01. - Anthrop Anz 54/2 (in press); **Huckenbeck, W., Scheil, H.-G., Kaiser, A., Stancu, V., Bonte, W.**, 1996: Northrhine Westphalian data on the locus F13B. - Anthrop Anz 54/2 (in press); **Huckenbeck, W., Demir, K., Scheil, H.-G., Alt, K.W.,Bonte, W.**, 1996: Düsseldorf Data on the PCR-based locus HumFES/FPS. - Gene Geography (submitted); **Huckenbeck, W., Scheil, H.-G., Stancu, V., Bonte, W.**, 1996: VNTR Locus D1S80: Allele frequencies and genotype distribution in the region of Düsseldorf. Anthrop Anz 54/1 (in press); **Kimpton, C., Fisher, D., Watson, S., Adams, M., Urquhart, A., Lygo, J., Gill, P.**, 1994: Evaluation of an automated DNA profiling system employing multiplex amplification of four tetrameric STR loci. - Int. J. Leg. Med. 106: 302-311; **Krüger, J., Fuhrmann, W., Lichte, K.-H., Steffens, C.**, 1968: Zur Verwendung des Polymorphismus der sauren Erythrocytenphosphatase bei der Vaterschaftsbegutachtung. - Dtsch. Z. Gerichtl. Med. 64, 127-146.; **Möller, A., Meyer, E., Brinkmann, B.**, 1994: Different types of structural variation in STR's: HumFES/FPS, HumVWA and HumD21S11. - Int. J. Leg. Med. 106: 319-323; **Möller, A., Wiegand, P., Grüschow, C., Seuchter, S.A., Baur, M.P., Brinkmann, B.**, 1994: Population data and forensic efficiency values for STR systems Hum VWA, Hum MBP and Hum FABP. - Int. J. Leg. Med. 106, 183-189. **SERAC**, 1994: FK01 (HumTH01) Instruction Manual, Fa. SERAC, Bad Homburg, Germany; **SERAC**, 1994: FK02 (HumVWA) Instruction Manual, Fa. SERAC, Bad Homburg, Germany; **SERAC**, 1994: FK03 (HumFES) Instruction Manual (SERAC, Bad Homburg, Germany); **SERAC**, 1994: FK04 (HumF13B) Instruction Manual, Fa. SERAC, Bad Homburg, Germany; **Skowasch, K., Wiegand, P., Brinkmann, B.**, 1992: pMCT 118 (D1S80): a new allelic ladder and an improved electrophoretic separation lead to the demonstration of 28 alleles. - Int. J. Leg. Med. 105, 165-168; **Wiegand, P., Budowle, B., Rand, S., Brinkmann, B.**, 1993: Forensic validation of the STR systems SE33 and TC11. - Int. J. Leg. Med. 105, 315-320

D1S80 alleles in the Wielkopolska (Poland) population

Jaroszewski J[1], Schütte U[2], Schurenkamp M[2], Krajewski P[3], Kempa J[1], Przybylski Z[1], Rand S[2] ,Depts of Radiobiology,Cell Biology and Forensic Medicine,Medical School in Poznań, Święcickiego 6, Poland[1] Institut für Rechtsmedizin, Westfälische Wilhelms-Universität,Von-Esmarch-Strasse 86, Münster, FRG[2] Institute for Plant Genetics, Polish Academy of Scie3nces, Poznań, Poland[3]

METHODS

Samples of venous blood were taken on EDTA from unrelated blood donots.
DNA was extracted using phenol-chloroform technique.DNA content was estimated by agarose gel electrophoresis by comparison with DNA standard and
adjusted to 1 ng/μl using bidestilled water. Amplification (Rand et al 1992)
of the D1S80 locus was carried out using 1-2 ng template and the primers
described by Budowle et al (1991). Temperature profile: denaturation 95°C,
60 s, extension 72°C, 240 s, annealing 65°C, 60 s, 27 cycles in Triothermoblock (Biometra). Separation of the fragments was accomplished using
discontinuous gel electrophoresis (Allen et al 1989). The amplified alleles
were visualised by silver staining. The allelic ladder consisted of 20 alleles and was run every third electrophoretic lane. The obtained allele frequencies were compared with those for other populations, obtained using
a similar technique (Skowasch et al 1992, Deka et al 1994, Kloosterman et
al 1993, Miścicka-Śliwka et al 1994, Nu En Huang et al 1994, Huber and Holz
1994, Martinez-Jaretta et al 1994, Pawłowski 1995). In the cases where
the results were published in the graph form, counts of alleles of individual types were calculated on the basis of allele frequencies and the total
numbers of analysed alleles. The allele counts were analysed by the correspondence analysis (Greenacre 1984) and by the hierarchical grouping of
populations using the method of group averages, on the basis of the Bhatta-
charyya distances among populations (Mardia, Kent and Bibby,1979). Hardy-
-Weinberg equilibrium in the examined Wielkopolska population was tested
using the allele grouping method (Skowasch et al 1992).

RESULTS

A total of 348 individuals were examined. Like in other populations in Europe the alleles 18 and 24 were most frequent. The allele frequency distribution conformed with expectations of Hardy-Weinberg equilibrium. Almost 7%
alleles involved cathodic or anodic variants of the standards included in
the allelic ladder and the off-ladder variants-similarly to results of Skowasch et al (1992) and those of Kloosterman et al (1993) - were particular-

ly frequent beyond the two main allelic peaks. Out of 696 alleles, 79.6% were observed in heterozygous combination. While distribution of D1S80 alleles was remarkably similar in populations of Europe, differences were noted between distant populations. In correspondence analysis Dogrib Indians and Kachari populations proved clearly distinct from two groups of populations, one including European populations and the other:China, Pehuenche Indians and Samoans. The amount of information about variability of populations represented in the pattern obtained in the coordinate system of first principal axes was equal to 34.40 + 23.08 =57.48% of total variability. Hierarchical grouping distinguished three groups of populations: European populations, China+Pehuenche Indian populations and Samoan populations.

Allele	Frequency	No of alleles
17	0.14%	1
18	21.84%	152
19 n	0.29%	2
20	1.29%	9
21	1.01%	7
22	4.45%	31
23	1.15%	8
24	36.78%	256
25	7.90%	55
26	2.30%	16
27	0.43%	3
28	5.46%	38
29	3.88%	27
30	0.86%	6
31	7.90%	55
32	0.14%	1
33	0.43%	3
35	0.15%	1
36	1.15%	8
37	1.87%	13
41	0.43%	3
41	0.14%	1

DISCUSSION

D1S80 allele frequency distribution in Wielkopolska, Poland has been found to resemble respective distributions in other European populations but to differ from those for geographically more distant populations.

Origin of data: D1S80 allele frequency distributions for Highlanders, New Guinea, Pehguenche Indians, Chile, Dogrib Indians, Canada, American and Western Samoas, Kacharis of North-East India and German Caucasians originate from Deka et al (1994), for population of China ffom Nu En Huang et al (1994), on population from Asturia from Martinez-Jareta et al (1994), for population of Holland from Kloosterman et al (1993), on samples of German population from Bonn from Huber and Holtz (1994) and of Münster from Skowasch et al (1992) on samples of Polish populations in Gdansk from Pawlowski (1995) and in Bydgoszcz from Miścicka-Śliwka (1994).

REFERENCES: Allen RC, Graves G, Budowle B, (1989) Polymerase chain reaction amplification products separated on rehydrable polyacrylamide gels and stained wizth silver. Biotechniques 7:736-744.Budowle B, Chakraborty R ET ALś(1991) Analysis of the variable number of tandem repeat locus D1S80 by the PCR followed by high resolution PAGE. Am.J. Hum.Genetics 48:137-144, Deka R, DeCroo S, Li Jin et al (1994), Population genetic characteristics of the D1S80 locus in seven human populations. Hum.Genet.94:252-258, Greenacre MJ (1984),

Theory and applications of correspondence analysis, Academic
Press, London, Kloosterman AD, Budowle B, DAselaar P (1993),
PCR amplification and detection of the human D1S80VNTR locus.
Int J Leg Med 105:257-264, Mardia KV, Kent JT, Bibby JM (1979),
Multivariate analysis. Academic Press, London. Martinez-Jarreta
B, Almuzara I, et al (1994), AMPFLP analysis in the VNTR locus
D1S80 in Asturias (North-Werst Spain).Acta Med Leg 44:67-69.
Miścicka-Śliwka D, Syroczyńska A et al,(1994),Investigation of
D1S80 VNTR locus in a Polish population, Acta Med Leg 44:72-73.
Nu En Huang, Chakraborty R et al (1994), D1S80 allele frequen-
cies in a Chinese populations. Int J Leg Med 107:118-120. Pawłow-
ski et al (1995), private communication. Rand S, Puers C et al
(1992), Population genetics and forensic efficiency data for
4 AMPFLP´s. Int J Leg Med 104:329-333, Skowasch K, Wiegand P,
Brinkmann B (1992), pMCT118 (D1S80): a new allelic ladder and
an improved electrophoretic separation lead to the demonstration of 28 alleles.Int J Leg Med 105: 165-168.

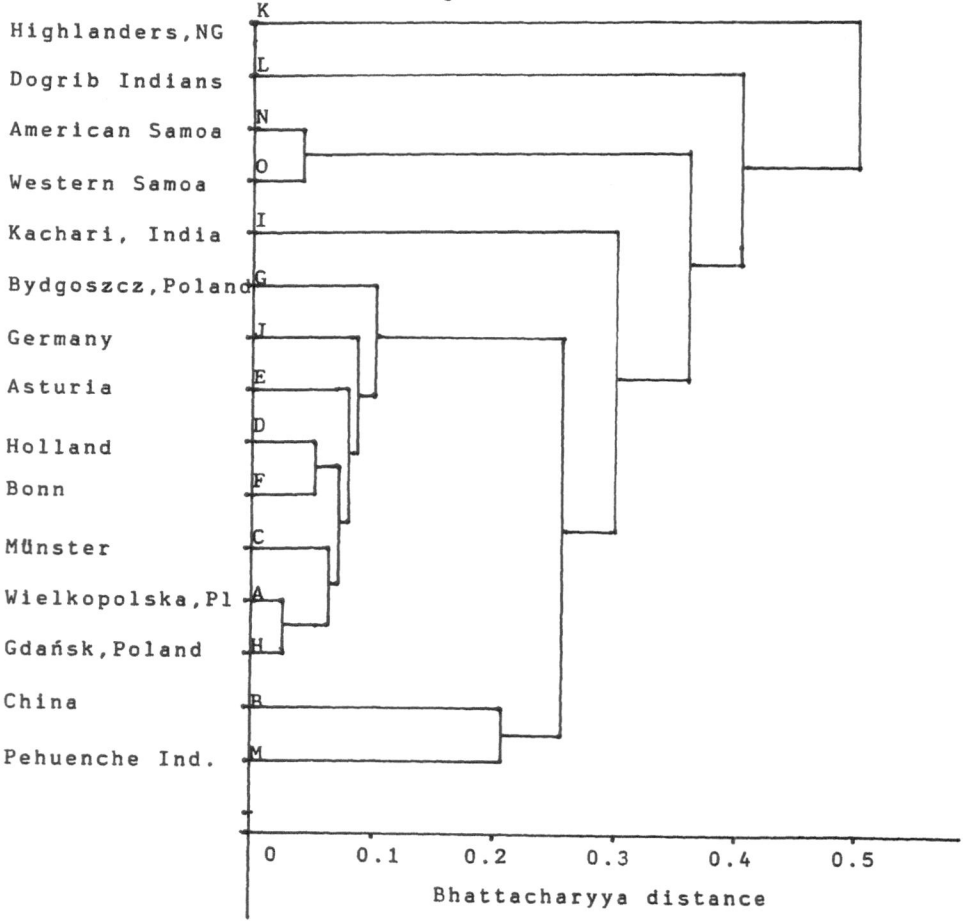

Result of hierarchical groupping of populations
using the method of group averages.

A STUDY ON THE SHORT TANDEM REPEAT SYSTEM ACTBP2 (SE33) IN AN AUSTRIAN POPULATION SAMPLE USING NON-DENATURING ELECTROPHORESIS AND A SEQUENCED ALLELIC LADDER

M. Klintschar, R. Crevenna

Institut für Gerichtliche Medizin, Karl Franzens Universität Graz, Austria

System and locus: SE33 (ACTBP2) (Polymeropoulos et al.1992)

Population and sample size: Austria, 100 individuals.

MATERIALS AND METHODS:

Amplification and electrophoresis were performed according to Wiegand et al 1993. Typing was performed by comparison with a sequenced allelic ladder (Möller and Brinkmann 1994)
As suggested by Rand et al. 1992 the alleles were pooled into 4 groups before testing for Hardy-Weinberg equilibrium using chi^2 tests. The mean exclusion chance (ME) was calculated according to Krüger et al. 1968 and the discriminating power was calculated as 1-S (expected phenotype frequencies)^2 (Fisher 1951).

RESULTS:

A total of 70 genotypes corresponding to 21 alleles (Table 1) were found in the 100 subjects tested. 25 alleles migrated differently from the alleles in the ladder. Accordingly they were assigned the letter "A" if migrating anodal, or "C" if migrating cathodal of the closest allele. The inclusion of these interalleles resulted in a summ of 79 genotypes (Table 2). No significant deviations from Hardy Weinberg deviations were found. The heterocygosity rate was 97%, the mean exclusion chance (ME) was 0.87, and the discriminating power (PD) was 0.98. exclusion chance (ME) was calculated according to Krüger et al. 1968 and the discriminating power was calculated as 1-S (expected phenotype frequencies)2 (Fisher 1951).

Allele	Frequency	Allele	Frequency	Allele	Frequency	Allele	Frequency
12	0,011	18	0,113	24	0,016	29	0,086
13	0,022	19	0,016	25	0,048	30	0,043
14	0,048	20	0,022	26	0,065	31	0,043
15	0,027	21	0,038	27	0,081	32	0,016
16	0,065	22	0,027	28	0,091	33	0,000
17	0,097	23	0,027				

Tab 1. Allele frequencies in percent

Gen.	Obs.	Gen.	Obs.	Gen.	Obs.	Gen.	Obs.
13//17	1	17//18	3	19//28	2	24//31	1
13//20	1	17//19	1	19//28C	1	24A//31A	1
13//24	1	17//21	1	19//28A	1	25//26	1
14//17	1	17//22	1	19//29	4	25A//29A	1
14//17	1	17//23	2	19//30	2	25//29	1
14//19	1	17//28	1	19//30A	2	26//28	1
14//30	1	17//31	2	20//26	1	26//29	1
14//31A	1	17A//32	1	20//27	1	26//31A	1
15//18	2	18//19	2	20//30A	1	27//28C	1
15//19	1	18//22	1	21//27	1	27//29	2
15//27	2	18//26A	1	21//29	2	27//29A	1
15//28	1	18//27	2	22//27	1	28//29	2
15//30A	1	18//28	2	22//29	1	28//30A	1
15//32	1	18//28A	2	22//31	2	29//30A	1
15//33	1	18//29A	1	22//31A	1	30//30	1
16//18	1	18//30	2	23//26	1	30//32	1
16//19	1	18//30A	1	23A//28	1	30//33	1
16//27	1	19//19	1	23A//29	1	31//33	1
16//28	1	19//24	1	23A//30	1	32//32	1
16//32	1	19//26	1	24A//26	1		

Table 2. Observed genotypes

COMMENTS:

Despite-or because-of its outstanding polymorphicity, the STR system ACTBP2 (Se33) is problematic due to difficulties in typing, influence of the electrophoretic setup, or the allelic ladder used. This is confirmed by the fact that, as opposed to several other STRs, no commercial kits are available at the moment. The usage of a sequenced allelic ladder allows a nomenclature corresponding to the number of repeats (Möller and Brinkmann 1994). However, a standardized electrophoretic system would be necessary to allow inter-laboratory controls for such a complicated STR system.

REFERENCES:

Fisher R (1951) Standard calculations for evaluating a blood group system. Heredity 5: 95-102
Krüger J, Fuhrmann W, Lichte KH, Steffens C (1968) Zur Verwendung des Polymorphismus der sauren Erythrocytenphosphatase bei der Vaterschaftsbegutachtung. Dtsch Z Gerichtl Med 64: 127-146
Möller A, Brinkmann B (1994) Locus ACTBP2 (Se33) Sequencing data reveal considerable polymorphism Int J Leg Med 106: 262-267
Polymeropoulos MJ, Rath DS, Xiao H, Merril CR (1992) Tetranucleotide repeat polymorphism at the human beta-actin related pseudogene H-beta-Ac-psi-2 (ACTBP2). Nucleic Acids Res 20: 1432
Rand S, Puers C, Skowasch K, Wiegand P, Budowle B, Brinkmann B (1992) Population genetics and forensic efficiency data of 4 AMPFLΩs. Int J Leg Med 104: 329-333
Wiegand P, Budowle B, Rand S, Brinkmann B (1993) Forensic validation of the STR systems SE33 and TC11 Int J Legal Med 105:315-320

HLADQA1 ALLELE-FREQUENCIES IN THE WORLD USING A BIPLOT TO VISUALISE ALLELES AND POPULATIONS SIMULTANEOUSLY

A.D. Kloosterman[*], M. Sjerps[*], D. Eerhart[*] and N. Dimo[**]

Gerechtelijk Laboratorium, Ministerie van Justitie, Rijswijk, NL[*]
Institute Med Légale, Université de Lausannne, Switzerland[**]

INTRODUCTION

Population genetic studies show differences within and between racial groups for the HLADQA1 locus[1][2]. The chi-square test is a relatively simple test which is often used when comparing population samples. However, when a large number of samples are compared, it is difficult to get a clearly structured overall picture. A quick overview of the distances between populations and deviant allele frequencies can be obtained from a so-called biplot [3]. This type of plot is related to principal components analysis and has many variants, which are increasingly used in anthropometric and genetic analyses Using the biplot graphic display we analysed the HLADQA1 allele-frequency data of 31 population samples [4][5][6][7][8][9][10][11][12][13][14][15][16][17][18][19].

STATISTICAL METHODS

Table 1 gives the overview of the 31 populations that were compared. A biplot [1] is used to visualise the allele frequency data table which consists of rows (populations) and columns (alleles). The type of plot we use is obtained from relative allele frequencies by subtracting column means and scaling of row factors with the singular values. The data analysis was performed using the software Spectramap[20]. The biplots are interpreted in the following way. Alleles are represented by squares, and populations by circles. Populations that are close together in the plot have similar allelic compositions, in contrast to populations that are far apart. The population frequencies of any allele a can be compared by perpendicular projection of the populations on a line drawn through allele "a" and the origin (Fig.1). The horizontal and vertical direction in the biplot each account for a certain fraction of the total information (e.g., the total variance of the allele frequencies). These fractions are reported in the figure legend

RESULTS

In the biplot of all examined populations (Fig.1), the Caucasians appear a relatively homogeneous group, and so do the Black populations. The Asian populations are scattered over the plot, indicating heterogeneity. By perpendicular projection of the population points on the axis drawn through the centre of the plot (+) and allele 3, it can be seen that the Japanese sample shows an exceptionally high frequency for this allele, whereas the Indonesian sample scores very low. Other differences can be detected in a similar way.

SPECTRAMAP

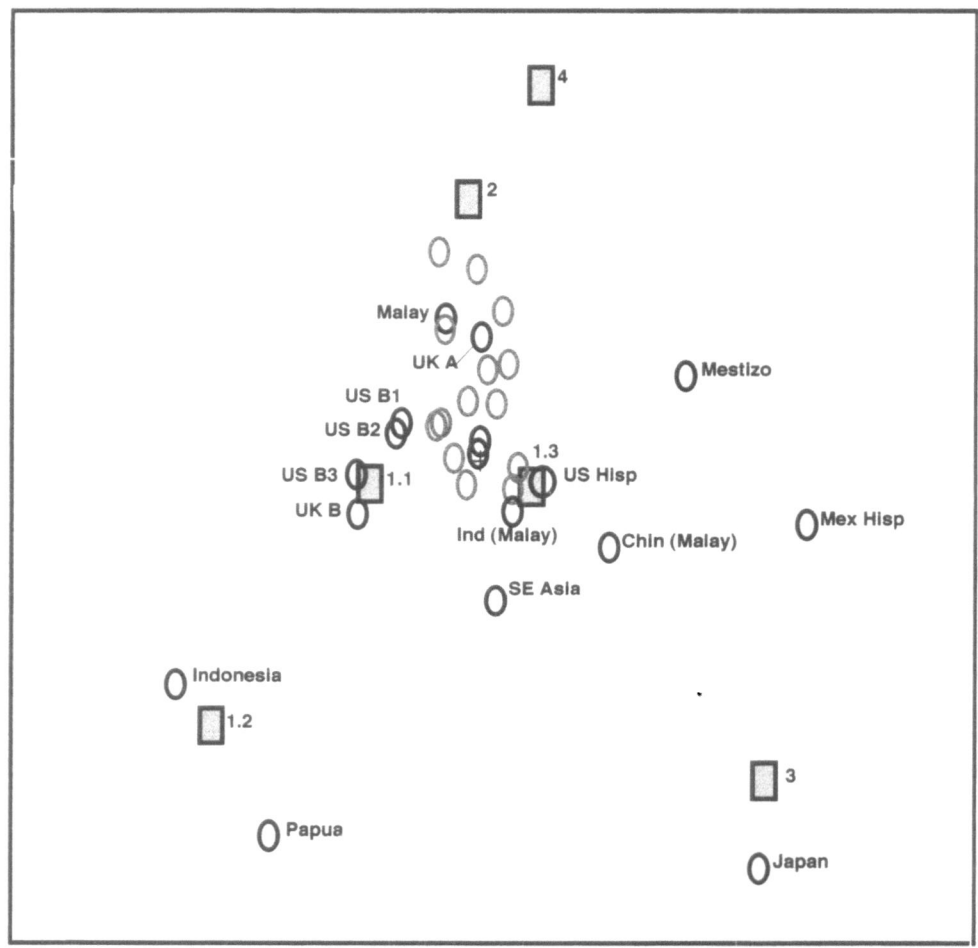

Fig 1 Biplot of the HLADQA1-locus for all populations investigated (abbreviations as in Table 1). The biplot graphic display accounts for 73% of the total variance (horizontal and vertical direction 46% and 27% resp).
The Caucasian-population samples which appear a relatively homogeneous group are given by grey circles and not further specified.

CONCLUSIONS

The biplot allows a quick overview of similarities and differences between the allele frequency distributions when many samples are analysed. A nice feature of the plot is that it visualises both alleles and populations in the same plot. It should be noted, however, that some of the information is lost because the biplot reduces a high dimensional space to only two dimensions. Nevertheless, the biplots in this paper reproduce 73% of the total variation, hence most of the information is retained.

Table 1 Overview of the analysed population-samples

Country	Racial group	N ind	Ref	Biplot code	Country	Racial group	N ind	Ref
US	Black	224	1	US B1	US	Cauc	413	1
US	Black	172	1	US B2	Italy	Cauc	103	18
Marion US	Black	203	8	US B3	Lisboa Port	Cauc	106	5
UK	Asian	191	11	UK A	Porto Port	Cauc	325	6
Japan	Asian	92	1	Japan	Andalusia Sp.	Cauc	174	7
Mexico	Mestizo	100	1	Mestizo	Marion US	Cauc	185	8
Mexico	Hispanic	169	1	Mex. Hisp	US	Cauc	174	1
US	Hispanic	146	1	US Hisp	Bavaria Ger.	Cauc	213	9
SE Asia	Asian	87	1	SE Asia	S-W Swit	Cauc	237	19
Indonesia	Asian	144	1	Indonesia	NL	Cauc	157	15
NW Guinea	Papua	134	1	Papua	Germany	Cauc	212	10
Malaysia	Asian Malay	130	17	Malay	Finland	Cauc	112	12
Malaysia	Asian Chinese	125	17	Chin (Malay)	Australia	Cauc	280	16
Malaysia	Asian Indian	137	17	Ind (Malay)	Switzerland	Cauc	200	13
UK	Black	202	11	UK B	Spain	Cauc	120	14
					UK	Cauc	201	11

REFERENCES

1 R. Helmuth et al (1990); HLADQA1 allele and genotype frequencies in various human populations; Am J Hum Genet 47:515-523
2 A Piazza A et al (1980); The HLA-A,B gene frequencies in the world: migration or selection? Hum Immunol 1:297-304
3 Gabriel KR (1971) The biplot graphic display of matrices with applications to principal components analysis. Biometrika 58: 453-467
4 Cavalli-Sforza LL, Menozzi P, Piazza A (1994). The history and geography of human genes. Princeton University Press, New Jersey.
5 R Espinheira et al; Adv For Haemogen 5:499-501
6 MF Pinheiro et al; Adv For Haemogen 5:559-561
7 P Sanz et al. Adv For Haemogen 5:572-574
8 MA Tahir et al; Adv For Haemogen 5:596-598
9 GM Weichold et al; Adv For Haemogen 5:599-602
10 PM Schneider et al (1991); Arch Krimino 188:167-174
11 KM Sullivan et al (1992; Int J Leg Med 105:17-20
12 A Sajantila et al (1991); Int J Leg Med 104:181-184
13 MN Hochmeister et al The application of PCR to forensic science. Birkhauer Verlag, Basel
14 JA Lorente et al (1992); Proceedings Promega Int Symp Human Identification
15 AD Kloosterman et al (1993); Int J Leg Med 105:233-238
16 CS Harrington et al (1991); Forensic Sc Int 51:147-157
17 Chong-Lek Koh et al (1994); Hum Hered 44:150-155
18 A. Tagliabracci et al (1992); Int J Leg Med 105:161-164
19 N. Dimo (1995), personal communication
20 Smit Consult, Drunen, The Netherlands; Spectramap for biplot analysis

EFFICIENCY OF 6 STR SYSTEMS, HLADQα AND THE POLYMARKER SYSTEMS (PM) IN PATERNITY TESTING

Kratzer A. and Bär W.

Institute of Legal Medicine, University of Zürich, Winterthurerstr.190, CH-8057 Zürich, Switzerland

Introduction

In order to test the efficiency of PCR based DNA systems in paternity testing the following 12 systems were selected: the 6 STR systems SE33, D21S11, HUMTHO1, HUMVWA, HUMF13A1 and HUMFES, HLADQα and the 5 Polymarker systems (PM) LDLR, GYPA, HBGG, D7S8 and GC. This study presents the results of 47 cases of disputed paternity (26 nonexclusion and 21 exclusion cases) which were examined with the 12 PCR systems. The results were compared with the efficiency of the 4 single locus VNTR systems MS43A, MS31, G3 and yNH24 routinely used in paternity cases since 1991.

Methods

a) STR-Systems:

Primers: SE 33 (Polymeropoulos et al. 1992), D21S11 (Sharma and Litt 1991), HUMTHO1 (Edwards et al. 1991), HUMVWA (Kimpton et al. 1992), HUMF13A1 (Polymeropoulos et al. 1991), HUMFES (Polymeropoulos et al. 1991).

Amplification conditions (Thermocycler: Biometra Triothermoblock):
SE33 and HUMTHO1: 94°C - 45 sec., 60°C - 30 sec., 72°C - 30 sec; 30 cycles.
D21S11, HUMVWA, HUMF13A1, HUMFES: 94°C - 45 sec., 55°C - 30 sec., 72°C - 30 sec.; 30 cycles.

Analysis and fluorescent detection: The PCR-products were analyzed and detected on an ABI 373A automated DNA sequencer (ABI GeneScan 672). The electrophoresis was carried out on 6 % denaturing polyacrylamide gels according to the ABI protocol (running conditions: 1600 V, 24mA,7-8hs). Allele designations were determined by comparison with an allelic ladder.

b) HLA DQ α and PM Systems:

Amplification and typing reactions were performed according to the Cetus Protocol (HLA DQα Forensic DNA Amplification & Typing Kit, AmpliType PM PCR Amplification and Typing Kit).

c) RFLP:

Paternity investigations using the four single locus probes MS43A, MS31, G3 and yNH24 has been published previously (Bär and Kratzer 1992).

Results

1. Nonexclusions

26 cases were analysed. The biostatistical evaluation of a nonexclusion was performed according to Essen-Möller (1938). Table 1 shows the calculated W-values using different sets of combinations of PCR based systems in comparison to 4 SLPs. The results demonstrate that all 12 investigated PCR systems are usually necessary to reach a conclusive probability of above 99.8 % in all cases, whereas DNA analysis with 4 single locus systems led to W-values of above 99.8 % in all cases.

The average contribution of each system is expressed in the average EM-value which is shown in table 2 and 3. The results show that the STR system SE33 is comparable with any of the single locus system.

Table 1:
W-Values resulting after applying different test batteries of VNTRs in 26 cases

W-Value	4 STRs* PM, DQα	6 STRs*	6 STRs* PM, DQα	4 SLP
< 99.8 %	15	3	0	0
≥ 99.8 %	11	23	26	26

*4 STRs: THO1, VWA, F13A1, FES
*6 STRs: SE33, D21S11, THO1, VWA, F13A1, FES

Table 2: Average EM-Values of 12 PCR systems (N = no of cases)

System	SE33	D21S11	THO1	VWA	F13A1	FES	DQα	PM
EM	8.055	9.3085	9.5775	9.5468	9.4116	9.6734	9.5520	9.3694
N	27	27	27	28	28	28	37	27

Table 3: Average EM-Values of the single locus systems (N = no of cases)

System	MS43A	MS31	G3	yNH24
EM	9.0101	8.9869	8.9175	9.1044
N	105	105	104	104

2. Exclusions

21 exclusion cases were analysed with the above described 12 PCR systems. Table 4 and 5 show the results of the exclusion efficiency in comparison with the single locus systems. The power of exclusion differs considerably and does not reach the high efficiency of any single locus systems.The highest value was observed for the STR system SE33. Multiple exclusions (3 and more exclusions per case) were only obtained using all 12 PCR systems whereas DNA analysis with 4 single locus probes always led to multiple exclusions (≥ 3).

Table 4: Average power of exclusion (PE)

PCR	SE33	D21S11	THO1	VWA	F13A1	FES	DQa	PM
PE	79%	62.5%	71%	57%	52%	43%	53%	61%

SLP	MS43A	MS31	G3	yNH24
PE	90%	95%	89%	96%

Table 5: Number of exclusions (Excl.) per case (N = 21)

Systems	no Excl.	1 Excl.	2 Excl.	3 Excl.	≥ 4 Excl.
PM	9	10	2	0	0
PM+DQα	2	12	6	1	0
6 STR's	0	1	3	5	12
6 STR's,PM,DQα	0	0	0	4	17
4 SLP	0	0	0	1	20

Discussion

With the exception of the STR system SE33 all PCR systems studied have a considerable smaller efficiency than each of the 4 single locus VNTR systems. SE33 is comparable with a single locus VNTR system. For paternity testing at least 12 PCR systems must be applied to obtain a comparable efficiency as with a battery of the 4 single locus VNTR systems.

The PCR systems are useful and reliable marker systems for paternity testing with many advantages: e.g. discrete alleles, high sensivity and the technique is rapid and less expensive. However only a considerable number of PCR systems are capable to match the high efficiency of the polymorphic single locus systems. In a intermediate phase combinations of SLP and PCR systems are useful.

Acknowledgments: The authors thank B. Blattmann and M. Stadler for excellent technical assistance.

References:

1. Bär W and Kratzer A (1992): Paternity investigations based on DNA analysis only. In: Advances in Forensic Haemogenetics 4, Springer Verlag Berlin Heidelberg 1992, pp. 123-125

2. Edwards A, Civitello A, Hammond HA, Caskey CT (1991): DNA typing and genetic mapping with trimeric and tetrameric tandem repeats. Am J Hum Genet 49: 746 - 756

3. Essen-Möller E (1938): Die Beweiskraft der Aehnlichkeit im Vaterschaftsnachweis. Theoretische Grundlagen. Mitteil Anthropol Gesell Wien 68: 9-53

4. Kimpton CP, Walton A, Gill P (1992): A further tetranucleotide repeat polymorphism in the vWF gene. Hum Mol Gen 1: 287

5. Polymeropoulos MH, Rath DS, Xiao H, Merril CR (1991): Tetranucleotide repeat polymorphism at the human coagulation factor XIII A subunit gene (F13A1). Nucleic Acids Res 19: 4036

6. Polymeropoulos MH, Rath DS, Xiao H, Merril CR (1991): Tetranucleotide repeat polymorphism at the human c-fes/fps proto-oncogene (FES). Nucleic Acids Res 19, 4018

7. Polymeropoulos MH, Rath DS, Xiao H, Merril CR (1992): Tetranucleotide repeat polymorphism at the human beta-actin related pseudogene H-beta-Ac-psi-2 (ACTBP2). Nucleic Acids Res 20, 1432

8. Sharma V and Litt M (1991): Tetranucleotide repeat polymorphism at the D21S11 locus. Human Molecular Genetics 1, 67

SWISS POPULATION DATA FOR THE STR SYSTEMS HUMVWA HUMF13A1 AND HUMFES

Kratzer A. and Bär W.

Institute of Legal Medicine, University of Zürich,
Winterthurerstr.190, CH-8057 Zürich, Switzerland

Systems and loci: HUMVWA (12p12-12pter), HUMF13A1 (6p25-p24) and HUMFES (15q25-qter).

Population and sample size: Swiss population sample, N = 386 for HUMVWA, N = 425 for HUMF13A1 and N = 370 for HUMFES.

Methods:

HUMVWA Primers (Kimpton et al. 1992), HUMF13A1 Primers (Polymeropoulos et al. 1991), HUMFES Primers (Polymeropoulos et al. 1991).

Amplification conditions (Thermocycler: Biometra Triothermoblock):
94°C - 45 sec., 55°C - 30 sec., 72°C - 30 sec.; 30 cycles. HUMVWA and HUMF13A1 were coamplified.

Analysis and fluorescent detection: The PCR-products were analyzed and detected on an ABI 373A automated DNA sequencer (ABI GeneScan 672). The electrophoresis was carried out on 6 % denaturing polyacrylamide gels according to the ABI protocol (running conditions: 1600 V, 24mA, 8hs). Allele designations were determined by comparison with an allelic ladder.

HWE-Analysis: The Hardy-Weinberg equilibrium hypothesis was tested using the software HWEANA17.EXE (HWE-Analysis, Version 3.0) developed and refined by Puers (1994/95).

Results:

HUMVWA: Observed genotypes

Gen.	Obs.	Gen.	Obs.	Gen.	Obs.	Gen.	Obs.
13-14	1	15-15	1	16-18	36	18-19	18
14-14	3	15-16	17	16-19	11	18-20	2
14-15	6	15-17	16	16-20	1	19-19	3
14-16	16	15-18	18	17-17	21	19-20	4
14-17	21	15-19	4	17-18	48	19-21	1
14-18	13	15-20	2	17-19	26		
14-19	2	16-16	16	17-20	2		
14-20	1	16-17	57	18-18	19		

HUMVWA: Allele frequencies

Allele	Frequency	Allele	Frequency	Allele	Frequency
13	0.001	16	0.220	19	0.093
14	0.085	17	0.275	20	0.016
15	0.084	18	0.224	21	0.001

HUMF13A1: Observed genotypes

Gen.	Obs.	Gen.	Obs.	Gen.	Obs.	Gen.	Obs.
3-3	2	4-7	7	5-15	4	6-19	1
3-4	2	4-8	1	5-16	3	7-7	48
3-5	13	4-12	1	6-6	44	7-13	1
3-6	19	4-14	1	6-7	91	7-15	7
3-7	27	4-15	1	6-8	1	7-16	4
3-15	3	5-5	8	6-12	1	15-15	1
3-16	2	5-6	48	6-13	1	15-17	1
4-4	1	5-7	57	6-14	2		
4-5	5	5-12	1	6-15	4		
4-6	9	5-13	1	6-16	2		

HUMF13A1: Allele frequencies

Allele	Frequency	Allele	Frequency	Allele	Frequency
3	0.082	8	0.002	16	0.013
4	0.034	12	0.004	17	0.001
5	0.174	13	0.004	19	0.001
6	0.314	14	0.004		
7	0.341	15	0.026		

HUMFES: Observed genotypes

Gen.	Obs.	Gen.	Obs.	Gen.	Obs.	Gen.	Obs.
8-9	1	9-11	1	10-13	9	12-13	6
8-10	1	9-12	1	11-11	53	12-14	1
8-11	7	10-10	35	11-12	66		
8-12	1	10-11	103	11-13	9		
9-10	1	10-12	59	12-12	16		

HUMFES: Allele frequencies

Allele	Frequency	Allele	Frequency	Allele	Frequency
8	0.014	11	0.396	14	0.001
9	0.005	12	0.224		
10	0.327	13	0.032		

Forensic efficiency

	VWA	F13A1	FES
Mean paternity exclusion chance (MEC)	0.6117	0.5223	0.4165
Mean exclusion probability (MEP)	0.6057	0.5041	0.4066
Polymorphism information content (PIC)	0.7743	0.7054	0.6240
Probability of match (pM)	0.0730	0.1091	0.1679
Discrimination power (D)	0.9271	0.8909	0.8321

Comments:

A Swiss population database has been established for the 3 PCR based STR loci HUMVWA, HUMF13A1 and HUMFES. For all 3 systems the Hardy-Weinberg equilibrium was tested using the HWE-Analysis computer programm of Puers (1994/95) which performs the following HWE-analyses: the exact test, chi-square and logarithmic likelihood ratio test, test of HWE hypothesis by comparison of the observed heterozygosity/homozygosity with the unbiased estimate of the expected heterozygosity/homozygosity, the Random-shuffling-exact-, the chi-square- and G-Test. All 3 loci showed no significant deviations from assumed Hardy-Weinberg equilibria.

The distributions of allele frequencies in the Swiss population sample are similiar to those observed in other Caucasians, e.g. in Germany (Möller et al. 1994), in Italy (Buscemi et al.1995), in the UK (Kimpton et al. 1993) and in France (Pfitzinger et al. 1995).

The 3 investigated polymorphic STR systems HUMVWA, HUMF13A1 and HUMFES are reliable and sensitive marker systems that are well suited for use in forensic casework.

Acknowledgments: The authors thank M. Stadler for excellent technical assistance.

References:
1. Buscemi L, Cucurachi N, Mencarelli R, Tagliabracci A, Wiegand P, Ferrara SD (1995): PCR analysis of the short tandem repeat (STR) system HUMVWA31. Allele and genotype frequencies in an Italian population sample. Int J Leg Med 107: 171-173

2. Kimpton CP, Walton A, Gill P (1992): A further tetranucleotide repeat polymorphism in the vWF gene. Hum Mol Gen 1: 287

3. Kimpton CP, Gill P, Walton A, Urquhart A, Millican ES, Adams M (1993): Automated DNA profiling employing multiplex amplification of short tandem repeat loci. PCR Methods and Applications 3: 13-22

4. Möller A, Wiegand P, Grüschow C, Seuchter SA, Baur MP, Brinkmann B (1994): Population data and forensic efficiency values for the STR systems HumVWA, HumMBP and HumFABP. Int J Leg Med 106: 183-189

5. Pfitzinger H, Rousselet F, Mangin P (1995): French experience in STR systems: Caucasian Population data bases, automated fluorescent quadruplex typing and forensic applications for HUMFESFPS, HUMTHO1, HUMVWA31/A and HUMF13A1 Loci. In: Proceedings from the Fifth International Symposium on Human Identification 1994. Promega Corporation, Madison, USA, pp85-94

6. Polymeropoulos MH, Rath DS, Xiao H, Merril CR (1991): Tetranucleotide repeat polymorphism at the human coagulation factor XIII A subunit gene (F13A1). Nucleic Acids Res 19: 4036

7. Polymeropoulos MH, Rath DS, Xiao H, Merril CR (1991): Tetranucleotide repeat polymorphism at the human c-fes/fps proto-oncogene (FES). Nucleic Acids Res 19, 4018

8. Puers C (1994/95): Manual for the software HWE-Analysis, Version 3.1, Institute of Legal Medicine, University of Münster, Germany, copyright 1994/95

STUDIES ON THE HUMTH01 AND HUMVWA POLYMORPHISMS IN A SOUTH WEST GERMAN POPULATION

K. Leim, S. Degenhartt, W. Reichert, R. Mattern

Institut of Legal Medicine, Heidelberg University, Germany

System and locus: HUMTH01 (11p15.5-p15)

Population and sample size: South West Germany. N = 305

Methods:

DNA was extracted from EDTA-blood using 5 % Chelex 100 [1]

Primers: 5' GTG GGC TGA AAA GCT CCC GAT TAT 3'
             5' GTG ATT CCC ATT GGC CTG TTC CTC 3' [2]

PCR amplification conditions: The amplification mix contained 10-30 ng template DNA, 1 U Taq-polymerase (Pharmacia), 5 µl 10 x buffer (Pharmacia), 0,2 mM dNTP mix (Pharmacia), 0,25 µM of each primer (Biometra), 0,16 µg/µl BSA (Boehringer) and was diluted to a final volume of 50 µl with distilled water. The reaction mixture was overlayed with 20 µl mineral oil.

After a first denaturation for 5 min at 94°C a total of 30 cycles for 45 sec at 94°C, 30 sec at 60°C, 30 sec at 72°C was carried out, followed by a last extension for 7 min at 72°C (Thermocycler: Biometra TRIO-Thermoblock)

Electrophoretic methods: Electrophoretical separation of the PCR products was performed in polyacrylamid gels (7,2% T, 3% C, 750 µm thick, horizontal) with piperazin diacrylamid as cross-linker using a discontinuos buffer system [4]. Gels were run at
1000 V, 40 mA,   5 W for 90 min
1000 V, 40 mA, 10 W for 60 min
1000 V, 40 mA, 15 W until the bromphenol blue front had reached the anode. The seperationdistance was 20 cm. Gels were silver stained using a standard protocol [5].
The allels were typed by side to side comparison with an allele ladder (Serac), composed of the allels 5,6,7,8,9,9.3 and 10.

Results:

Observed genotypes

Gen.	Obs.	Gen.	Obs.	Gen.	Obs.	Gen.	Obs.
5-5	0	6-6	13	7-8	12	8-10	1
5-6	3	6-7	16	7-9	15	9-9	13
5-7	0	6-8	14	7-9.3	36	9-9.3	38
5-8	0	6-9	22	7-10	4	9-10	2
5-9	0	6-9.3	47	8-8	2	9.3-9.3	21
5-9.3	0	6-10	2	8-9	11	9.3-10	2
5-10	0	7-7	9	8-9.3	21	10-10	1

Chi-square = 8.22, d.f. = 14, $0.70 < p < 0.90$
Cells with expected values of less than five were calculated together

Allele frequencies

Allele	Frequency	Allele	Frequency
5	0.0049	9	0.1869
6	0.2131	9.3	0.3049
7	0.1656	10	0.0213
8	0.1033		

System and locus: HUMVWA (12p12-12pter)

Population and sample size: South West Germany. N = 206

Methods:

Primers: 5' CCC TAG TGG ATG ATA AGA ATA ATC AGT ATG 3'
             5' GGA CAG ATG ATA AAT ACA TAG GAT GGA TGG 3' [3]

PCR amplifation conditions were the same as for HUMTH01 with the exception that a total of 35 cycles was carried out.

Electrophoretic methods were identical with that of HUMTH01.

Typing was performed by side to side comparison with an allele ladder (Serac), composed of the alleles 13 - 21.

Results:
Observed genotypes

Gen.	Obs.	Gen.	Obs.	Gen.	Obs.	Gen.	Obs.
13-13	0	14-15	11	15-18	5	17-18	24
13-14	0	14-16	6	15-19	4	17-19	6
13-15	0	14-17	16	15-20	0	17-20	2
13-16	0	14-18	9	16-16	9	18-18	10
13-17	2	14-19	0	16-17	26	18-19	9
13-18	0	14-20	0	16-18	24	18-20	1
13-19	0	15-15	0	16-19	13	19-19	0
13-20	0	15-16	8	16-20	1	19-20	1
14-14	2	15-17	10	17-17	7	20-20	0

Chi-square = 13.78, d.f. = 15, 0.50 < p < 0.70
Cells with expected values of less than five were calculated together

Allele frequencies

Allele	Frequency	Allele	Frequency
13	0.0049	17	0.2427
14	0.1117	18	0.2233
15	0.0922	19	0.0801
16	0.2330	20	0.0121

Comments:

The oberved HUMTH01 and HUMVWA genotype frequencies are in a good agreement with the expected distribution under the Hardy-Weinberg law. Heterozygosity : HUMTH01 80.6% (81.73 expected), HUMVWA 86.4% (83.21% expected). Discrimination power: HUMTH01 72.5%, HUMVWA 75.5%.
With the nondenaturating polyacralamid gels used in our experiments a clear-cut decision between allele HUMTH01 9.3 and 10 could not be made on each gel. A small sample of 40 true family trios showed for both systems normal segregation with no examples of mutation or non-Mendelian inheritance.

References:

[1] Walsh P S, Metzger D A, Higuchi R, Bio Tech 1991; 10: 506-513
[2] Gill P, Kimpton C, D'Aloja E, Andersen J F, Bär W, Brinkmann B, Holgersson S, Johnsson V, Kloostermann A D, Lareu M V, Nellemann L, Pfitzinger H, Phillips C P, Schneider P M, Stenersen M, Forensic Sci Int 1994; 65: 51-59
[3] Kimpton C, Walton A, Gill P, Hum Molecular Genet 1992; 1: 287
[4] Budowle B, Chakraborty R, Giusti A M, Esenberg A J, Allan R C, Am J Hum Genet 1991; 48: 137-144
[5] Allen RC, Graves G, Budowle B, Bio Tech; 7: 736-744
[6] Nei M, Roychoudhury A K, Genetics 1974; 76: 379-390

SPANISH POPULATION DATA ON SEVEN LOCI (D1S80, D17S5, HUMTH01, HUMVWA, ACTBP2, D21S11 and DQA1): EQUILIBRIUM AND INDEPENDENCE

M. Lorente[1], J.A. Lorente[1], J.C. Alvarez[1], B. Budowle[2] &
E. Villanueva[2]

[1] University of Granada, Dept. of Forensic Medicine, Granada, Spain

[2] FSRTC - Research Unit. Laboratory Division. FBI Academy, Quantico, Va, USA.

INTRODUCTION

Amplification by the Polymerase Chain Reaction (PCR) and subsequent electrophoresis of the amplified products have become a useful approach for typing variable number of tandem repeats (VNTR) loci. Currently there is an increasingly number of data on VNTR and especially on the STR loci (i.e., Edwards et al, 1992), regarding their allele frequencies and genotype distribution in various population.

For the genetics markers, such as VNTRs & STRs, in identity testing, it is desirable to collect allele/genotype data from relevant populations, so that the forensic scientist can provide a guideline to estimate of the rarity of a genetic profile.

MATERIALS AND METHODS

Population: 120 unrelated Spanish Caucasians from Andalucia (South of Spain)
Statistical tests:
1. Hardy-Weinberg equilibrium:
1.1. Goodness-of-fit chi-square test, based on the total number of homozygotes and heterozygotes
1.2. Likelihood ratio test, comparing the frequencies of each specific genotype with their expectations under the Hardy-Weinberg assumptions.
1.3. Guo-Thompson's exact test, 1000 replications.
2. Gametic phase equilibrium:
2.1. Interclass correlation test (Karlin et al, 1991)
2.2. Test of the observed variance (Sk^2) of the number of heterozygotes classes.

RESULTS AND DISCUSSION

Interclass correlation test (Karlin et al, 1981)

	RHO	P
D1S80-HUMTH01	0.045760	0.323
D1S80-D17S5	-0.214510	0.644
D1S80-ACTBP2	-0.037771	0.436
D1S80-HUMVWA	-0.023085	0.605
D1S80-D21S11	0.011053	0.786
HUMTH01-D21S11	-0.029091	0.527
HUMTH01-ACTBP2:	-0.040358	0.363

Interclass correlation test (continuation)

HUMTH01-VWA:	-0.012521	0.784
HUMTH01-D17S5:	0.014939	0.764
D17S5-D21S11:	0.025888	0.558
D17S5-ACTBP2:	-0.183110	0.704
D17S5-HUMVWA:	-0.051937	0.256
DQA1-D1S80:	-0.022010	0.615
DQA1-D17S5:	-0.017704	0.692
DQA1-D21S11:	0.010995	0.835
DQA1-ACTBP2:	-0.002433	0.958
DQA1-HUMTH01:	-0.014330	0.753
DQA1-HUMVWA:	0.007176	0.881
ACTBP2-HUMVWA:	0.061216	0.183
ACTBP2-VWA:	0.061216	0.183
ACTBP2-D21S11:	-0.008573	0.856
HUMVWA-D21S11:	-0.005315	0.906

Results of tests used for Hardy-Weinberg equilibrium

	Chi-square	Likelihood	Guo-Thompson
HUMTH01	0.225	0.097	0.070
HUMVWA	0.005	0.434	0.349
ACTBP2	0.017	0.840	0.008
D21S11	0.547	0.008	0.115
HLA-DQA1	0.554	0.458	0.597
D1S80	0.708	0.999	0.508
D17S5	0.249	0.394	0.352

Parameters of Forensic interest:

	Discrim.Pow.	# combinat.	Pater. Ind.
HUMTH01	0.9333	2380	74.28%
HUMVWA	0.9415	1281	75.03%
ACTBP2	0.9928	279577	90.48%
D21S11	0.9307	4068	74.47%
HLA-DQA1	0.9343	1281	74.46%
D1S80	0.9208	83385	79.44%
D17S5	0.9676	4068	82.89%
Total	0.999999	-	99.90

According to these results, all but one loci (ACTBP2) are in equilibrium and independent in all cases. A test for independence for ACTBP2 can be problematic because of the allele designation strategy studied. The even numbered alleles generally represent discrete data, while the odd numbered alleles are drived from binned data.

Classical tests are more prone to be affected by the sample characteristics. In this study, chi-square test is significative for the HUMVWA locus because the ratio homozygotes/heterozygotes is higher than expected. Nevertheless, both the likelihood ratio test amd the Guo-Thompson's one are not significative. Therefore, we strongly recommend to use more than one test to check the Hardy-Weinberg equilibrium and the gametic phase equilibrium.

In conclussion, these seven loci are useful for identity testing in criminalistic and paternity cases.

REFERENCES

Chakraborty R, Fornage M, Guegue R. Boerwinkle E (1991) Population genetics of hypervariable loci: analysis of PCR-based VNTR polymorphism within a population. In: T. Burke, G. Dolf, A.J. Jeffreys, and R. Wolff (eds.), DNA fingerprinting: approaches and applicatios, Birkhauser Verlag, Berlin, pp. 127-143

Edwards A, Hammond H, Jin L, Caskey CT, Chakraborty R (1992) Genetic variation at five trimeric and tetrameric loci in four human population groups. Genomics 12: 241-253

Guo SW, Thompson EA (1992) Performing the exact test of Hardy-Weinberg proportion for multiple alleles. Biometrics 48: 361-372

Karlin S, Cameron EC, Williams PT (1981) Sibling and parent-offspring correlation estimation with variable family size. Proc. Natl. Acad. Sci. U.S.A. 78: 2664-2668

Nei M, Roychoudhury AK (1974) Sampling variances of heterozygosity and genetic distance. Genetics 76: 379-390

Nei M (1978) Estimation of average and genetic distance from a small number of individuals. Genetics 89: 583-590

Weir BS (1992) Independence of VNTR alleles defined by fixed bins. Genetics 130: 873-887

This work was supported by a grant of the Spanish Ministry of Education and Science (DGICYT) PB93-1155

TWO HIGHLY POLYMORPHIC VNTR LOCI D5S110 (LH1) AND D4S139 (PH30): ANALYSIS, FORMAL AND POPULATION GENETIC DATA.

C. Luckenbach*, A. Luckenbach*,V. Almeida**, M. Mainka*, J. Jung*, H. Ritter*

* Inst. f. Anthroplogie und Humangenetik, Wilhelmstr. 27, 72074 Tübingen, FRG
**Inst. Anthropologia, Universidade Porto, 4000 Porto, Portugal

Summary
The experimental technique is described that enable RFLP typing with the two hypervariable VNTR loci D5S110 (LH1) and D4S139 (pH30). Population and formal genetic studies were performed using HaeIII restricted DNA from 450 unrelated individuals (SW-Germany) and 35 families with 172 children (NW-Portugal). Both loci reveal more than 70 alleles ranging between 0.8 kb and 9.5 kb at D5S110 (LH1) and between 1.5 kb and 19.5 kb at D4S139 (pH30). In 172 meioses analysed, one recombination event was observed at the D4S139 locus (recombination frequency of 0.0058) and none at the locus D5S110. Allele frequency distributions were determined for each of the two loci. Heterozygosity calculation results in 93.01% for LH1 and 96.62% for ph30.
The findings show that these loci represent further genetic markers which are very informative for identity tests as well as for parentage analysis.

1. Introduction
The most evident genetic markers for discrimination among individuals are the highly polymorphic variable number of tandem repeats (VNTR) loci. The technology to use these markers is the well-characterized restriction fragment length polymorphism (RFLP) analysis. In this study we describe two loci, D5S110 (LH1), Armour et al. (1990), and D4S139 (pH30), Milner et al. (1989), which are compatible with the restriction enzyme HaeIII used with other known VNTR loci like D2S44 (YNH24), D10S28 (TBQ7) and D17S26 (EFD52). Furthermore we present the frequency distributions of the alleles, the heterozygosity and the mutation rates for both loci.

2. Materials and methods

2.1. Experimental technique
DNA-Isolation: 5 ug human genomic DNA and cell-line K562 DNA according to the protocol of Miller et al. (1988).
RE-Digest: 50 U Hae III (Boehringer Mannheim / FRG).
Molecular weight marker: NICE^{TM} DNA Analysis Ladder (GIBCO BRL, Eggenstein/FRG) with fragment sizes ranging from 22.621 kb to 0.526 kb.
Electrophoresis: 0.8% agarose gel (TBE buffer), 40V, 30hrs.
Transfer: Vacuum blotting with 50 mbar
Hybridization: Alkaline phosphatase-conjugated single-locus probe LH1 and pH30 (Gibco BRL) and the molecular weight marker probe MW100 (Gibco BRL)
Detection: Chemiluminescent with CSPD (Promega)

2.2. Image analysis and molecular weight calculation
according to Luckenbach et al. (1994)

2.3. Allele frequencies
Allele sizes are stored in a multi-user relational database and frequencies were analysed according to the classical mathematical rounding procedure (0.05kb-0.14kb = 0.1kb). 450 unrelated individuals from SW-Germany and 35 families with 172 children from N-Portugal were tested.

2.4. Statistical evaluations
We selected some common statistical paramters, i. e. arithmetic mean (AM), standard

deviation (SD) and coefficient of variation (CV) to check the precision of our analysis method. Thus we have made serial intergel measurements of the two K562 DNA fragments separated on 35 gels and hybridized to LH1 and pH30.

3. Results and Discussion

3.1. Gel Image
Figure 1 shows examples of the fragment patterns of HaeIII restricted DNA from 16 individuals and the cell-line K562 DNA, detected by LH1 and pH30; the molecular weight markers run in lane 1, 10 and 19. These profiles represent sharp bands ranging from 6 kb to 1kb (LH1) and from 15 kb to 3 kb (pH30). Each person is heterozygous with only one exception.

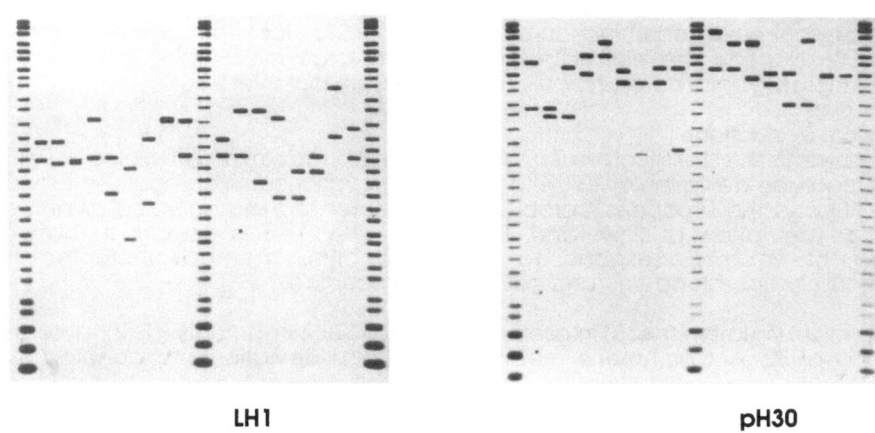

LH1   **pH30**

Fig.1: Image pattern of HaeIII restricted DNA from 16 individuals, (lanes 2-9, 11-18), the K562 cell-line (lane 19), detected by LH1and pH30, molecular weight marker MW100 (lanes 1,11,20).

3.2. Allele frequencies
Figure 2 summarizes the allele frequency distributions at the loci D5S110 (LH1) and D4S139 (pH30) from 450 unrelated individuals (SW-Germany).

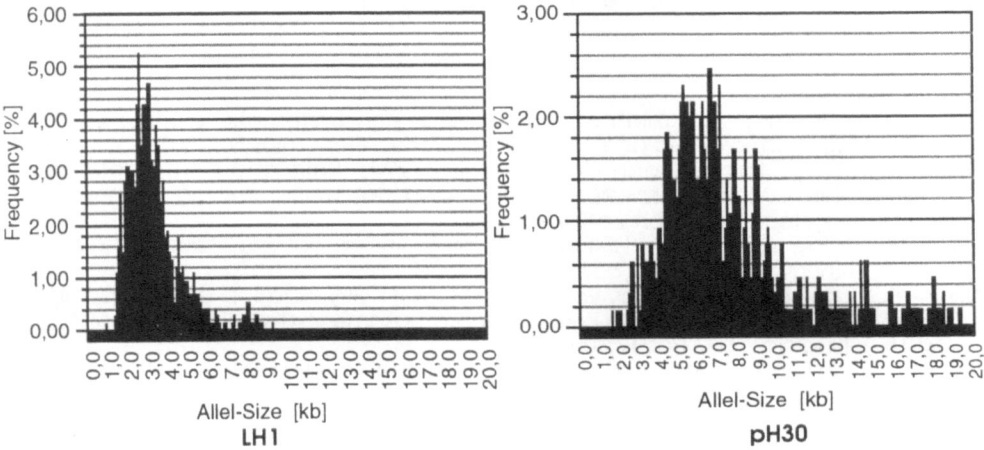

Fig.2: Allele frequency distribution revealed by LH1 and pH30, (n = 450 unrelated individuals)

Major allele clusters were detected by LH1 at 2.6 kb with 5.24%, at 3.1 kb with 4.7% and finally at 2.5 kb and 2.9 kb with 4.3%; pH30 shows 20 peaks, which are broadly distributed between 4 kb and 9 kb with a maximum frequency of 2.45% at 6.7 kb. It is an important and unusual fact that the alleles revealed by pH30 range from 1.5 kb to 19.5 kb with frequencies between 0.002% and 2.5%. The heterozygosity for the locus D5S110 (450 indivduals) and locus D4S139 (450 individuals) was found to be 93.01% and 96.62%, respectively.

The allele frequencies revealed in the small sample of 70 unrelated individuals from N-Portugal were similar to the data determined in SW-Germany, but further studies must be performed to verify these results.

3.3. Mutation rates

We analysed 35 families with 172 children and didn't observe any mutation at the D5S110 locus, but one recombination event at the D4S139 locus, i.e. a recombination rate of 0.0058. Normally the recombination rate will enlarge investigating more families, because it increases with heterozygosity which is at both loci over 93%.

3.4. Statistical evaluations

Table 1 represents the statistical results. We calculated a maximum 3 SD value of 0.0569 or in a percentage deviation of 1.55% for the intergel variation. In comparison to these data the FBI and the Lifecodes Corporation calculated a fixed SD value given as a percentage deviation of 2.5% and 1.8% (Weir, 1992). It is apparent that low measurement errors correspond to precise analysis methods including the experimental, image-processing and calculation procedure.

Table 1: Intergel variation (n=35) in allele sizing of two K562 fragments (f1,f2), detected by LH1 and pH30. AM arithmetic mean; SD standard deviation; CV coefficient of variation.

	LH1		pH30	
	f1	f2	f1	f2
AM (kb)	3,691	2,922	6,435	3,424
SD	0,019	0,010	0,028	0,016
CV (%)	0,515	0,338	0,433	0,463
3 CV (%)	1,545	1,014	1,299	1,389

Summarizing all results we conclude that the single-locus probes LH1 and ph30 are valuable complements to the well-established probe-systems like YNH24, EFD52 or TBQ7.

References

Armour JA, Povey S, Jeremiah S, Jeffreys AJ (1990) Systematic cloning of human minisatellites from ordered array charomid libraries. Genomics 8(3):501-512

Luckenbach C, Luckenbach A, Ritter H (1994) Restriction fragment length polymorphism: Molecular weight analysis and calculation with a scanner-based computer system. Electrophoresis 15:149-152

Miller SA, Dykes DD, Polesky HF (1988) A simple salting out procedure for extracting DNA from human nucleated cells. Nucleic Acids Res 16:1215

Milner EC, Lotshaw CL, Willems van Dijk K et al. (1989) Isolation and mapping of a polymorphic DNA sequence pH30 on chromosome 4 (HGM provisional number D4S139). Nucleic Acids Res 17:4002

Weir EC (1992) Independence of VNTR alleles defined as fixed bins. Genetics 130(4):473-887

ALLELE FREQUENCY DISTRIBUTION OF FIVE VNTR LOCI AND PATERNITY TESTING IN NORTH-EAST OF SPAIN

J.A.Luque, P.García, R.M.Fernández, M.Crespillo, E.Ramírez and J.L.Valverde.

Sección de Biología. Instituto Nacional de Toxicología. Ministerio de Justicia e Interior. Merced 1, 08002 Barcelona, Spain.

System and locus: MS1 / Hinf I (D1S7)
MS31 / HinfI (D7S21)
MS43a /Hinf I (D12S11)
MS8 / Hinf I (D5S43)
YNH24 / Hinf I (D2S44)

Population and sample size: Catalonia (N.E. of Spain). N=208

Methods:
Extraction method: proteinase K/SDS, phenol/chloroform [1]
Restriction enzyme: Hinf I (Promega)
Electrophoresis and blotting: The gels (0.7% agarose in TBE buffer) were electrophoresed and Southern blotted in a nylon membrane according to the EDNAP group protocol and recommendations [2]. NICE DNA analysis ladder (BRL) was used as size marker and K562 DNA as genomic control.
Hybridization: The membranes were sequentially hybridised with the YNH24 (Promega), MS8, MS43a, MS31 and MS1 (Cellmark) alkaline phosphatase labelled probes, following Cellmark protocol.
Size measurement and data analysis: DNA band size was measured following Elder & Southern method [3] with a computerised analytical imaging system (BioImage). Frequency distribution was analysed using sliding window approach [4] with 5 base pairs (bp) intervals and a 5.6% window. Within and between sample comparisons have been made (intergel comparison of the genomic control (K562 DNA) bands, intergel comparison of duplicated sample analysis and inter/intragel comparison between mother/child shared bands).

Results:

Table 1. Data from repeated sizing of the genomic control.

	MS1		MS31		MS43a		MS8		YNH24	
	HMW	LMW	HMW	LMW	HMW	LMW	HMW	LMW	HMW	LMW
Number of bands	78	78	85	85	74	74	64	64	70	70
Mean	4814	4465	7814	6957	13448	5259	5532	4770	4008	2898
Maximum	4885	4525	7934	7056	13779	5327	5583	4823	4052	2942
Minimum	4766	4421	7728	6897	13169	5203	5446	4728	3967	2868
SD	26	21	46	31	133	25	25	21	17	14
Maximum difference	2.46%	2.33%	2.65%	2.28%	4.54%	2.35%	2.47%	1.99%	2.13%	2.55%

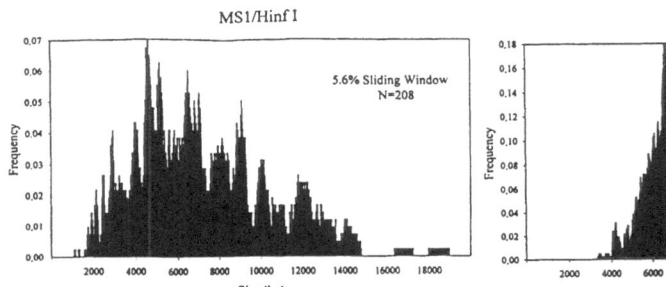

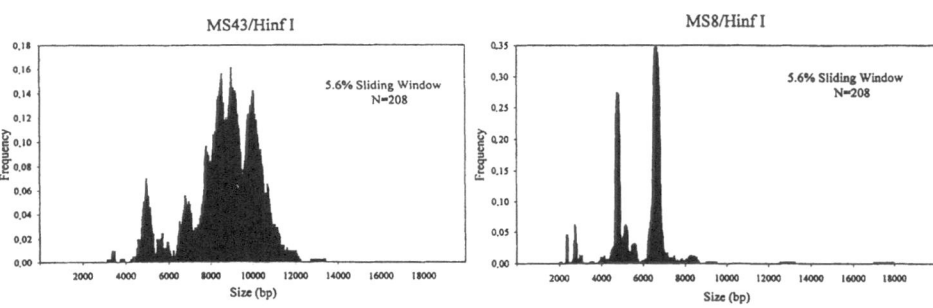

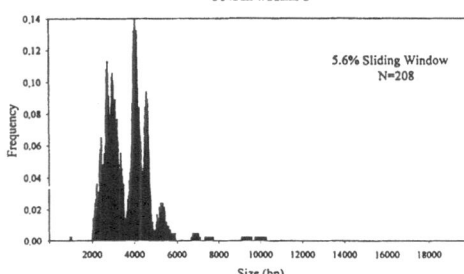

	Heterozygosity	Allele size range (Kb)	Most common size	
			Size(bp)	Frequency
MS1	94.2%	1.1->20	4745±2.8%	0.070
MS31	90.2%	3.4-11.0	6725±2.8%	0.180
MS43a	92.7%	3.2-13.1	8995±2.8%	0.160
MS8	79.5%	2.1-17.5	6615±2.8%	0.351
YNH24	94.2%	1.0-10.0	4085±2.8%	0.140

Figure 1. Allele frequency distribution for the five VNTR loci (D1S7, D7S21, D12S11, D5S43 and D2S44) using sliding window method and data summary.

Table 2. Intra and intergel comparisons between the mother/child shared bands from paternity testing and between bands of the same individual analysed in different gels.

	Mother/child shared band		Duplicated sample
	Intragel	Intergel	Intergel
Number of band comparisons	531	536	1593
Mean of deviation	0.38%	0.87%	0.82%
Maximum deviation	1.96%	4.17%	5.08%
Percentage of match in ±2.8% guideline	100%	98.5%	98.6%

Comments:

The allele frequency distribution of the five VNTR loci in north-east of Spain is similar to others Caucasian populations [5, 6, elsewhere].

In the intra and intergel comparisons, it seems that there is not correlation between deviation and band size. However, over 12000 bp the deviation is higher. The deviation intergel is similar in mother/child and within person comparisons, and lower in the mother/child intragel comparisons. In this one, 100% of comparisons fall into the 2.8% match criterion (max. 1.96%), thus, mother-child-alleged father samples in paternity testing must be coelectrophoresed if it is possible. In the intergel comparisons 98.5% and 98.6% of samples match within 2.8% range. Reviewing the data, most of the samples over 2.8% range are maternal mutation (mainly with MS1 probe), molecular weight over 12000 bp or distorted bands.

References:

1. Sambrook J, Fritsch EF, Maniatis T (1989) Molecular Cloning: A Laboratory Manual, 2nd edn. Cold Spring Harbor Laboratories Press, Cold Spring Harbor
2. DNA Commission of the ISFH (1992) Second DNA recommendations. Int J Leg Med 104:361-364
3. Elder JK, Amos A, Southern EM, Shippey GA (1983) Measurement of DNA length by gel electrophoresis. Anal Biochem 128:223-226
4. Gil P, Evett IW, Woodroffe S, Lygo JE, Millican E, Webster M (1991) Databases, quality control and interpretations of DNA profiling in the Home Office Forensic Science Service. Electrophoresis 12:204-209
5. Buffery C, Burridge F, Greenhalgh M, Jones S, Willott G (1991) Allele frequency distributions of four variable number tandem repeat (VNTR) loci in the London area. Forensic Sci Int 52:53-64
6. Albarran C, Alonso A, Martin P, Sancho M (1994) Allele frequency distributions of five VNTR loci (D1S7, D7S21, D12S11, D5S43 and D2S44) in Spain. In: Bär W, Fiori A, Rossi U (eds) Advances in Forensic Haemogenetics. Springer-Verlag, Berlin, pp 463-465

SPANISH POPULATION DATA ON 13 PCR-BASED SYSTEMS

P. Martín*, A. Alonso*, B. Budowle**, C. Albarrán*, O. García*** and M. Sancho*

* Sección de Biología. Instituto de Toxicología. M° de Justicia e Interior. Madrid. SPAIN.
** Forensic Science Research and Training Center, FBI Academy, Quantico, Virginia. USA.
*** Laboratorio UTAP.Departamento de Interior. Gobierno Vasco. Bilbao. SPAIN.

INTRODUCTION

The enzymatic amplification of polymorphic DNA-loci by PCR (Saiki et al. 1985) offers a number of distinct advantages in forensic DNA typing. First a rapid and specific typing of genetic markers. Second, amplification and detection of target sequences may allow reliable typing results from very small amounts of even degraded DNA. These advantages make the PCR-based typing one of the methods of choice for forensic identification of body fluids and human remains and for paternity testing.

This study presents allele/genotype frecuency data in a Spanish population sample (n=187-244) for 7 Short Tandem Repeat (STR) loci and 6 sequence polymorphism loci. The loci are: FES/FPS (15q25-qter), VWA (12p12-pter), TH01 (11p15.5), F13B (1q31-q32.1), CSF1PO (5q33.5-q34), F13A1 (6p24-p25), TPOX (2p13), HLA-DQA1 (6p21.3), LDLR (19p13.1-p13.3), GYPA (4q28-q31), HBGG (11q), D7S8 (7cen-q22) and Gc (4q11-q13).

MATERIALS AND METHODS

Population Sample and Sample Preparation

EDTA-blood samples were collected from a total of 244 unrelated Spanish individuals living predominantly in the Communities of Madrid, Castilla-La Mancha, Castilla-León (Central-Spain) and Valencia (Eastern-Spain). The DNA was extracted by the standard phenol/chloroform extraction procedure.

PCR and Typing

The amplification of HUMFES/FPS, HUMVWA, HUMTH01, HUMF13B, HUMCSF1PO, HUMF13A1 and HUMTPOX was performed separately according to the manufacturer's recomendations using the Gene Print STR system (Promega Corporation, Madison, WI, USA) in a 480 Perkin-Elmer thermal cycler. PCR products were typed by denaturing polyacrylamide gel electrophoresis and stained with silver as described previously (Budowle et al. 1991).

The amplification and typing of HLA-DQA1 and PM systems were performed according to the manufacturer's recomendations using the amplitype PM and HLA-DQA1 forensic DNA amplification and Typing kits (Perkin-Elmer Corporation, Norwalk, CT).

Statistical Analysis

The frecuency of each allele for each locus was calculated from the numbers of each genotype in the sample. Unbiased stimates of expected heterozygosity were computed as described by Edwards et al. (1992). The expected numbers of distinct homozygous and heterozygous genotypes and their standard errors (SE) were calculated according to the method described by Chakraborty et al. (1988, 1991). Possible divergence from Hardy-weinberg expectations (HWE) was determined by calculating the unbiased estimate of the expected homozygote/heterozygote frequencies (Chakraborty et al. 1988; Nei et al. 1974; Nei et al. 1978), the likelihood ratio test (Edwards et al. 1992; Chakraborty et al.

1991; Weir 1992) and the exact test (Guo et al. 1992). An interclass correlation criterion (Karlin et al. 1981) for two-locus association was used for detecting disequilibrium between loci. Independence across all loci was determined by examining whether or not an observed variance of the number of heterozygous loci in the population sample is outside its confidence interval under the assumption of independence (Brown et al. 1980; Chakraborty 1984; Chakraborty et al. 1994). When appropiate, the Bonferroni procedure was used to correct for multiple analysis to determine whether or not HWE or equilibrium between loci holds in the population.

RESULTS AND DISCUSSION

The observed allele frequencies for 13 PCR-based systems in the Spanish population sample are shown in Table 1. The results of the different test procedures for testing the correspondence of the genotype frequencies with their HWE expected proportions are shown in Table 2. Except for LDLR (p=0.02), the genotype frequency distributions for the loci do not deviate from HWE based on the homozygosity test, the likelihood ratio test and the exact test. The departure from HWE for LDLR, which is not highly significant, is most likely due to sampling variance, and the difference in LDLR genotype estimates using the product rule or the counting method is small. This suggests that the use of the product rule for estimating LDLR genotype frequencies would still provide a valid estimate for forensic or human identity purposes. These data also show that departures from HWE generally have little impact on genotype frequency estimates when independence is assumed.

An analysis was performed to determine whether or not there were any detectable associations between any of the 13 PCR-based loci. An interclass correlation test analysis demonstrated that there were only 3 departures out of 78 tests (F13B/CSF1PO, p=0.015; LDLR/Gc, p=0.037; and TH01/HLA-DQA1, p=0.043), this is less than 5% of the observations. Thus, the amount of departures was no more than expected. Also, with a Bonferroni correction (used for correcting when multiple tests are performed on a population sample), there was no evidence for departures from expectations for pair-wise comparisons of PCR-based loci.

In conclusion, a Spanish population database has been established for 13 PCR-based loci and it has been shown that the allele frequency data can be used in identity testing to estimate the frequency of a multiple PCR-based DNA profile in the Spanish population.

REFERENCES

Brown AHD, Feldman MW, Nevo E (1980) Genetics 96: 523-536
Budowle B, Chakraborty R, Giusti AM, Eisenberg AJ, Allen RC (1991) Am J Hum Genet 48: 137-144
Chakraborty R (1984) Genetics 108: 719-731
Chakraborty R, Fornge M, Guegue R, Boerwinkle (1991) In: Burke T, Dolf G, Jeffreys AJ, Wolff R (eds) DNA fingerprinting: approaches and applications. Birkhauser, Berlin, pp 127-143
Chakraborty R, Smouse PE, Neel JV (1988) Am J Hum Genet 43: 709-725
Chakraborty R, Zhong Y, Jin L, Budowle B (1994) Am J Hum Genet 55: 391-401
Edwards A, Hammond HA, Jin L, Caskey CT, Chakraborty R (1992) Genomics 12: 241-253
Guo SW, Thompson EA (1992) Biometrics 48: 361-372
Karlin S, Cameron EC, Williams PT (1981) Proc Natl Acad Sci USA 78: 2664-2668
Nei M (1978) Genetics 89: 583-590
Nei M, Roychoudhury AK (1974) Genetics 76: 379-390
Saiki RK, Scharf S, Faloona T, Mullis KB, Horn GT, Erlich HA, Arnheim N (1985) Science 230: 1350-1354
Weir BS (1992) Genetics 130: 873-887

Table 1. Allele frequencies for 13 PCR-based systems in a Spanish population sample.

HLA-DQα (n=474) Allele / Freq.	FES/FPS (n=382) Allele / Freq.	VWA (n=444) Allele / Freq.	TH01 (n=488) Allele / Freq	F13B (n=392) Allele / Freq.	CSF1PO (n=374) Allele / Freq.	F13A1 (n=398) Allele / Freq.	TPOX (n=436) Allele / Freq.
1.1 / 0.116	8 / 0.008	14 / 0.106	6 / 0.217	6 / 0.115	8 / 0.003	3.2 / 0.085	6 / 0.002
1.2 / 0.162	9 / 0.003	15 / 0.144	7 / 0.176	7 / 0.010	9 / 0.011	4 / 0.043	8 / 0.546
1.3 / 0.063	10 / 0.319	16 / 0.227	8 / 0.166	8 / 0.250	10 / 0.267	5 / 0.206	9 / 0.096
2 / 0.154	11 / 0.382	17 / 0.286	9 / 0.178	9 / 0.189	11 / 0.275	6 / 0.256	10 / 0.060
3 / 0.133	12 / 0.246	18 / 0.149	9.3 / 0.256	10 / 0.431	12 / 0.374	7 / 0.372	11 / 0.268
4 / 0.371	13 / 0.039	19 / 0.074	10 / 0.006	11 / 0.005	13 / 0.067	8 / 0.013	12 / 0.028
	14 / 0.003	20 / 0.014			14 / 0.003	13 / 0.013	
						14 / 0.005	
						15 / 0.008	

LDLR (n=404) Allele / Freq.	GYPA (n=404) Allele / Freq.	HBGG (n=404) Allele / Freq.	D7S8 (n=404) Allele / Freq.	Gc (n=404) Allele / Freq.
A / 0.450	A / 0.527	A / 0.498	A / 0.564	A / 0.297
B / 0.550	B / 0.473	B / 0.493	B / 0.436	B / 0.163
		C / 0.010		C / 0.540

n = Number of alleles.

Table 2. HWE test for independence on 13 PCR-based systems in a Spanish population sample

	FES/FPS	VWA	TH01	F13B	CSF1PO	F13A1	TPOX
Obs. Homozygosity	30.9%	16.2%	22.5%	28.1%	28.9%	24.1%	36.7%
Exp. Homozygosity [a]	30.8%	19.2%	20.2%	29.6%	29.0%	25.4%	38.2%
Homozygosity Test [b]	0.989	0.266	0.354	0.648	0.967	0.677	0.644
Likehood Ratio Test [b]	0.757	0.443	0.288	0.695	0.371	0.406	0.713
Exact Test [b]	0.634	0.392	0.296	0.763	0.550	0.282	0.373

	HLA-DQAα	LDLR	GYPA	HBGG	D7S8	Gc
Obs. Homozygosity	19.4%	58.4%	53.0%	42.6%	52.5%	42.1%
Exp. Homozygosity [a]	22.2%	50.4%	50.0%	48.9%	50.7%	40.5%
Homozygosity Test [b]	0.310	0.022	0.402	0.072	0.615	0.639
Likehood Ratio Test [b]	0.695	0.027	0.478	0.194	0.675	0.920
Exact Test [b]	0.817	0.018	0.478	0.142	0.675	0.877

a- Expected homozygosity is an unbiased estimate
b- These values are probability values

ALLELE FREQUENCIES OF D1S80, LDLR, GYPA, D7S8, GC, HBGG AND SE 33 IN POLISH POPULATION SAMPLE

Miścicka-Śliwka D., Śliwka K., Syroczyńska A., Grzybowski T., Baranowska B., Berent J.A.

Forensic Medicine Institute, The Ludwik Rydygier's University School of Medical Sciences in Bydgoszcz, ul. M. Skłodowskiej-Curie 9, 85-094 Bydgoszcz, Poland

INTRODUCTION

The application of any new genetic system in forensic casework requires a sufficiently large data base of population. In the present study, we report the allele frequency distribution for seven different loci in the Polish population of Pomerania-Kujawy Region. Five of these markers are coamplified simultaneously using the Amplitype PM kit (Perkin-Elmer): low density lipoprotein receptor (LDLR), glycophorin A (GYPA), hemoglobin G gammaglobin (HBGG), D7S8 linked to cystic fibrosis locus and Group specific Component (GC). The other two loci are VNTR D1S80 (Nakamura 1988) and STR ACTBP2 (SE33) (Polymeropoulos 1992). In addition, we have sequenced selected SE 33 alleles to determine possible sequence structure variations which may cause the allele designation difficult.

MATERIALS AND METHODS

DNA EXTRACTION

Blood samples were obtained from unrelated individuals. Sample sizes were 306 for D1S80, 187 for PM and 31 for SE 33 analysis. DNA was isolated by Proteinase K/Phenol/Chloroform extraction method followed by absolute ethanol precipitation.

PCR AMPLIFICATION

PCR reactions for D1S80 and PM were performed with commercial kits and procedure. SE 33 amplification was performed using 5 ng template in a 10 μl reaction volume comprising 1x Promega buffer, 1.5 mM $MgCl_2$, 200 μM of each dNTP (Perkin-Elmer), 0.7 μM of each primer and 0.5 U of Taq DNA Polymerase (Promega). Primer sequences were used according to Polymeropoulos (1992). Samples were amplified for 10 cycles of 10 s at 94^0 C, 66^0 C and 72^0 C and then the same denaturing and extension conditions, but an annealing temperature of 64^0 C for an additional 20 cycles on a 9600 thermal cycler.

PCR PRODUCTS VISUALISATION

The analysis of PM alleles was based on reverse dot blot reactions with oligonucleotide probes. D1S80 alleles were separated by electrophoresis on ultrathin layer horizontal polyacrylamide gels 12% T, 3% C with DATD as a crosslinker. Gels were run at constant temperature of 10^0 C and constant current 15 mA. SE 33 alleles were diagnosed by vertical electrophoresis in 0.8 mm thick 8% Tris-sulfate polyacrylamide gels run at a constant 500 V. Typing was performed by comparison with a sequenced allelic ladder kindly donated by Prof. B. Brinkmann (Institute of Legal Medicine, Munster). Bands were visualised by silver staining (Allen 1989) and recorded by computer imaging.

CYCLE SEQUENCING

For sequencing reactions, DNA (100 ng) was amplified in a volume 100 μL consisting of 1x Promega buffer, 0.7 mM $MgCl_2$, 200 μM of each dNTP, 0.5 μM of each primer and 2 U Taq DNA Polymerase. To increase the size of PCR products, new primer sequences were designed: F: 5' GAG CCG AGG TCA TGC CAT TG 3' ; R: 5' GAC GAC GAG CGC GGT GAT AG 3'. After the Hot Start at 94^0 C for 2 minutes samples were amplified for 29 cycles of 30 s at 94^0 C, 30 s at 64^0 C and 90 s at 72^0 C (Perkin-Elmer 9600). Cycle sequencing reactions were carried out using the AutoCycle Sequencing Kit (Pharmacia), 160-180 ng PCR template and 0.5 μM internal (nested) sequencing primer (ACTBP2-primer 1: 5' AAT CTG GGC GAC AAG AGT GA 3'), fluorescently labelled at 3' end (Markiewicz 1992). Amplification conditions were: Hot Start at 94^0 C-2 min, 94^0 C-15 s, 64^0 C-15 s, 72^0 C-40 s; 36 cycles, followed by final elongation at 72^0 C-10 min. The sequencing products were separated in a 6% 0.35 thick denaturing gel which was run for 200 min at 1500 V, 40 mA and 40 W on the A.L.F. DNA Sequencer (Pharmacia).

RESULTS AND DISCUSSION

POPULATION DATA

Allele frequency distribution of **PM** loci is given in Fig. 1. The most common alleles were LDLR B (f = 0.623) and D7S8 A (f = 0.591). Our results have shown that in locus LDLR, AB and AA genotypes are the most and the least frequent, respectively. In GYPA, HBGG and D7S8 markers the most frequent genotype was AB. It clearly corresponds to earlier data obtained for Swiss, U.S. Caucasian and U.S. Hispanic populations (Hochmeister 1994; kit leaflet by Roche Molecular Systems). In locus GC however, we have found AC genotype being the most frequent. It correlates with the data obtained for Swiss and U.S. Caucasian population samples, but differs from U.S. Hispanic frequencies. What is more interesting, results obtained for Portugal population sample (n = 115) (Pinheiro 1994) also indicate, as in the case of our data, AC as the most frequent genotype in GC locus. We hope that further interlaboratory comparisons and validation experiments will explain this striking difference. Heterozygosity Index (HI) for these markers was in the range of 0.51-0.79 and the combined power of discrimination (PD) value was approximately 0.94. The genotype distribution was in Hardy-Weinberg equilibrium for all the five loci. These findings, if followed by estimation of mutation rates and level of sensitivity of the system in the cases when heavily degraded DNA is available, seem to validate PM loci for paternity and forensic casework.

In our **D1S80** population study 21 alleles were observed. Fig. 2 shows their frequency distribution. The most common were 18 (f = 0.209) and 24 (f = 0.322). It clearly corresponds to our previous studies. The comparison of our allele frequencies to population data from Western Europe shows certain similarities. Some existing differences are probably caused by the size of the samples, but it is confirmed that 18 and 24 alleles are the most frequent in D1S80 system. In addition to expected PCR products, the "interalleles" (19^m, 20^m, 22^m, 24^m) were found. The distribution of observed and expected D1S80 phenotypes is in Hardy-Weinberg equilibrium. The observed heterozygosity was 0.80 (expected 0.97) and power of discrimination value was 0.95. The high level of polymorphism and high HI and PD values make this marker very useful in forensic blood identification and alleged paternity examination.

SE 33 allele frequencies are given in Fig. 3. Seventeen different alleles were observed. The most common were 19 (f = 0.145), 26 and 28 (f = 0.113). In our population sample, 28 genotypes were observed with the genotypes 23/28 and 26/28 being the most frequent (f = 0.065). Heterozygosity Index was 0.94 in comparison with expected heterozygote frequency h = 0.966. The population data clearly corresponds to those obtained by Polymeropoulos (1992) for small U.S. population (n = 39) but show a striking difference to data from German sample (Wiegand 1993). Different sizes in both studies (n = 31 and n = 180) probably could explain the differences observed. Power of discrimination for our sample was 0.96. It confirmed the value of this STR system as highly polymorphic and sensitive marker for human identification.

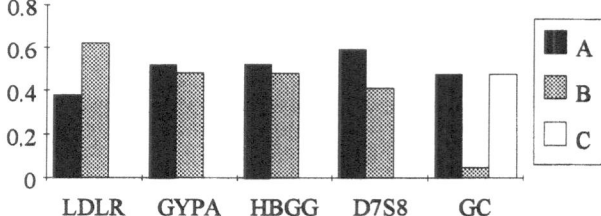

Fig. 1. Frequencies of PM alleles in population of Pomerania-Kujawy region of Poland.

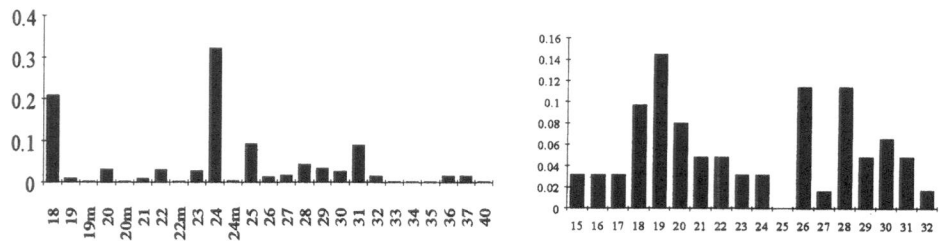

Fig. 2. (left) Frequencies of D1S80 alleles in population of Pomerania-Kujawy region of Poland.
Fig. 3. (right) Frequencies of SE33 alleles in population of Pomerania-Kujawy region of Poland.

SEQUENCING DATA

To determine possible sequence structure variation of the complex STR system SE 33, we selected three alleles which had not been succesfully designed in our previous routine forensic practice, and sequenced them using the cycle sequencing strategy. Prior to sequencing, we had generated longer PCR template by redesigning the primer sequences based on the HUMACTBP2 sequence published by Moos (1983). In the cycle sequencing reactions we used the forward SE 33 primer as internal (nested) sequencing primer. In two of the alleles, we found the common sequence structure $(AAAG)_m$ $(AAAAAG)$ $(AAAG)_n$, which had been previously described by Moos (1983), Urquart (1993) and Moller (1994). In the third allele however, in 5' flanking region of regular repeats AAAG, we observed two hexanucleotide units AAAAAG (positions 29-34 and 39-44) as described by Moos (1983) and two types of irregular repeats: three AG insertions in positions 77-82 followed by AAG motif (positions 83-85). Furthermore one AG insertion occurred also in regular AAAG repeats region (positions 90-91). The region with variable sequence structure is shown in Fig. 4. Our preliminary sequence data suggests that more SE 33 sequence structures may exist than it has been described by Urquart (1993) and Moller (1994). STR length polymorphism, combined with sequence polymorphism may lead to higher possibilities of human identification but further validation and sequencing experiments are required.

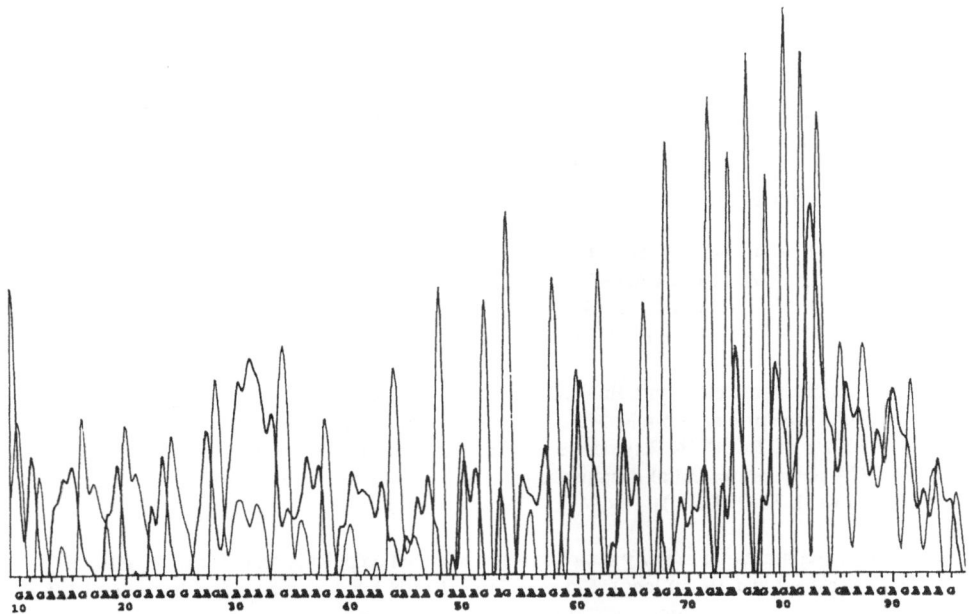

Fig. 4. Hypervariable region sequence of one of the SE 33 alleles.

REFERENCES

Allen R, Graves G, Budowle B (1989) Polymerase chain reaction amplification products separated on rehydratable polyacrylamide gels and stained with silver. Bio Tech 7: 736-744

Hochmeister MN, Budowle B, Barrer UV, Dimhofer R (1994) Swiss population data on the loci HLA DQ alpha, LDLR, GYPA, HBGG, D7S8, GC and D1S80. J Forensic Sci 67: 175-184

Markiewicz WT, Groger G, Rosch R, Zebrowska A, Seliger H (1992) A new method of synthesis of fluorescently labelled oligonucleotides and their application in DNA sequencing. Nucleosides Nucleotides 11: 1703-1711

Moller A, Brinkmann B (1994) Locus ACTBP2 (SE33). Sequence data reveal considerable polymorphism. Int J Leg Med 106: 262-267

Moos M, Gallwitz D (1983) Structure of two human beta-actin-related processed genes one of which is located next to simple repetitive sequence. EMBO J 2: 757-761

Nakamura Y, Carlson M, Krapcho K, White R (1988) Isolation and mapping of polymorphic DNA sequence (pMCT 118) on chromosome 1p (D1S80). Nucl Acids Res 16: 9364

Pinheiro MF, Pontes ML, Costa P (1994) Use of the Amplitype PM coamplification system on forensic analysis. In: Mangin P, Ludes B (eds) Acta Medicinae Legalis, vol XLIV. Springer, Berlin Heidelberg New York p 81

Polymeropoulos MJ, Rath DS, Xiao H, Merril CR (1992) Tetranucleotide repeat polymorphism at the human beta-actin related pseudogene H-beta-Ac-psi-2 (ACTBP2). Nucl Acids Res 20: 1432

Urquart A, Kimpton CP, Gill P (1993) Sequence variability of the tetranucleotide repeat of the human beta-actin related pseudogene H-beta-Ac-psi-2 (ACTBP2). Hum Genet 92: 637-638

Wiegand P, Budowle B, Rand S, Brinkmann B (1993) Forensic validation of the STR systems SE33 and TC11. Int J Leg Med 105: 315-320

HAPLOTYPE FREQUENCIES OF TWO STRs OF THE CHROMOSOME 8q: D8S344 AND D8S323

S. Mourelo, S. Dios, B. Caeiro

Section of Anthropology. Faculty of Biology. University of Santiago de Compostela. Galicia (Spain).

At the Region I of chromosome 8q, two synthenic tetranucleotide repeats, D8S323 (Lu 1993) and D8S344 (Ward 1993), are adscribed. In this work, a diplex amplification of both STRs is described, and the technical conditions in a population study are applied. On the basis of allele and haplotype frequencies, the utility of both systems in human genetic profiling is discused.

MATERIALS AND METHODS

DNA was extracted from 209 individuals from Galician population (NW Spain) by using the standard phenol-clhoroform (Maniatis 1982) or chelating resins (Singer-Sam 1989).

The sequences of the primers were as discused (Lu 1993) and (Ward 1993) for D8S344 and D8S323 respectively:

D8S344   1: 5' -CCA CCT TCC TGT CCA GTC GCA AG -3'
                  2: 5' -AAA CAA AAA TAG CTG GGC ATG GTG A -3'
D8S323   1: 5' -CAC CAC TAC ACT CCA GCC TGT AA -3'
                  2: 5' -ACT CTT ACA TTC CCA CAC CCC CAT A -3'

The PCR reactions parameters, in a final volume of 12.5 µL, consisted of: 20-50 ng of DNA, 200 µM dNTPs, 0.5 µM each primer, 2.5 mM $MgCl_2$, the reaction buffer (200 mM Tris-HCl pH 8.4, 500 mM KCl), 0.325 units of Taq DNA Polymerase (Gibco BRL) specifically bound to a monoclonal antibody anti Taq DNA polymerase. Initial denaturation was at 95°C for 5 min, followed by 30 cycles of 94°C (30 s), 59°C (30 s), 72°C (1 min).

Electrophoretic separation of amplify samples, was performed on polyacrylamide native gels (6% T, 5% C, 0.4 mm thickness and 19 cm long). 375 mM Tris-HCl pH 8.8 was used as gel buffer and 125 mM Tris-Glycine pH 8.8 for the bridge. Electrophoresis was accomplished in horizontal plates at constant V= 300 for 2 h at 18°C. Alleles were visualised using the silver staining method (Budowle 1991).

RESULTS AND DISCUSSION

Phenotype patterns diplex amplification of D8S323 and D8S344 are displayed in Fig. 1. Given that the alleles of both STRs differ between each other around 100 bp, a co-migration without overlapping is perfectly feasible. However, special attention has to be paid to the size of the pore, length of gel and temperature of electrophoretic running. With regard to PCR co-amplification, we have observed that the most critical parameter lies in the temperature of annealing; so, higher temperatures than 59°C lead us to non-specific amplification bands for D8S344, and lower temperatures than 57°C produce a decrease in the efficiency of amplification for D8S323 (Fig. 2). Even so, the use of monoclonal antibodies to Taq DNA polymerase (Kellogg 1994) is advisable in order to clarify the banding pattern.

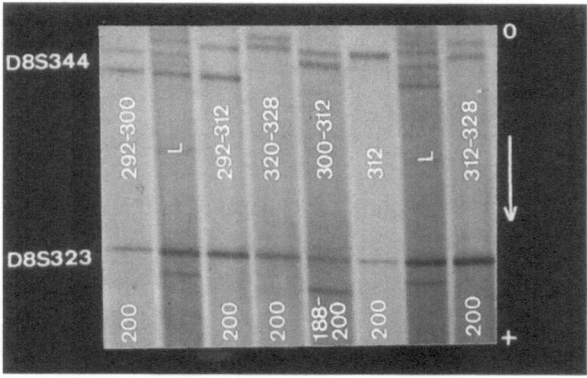

Figure 1. Electrophoretic patterns of the diplex amplification. Ladder consists of alleles of 192, 200, 292, 296, 300, 320, 328 bp.

An initial survey in the Galician population displays 8 alleles for D8S344 which configure values of H= 0.621 and PIC= 0.590. With regard to D8S323, up to 4 alleles were found and values of unbiased H= 0.449 and PIC= 0.352. Allele frequencies for both markers are shown in Table 1. No significant statistical departures from the Hardy-Weinberg proportions were observed either loci. Given that both loci are found in the same chromosome region (8q Region I), a genetic characterization in terms of haplotype frequencies would be feasible. Notwithstanding, no significant evidence of association of phenotypes for both STRs (p> 0.10), were observed (Table 2), which allows us to consider each system independently when carrrying out the statistical calculations.

Table 1. D8S344 and D8S323 allele frequencies in 209 unrealated Galicians.

	D8S344	**D8S323**	
Size (bp)	Frequency ± s.e.	Size (bp)	Frequency ± s.e.
328 bp	0.0167 ± 0.0062		
324 bp	0.0694 ± 0.0124		
320 bp	0.0598 ± 0.0116	200 bp	0.6651 ± 0.0231
312 bp	0.5789 ± 0.0241	196 bp	0.0024 ± 0.0024
308 bp	0.0120 ± 0.0053	192 bp	0.3301 ± 0.0230
300 bp	0.1531 ± 0.0176	188 bp	0.0024 ± 0.0024
296 bp	0.0024 ± 0.0024		
292 bp	0.1077 ± 0.0152		
H= 0.621	PIC= 0.590	H= 0.449	PIC= 0.392

In conclusion, multiplexing of D8S344 and D8S323 allows for a clear diagnosis of the phenotype patterns of both STRs. The relatively good relation between the degree of polymorphism and the number of alleles displayed, expresses the interest of the use of these systems in genetic characterization studies.

Table 2.Estimated haplotype frequencies according to the maximum-likelihood procedure outlined by Hill (1974). The most common allele of each marker was treated as one allele, and the remaining ones were combined (AC). D= linkage disequelibrium coefficient, D'= percentage of maximal disequilibrium, $\chi^2{}_G$= the goodness-of-fit statistic.

A4-A1	A4-AC	AC-A1	AC-AC
0.4137	0.1652	0.2514	0.1697

D= 0.0287
D'= 14.8 %
$\chi^2{}_G$= 3.17
p> 0.10

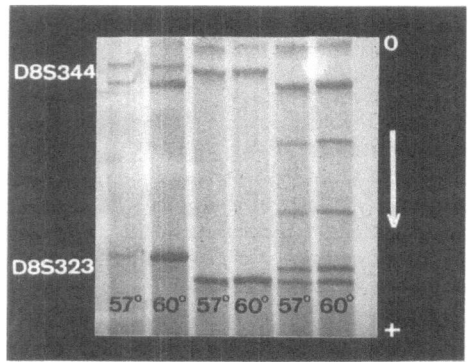

Figure 2. Effect of the annealing temperature (°C) in the efficiency of the amplification.

REFERENCES

Budowle B, Chakraborty R, Giusti AM, Eisenberg AJ, Allen LC (1991) *Am. J. Hum. Genet. 48*:137-144

Hill WG (1974) Estimation of linkage disequilibrium in randomly mating populations. *Heredity 33*:229-239

Kellogg DE, Rybalkin Y, Chen S, Mukhamedova N, Vlasik T, Siebert PD, Chenchik A (1994) TaqStart Antibody: hot start PCR facilitated by a neutralizing monoclonal antibody directed against Taq DNA polymerase. *Bio Techniques 16*:1134-1137

Lu J, Riley R, Robertson M, Nelson L, Ward K (1993) Tetranucleotide repeat polymorphism at the D8S342, D8S323, D8S345, D8S315 and D8S347 loci on 8q. *Hum. Mol. Genet. 2*:1743

Maniatis T, Fritsch EF, Sambrook J (1982) Molecular Cloning: a laboratory manual.Cold Spring Harbor Laboratory, New York

Singer-Sam J, Tanguay RL, Riggs AD (1989) Use of chelex to improve the PCR signal from small number of cells. *Amplifications 3*:11

Ward K, Riley R, Lu J, Robertson M, Nelson L (1993) Tetranucleotide repeat polymorphism at the D8S344 locus. *Hum. Mol. Genet. 2*:1087

ACKNOWLEDGMENTS

This work was partially supported by grants from the Ministerio de Educación y Ciencia (CICYT SAF92-0557) and Xunta de Galicia (XUGA 20001B94).

Japanese population data on six STR loci

A. Nagai, S. Yamada, Y. Watanabe, Y. Bunai and I. Ohya

Department of Legal Medicine, Gifu University School of Medicine
40 Tsukasa-machi, Gifu 500, Japan

Loci: F13A01, F13B, LPL, TH01, TPOX and vWF

Population and sample size: 531 unrelated Japanese individuals living in Gifu Prefecture (central region of Japan). Number of individuals analyzed for each locus: 140 (F13A01), 357 (F13B), 276 (LPL), 531 (TH01), 314 (TPOX) and 362 (vWF)

Methods: PCR amplification for the six STR loci was performed using the *GenePrint*™ STR System (Promega). The amplified products were electrophoretically separated in 4% denaturing polyacrylamide gels (300 mm long and 1 mm thick) according to the *GenePrint*™ Technical Manual and visualized by silver staining [1]. Alleles were determined by comparison with the allelic ladders included in the kits. The chance of exclusion (CE) was calculated using the computer program described by Ohno et al. [2]. The power of discrimination, heterozygosity, and polymorphism information content were calculated as described by Fisher [3], Nei and Roychoudhury [4], and Botstein et al. [5], respectively.

Results:

Allele frequencies

F13A01		F13B		LPL	
Allele	Frequency	Allele	Frequency	Allele	Frequency
3.2	0.332	7	0.003	7	0.004
4	0.093	8	0.064	9	0.002
5	0.043	9	0.203	10	0.707
6	0.525	10	0.725	11	0.100
7	0.004	11	0.004	12	0.185
12	0.004			13	0.004

TH01		TPOX		vWF	
Allele	Frequency	Allele	Frequency	Allele	Frequency
6	0.243	8	0.463	13	0.004
7	0.289	9	0.111	14	0.181
8	0.049	10	0.037	15	0.039
9	0.377	11	0.344	16	0.196
9.3	0.031	12	0.040	17	0.275
10	0.011	14	0.005	18	0.214
				19	0.076
				20	0.015

Statistical evaluations

Loci	CE	PD	h	PIC
F13A01	0.34	0.77	0.61	0.53
F13B	0.22	0.62	0.43	0.38
LPL	0.24	0.66	0.46	0.41
TH01	0.46	0.86	0.71	0.66
TPOX	0.39	0.82	0.65	0.59
vWF	0.60	0.93	0.80	0.77
Combined	0.95	0.99994		

CE: chance of exclusion, PD: power of discrimination, h: Heterozygosity, PIC: polymorphism information content

Comments: Conventional χ^2 test between observed and expected genotype frequencies showed all loci conformed to Hardy-Weinberg equilibrium. The results of this study demonstrate that TH01, TPOX and vWF are more useful for forensic investigations in the Japanese population than the other 3 loci.

References

1. Budowle B, Chakraborty R, Giusti AM, Eisenberg AJ, Allen RC (1991) Analysis of the VNTR locus D1S80 by the PCR followed by high-resolution PAGE. Am J Hum Genet 48: 137-144
2. Ohno Y, Sebetan IM, Akaishi S (1982) A simple method for calculating the probability of excluding paternity with any number of codominant alleles. Forensic Sci Int 19: 93-98
3. Fisher RA (1951) Standard calculations for evaluating a blood group system. Heredity 5: 95-102
4. Nei M, Roychoudhury AK (1974) Sampling variances of heterozygosity and genetic distance. Genetics 76: 379-390
5. Botstein D, White RL, Skolnick M, Davis RW (1980) Construction of a genetic linkage map in man using restriction fragment length polymorphisms. Am J Hum Genet 32: 314-331

Forensic Application of STR Polymorphic Markers

S. Nakamura, T. Sawaguchi and A. Sawaguchi

Department of Legal Medicine, Tokyo Women's Medical
College, Tokyo 162, Japan

Introduction

STR (short tandem repeat) polymorphisms are powerful tools for human identification, paternity analysis and genetic mapping. STR loci consist of short, repetitive sequence elements of 3 to 7 bases pairs in length, and may be amplified using the polymerase chain reaction (PCR).
In the present study, we analysed 6 STR systems CSF1PO, FESFPS, F13B, TH01, TPOX and vWF to obtain allele frequency data for a Japanese population living in Tokyo. The efficiency of these STR systems in paternity testing including postmortem paternity cases was also analysed.

Materials and methods

Blood samples were obtained from 150 healthy Japanese individuals living in Tokyo. DNA was isolated from EDTA-treated blood samples by proteinase K / phenol / chloroform extraction. Polymorphic STR loci tested in the present study were indicated in Table 1. PCR amplification was performed using the GenePrint™ STR Systems (Promega Corporation, USA) and technical manual #TMD004 provided by the manufacturer. The electrophoresis was carried out on 4% denaturing polyacrylamide gels with the Sequi-Gen II system (BIO-RAD, USA) at constant voltage of 1,500V. The bands were visualized by silver staining with Silver Stain Plus Kit (BIO-RAD, USA). The alleles were determined with the allelic ladder provided in the GenePrint™ STR Systems from Promega Corporation.

Table 1 Polymorphic STR Loci tested in the Present Study

Locus	Gene (Chromosomal Location)	Rpeat Sequence	Allele Size Range (bases)
CSF1PO	Human c-fms proto-oncogene (5q33.5 - p34)	AGAT	299 - 323
FESFPS	Human c-fes/fps proto-oncogene (15q25-qter)	AAAT	222 - 250
F13B	Human coagulation factor XIII B subunit (1q31-q32.1)	AAAT	169 - 185
TH01	Human tyrosine hydroxylase (11p15.5)	AATG	179 - 203
TPOX	Human thyroid peroxidase (2p13)	AATG	232 - 248
vWF	Human von Willebrand factor (12p12-qter)	AGAT	139 - 167

Results and discussion

In 150 Japanese subjects, a total of 8 alleles for CSF1PO, 6 alleles for FESFPS, 5 alleles for F13B, 6 alleles for TH01, 6 alleles for TPOX and 8 alleles for vWF was observed.

The most common alleles were 12 for CSF1PO, 11 for FESFPS, 10 for F13B, 9 for TH01, 8 for TPOX and 17 for vWF. The distribution of 6 STR allele frequencies, heterozygosities, polymorphism information contents (PIC) and matching probabilities (pM) were indicated in Table 2. The combined matching probability of 6 STR systems was estimated as 9.2×10^{-6} and the combined power of discrimination was therefore 99.99908%. The combinational resolution of these 6 STR systems has been shown to be a powerful tool in personal identification.

The distribution of 6 STR allele frequencies in the various populations were compared. Allele frequency profiles for CSF1PO, FESFPS, TPOX and vWF in the present study were essentially the same as those indicated in Caucasians (Hammond et al. 1994; Puers et al. 1993a; Kimpton et al. 1992), and the allele frequency profiles for CSF1PO, FESFPS and TH01 from the present study showed a good agreement with Asians data obtained from Hammond et al. (1994) and Puers et al. (1993b). In F13B system the frequency of allele 10 obtained from the present study was higher than that obtained from Caucasian (Nishimura and Murray 1992), and the variant allele 9.3 in TH01 system was a rare allele in the Japanese and also in Asian whereas this allele was the most common in Caucasian (Puers et al. 1993b).

A postmortem paternity case was analysed by conventional systems and DNA profiling. The results were presented in Table 3. Routine paternity testing consisted of the conventional serological analysis of the red cell antigen systems ABO, MNSs, Rhesus, P, Duffy, Kidd and Lewis, the serum proteins GC, HP, BF, IF, C1R, C2, C6, C7, C81 and PLG, the red cell enzymes ACP, PGM1, ESD, GPT and PGD, and leucocyte antigens HLA-A, -B, -C by means of standard techniques. The probability of fatherhood by means of conventional systems was calculated as 83.25%. The simultaneous analysis of 4 STR systems following separate amplifications was presented in Fig. 2. From DNA profiling, the cumulative probability of fatherhood was calculated as 99.85%. An unequivocal conclusion was obtained.

From the present study, these STR systems are useful genetic markers for paternity tests and individual identification in forensic analysis.

Table 2 Analysis of Japanese population with six STR loci

Locus	CSF1PO	FESFPS	F13B	TPOX	TH01	vWF
			Allele frequency (%)			
Allele 6	-	-	-	-	20.16	-
Allele 7	0.97	-	0.33	-	29.84	-
Allele 8	2.43	-	4.68	48.64	4.65	-
Allele 9	6.80	1.39	20.33	5.78	41.09	-
Allele 9.3	-	-	-	-	2.71	-
Allele 10	26.21	13.89	74.33	3.06	1.55	-
Allele 11	17.96	33.33	0.33	36.06	-	-
Allele 12	35.44	30.56	-	4.76	-	-
Allele 13	9.22	18.06	-	1.70	-	0.47
Allele 14	0.97	2.77	-	-	-	17.67
Allele 15	-	-	-	-	-	4.65
Allele 16	-	-	-	-	-	18.60
Allele 17	-	-	-	-	-	28.83
Allele 18	-	-	-	-	-	22.79
Allele 19	-	-	-	-	-	6.06
Allele 20	-	-	-	-	-	0.93
Hetero-zygosity (%)	75.95	74.26	40.40	62.66	69.83	79.32
PIC	0.72	0.70	0.36	0.56	0.65	0.76
pM	0.094	0.110	0.404	0.206	0.144	0.074

591

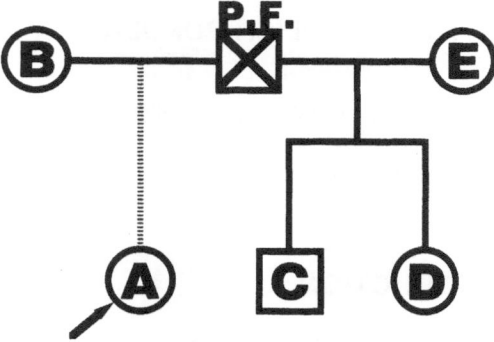

Fig. 1 Paternity testing with six STR loci in postmortem paternity case.

Table 3 Results of paternity testing

Markers	Probability of Fatherfood
Conventional Markers	0.8325
D1S80	0.7866
CSF1PO	0.7298
FESFPS	0.6923
F13B	0.5140
TH01	0.6729
TPOX	0.5069
vWF	0.7293
Cumulative	0.9985

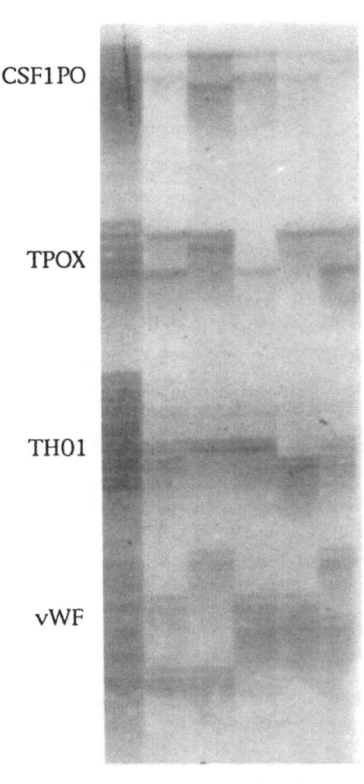

CSF1PO

TPOX

TH01

vWF

L A B C D E

Fig. 2 Silver detection of 4 STR Loci.

References

Hammond HA, Jin L, Zhong Y, Caskey CT and Chakraborty R (1994) Evaluation of 13 short tandem repeat loci for use in personal identification applications. Am J Hum Genet 55: 175-189.

Kimpton C, Walton A and Gill P (1992) A further tetranucleotide repeat polymorphism in the vWF gene. Hum Mol Genet 1: 287.

Nishimura DY and Murray JC (1992) A tetranucleotide repeat for the F13B locus. Nucl Acids Res 20: 1167.

Puers C, Lins AM, Sprecher CJ, Brinkmann B and Schumm JW (1993a) Analysis of polymorphic short tandem repeat loci using well-characterized allelic ladders. Proceedings from the fourth international symposium on human identification 1993. Promega Corporation, p 161-172.

Puers C, Hammond HA, Jin L, Caskey CT and Schumm JW (1993b) Identification of repeat sequence heterogeneity at the polymorphic short tandem repeat locus HUMTH01[AATG]n and reassignment of alleles in population analysis by using a locus-specific alleleic ladder. Am J Hum Genet 53: 953-958.

POPULATION STUDIES OF TWO AMPFLPs AND TWO STRs SYSTEMS IN A NORTH POLISH POPULATION.

R. Pawłowski, A. Welz, A. Maciejewska, R. Paszkowska

Institute of Forensic Medicine, Medical University of Gdańsk, Poland.

INTRODUCTION

Analysis of variable number of tandem repeats (VNTR) is widely used in forensic testing. PCR amplification of many polymorphic VNTR regions has been described. The most commonly amplified fragment length polymorphisms (AMPFLPs) loci, are D1S80, ApoB, D17S5 and COL2A1. Recently, a number of short tandem repeats (STRs) loci, have been described and applied to the forensic practice.

We describe here the results of population studies of two AMPFLPs and two STR systems investigated in the North Poland, Gdańsk area.

The aims of this investigation were following: 1) to obtain allele frequencies for Polish population, 2) to test whether the allele frequencies conform to Hardy-Weinberg expectations and 3) to compare results with other population samples.

MATERIALS AND METHODS

Blood samples were taken from persons of both sexes living in the North Poland (Gdańsk area). DNA was isolated from blood samples obtained from unrelated persons using non-organic and non-enzymatic method (Lahiri et al. 1992). The analyzed VNTR systems and PCR conditions are shown in Table 1. PCR was carried out in $20\mu l$ reaction volumes, using 2-10ng of template DNA, 1 U Taq-DNA-polymerase (Biometra), 200mM of each dNTPs, 1 mM of each primer and $2\mu l$ reaction buffer.

Table 1. VNTR loci studied.

Locus	Chromosome location	Chromosomes tested (n)	Primer sequences	Amplification conditions
D1S80	1p36-p35	414	Kasai at al. (1990)	Kloosterman et al. (1993)
D17S5	17p13.3	408	Horn et al. (1989)	Rand et al. (1992)
HUMTH01	11p15.5-p15	406	Edwards et al.(1991)	Wiegand et al. (1993)
HUMVWA	12pter-p12	370	Kimpton et al. (1992)	Möller et al. (1994)

Electrophoretic separation of PCR products was performed by high resolution polyacrylamide gel electrophoresis according to Allen et al. (1989). Gels were silver stained using the modified Bassam (1991) method.

RESULTS AND DISCUSSION

For D1S80 19 different alleles and 59 genotypes were observed. In a sample of 204 persons 13 alleles and 53 genotypes were observed for the D17S5 locus.

For HUMVWA 8 alleles and 27 genotypes were observed and for HUMTH01 7 alleles and

Table 2. Allele frequencies of D1S80 in the Polish population (N=207).

Allele	Frequency	Allele	Frequency	Allele	Frequency	Allele	Frequency
18	0.2005	23	0.0386	28	0.0507	33	0.0024
19	0.0024	24	0.3623	29	0.0459	36	0.0072
20	0.0266	25	0.0628	30	0.0121	37	0.0121
21	0.0072	26	0.0290	31	0.0604	41	0.0024
22	0.0459	27	0.0169	32	0.0145		

Chi-square = 17.178, df=13, 0.2>P>0.1

Table 3. Allele frequencies of D17S5 in the Polish population (N=204).

Allele	Frequency	Allele	Frequency	Allele	Frequency	Allele	Frequency
1	0.0515	5	0.0613	9	0.0539	13	0.0074
2	0.1324	6	0.0490	10	0.0539		
3	0.1961	7	0.0171	11	0.0759		
4	0.2672	8	0.0490	12	0.0098		

Chi-square = 15.75, 0.3<P<0.5 , df=13

Table 4. Allele frequencies of HUMVWA in the Polish population (N=185).

Allele	Frequency	Allele	Frequency	Allele	Frequency	Allele	Frequency
13	0.0054	15	0.0972	17	0.2864	19	0.0945
14	0.0648	16	0.1945	18	0.2324	20	0.0243

Chi-square = 15.867, df=14, 0.5>P>0.3

Table 5. Allele frequency of HUMTH01 in the Polish population (N=203)

Allele	Frequency	Allele	Frequency	Allele	Frequency	Allele	Frequency
5	0.0024	7	0.1256	9	0.1847	10	0.0123
6	0.2487	8	0.1206	9.3	0.3054		

Chi-square= 11.224, df=12, 0.5<P<0.7

Table 6. Forensic value of the four analysed systems in the Polish population.

System	H obs.	H exp±SE	DP	DI	PIC	pM
D1S80	0.802	0.812±0.027	0.935	0.071	0.793	0.065
D17S5	0.804	0.853±0.025	0.950	0.069	0.836	0.050
HUMVWA	0.789	0.804±0.029	0.932	0.080	0.775	0.068
HUMTH01	0.782	0.782±0.029	0.916	0.087	0.746	0.084

19 genotypes were observed. Tables 2, 3, 4 and 5 show allele distribution of the analyzed systems. The Chi-square test was carried out to estimate if the population sample conforms to the Hardy-Weinberg (H-W) equilibrium. The Polish population meets H-W expectations for D1S80, D17S5, HUMVWA and HUMTH01. Table 6 shows forensic value of the analysed systems expressed as various statistical parameters. Comparison of allele distributions for different populations was done using the 2-way RXC contingency table.

For D1S80 locus, a comparison of the Polish data with the Danish (Thymann et al. 1993), German (Schnee et al. 1993), and Swiss (Hochmeister et al. 1994) populations showed no statistical differences. On the other hand, the general Polish D1S80 distribution was statistically different from the Spanish (Lareu et al. 1993) and Dutch (Kloostermann et al. 1993) at P<0.005. Comparison of allele distribution for D17S5 showed no statistical differences between the Polish and American (Batanian et al. 1990) populations. However there were statistically significant differences between the Polish and Spanish (Gene et al 1995) populations (P=0.001), Polish and Italian (Buscemi et al. 1994; P=0.05), and Polish and German (Rand et al. 1992) populations (P=0.031). For HUMVWA we did not observe statistical differences in alleles distribution between the Polish and German (Möller et al. 1994) and Polish and English (Drozd et al. 1994) populations. Statistically significant differences were observed between the Polish and Finnish (P<0.05; Sajantila et al. 1994), and Polish and Spanish (P<0.001; Pestoni et al. 1995) populations. We have shown that there is no significant difference in the allele frequencies at the HUMTH01 locus between the Polish and German (Wiegand et al. 1993), Swiss (Hochmeister et al. 1994) and Spanish (Pestoni et al. 1995) populations. However, these distributions in the Polish and Danish populations differed significantly (P=0.001).

In conclusions, this study shows that the analyzed loci are highly polymorphic in the Polish population, and could be used as a powerful DNA typing systems.

REFERENCES

Allen RC., G. Graves, B Budowle (1989) BioTechniques 1989, 7, 736.
Bassam BJ, Caetano-Anolles G, Gresshoff PM (1991) Anal Biochem 80:81-84.
Batanian JR, Ledbetter SA, Wolff RK, Nakamura Y, White R, Dobyns WB (1990) Hum Genet 85: 555.
Buscemi L, Cucurachi N, Mancarelli R, Sisti B, Tagliabracci A, Ferrara SD (1994) Int J Leg Med 106:200.
Drozd MA, Archard L, Lincoln PJ, Morling N, Nellemann, Phillips C, Soteriou B, Syndercombe Court D (1994) Forensic Sci Int 69: 161-170.
Edwards A, Civitello A, Hammond HA, Caskey CT (1991) Am J Hum Genet 49:746-756.
Hochmeister M, Budowle B, Borer UV, Dirnhofer R (1994) For Sci Int, 67, 175-184.
Hochmeister M, Jung J, Budowle B, Borer UV, Dirnhofer R (1994) Int J Leg Med 107:34-36
Horn GT, Richards B, Klinger KW (1989) Nucleic Acids Res 17:2140
Gene M, Huguet E, Sanchez-Garcia C, Moreno P,Corbella, Mezquita (1995) Int J Leg Med 107:222.
Kasai, K., Nakamura, Y., R. White. J Forensic Sci, 1990,35,1196.
Kimpton CP,Walton A, Gill P (1992) Hum Mol Genet 1: 287-289.
Kloosterman AD, Budowle B, Daselaar P (1993) Int J Legal Med 105: 257-264.
Lahiri DK,Bye S, Numberger Jl,Hodes ME, Crisp M (1992) J Biochem Biophys Methods 25: 193-205.
Lareu MV, Munoz I, Pestoni C, Rodriguez MS, Vide C, Carracedo A (1993) Int J Leg Med 106,124-128.
Möller A, Wiegand P, Grüschow C, Seuchter S, Baur M, Brinkmann B (1994). Int J Legal Med 106:183.
Nellemann LJ, Moller A, Morling N (1994) Forensic Sci Int 68: 45-51.
Pestoni C, Lareu MV, Rodriguez MS, Munoz I, Barros F, Carracedo A (1995) Int J Leg Med 107:283-290.
Rand S, Puers C, Skowasch K, Wiegand P, Budowle B, Brinkmann B (1992) Int J Legal Med 104:329-333.
Sajantila A, Pacek P, Lukka M, Syvanen A, Nokalainen P, Sistonen P, Peltonen L, Budowle B (1994) Forensic Sci Int (1994) 68:91-102.
Schnee J, Blass G, Herrmann S, Schneider HR, Forster R, Bassler, Pflug W (1993) Forensic Sci Int 59:131.
Thymann M, Nellemann L, Masuba G, Irgens-Moller L, Morling N (1993) Forensic Sci Int 60, 47-56.
Wiegand P, Budowle B, Rand S, Brinkmann B (1993) Int J Leg Med 105:315

ALLELE FREQUENCY DISTRIBUTION OF 15 PCR-BASED DNA POLYMORPHISMS IN THE POPULATION OF GALICIA (NW SPAIN)

C. Pestoni, A. García-Rivero, S. Bellas, M.V. Lareu, M.S. Rodríguez-Calvo, F. Barros, I. Muñoz and A. Carracedo.
Institute of Legal Medicine. Faculty of Medicine. 15705 Santiago de Compostela. Galicia. Spain.

Systems and loci: HLA DQA1 (6p21.3), LDLR (Cr 19), GYPA (Cr 4), HBGG (Cr 11), D7S8, GC (Cr 4), pMCT (D1S80), YNZ22 (D17S5), COL2A1 (12q14.3), 3'ApoB (Cr 2), HUMTH01 (11p15.5-p15), HUMVWA31/A (12p12-12pter), HUMF13A1 (6p24-25), HUMFES/FPS (15q25-qter), HUMLPL (8q22).

Population and sample size: 140 to 250 unreleated people from Galicia (NW Spain).

Methods:
Primers and PCR amplification conditions: HLA DQA1 and pMCT (Lareu et al. 1993), LDLR, GYPA, HBGG, D7S8 and GC (AmpliType PM PCR Amplification and Typing kit (Perkin Elmer)), YNZ22 (Rand et al. 1992), COL2A1 (Wu et al. 1990), 3'ApoB (Boerwinkle et al. 1989), HUMTH01, HUMVWA31/A, HUMF13A1, HUMFES/FPS and HUMLPL (Pestoni et al. 1995).
Method of detection: HLA DQA1, LDLR, GYPA, HBGG, D7S8 and GC (Dot-blot with ASO probes - AmpliType HLA DQα and PM kits (Perkin-Elmer)), pMCT and YNZ22 (PAGE (PhasGels 8-25, Pharmacia) followed by silver-staining), COL2A1, 3'ApoB, HUMTH01, HUMVWA31/A, HUMF13A1, HUMFES/FPS and HUMLPL (ALF DNA sequencer, Pharmacia).

Results:
Allele frequencies:

HLA DQA1 (n=178)

Allele	Frequency	Allele	Frequency	Allele	Frequency
0101	0.1826	0103	0.0955	0301	0.0871
0102	0.1966	0201	0.1039	0501	0.3343

χ^2: 13.3124; p:0.5781

POLYMARKER (n=143)

Locus	Allele	Frequency	Locus	Allele	Frequency	Locus	Allele	Frequency
LDLR	A	0.3986	GYP	A	0.4825	D7S8	A	0.5594
	B	0.6014		B	0.5175		B	0.4406

χ^2:0.009; p:0.924 χ^2:0.188; p:0.665 χ^2:0.007; p:0.934

Locus	Allele	Frequency	Locus	Allele	Frequency
HBGG	A	0.5909	GC	A	0.2762
	B	0.3986		B	0.1748
	C	0.0105		C	0.5490

χ^2:1.861; p:0.602 χ^2:0.553; p:0.907

D1S80 (n=149)

Allele	Frequency	Allele	Frequency	Allele	Frequency
16	0.0034	23	0.0235	30	0.0101
17	0.0067	24	0.3557	31	0.0403
18	0.2617	25	0.0302	32	0.0034
19	0.0034	26	0.0034	33	0.0101
20	0.0336	27	0.0201	34	0.0067
21	0.0302	28	0.0268	36	0.0101
22	0.0436	29	0.0738	37	0.0034

Exact test: p:0.193

YNZ22 (n=137)

Allele	Frequency	Allele	Frequency	Allele	Frequency
1	0.0365	5	0.0438	9	0.1058
2	0.1934	6	0.0511	10	0.0620
3	0.1934	7	0.0146	11	0.0182
4	0.2518	8	0.0255	12	0.0036

Exact test: p:0.168

COL2A1 (n=164)

Allele	Frequency	Allele	Frequency	Allele	Frequency
11	0.1311	13	0.5579	15	0.0244
12	0.0366	14	0.2409	16	0.0091

Exact test: p:0.674

3'ApoB (n=183)

Allele	Frequency	Allele	Frequency	Allele	Frequency
25	0.0027	35	0.2322	43	0.0191
29	0.0055	36	0.0027	45	0.0574
30	0.0055	37	0.3852	47	0.0956
31	0.0765	39	0.0301	49	0.0109
33	0.0574	41	0.0191		

Exact test: p:0.124

HUMTH01 (n=234)

Allele	Frequency	Allele	Frequency	Allele	Frequency
5	0.0021	7	0.1731	9	0.1774
6	0.2115	8	0.1325	9.3	0.3034

Exact test: p:0.928

HUMVWA31/A (n=158)

Allele	Frequency	Allele	Frequency	Allele	Frequency
14	0.1297	17	0.2247	20	0.0095
15	0.1108	18	0.2247		
16	0.2595	19	0.0411		

Exact test: p:0.857

HUMF13A1 (n=143)

Allele	Frequency	Allele	Frequency	Allele	Frequency
3.2	0.0874	7	0.3671	12	0.0035
4	0.0385	8	0.0070	15	0.0175
5	0.1748	10	0.0035	16	0.0070
6	0.2832	11	0.0035	17	0.0070

Exact test: p:0.708

HUMFES/FPS (n=124)

Allele	Frequency	Allele	Frequency	Allele	Frequency
8	0.0121	10	0.3306	12	0.1815
9	0.0081	11	0.4193	13	0.0484

Exact test: p:0.723

HUMLPL (n=113)

Allele	Frequency	Allele	Frequency	Allele	Frequency
1	0.0885	3	0.2611	5	0.0796
2	0.3717	4	0.1903	6	0.0088

Exact test: p:0.695

Comments: All the systems were in Hardy-weinberg equilibrium. No significant differences with other caucasian populations were found except for HLA DQA1. No mutations were found for any of the systems in a total of 95 paternal meioses and 120 maternal meioses. Anomalous electrophoretic mobility was observed for HUMF13A1 and 3'ApoB systems in non-denaturing PAGE.

Systems	h	PD	CE	Systems	h	PD	CE
HLADQA1	0.7914	0.9211	0.5932	YNZ22	0.8427	0.9453	0.6828
LDLR	0.4755	0.6141	0.1823	COL2A1	0.6133	0.7946	0.3689
GYPA	0.5174	0.6247	0.1873	HUMTH01	0.7859	0.9195	0.5737
HBGG	0.5454	0.6307	0.1960	HUMVWA31/A	0.8033	0.9308	0.6052
D7S8	0.4895	0.6214	0.1857	HUMF13A1	0.7475	0.8956	0.5226
GC	0.5944	0.7643	0.3174	HUMFES/FPS	0.6821	0.8392	0.4172
D1S80	0.7936	0.9342	0.6189	HUMLPL	0.7465	0.8932	0.5160
3'ApoB	0.7764	0.9238	0.5889				

REFERENCES

Boerwinkle E, Xiong W, Fourest E, Chang L (1989) Rapid typing of tandemly repeated hypervariable loci by the polymerase chain reaction: application to the apolipoprotein B 3′ hypervariable region. Proc Natl Acad Sci USA 86:212-216

Lareu MV Muñoz I, Pestoni C, Vide MC, Carracedo A (1993) The distribution of HLA DQA1 and D1S80 (pMCT118) alleles and genotypes in the population of Galicia and Central Portugal. Int J Leg Med 106: 124-128.

Pestoni C, Lareu MV, Rodríguez MS, Muñoz I, Barros F, Carracedo A (1995) The use of the STRs HUMTH01, HUMVWA31/A, HUMF13A1, HUMFES/FPS, HUMLPL in forensic application: validation studies and population data for Galicia (NW Spain). Int J Leg Med 107:283-290.

Rand S, Puers C, Skowasch K, Wiegand P, Budowle B, Brinkmann B (1992) Population genetics and forensic efficiency data of 4 AMPFLP's. Int J Leg Med 104:329-333

Wu S, Seino S, Bell GI (1990). Human collagen, type II, alpha 21, (COL2A1) gene: VNTR polymorphism detected by gene amplification. Nucleic Acids Res 18:3102

THE ALLELIC DISTRIBUTION OF 5 STR SYSTEMS IN A NORTH ITALIAN POPULATION.

A. Piccinini, S. Rand*, B. Brinkmann*.

Institute of Legal Medicine. University of Milan.
Milano, Italy.

* Institute of Legal Medicine. University of Muenster.
Muenster, Germany.

Systems and loci: HUMFES/FPS (15q25-qter); HUMVWA (12p12-pter); HUMF13B (1q31-q32.1); SE33 (ACTBP2); HUMD21S11.

Population sample size: North Italy (Milano residents). HUMFES/FPS: N=115; HUMVWA: N=118; HUMF13B: N=119; HUMACTBP2: N=118; HUMD21S11: N=119.

Methods: Primers: HUMFES/FPS (Polymeropoulos et al., 1991), HUMVWA (Kimpton et al., 1992), HUMF13B (Nishimura and Murray, 1992), HUMACTBP2 (Polymeropoulos et al., 1992), HUMD21S11(Sharma and Litt, 1992).

PCR and electrophoretic conditions: HUMFES/FPS, HUMVWA, HUMD21S11 (Moeller et al., 1994); HUMF13B (Alper et al., 1995a); HUMACTBP2 (Wiegand et al., 1993).

Statistical analyses: the statistical evaluations were carried out using the programme HWE Analysis ver. 3 provided by C. Puers (Muenster, Germany). The programme checks the Hardy-Weinberg equilibrium by the Chi-Squared test, the logarithmic likelihood ratio (G) test, and the exact test by randomly shuffling the observed alleles 5000 times, as well as other statistical parameters. The frequency profile comparison between Italians, Germans and Turks was performed using a dedicated software for genetic heterogeneity (RxC contingency table; G. Carmody, Ottawa - Canada).

Results and discussion
The allele frequency distributions for the 5 systems investigated in the Italian population were compared to German (B.Brinkmann personal communication) and Turkish data (Alper et al,1995a; Alper et al., 1995 b). Relevant statistical data for each system are summarised in Table 1. No deviation from Hardy-Weinberg equilibrium was found for each locus studied in the Italian population.
The distribution patterns were similar in Italians, Germans and Turks. However, some statistical significant differences exist in some systems (HUMFES/FPS: Germans-Turks Chi-squared P value = 0.002 ±0.0014 Standard Error (SE); F13B: Italians-Turks Chi-squared P value = 0.000, German-Turks = 0.001 ±0.0010 SE; HUMACTBP2: Italians-Germans Chi-squared P value = 0.004 ±0.002 SE, Italians-Turks = 0.005 ±0.0022 SE, Germans-

Turks 0.001 ±0.001 SE; HUMD21S11: Italians-Turks Chi-squared P value = 0.003 ±0.0017 SE, Germans-Turks = 0.000).

For medium polymorphic systems (HUMFES/FPS, HUMF13B, HUMD21S11)the main differences seem to be a higher frequency for one allele in one population (e.g. allele 12 in Turks for HUMFES/FPS, allele 10 in Italians for HUMF13B, allele 32.2 in Turks for HUMD21S11). Remarkably, the results of HUMVWA typing showed no significant differences among the populations. For the most polymorphic system HUMACTBP2 the differences seem to lie at the extremes of the allelic ladder, even though the lower molecular weight gaussian peak of the frequency distribution seems to show significant differences in the German population when compared to the Italian and Turkish ones.

Conclusions

The allele frequency distributions of 5 STR systems in an Italian population are presented and compared with 2 other Caucasian populations (Germans and Turks) pointing out some statistical differences between them. These differences may be caused first of all by the size of the populations studied or could be due to actual interpopulation differences, related to one allele for the medium polymorphic systems (HUMFES/FPS, HUMF13B, HUMD21S11). It is not surprising for the system HUMACTBP2 to show statistically significant differences: this can be due to its higher degree of polymorphism.

These data strongly suggest that in the European populations some differences do exist and therefore local population databases are needed to perform biostatistical calculations in routine forensic casework.

References

Alper B, Schuerenkamp M, Meyer E (1995a) HumFES/FPS and HumF13B: population genetic study on a Turkish and German population survey. Int J Legal Med - In press.

Alper B, Wiegand P, Brinkmann B (1995b) Population genetic study from a Turkish population survey using 3 STR systems. Int J Legal Med - In press.

Kimpton C, Walton A, Gill P (1992) A further tetranucleotide repeat polymorphism in the vWF gene. Hum Mol Genet 1: 287.

Moeller A, Meyer E, Brinkmann B (1994) Different types of structural variation in STRs: HumFES/FPS, HumVWA and HumD21S11. Int J Legal Med 106: 319-323.

Nishimura DY and Murray JC (1992) A tetranucleotide repeat for the F13B locus. Nucleic Acid Res 20: 1167.

Polymeropoulos MH, Rath DS, Xiao H, Merril RM (1991) Tetranucleotide repeat polymorphism at the human c-fes/fps proto-oncogene (FES). Nucleic Acids Res 19: 4018.

Polymeropoulos MH, Rath DS, Xiao H, Merril CR (1992) Tetranucleotide repeat polymorphism at the human beta-actin related pseudogene H-beta-Ac-psi-2 (ACTBP2). Nucleic Acids Res 20: 1432.

Sharma V, Litt M (1992) Tetranucleotide repeat polymorphism at the D21S11 locus. Hum Mol Genet 1: 67.

Wiegand P, Budowle B, Rand S, Brinkmann B (1993) Forensic validation of the STR systems SE33 and TC11. Int J Legal Med 105: 315-320.

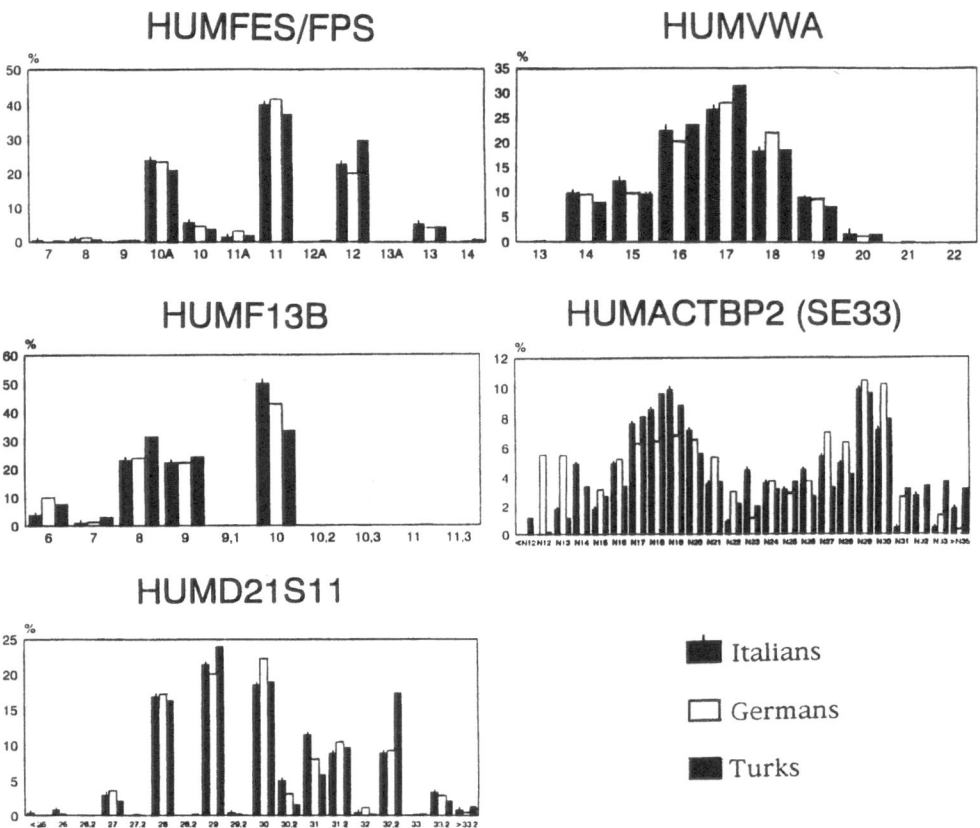

Fig. 1.
Comparative results of the allele frequency distribution for the 5 systems
investigated in the Italian, German and Turkish populations.

System	Observed Heterozyg.	Mean Excl. Chance	Polym.info content	Prob. of match	Discrim. power
FES/FPS	0.6870	0.5024	0.6892	0.1155	0.8845
VWA	0.7966	0.6282	0.7862	0.0653	0.9346
F13B	0.5882	0.3842	0.5876	0.1787	0.8213
ACTBP2	0.9182	0.8564	0.9352	0.0165	0.9835
D21S11	0.8103	0.7074	0.8397	0.0427	0.9573

Table 1.
Statistical evaluations relevant to the STR systems studied in the Italian
population.

POPULATION STUDY OF 3 STR LOCI IN THE NORTH OF PORTUGAL

M. F. Pinheiro[1,2], M.L.Pontes[1], M. Gené[3], E. Huguet[3] and J. Pinto da Costa[1,2]

1 Medico-Legal Institute, 4050 PORTO, PORTUGAL
2 Biomedical Sciences Institute "Abel Salazar", University of Oporto
3 Forensic Genetics Laboratory. School of Medicine University of Barcelona (UB).
  28028 BARCELONA, SPAIN

SYSTEMS AND LOCI: HUMVWA31A (12 p 12-12 pter)
                        HUMTH01 (11 p 15.5 - p 15)
                        HUMFES/FPS (15 q 25-qter)

POPULATION AND SAMPLE SIZE:

HUMVWA31A n=263. HUMTH01 n=319. HUMFES/FPS n=307

METHODS:

Primers :
            HUMVWA31A (Kimpton et al. 1992)
            HUMTH01 (Polymeropoulos et al. 1991)
            HUMFES/FPS (Polymeropoulos et al. 1991)

PCR amplification conditions:
 Singleplex amplifications in a Perkin Elmer 480 according to EDNAP recommendations
(Kimpton et al. 1995).

Electrophoretic methods:
Short 5% Long Ranger gel electrophoresis. The gels were run for 2 h at 1000 V, 35 mA,
25 W, 50°C and laser power at 3 mW on the ALF DNA sequencer. The allelic ladders
were constructed with alleles of known size from each locus. STR products were
automatically sized by the Fragment Manager software (Pharmacia TM), using internal
standard sizers with 100 and 300 bp (Pharmacia TM) and an external ladder with 50-
500bp (Pharmacia TM).

RESULTS:

Table 1. Observed genotypes in a sample population of the North of Portugal

HUMVWA31A		HUMTH01		HUMFES/FPS	
Gen.	Obs.	Gen.	Obs.	Gen.	Obs.
13-14	1	6-6	9	8-10	4
13-16	1	6-7	25	8-11	1
13-17	1	6-8	20	8-12	2
14-14	2	6-9	30	8-13	1
14-15	13	6-9.3	41	10-10	31
14-16	8	6-10	2	10-11	66
14-17	13	7-7	6	10-12	52
14-18	11	7-8	19	10-13	6
14-19	10	7-9	17	10-14	2
15-15	6	7-9.3	27	11-11	49
15-16	17	8-8	2	11-12	48
15-17	15	8-9	17	11-13	15
15-18	11	8-9.3	24	12-12	26
15-19	2	8-10	2	12-13	4
16-16	8	9-9	12		
16-17	33	9-9.3	32		
16-18	20	9-10	2		
16-19	7	9.3-9.3	32		
16-20	5				
17-17	20				
17-18	23				
17-19	11				
17-21	2				
18-18	9				
18-19	9				
18-20	3				
19-19	2				
$X^2=39.63$		$X^2=15.86$		$X^2=18.23$	
d.f.=36		d.f.=15		d.f.=15	
$0.350>p>0.300$		$0.400>p>0.350$		$0.260>p>0.250$	

Table 2. Allele frequencies in a sample population of the North of Portugal

HUMVWA31A		HUMTH01		HUMFES/FPS	
Allele	Frequency	Allele	Frequency	Allele	Frequency
13	0.0057	6	0.2131	8	0.0130
14	0.1141	7	0.1567	10	0.3127
15	0.1331	8	0.1348	11	0.3713
16	0.2034	9	0.1912	12	0.2573
17	0.2623	9.3	0.2947	13	0.0423
18	0.1806	10	0.0094	14	0.0033
19	0.0817				
20	0.0152				
21	0.0038				

Table 3. Statistical parameters

	HUM VWA31A	HUM TH01	HUM FES/FPS
Heterozygosity Index (HI	0.8213	0.8088	0.6547
Power of discrimination (PD)	0.9429	0.9223	0.8483
Chance Exclusion (CE)	0.6410	0.5810	0.4290
Essen - Möller mean value (EM)	9.49	9.57	9.69

COMMENTS:

The high number of alleles and the statistical parameters obtained make these markers good tools for forensic analysis. The described automated typing protocol is presently employed in our routine paternity testing and in some criminal cases.

REFERENCES:

Kimpton C, Walton A, Gill P, (1992) A further tetranucleotide repeat polymorphism in the VWF gene. Hum Mol Genet 1:287

Kimpton C, Gill P, D'Aloja E, Andersen JF, Bar W, Holgersson S, Jacobsen S, Johnsson V, Kloosterman AD, Lareu MV, Nellemann L, Pfitzinger H, Phillips CP, Rand[m] S, Schmitter H, Schneider PM, Sternersen M, Vide MC (1995) Report on the second EDNAP collaborative STR exercise. Forensic Sci Int 71:137-152

Polymeropoulos MH, Xiao H, Rath DS, Merril CR (1991) Tetranucleotide repeat polymorphism at the human tyrosine hydroxylase gene (TH). Nucleic Acids Res 19:4018

Population genetics of the STRs TPO, TH01 and VWFA31/A in S.Tomé e Príncipe

M.J. Prata, A. Amorim, L. Gusmão and M. J. Trovoada

Inst. Antropologia, Univ.Porto and IPATIMUP, 4050 Porto, Portugal

Systems and loci
TPO, repeat (AATG), intron 10 of thyroid peroxidase gene (2p23-pter)
TH01, repeat (TCAT), intron 1 of tyrosine hydroxylase gene (11p15.5-p15)
VWFA31/A, repeat (TCTR), intron 40 of von Willebrand factor gene (12p12-pter).

Population and sample sizes
S.Tomé e Príncipe (Gulf of Guinea)
TPO: N=147
TH01: N=143
VWFA31/A: N=133

Methods: Samples: blood from unrelated newborns; DNA extraction: method of Lareu *et al.* (1994); electrophoresis according to Luis and Caeiro (1995). Silver staining: Budowle *et al.* (1992);
TPO: primers (Anker *et al.*, 1992); amplification conditions: 5 min at 93°; 94°: 1 min; 63°: 0.5 min; 72°: 1.5 min; 27-35 cycles
TH01: primers (Gill *et al.*, 1994); amplification conditions: 5 min at 93°; 94°: 1 min; 54°: 1 min; 72°: 1 min; 27-35 cycles
VWFA31/A: primers (Kimpton *et al.*, 1992); amplification conditions: the same as for TH01.

Results:

Allele frequencies

TPO allele	Freq.	TH01 allele	Freq.	VWFA31/A allele	Freq.
6	0.065	6	0.091	13	0.026
7	0.034	7	0.357	14	0.083
8	0.388	8	0.346	15	0.184
9	0.197	9	0.150	16	0.286
10	0.075	9.3	0.049	17	0.199
11	0.214	10	0.007	18	0.135
12	0.027			19	0.056
				20	0.030

Observed genotypes

TPO genotypes	Obs.	TH01 genotypes	Obs.	VWFA31/A genotypes	Obs.
6-8	10	6-6	1	13-14	1
6-9	7	6-7	4	13-15	1
6-10	1	6-8	14	13-16	2
6-11	1	6-9	5	13-17	1
7-8	6	6-9.3	1	13-18	2
7-9	2	7-7	18	14-14	1
7-11	1	7-8	38	14-15	4
7-12	1	7-9	17	14-16	6
8-8	17	7-9.3	6	14-17	6
8-9	26	7-10	1	14-18	3
8-10	12	8-8	15	15-15	7
8-11	22	8-9	13	15-16	9
8-12	4	8-9.3	4	15-17	10
9-9	6	8-10	1	15-18	10
9-10	4	9-9	2	15-19	1
9-11	4	9-9.3	3	16-16	15
9-12	3	9-10	1	16-17	16
10-10	2			16-18	5
10-11	1			16-19	6
11-11	17			16-20	2
				17-17	3
				17-18	8
				17-19	4
				17-20	2
				18-18	2
				18-19	2
				18-20	2
				19-19	1
				20-20	1
see Comments section		P=0.73		P=0.49	

Comments:

Genotype distribution for TPO system is not in accordance with Hardy-Weinberg expectations. Sequential statistical analysis for each allele (Rand *et al.*, 1992) has demonstrated that only TPO*11 distribution is abnormal, with a large excess of homozygotes (χ^2 =25.2, 1d.f., P<0.001). Since another sample studied by us (N.Portugal) is in equilibrium, this finding is probably due to a specific feature of this locus in this population. Sequencing of a subsample is under progress. A new allele (7) was found, and allele 6, which is rare in Caucasians, has a rather high frequency in this sample; no other data on Blacks are available for comparisons.

Concerning TH01, a very low frequency for the allele 9.3 (still lower than in USA Blacks) was found; on the other hand, allele 8 exhibits a very high frequency.

In VWFA31/A system alleles 12 and 21 were not observed but allele 13, a rare allele both in Caucasians and USA Blacks, reached polymorphic proportions (2.6%).

References

Anker R, Steinbrueck T, Donis-Keller H (1992) Tetranucleotide repeat polymorphism at the human thyroid peroxidase (hTPO) locus. Hum Mol Genet 1: 137

Budowle B, Chakraborty R, Giusti AM, Eisenberg AJ, Allen RC (1991) Analysis of the VNTR locus D1S80 by the PCR followed by high-resolution PAGE. Am J Hum Genet 48: 137-144

Gill P, Kimpton C, D'Aloja E, Andersen JF, Bar W, Brinkmann B, Holgersson S, Johnson V, Kloosterman AD, Lareu MV, Nellemann L, Pfitzinger H, Phillips CP, Schmitter H, Schneider PM, Stenersen M (1994) Report of the European DNA profiling group (EDNAP) towards standardisation of short tandem repeat (STR) loci. Forensic Sci Int 65: 51-59

Kimpton C, Walton A, Gill P (1992) A further tetranucleotide repeat polymorphism in the vWF gene. Hum Mol Genet 1: 287

Lareu MV, Phillips CP, Carracedo A, Lincoln PJ, Court DS, Thomson JA (1994) Investigation of the STR locus HUMTH01 using PCR and two electrophoresis formats: UK and Galician Caucasian population surveys and usefulness in paternity investigations. Forensic Sci Int 66: 41-52

Luis JR, Caeiro B (1995) Application of two STRs (VWF and hTPO) to human population profiling. A survey in Galicia. Human Biology (in press)

Rand S, Puers C, Skowasch K, Wiegand P, Budowle B, Brinkmann B (1992) Population genetics and forensic efficiency data of 4 AMPFLPs. Int J Legal Med 104: 329-333

Acknowledgements This work was partially supported by JNICT (Junta Nacional de Investigação Científica e Tecnológica, BD/2849/93-ID and PBIC/C/CEN/1174/92) and CNCDP (Comissão Nacional para as Comemorações dos Descobrimentos Portugueses, research contract nº 70).

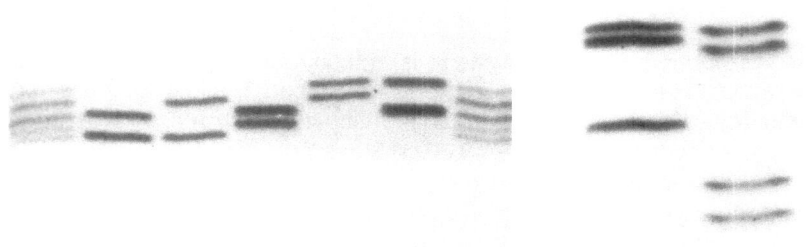

Fig.1. TH01 genotypes
From left to right: lane 1: ladder; lane 2: 8-9.3; lane 3: 7-9.3;lane 4: 8-9; lane 5: 6-7;lane 6: 6-8;lane 7: ladder.

Fig.2. Distinction of TH01 9, 9.3 and 10 alleles and heteroduplex analysis.
From left to right: lane 1: 9-9.3; lane 2: 9-10

AUTOMATED ANALYSIS OF 5 STR LOCI: ALLELE FREQUENCIES AND FAMILY STUDIES IN THE GERMAN POPULATION

J. Reinhold, J. Arnold
Institut für Labormedizin
Haugerkirchgasse 7, D-97070 Würzburg

Introduction

Analysis of polymorphic DNA loci by the polymerase chain reaction (PCR) technique is a very powerful tool not only in the field of criminal investigation but also in paternity testing. Compared to VNTR systems typed by Southern Blot hybridisation, STR elements offer considerable advantages concerning sensitivity, precision and reproducibility of fragment size estimates and biomathematical evaluation.

However, to reach the discrimination power of highly informative RFLP systems, at least the 2-fold number of STR loci has to be analyzed. Thus for both technical and economic reasons, an automated analysis / evaluation system is desirable for routine paternity testing. The Applied Biosystems 373A sequencer used in our laboratory allows the simultaneous electrophoretic separation and detection of the 5 STR loci HUMTH01, HUMFES/FPS, HUMvWF, D21S11 and ACTBP2 (also named SE33). We set up databases in order to establish reliable allele frequency distributions for the German population. Extensive family studies demonstrated autosomal codominant inheritance of segregating alleles at a very low rate of mutational events.

Material and Methods

Human genomic DNA was prepared from peripheral blood by a standard salting out procedure. [Miller, 1988]

PCR reactions were carried out in the the presence of 5'-fluorescence labelled primers. Mixtures contained: 5 ng template DNA, 2,5 µl 10 x PCR buffer (GeneAmp, ABI), 200 µM dNTPs, 0,25 µM primer a and b, 1,5 mM $MgCl_2$ and 1U Taq polymerase (AmpliTaq, ABI).

Primers: primer sequences as described by Kimpton (1993) 1. HUMTH01, GTG-strand 6-FAM labelled 2. HUMFES/FPS, GGG-strand TAMRA labelled 3. HUMvWF, CCC-strand HEX labelled 4. D21S11, TGT-strand 6-FAM labelled 5. ACTBP2, AAT-strand HEX/TAMRA labelled.

Amplification: 94°C - 15 sec, 55°C - 30 sec, 72°C - 60 sec, 30 cycles (primers 1-4); 94°C - 15 sec, 60°C - 30 sec, 72°C - 60 sec, 30 cycles (primers 5); Thermocycler: Perkin Elmer 9600

Electrophoresis and detection: Pooled PCR products were analyzed by an ABI 373A DNA sequencer using ABI 672 GeneScan analysis and collection software. Separation was carried out on 6% denaturing polyacrylamide gels (2000 V, 20 mA, 30 W, 8 h). Internal standard: GS 2500 ROX (ABI); ACTBP2 allelic ladder (HEX labelled) was reamplified from a 1:10.000 dilution of pooled DNA samples.

Results

Automated analysis of fluorescent PCR products amplified from HUMTH01, HUMvWF, HUMFES/FPS and D21S11 loci is a straightforward and highly reproducible method. Standard deviation of fragment size estimates within gels ranged from 0,04 bp (HUMTH01, allele 9,3) to 0,09 bp (D21S11, allele 50). Similar results were obtained for between-gel reproducibility. For these systems typing of individual alleles can therefore solely rely on fragment size estimates without using an allelic ladder. In contrast, the complex ACTBP2

Power of discrimination

Of the 5 loci under consideration, ACTBP2 is the most polymorphic one displaying at least 38 different alleles. Heterozygosity rates, power of exclusion and average probability of paternity are summarized in Table 2. The combined power of exclusion is 99,7%. This value is equivalent to the discrimination power of 2 -3 highly informative single locus systems.

At present we are validating a set of 7 STR loci markers (FGA and D18S51 as additional loci) with a discrimination power corresponding to 4 SLS. We speculate that in the near future automated PCR analysis will completely replace RFLP methodology in routine paternity cases .

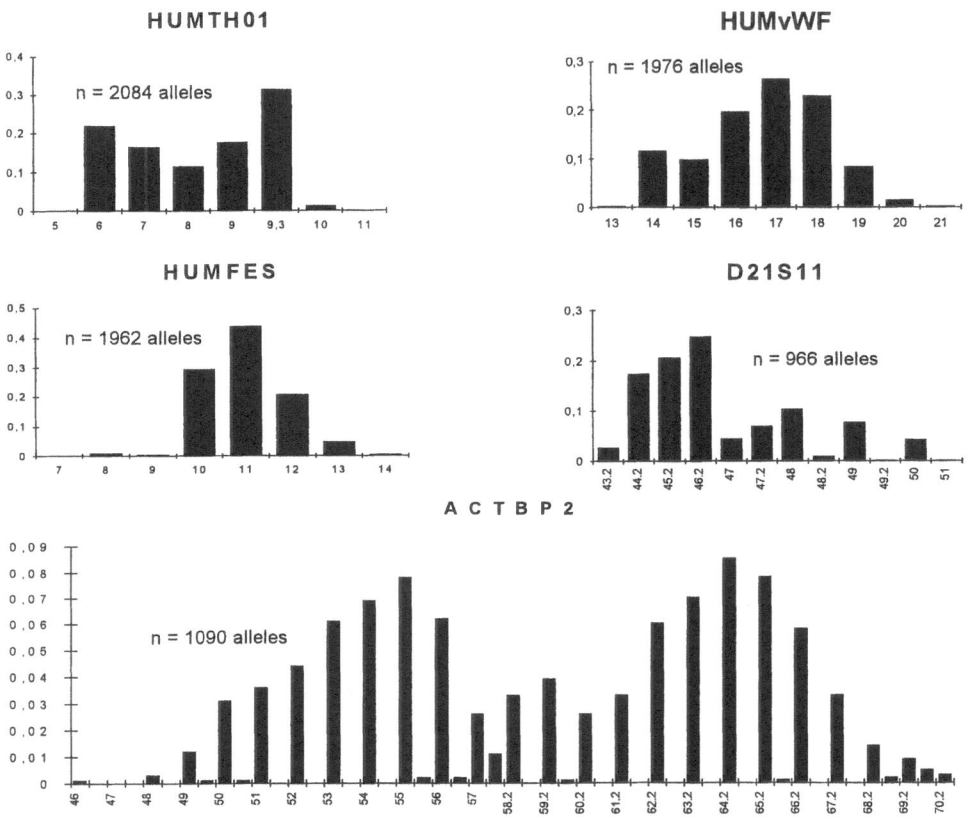

Figure 2: Allelic distribution at 5 STR loci. Nomenclature for HUMTH01, HUMFES/FPS and HUMvWF is based on sequencing data; nomenclature for D21S11 and ACTBP2 refers to Schmitter (1995) / personal communication.

References

Kimpton C. P., Gill P., Walton A., Urquhart A., Millican E. S. and Adams M. (1993). PCR Methods and Applications. **3**: 13 - 22

Miller S. A., Dykes D. D. and Polesky H. F. (1988). A salting out procedure for extracting DNA from human nucleated cells. Nucleic Acids Res. **16**: 1215

Schmitter H., Sonntag M.-L. (1995). Proposal for general rules for the denominations of alleles of STR-loci based on the electrophoretic mobilities of their fragments. Klin. Lab. **41**: 173 - 176

locus demonstrates a consistently higher standard deviation (up to 0,19 bp within gels and 0,61 bp between gels), so that identification of alleles differing by just 1 bp was not possible in each case. We therefore decided to use an allelic ladder as additional internal standard. DNA samples were labelled with TAMRA, the ladder labelled with HEX. Difference in electrophoretic mobility due to different dyes was in the range of 0,1 - 0,2 bp for a given fragment. As sizing errors within a single lane affect both ladder and sample to the same extent, this method allows identification of ACTBP2 alleles with very high precision (Figure 1). Very rare events of overlapping ACTBP2/FES alleles can be simply clarified by separate analysis of the respective fragments.

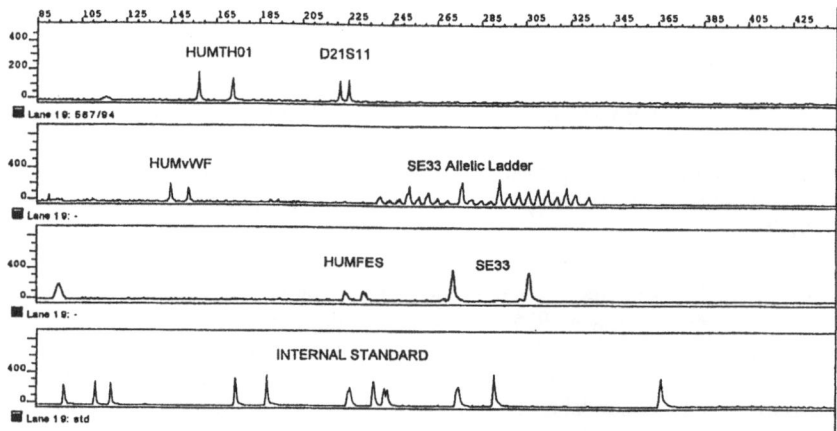

Figure 1: Electrophoretogram display of PCR-products of 5 STR systems run in the same gel lane

For all STR systems we set up data bases with a large population sample originating from southern and middle Germany. Allelic distributions (n = 966 - 2084 fragments) are shown in Figure 2. Chi square tests performed with all systems indicated that there is no significant deviation from the assumed Hardy-Weinberg equilibrium (data not shown).

Family studies

With regard to paternity testing, genetic stability of polymorphic DNA loci is of major interest. As a guideline, de novo mutation rates should not exceed 1%. We carried out extensive family studies consisting mainly of paternity cases investigated parallel to 12 conventional bloodgroup markers. Altogether 435 - 938 parent / child combinations were investigated for each system. Table 1 shows the individual mutation rates associated with the 5 loci. We conclude that these 5 STR loci are genetically stable and do not give rise to false exclusions as seen with some single locus systems.

Table 1: Genetic stability of STR loci

System	meiosis	mutat. events	rate
HUMTH01	938	0	< 0,11
HUMFES	870	0	< 0,12
HUMvWF	862	0	< 0,12
D21S11	435	0	< 0,23
ACTBP2	481	1	0,21

Table 2: Discrimination power of 5 STR systems

System	Hetero-zygosity	Power of exclusion	Mean EM value
HUMTH01	78,3%	57,0%	9,6335
HUMFES	67,8%	46,7%	9,7267
HUMvWF	81,1%	61,8%	9,5821
D21S11	83,9%	67,5%	9,5119
ACTBP2	94,7%	89,0%	9,0414
Combined		99,7%	7,4956

SOUTHERN SPAIN POPULATION FREQUENCIES OF THE LOCI LDLR, GYPA, HBGG, D7S8 AND Gc. A COMPARISON BETWEEN ANDALUSIAN AND CANARY ISLANDS FREQUENCIES.

PRIETO V, ANDRES MI, FLORES IC, SANZ P.

National Institute of Toxicology. Seville. Spain.

Introduction

The AmpliType® PM PCR Amplification and Typing Kit was developed by Roche Molecular Systems USA. It simultaneously coamplifies HLA DQα, LDLR (Low density lipoprotein receptor), GYPA (Glycophorin A), HBGG (hemoglobin G gammaglobin), D7S8 and Gc (group specific component) and types the last five loci in a single reverse dot blot strip. Its use is widespread and it was proved to be specially useful due to its high sensitivity, very close to that obtained with the HLA-DQα system (Espinheira 1994; Pinheiro 1994; Reena 1995; Budowle 1995).

Before a genetic marker can be used for the analysis of evidentiary samples its forensic applicability should be evaluated. This multiplex Amplification and Typing kit has been widely validated (Herrin 1994; Budowle 1995; Reena 1995; Fildes 1995; Sanz 1994). In addition, the routine use in identity testing, both in forensic casework and paternity testing, needs statistical evaluation, therefore a reference population database must be established by each laboratory. Since the routine work in our laboratory, located in Southern Spain, involves populations of Andalusia and the Canary Islands, we have undertaken a comparison between the two populations in order to assess the applicability of common or separate databases. The correspondence between PCR genotyping and IEF phenotyping results for Gc, including individuals showing rare migrating protein patterns, is also reported.

Material and Methods

Blood samples were taken from 158 individuals (106 Andalusian and 52 from the Canary Islands) from our casework and staff. DNA extraction was achieved using Chelating Agent (Sigma) according to Perkin Elmer Cetus Corporation protocols. Amplification and Typing was performed with the AmpliType PM kit (Perkin Elmer®) and according to protocols provided by the manufacturer. The cycling reaction was carried out in a Perkin Elmer 480 Thermocycler.

Statistical Analysis

The frequency of each allele for each locus was calculated from the numbers of each genotype in the sample set. Possible divergence from Hardy-Weinberg equilibrium was determined by the Chi-square test. Comparison between populations were also carried out by the Chi-square test. Estimates of heterozygosity and combined power of discrimination (PD) and a priori chance of exclusion (CE) were calculated.

Results

Table 1

Locus	Genotype	ANDALUSIA Observed N	%	All. Freq.	CANARY ISLANDS Observed N	%	All. Freq.
LDLR	AA	28	26.41	A=0.4953	12	23.08	A=0.4231
	AB	49	46.23	B=0.5047	20	38.46	B=0.5769
	BB	29	27.36	X^2=0.6039	20	38.46	X^2=2.3357
				df=1 p=0.4371			df=1 p=0.1264
GYPA	AA	28	26.41	A=0.5094	12	23.08	A=0.4615
	AB	52	49.06	B=0.4906	24	46.15	B=0.5385
	BB	26	24.53	X^2=0.0362	16	30.77	X^2=0.2649
				df=1 p=0.8490			df=1 p=0.6068
D7S8	AA	35	33.02	A=0.5849	9	17.31	A=0.4712
	AB	54	50.94	B=0.4151	31	59.61	B=0.5288
	BB	17	16.04	X^2=0.2551	12	23.08	X^2=2.0027
				df=1 p=0.6135			df=1 p=0.1570
HBGG	AA	27	25.47	A=0.4953	14	26.92	A=0.5481
	AB	51	48.11	B=0.4906	27	51.92	B=0.4327
	AC	0	- *	C=0.0142	2	3.58*	C=0.0192
	BB	25	23.58	X^2=0.0538	9	17.31	X^2=1.1435
	BC	3	2.83*	df=1 p=0.8167	0	- *	df=1 p=0.2849
	CC	0	- *		0	- *	
Gc	AA	12	11.32*	A=0.3160	3	5.77*	A=0.2212
	AB	12	11.32	B=0.1840	4	7.69*	B=0.2115
	AC	31	29.24	C=0.5000	13	25.00	C=0.5673
	BB	2	1.89*	X^2=0.8353	3	5.77*	X^2=0.0296
	BC	23	21.70	df=2 p=0.6586	12	23.08	df=1 p=0.8634
	CC	26	24.53		17	32.69	

*pooled classes

Table 2 Comparison between the two populations

	LDLR	GYPA	D7S8	HBGG	Gc
X^2	2.9396	0.3011	2.2578	1.1973	0.8649
df	4	4	4	6	6
p	0.5680	0.9897	0.6885	0.9770	0.9902

No statistically significant differences were found between them

Table 3 Allelic frequencies and heterozygosity of both populations

	LDLR	GYPA	D7S8	HBGG	Gc
Allele Frequency	A=0.4715 B=0.5285	A=0.4937 B=0.5063	A=0.5475 B=0.4525	A=0.5127 B=0.4715 C=0.0158	A=0.2848 B=0.1930 C=0.5221
Heterozygosity (%)	43.67	48.10	53.80	52.53	60.13

Combined Power of Discrimination = 0.9957

Combined Power of Exclusion = 0.7472

Genotyping of Gc variants

Rare migrating IEF patterns, occasionally encountered in our casework and typed according to the recommendations of the International Workshop of the Gc system held in 1978 (Westwood 1986), were submitted to genotyping with the PM AmpliType® kit which was considered to unambiguously type 2, 1F and 1S Gc alleles (Reynolds 1990). The following results were obtained: Gc IEF phenotyping   1S1C   1F1C   1S1A   1S1C

     Gc PM genotyping   BC   BB   CC   CC

Comments:

1.- Cathodic variants of Gc-1 were genotyped as B allele (1F) or C allele (1S). The first example corresponds to a paternity case where the child received the rare allele from the alleged father. PM genotyping alone would reduce paternity index.

2.- Anodic variant of Gc-1 resulted as C allele (1S) or, presumably, was undetected (not amplified or not hybridated).

References

- Budowle B, Lindsey JA, DeCou JA, Koons BW, Giusti AM, Comey CT (1995) Validation and Population Studies of The Loci LDLR, GYPA, HBGG, D7S8 and Gc (PM loci), and HLA-DQA1 Using a Multiplex Amplification and Typing Procedure. JFSCAS 40(1): 45-54

- Espinheira R, Ribeiro T, Geada H, Reys L (1994) Polymarker and HLA DQA1 Genetic Markers in Forensic Casework. In: Mangin P, Ludes B (eds) Acta Medicinae Legalis Vol. XLIV. Springer Berlin Heidelberg, New York, pp. 37-38

- Fildes N, Reynolds R (1995) Consistency and Reproducibility of AmpliType® PM Results Between Seven Laboratories: Field Trial Results. JFSCAS 40(2): 279-286

- Herrin G, Fildes N, Reynolds R (1994) Evaluation of the AmpliType® PM DNA Test System on Forensic Case Samples. JFSCAS 39(5): 1247-1253

- Pinheiro MF, Pontes ML, Pinto da Costa J (1994) Use of the AmpliType® PM Coamplification System on Forensic Analysis. In: Mangin P, Ludes B (eds) Acta Medicinae Legalis Vol. XLIV. Springer Berlin Heidelberg, New York, pp. 81-82

- Reena R, Reynolds R (1995) AmpliType® PM and HLA DQA1 Typing from Pap Smear, Semen Smear, and Postcoital Slides. JFSCAS 40(2): 266-269

- Reynolds RL, Sensabaugh GF (1990) Use of The Polymerase Chain Reaction for Typing Gc Variants. In: Polesky HF, Mayr WR (eds) Advances in Forensic Haemogenetics vol 3. Springer-Verlag, Berlin Heidelberg, pp 158-161

- Sanz P, Prieto V (1994) Application of the AmpliType® PM coamplification system to forensic casework. In: Mangin P, Ludes B (eds) Acta Medicinae Legalis Vol. XLIV. Springer Berlin Heidelberg, New York, pp. 85-86

- Westwood SA, Werrett DJ (1986) Group-Specific Component: A Review of The Isoelectric Focusing Methods and Auxiliary Methods Available for the Separation of its Phenotypes. For Sci Int 32: 135-150

ALLELE FREQUENCY DISTRIBUTION OF D2S44, D12S11, D7S21, D7S22 AND D5S43 LOCI IN SOUTHERN SPAIN.

G Repetto, IC Flores and P Sanz.

National Institute of Toxicology, P.O. Box 863, 41080 - Sevilla, Spain.

INTRODUCTION

DNA analysis of restriction fragment length polymorphisms (RFLP's) has become one of the most powerful methods in forensic science casework and paternity testing. Nearly all laboratories working in the field of paternity testing and stain analysis prefer single locus probes (SLP's) because these probes have a better sensitivity than multilocus probes and offer the possibility of building a database for the allele frequency. We have implemented in routine case work in our laboratory the use of 5 single locus probes and the results of DNA analysis are reported as frequency data.

The forensic use of this technique is regarded as valid and reliable (NRC, 1992; Lander and Budowle, 1994). However, interpretation of test results is highly dependent on the population genetics of the markers, and a sufficiently large database of the relevant population must be established. The purpose of this study was to develop a frequency database for five hypervariable loci (D2S44, D12S11, D7S21, D7S22 and D5S43) of the population of our area (S Spain).

MATERIALS AND METHODS

DNA from blood samples of 110 unrelated individuals of southern Spain was extracted according to the method of Gill et al (1987, 1991) using phenol/chloroform. Complete restriction of DNA was carried out with the enzyme Hinf I. DNA was then quantified using a Hoefer TKO100 DNA fluorometer.

Size separation of restricted DNA and K562 / Hinf I digest genomic control DNA was achieved by electrophoresis in a 0.7% agarose gel running in TBE buffer for 18 hours (Gill et al, 1992). Following denaturation the DNA was transferred onto a nylon membrane and the DNA was fixed by ultraviolet irradiation. Alkaline phosphatase conjugated single locus probes MS31, MS43a, G3, MS8 and MS43a from Cellmark Diagnostics and YNH24 from Promega Corporation were used sequentially.

All autoradiographs were analysed using a computerized digital image analysis system (Bioimage, Millipore Corp.) which utilised the Elder and Southern method (1987) for band size calculation with reference to molecular weight markers (BRL/NICE). Data points were recorded at 0.01 kb intervals and binned to 0.1 kb for generation of the histograms.

RESULTS AND DISCUSSION

Our findings on VNTR allele frequency distribution in the population of Southern Spain are presented in Fig. 1. A summary of data is also presented in Table 1.

The histograms generated by our data show good correlation with previously published, caucasian data collections where loci and restriction enzyme are in common (Gill et al. 1991; Brinkman et al. 1991; Odelberg et al. 1989; Valverde et al., 1992).

Table 1: Allele size range, most frequent size range, frequency of the most common size range and heterozigosity of the five VNTR-loci studied on the population of Southern Spain (N=110).

Genetic locus	D2S44	D12S11	D7S21	D7S22	D5S43
DNA-probe	YNH24	MS43a	MS31	G3	MS8
Allele size range (Kbp)	1.86-9.61	2.90-14.78	2.46-9.97	1.66-14.78	2.33-9.16
Most frequent size range (Kbp)	2.65-2.75	9.05-9.15 9.15-9.25	5.45-5.55	3.15-3.25	6.65-6.75
Frequency of most common size range (%)	11.7	12.08	6.43	4.76	12.08
Heterozygosity (%)	95.75	95.10	95.05	83.33	85.0

REFERENCES

Brinkmann B, Rand S and Wiegand P (1991) Population and family data of RFLP's using selected single and multilocus systems. Int J Leg Med 104: 81-86.

Elder JK and Southern EM (1987) Computer aided analysis of one dimensional restriction fragment gels. In: Bishop MJ and Rawlings CJ (eds) Nucleic acid and protein sequence analysis. IRL Press, Oxford, pp 165-172.

Gill P, Lygo JE, Fowler SJ and Werrett DJ (1987) An evaluation of DNA fingerprinting for forensic purposes. Electrophoresis, 8: 38-44.

Gill P, Woodroffe S, Lygo JE and Millican ES (1991) Population Genetics of Four Hypervariable Loci. Int J Leg Med 104: 221-227.

Gill P, Woodroffe S, Bär W, Brinkman B, Carracedo A, Eriksen B, Jones S, Kloosterman AD, Ludes B, Mevag B, Pascali VL, Rudler M, Schmitter H, Scneider PM and Thompson JA (1992) A report of an international collaborative experiment to demonstrate the uniformity obtainable using DNA profiling techniques. Forensic Science International 53: 29-43.

Lander ES and Budowle B (1994) DNA fingerprinting dispute laid to rest. Nature 371: 735-738.

NRC (1992). DNA technology in forensic science. National Research Council. National Academy Press, Washington DC.

Odelberg SJ, Plaetke R, Eldridge JR, Ballard L, O'Connell P, Nakamura Y, Leppert M, Lalouel JM and White R (1989) Characterization of eight VNTR Loci by Agarose Gel Electrophoresis. Genomics 5: 915-924.

Valverde E, Cabrero C, Diez A, Carracedo A and Borras T (1992) Allele frequency in the population of Spain using several single locus probes. Advances in Forensic Haemogenetics 4. Ed Rittner C, Schneider PM, Springer Verlag, Berlin, pp 187-189.

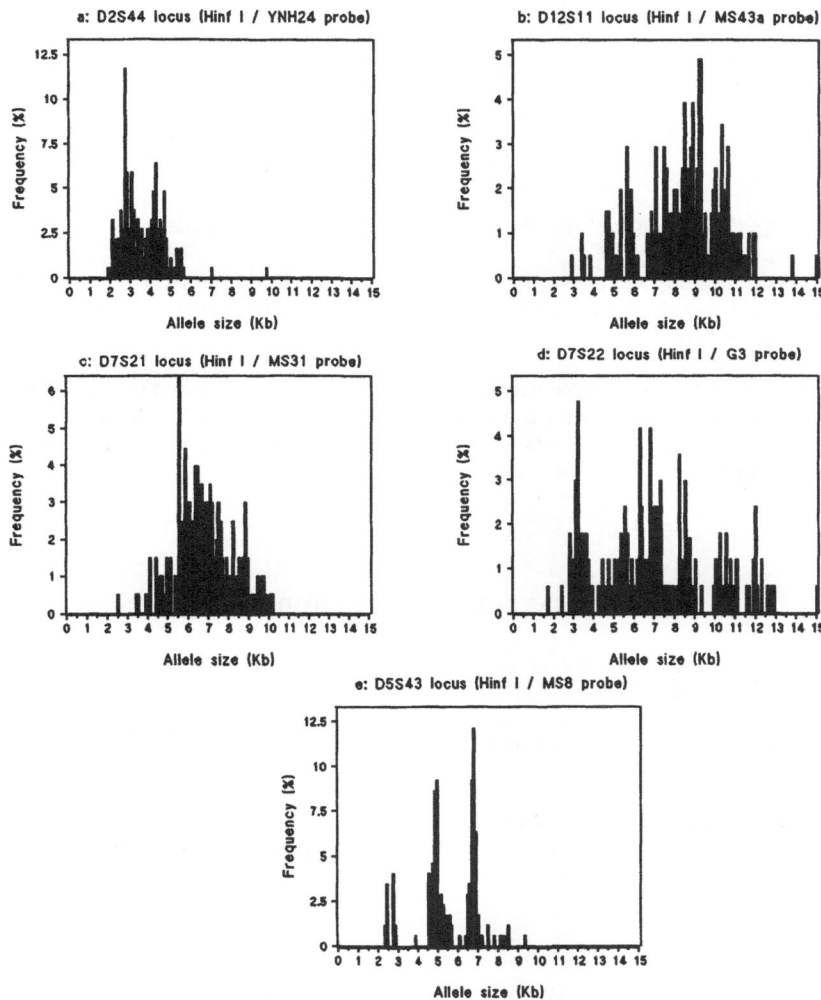

Figure 1: Distribution pattern of allele frequencies for D2S44 (a), D12S11 (b), D7S21 (c), D7S22 (d) and D5S43 (e) loci in the population of Southern Spain (N=110)

HLA-DQA1 POLYMORPHISM IN TWO PORTUGUESE POPULATION SAMPLES FROM LISBON AND THE SOUTH OF PORTUGAL

SM. Santos*, F. Simões**, A. Armada**, A. Clemente**, MC. Correia*.

*Forensic Science Laboratory, Polícia Judiciária, Lisboa, Portugal.
**INETI-Department of Biotechnology-BQ2, Queluz, Portugal.

INTRODUCTION

The HLA-DQA1 polymorphism provides a powerful tool to forensic analysis.

The purpose of this study was to analyse the HLA-DQA1 locus in view of its application in forensic casework, as recommended by the DNA Commission of the International Society for Forensic Haemogenetics (1992).

We describe the allele and genotype frequencies of two portuguese population samples from Lisbon and from the South of Portugal that have been investigated for HLA-DQA1 locus by the polymerase chain reaction (PCR), (Saiki et al, 1986; Comey et al,1991), using allele specific .oligonucleotides and reverse dot-blot methodology (Cetus).

MATERIAL AND METHODS

Blood samples from 120 unrelated individuals from Lisbon and 104 unrelated individuals from the South of Portugal were studied.

DNA was extracted from the blood stains using a chelating resin according to the method developed by Singer-Sam et al, (1989).

Amplification of the DNA samples and allele typing were performed using the Amplitype HLA-DQ Alpha Forensic Amplification and Typing Kit (Perkin-Elmer Cetus).

RESULTS AND DICUSSION

The distribution of observed and expected HLA-DQA1 genotypes and the allele frequencies for the two portuguese population samples are shown in Table 1, and no deviation from Hardy-Weinberg equilibrium was observed.

The similarity between the heterozygosity rate and the allelic diversity value (h) of both population samples is in good agreement with Hardy-Weinberg equilibrium (Table 2).

Table 1. Distribution of observed and expected HLA-DQA1 genotypes and allele frequencies.

GENOTYPE	LISBON (n=120)		SOUTH PORTUGAL (n=104)	
	observed	expected	observed	expected
1.1-1.1	6	4.22	1	1.88
1.1-1.2	4	4.69	4	4.58
1.1-1.3	0	4.50	2	3.23
1.1-2	6	6.37	6	5.25
1.1-3	9	6.19	5	3.90
1.1-4	14	14.81	9	7.27
1.2-1.2	1	1.31	3	2.78
1.2-1.3	4	2.50	5	3.92
1.2-2	2	3.54	8	6.38
1.2-3	3	3.44	4	4.74
1.2-4	10	8.23	7	8.83
1.3-1.3	0	1.20	2	1.38
1.3-2	6	3.40	5	4.50
1.3-3	4	3.30	5	3.35
1.3-4	10	7.90	3	6.23
2-2	3	2.41	2	3.66
2-3	6	4.68	6	5.44
2-4	8	11.20	10	10.13
3-3	2	2.27	0	2.02
3-4	7	10.86	9	7.53
4-4	15	13.00	8	7.01
χ^2 df=15	15.81 0.25<p<0.50		9.09 0.75<p<0.90	

ALLELES						
	1.1	1.2	1.3	2	3	4
Lisbon	0.1875	0.1042	0.1000	0.1417	0.1375	0.3291
South Portugal	0.1346	0.1635	0.1154	0.1875	0.1394	0.2596

Table 2. Statistical parameters.

	PD	h	Heterozygosity
Lisbon	0.931	0.800	0.775
South Portugal	0.942	0.824	0.846

The power of discrimination (PD) was estimated for Lisbon population sample (0.931), and for the South of Portugal population sample (0.942).

The data showed that for both samples the most frequent allele was HLA-DQA1*4 and the less frequent allele was HLA-DQA1*1.3. Differences in allele distributions were observed for the HLA-DQA1*1.1 allele (Lisbon= 0.1875; South Portugal=0.1346) and the HLA-DQA1*1.2 allele (Lisbon= 0.1042; South Portugal=0.1635)

The allele frequencies distribution of both population samples were similar to other Caucasian data, mainly from Portugal and Spain (Lareu et al, 1993; Martin et al, 1993; Pascal et al, 1993; Sanz et al, 1993).

Acknowledgements: The authors are grateful to the Department of Biology, Institute of Legal Medicine, University of Coimbra for providing useful information.

REFERENCES

Comey CT and Budowle B (1991) Validation Studies on the Analysis of the HLA-DQ Alpha Locus using polymerase Chain Reaction. Journal of Forensic Sciences 36: 239-249.

DNA Commission of the International Society for Forensic Haemogenetics (1992) Second DNA recommendations. Int. J. Leg. Med. 104:361-364.

Lareu MV, Munoz I, Pestoni C, Rodriguez MS, Vide C, Carracedo A (1993). The distribution of HLA-DQA1 and D1S80 (pMCT 118) alleles and genotypes in the population of Galicia and Central Portugal. Int J Leg Med 106:124-128.

Martin P, Garcia O, Alonso A, Albarran C, Aguirre A, Sancho M. (1993) HLA-DQA1 Subtyping by PCR Follwed by a Combined SSO/RFLP Method of Detection. Distribution of Alleles and Genotypes in Two Spanish Populations. In: Advances in Forensic Haemogenetics 5. Springer-Verlag, Berlin, Heidelberg, pp535-553.

Pascal O, Levayer T, Aubert D, Peneau A, Markey P, Moisan JP, (1993) French Population Data of 6 AMPLF'S. In: Advances in Forensic Haemogenetics 5. Springer-Verlag, Berlin, Heidelberg, pp542-544.

Sanz P, Repetto G, Prieto V, Flores I, HLA-DQA1 and D1S80 Polymorphism in the Population of Andaluzia (Southern Spain) In: Advances in Forensic Haemogenetics 5. Springer-Verlag. Berlin Heidelberg, pp.572-574.

Saiki RK, Bugawan GT, Horn GT, Mullis KB, Erlich HS. (1986) Analysis of enzymatically amplified B-globin and HLA-DQA1 DNA with allelic-specific oligonucleotide probes. Nature 324: 163-166.

Singer-Sam J, Tanguay RL, Riggs AD, (1989) Use of chelex to improve the PCR Signal from a small number of cells. Amplifications 3:11.

D1S80 LOCUS POLYMORPHISM IN A POPULATION SAMPLE FROM LISBON

SM. Santos*, F. Simões**, A. Armada**, A. Clemente**, MC. Correia*.

*Forensic Science Laboratory, Polícia Judiciária, Lisboa, Portugal.
**INETI-Department of Biotechnology-BQ2, Queluz, Portugal.

INTRODUCTION

The amplification of the D1S80 locus, a variable number of tandem repeats (VNTR) locus, by the polymerase chain reaction (PCR), (Saiki et al, 1985) is an effective tool to forensic analysis (Budowle et al, 1995).

The objective of this work was to analyse the polymorphism of D1S80 locus in order to apply the data in forensic casework, as recommended by the DNA Commission of the International Society for Forensic Haemogenetics (1992).

This study was performed on a portuguese population sample from Lisbon.

MATERIAL AND METHODS

Blood samples were collected from 110 unrelated individuals from Lisbon.

DNA was extracted from blood stains using a chelating resin according to the method developed by Singer-Sam et al, (1989).

Amplification of the DNA samples was carried out by following the recommended protocol of the D1S80 Forensic DNA Amplification Reagent Set (Perkin-Elmer Cetus). PCR products were separated on Phast Gels 10-15 (Pharmacia LKB) and visualised by silver staining according to the method described by Barros et al, (1992).

RESULTS AND DISCUSSION

In the Lisbon population sample, 20 different D1S80 alleles were found and the most common alleles were 24 (f=0.3409) and 18 (f=0.2273).

The distribution of the observed D1S80 genotypes and the allele frequencies for the Lisbon population sample are shown in Table 1 and Fig. 1. forty three different genotypes were found and the most frequent genotype was 18-24 (f= 0.1273). As there are a large number of possible genotypes, for determining whether or not this population sample is in Hardy-Weinberg equilibrium, any genotype with less than five observations, was pooled (X^2 =7.996; df=7; 0.25<p<0.50), (Budowle et al, 1991). This procedure was repeated with different allelic groups and no deviation was observed.

Table 1. Distribution of observed D1S80 genotypes from 110 individuals

Observed Genotypes	n	Observed Genotypes	n	Observed Genotypes	n	Observed Genotypes	n
16-24	1	18-29	6	22-24	2	24-36	1
17-24	1	18-31	2	22-25	1	25-27	1
18-18	6	18-33	1	22-29	1	25-28	2
18-20	1	18-37	1	22-31	1	25-29	1
18-21	2	19-22	1	24-24	16	25-30	1
18-22	3	20-29	1	24-25	4	28-29	1
18-24	14	20-34	1	24-27	2	28-30	1
18-25	1	21-24	3	24-28	5	29-29	3
18-26	2	21-25	1	24-29	4	29-37	1
18-27	1	21-26	1	24-31	5	31-36	1
18-28	4	21-29	1	24-32	1		

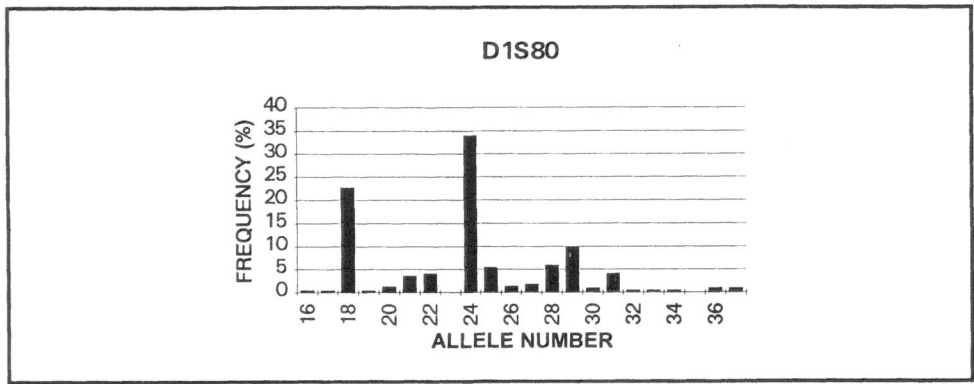

Figure 1. distribution of D1S80 alleles in a population sample from Lisbon (n= 110)

The observed heterozygosity (0.773) and the allelic diversity (h=0.814) for this sample are in agreement with Hardy-Weinberg equilibrium.

The discrimination power (PD) of D1S80 locus for this population sample was estimated as 0.9446.

A comparison between the allele frequencies distribution for Lisbon population sample and other Caucasians data, mainly from Portugal and Spain, showed only slight differences (Budowle et al, 1995; Lareu et al, 1993; Sanz et al, 1993).

Acknowledgements: The authors are grateful to the Department of Biology, Institute of Legal Medicine, University of Coimbra for providing useful information.

REFERENCES

Budowle B, Chakraborty R, Giusti AM, Eisenberg AJ, Allen RC (1991) Analysis of the VNTR Locus D1S80 by the PCR Followed by High Resolution PAGE. Am J Hum Genet 48:137-144.

Budowle B, Baechtel FS, Smerick JB, Presley KW, Giusti AM, Parsons G, Alevy MC, Chakraborty R (1995) D1S80 Population Data in African Americans, Caucasians, Southeastern Hispanics, Southwestern Hispanics, and Orientals Journal of Forensic Sciences 40:38-44.

Barros F, Lareu MV, Carracedo A (1992) Detection of Polymorphisms of Human DNA after polymerase chain reaction by minituarized SDS-PAGE. Forensic Sci Int 55:27-36.

DNA Commission of the International Society for Forensic Haemogenetics (1992) Second DNA recommendations. Int. J. Leg. Med. 104:361-364.

Lareu MV, Munoz I, Pestoni C, Rodriguez MS, Vide C, Carracedo A (1993). The distribution of HLA-DQA1 and D1S80 (pMCT118) alleles and genotypes in the population of Galicia and Central Portugal. Int J Leg Med 106:124-128.

Saiki RK, Scharf S, Faloona F, Mullis KB, Erlich HS, Arnheim R, (1985) Enzymatic amplification of betaglobin genomic sequences and restriction analysis for diagnosis of sickle cell anemia. Science 230: 1350-1354.

Sanz P, Repetto G, Prieto V, Flores I, HLA-DQA1 and D1S80 Polymorphism in the Population of Andaluzia (Southern Spain) In: Advances in Forensic Haemogenetics 5. Springer-Verlag. Berlin Heidelberg, pp.572-574.

Singer-Sam J, Tanguay RL, Riggs AD, (1989) Use of chelex to improve the PCR Signal from a small number of cells. Amplifications 3:11.

AMPFLP-TYPING OF THE D21S11 MICROSATELLITE POLYMORPHISM: ALLELE FREQUENCIES AND SEQUENCING DATA IN THE AUSTRIAN POPULATION

D.W.M.Schwartz, E.M.Dauber, B.Glock, W.R.Mayr

Clinical Department for Blood Group Serology,

University of Vienna

Waehringer Guertel 18-20/4I, A-1090 Vienna, Austria

INTRODUCTION

Human DNA microsatellite polymorphisms (Variable Number of Tandem Repeats, VNTR) with short repeat sizes (2-5bp) have become very useful markers in forensic haemogenetics in the last few years. For a number of reasons, typing for these markers is more and more preferred to conventional techniques in forensic casework:

- The large number, high polymorphism and thus the high information content of microsatellite markers
- The use of just one technique (PCR-Amplification Fragment Length Polymorphism, AMPFLP) for all markers
- The possibility to successfully employ these markers even for very low amounts of highly degraded stains

However, it must be stated that there are still some problems and restrictions with these systems. Typing by AMPFLP on polyacrylamide gels is not always very clear-cut, especially with certain markers (e.g. APOB, SE33) because of interalleles (variants with incomplete repeats or sequence variants with distinct electrophoretic mobility) and/or the limited resolution capability of electrophoresis. The allele frequency distribution in different populations has shown significant differences for certain systems, whereas other loci showed a more uniform distribution, at least in the populations studied so far. Since the amount of data is limited, especially for the microsatellites with short core repeat length (Short Tandem Repeats, STR) population studies are still required. Furthermore, detailed sequencing studies should also be performed for all markers in forensic use since only with this technique the polymorphism can be determined to the ultimate level. For routine use the AMPFLP technique will still stay the standard, but it is required that a marker consisting of alleles with known sequence is used with this technique [DNA comission of the ISFH, 1994]. In this work, we established optimized conditions for AMPFLP-typing of the tetranucleotide polymorphism at the D21S11 locus (Genbank M84567, [Sharma 1992]) and determined allele and genotype frequencies in our local (Austrian) population based on the alleles that could by resolved by AMPFLP. Sequencing studies were undertaken to define the alleles included in the marker and to identify sequence variants which have been previously reported for this locus [Moeller 1994].

MATERIAL AND METHODS

Population sample

A total of 200 healthy, unrelated indivduals (caucasians) of both sexes from Vienna were included in this study. Genomic DNA was extracted by standard techniques.

Primers

According to Sharma [1992] (Tab.2).

PCR

40ng template DNA, 0.4µM each primer, 2U polymerase (Dynazyme™, Finn Zymes Oy), 1x PCR buffer (50mM KCl, 10mM TrisCl pH=9.0 at 25°C, 0.1% Triton-X-100 and 1.5mM MgCl2) and 200µM of each dNTP, final volume 50µl overlaid with 50µl paraffine oil;
Hybaid Omnigene thermocycler;

first cycle	98°C 5min	62°C 10min	
26 cycles	94°C 60sec	62°C 60sec	72°C 75sec
last cycle	72°C 75sec		

Electrophoresis

PAGE was carried out as previously described [Schwartz 1994] on 6% native polyacrylamide gels (C=3%) in 112mM Tris-Acetic Acid rehydration buffer and 200mM Tris-Tricine electrode buffer.
running conditions: ramp: 1200V 12mA 10min
                      final   1200V 20mA
Subsequent silver staining was applied to visualize DNA [Bassam et al. 1991]. Typing was done by side-to-side comparison with the allelic ladder.

Allelic ladder

Single bands of heterozygous population samples, corresponding to distinct alleles, were eluted from the gel. DNA was purified using Wizard PCR Preps DNA Purification System (Promega, technical bulletin), diluted and reamplified. Equal concentrations of reamplification products were pooled to construct an allelic ladder.

Sequencing

Single strand sequence determination of the different alleles was performed using an automatic DNA-Sequencer (ALF™, Pharmacia LKB Technology) according to the protocol of the Pharmacia AutoRead™ Sequencing Kit (dye primers, T7 polymerase) on a 6% sequencing gel. A total of 37 alleles was sequenced including at least one sample for each distinct allele (as judged by AMPFLP). For each sample the sense and the antisense-strand were sequencend.

RESULTS AND DISCUSSION

AMPFLP typing

A total number of 12 alleles could be identified by PCR-AMPFLP in the population sample (Tab.1). These alleles were compared to the allelic ladder kindly provided by B. Brinkmann and designated according to the proposed nomenclature [Moeller 1994]. From the electrophoretic moblilty, it was not possible to clearly assign alleles 30.2, 31.2 and 32 (Fig.1). So two provisional designations were made: 30s and 31s (s=slow). Allele frequencies, mean paternity exclusion chance (MEC), mean exclusion probability (MEP) and polymorphism information content (PIC) are given in Tab.1. No significant deviation from Hardy-Weinberg expectations was observed.

Table 1: D21S11 allele frequencies (n=200)

allele designation	frequency (%)
25	0.3
26	0.3
27	2.8
28	21.5
29	19.8
30	23.8
30s	9.0
31	11.8
31s	0.8
32.2	5.5
33.2	4.3
34.2	0.5

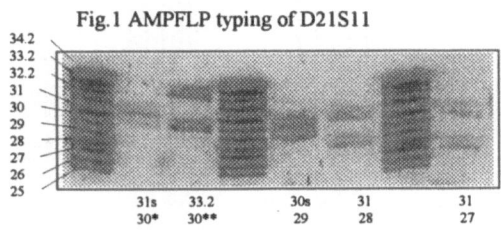

Fig.1 AMPFLP typing of D21S11

| 31s | 33.2 | 30s | 31 | 31 |
| 30* | 30** | 29 | 28 | 27 |

* variant 6-5-11
** variant 4-6-12 according to Tab.2

Mean paternity exclusion chance (MEC)   0.665
Mean exclusion probability (MEP)   0.661
Polymorphism information content (PIC)   0.809

Sequencing:

As already described [Moeller 1994], at the molecular level D21S11 actually contains 3 polymorphic regions (vrI-III, Tab.2). vrI consists of a (tcta)-tetranucleotide that shows a variation from 4-7 repeats. Just adjacent, vrII 2 shows either 3, 5 or 6 (tctg)-blocks. The most polymorphic part is vrIII that shows from 8-14 (tcta)-repeats. Additionally, in some alleles a constant block (ta tcta) is inserted at the 3'-end of vrIII which possibly represents an incomplete (tcta)2 repeat resulting from a dinucleotide deletion.

Table 2: D21S11 microsatellite sequence polymorphism

allele designation based on AMPFLP	sequence	size (bp)	constant region 1 (28bp)	constant region 2 (43bp)	insert	constant region 3 (66bp)	no. of alleles sequenced
24.2*	4-6-del-8	203	5' .....(tcta)4(tctg)6....	del (tcta)8		.......3'	0
C25	4-3-10	205	.....(tcta)4(tctg)3..	(tcta)10			1
C26	4-6-8	209	.....(tcta)4(tctg)6..	(tcta)8			1
27	4-6-9	213	.....(tcta)4(tctg)6..	(tcta)9			2
C27+	6-5-8	213	.....(tcta)6(tctg)5..	(tcta)8			3
C28	4-6-10	217	.....(tcta)4(tctg)6..	(tcta)10			2
C29***,+	4-6-11	221	.....(tcta)4(tctg)6..	(tcta)11			1
29	6-5-10	221	.....(tcta)6(tctg)5..	(tcta)10			3
30+	6-5-11	225	.....(tcta)6(tctg)5..	(tcta)11			1
C30+	6-5-11	225	.....(tcta)6(tctg)5..	(tcta)11			1
30+	4-6-12	225	.....(tcta)4(tctg)6..	(tcta)12			2
30.2+	5-6-10-ins	227	.....(tcta)5(tctg)6..	(tcta)10	ta tcta		1
30.2+	5-5-11-ins	227	.....(tcta)5(tctg)5..	(tcta)11	ta tcta		2
31**	5-6-12	229	.....(tcta)5(tctg)6..	(tcta)12			0
31**	6-5-12	229	.....(tcta)6(tctg)5..	(tcta)12			1
C31+	7-5-11	229	.....(tcta)7(tctg)5..	(tcta)11			5
31.2	5-6-11-ins	231	.....(tcta)5(tctg)6..	(tcta)11	ta tcta		1
32	6-5-13	233	.....(tcta)6(tctg)5..	(tcta)13			1
32+	5-6-13	233	.....(tcta)5(tctg)6..	(tcta)13			3
C32.2	5-6-12-ins	235	.....(tcta)5(tctg)6..	(tcta)12	ta tcta		3
C33.2	5-6-13-ins	239	.....(tcta)5(tctg)6..	(tcta)13	ta tcta		2
C34.2	5-6-14-ins	243	.....(tcta)5(tctg)6..	(tcta)14	ta tcta		

constant region 1: 5'- [gtg agt caa ttc ccc aag] tga att gcc t -3'

constant region 2: 5'- (tcta)3 ta (tcta)3 tca (tcta)2 tcca ta -3'

constant region 3 : 5'- tcg (tcta)2 tccag (tcta)2 cct cct att agt ctg tct ctg [gag aac att gac taa tac aac] - 3'

[] denotes primer target sequences

C25,26... Alleles included in allelic cocktail for AMPFLP typing

* Genbank sequence M 84567 shows a deletion of a 6 bp sequence (tcca ta) on the 3'-end of constant region 2

** alleles and variants described by Moeller et al.(1994)

+ alleles and variants described by Schwartz et al.(1995)

Several new sequence variants were identified (Tab.2). Remarkably, the Genbank M84567 sequence [Sharma 1992] shows another polymorphism so far only described on this occasion, namely a hexanucleotide deletion at the 5'-flank of vrIII. We suggest a new nomenclature for D21S11 alleles at the nucleotide level which allows the discrimination of all the so far described polymorphisms (Tab.2). Taking into account the relatively small number of alleles sequenced so far (compared to the observed polymorphism) it must be expected that even more variants will exist in the population. So, at the nucleotide level D21S11 represents one of the most polymorphic STR so far described and is therefore of high informative value in forensic haemogenetics when using DNA-sequencing. However, since the occurence of incomplete repeats is relatively common, this makes this locus difficult to type for with the AMPFLP-technique and the results should be interpreted with caution.

REFERENCES

Bassam BJ, Caetano Anolles G, Gresshoff PM: Fast and sensitive silver staining of DNA in polyacrylamide gels. Anal.Biochem.: 196: 80-83 (1991)

DNA comission of the ISFH: DNA recommendations - 1994 report concerning further recommendations of the DNA comission of the ISFH regarding PCR-based polymorphisms in STR (short tandem repeat) systems. Int.J.Leg.Med 107: 159-160 (1994)

Moeller A, Meyer E, Brinkmann B: Different types of structural variation in STRs: HumFES/FPS, HumVWA and HumD21S11. Int.J.Leg.Med 106: 319-323 (1994)

Schwartz DWM, Jungl EM, Krenek OR, Mayr WR: Simple and rapid typing for VNTR polymorphisms using high resolution electrophoresis of PCR products on rehydratable polyacrylamide gels. Advances in Forensic Haemogenetics 5: 170-172, Springer, Berlin, FRG (1994)

Sharma V, Litt M: Tetranucleotide repeat polymorphism at the D21S11 locus. Hum.Mol.Genet. 1: 67 (1992)

ACKNOWLEDGEMENTS

The authors are grateful to B. Brinkmann for providing an allelic ladder for standardisation and to H.Gnauer for his excellent technical assistance.

TYPING FOR THE HUMFES/FPS SHORT TANDEM REPEAT POLYMORPHISM IN AN AUSTRIAN CAUCASOID POPULATION SAMPLE

D.W.M.Schwartz, B.Glock, E.M.Dauber, E.M.Schwartz-Jungl, W.R.Mayr

Clinical Department for Blood Group Serology

University of Vienna

Waehringer Guertel 18-20/4I, A-1090 Vienna, Austria

SYSTEM AND LOCUS

HUMFES/FPS (intron 5 of the c-fes/fps proto-oncogene, 15q25-qter; Genbank Acession No.X06292 [Polymeropoulos 1991])

POPULATION AND SAMPLE SIZE: Vienna region (Austria). N=451

METHODS

primers [Moeller 1994]

A: 5'-ggg att tcc cta tgg att gg-3'
B: 5'-gcg aaa gaa tga gac tac at-3'

PCR

Amplification was carried out according to the protocol published by Moeller [1994] with some modifications:
reaction volume of 50μl
additional first denaturing step (5min - 98°C)
Hybaid Omnigene thermocycler

Electrophoresis

PAGE and silver staining was carried out on 6% native polyacrylamide gels in 112mM Tris/Acetic Acid and 200mM Tris/Tricine/0.55% SDS in horizontal mode as previously described [Schwartz 1994].

AMPFLP Typing

Typing was performed by side-to-side comparison with a sequenced allelic ladder, containing alleles 8 to 14, kindly provided by B. Brinkmann.

Sequencing

Automated single strand sequence determination of alleles corresponding to the ladder alleles was performed on an automatic DNA-Sequencer (ALF™, Pharmacia LKB Technology) according to the protocol of the Pharmacia AutoRead™ Sequencing Kit (dye primers, T7 polymerase) on a 6% sequencing gel. For each sample, the sense and the antisense strand were sequenced.

RESULTS AND COMMENTS

AMPFLP typing

AMPFLP Typing for the HumFES/FPS polymorphism in 451 healthy, unrelated Austrian Caucasoid individuals revealed 9 distinct alleles, corresponding to alleles 8-13 (including 10a and 11a; [Moeller 1994]) and an additional low frequency allele corresponding to 14 core repeats that has also been previously described [Hammond 1994]. Allele frequencies, together with the forensic statistical efficiency values are listed in Tab.1. The phenotype distribution showed no significant deviation from Hardy-Weinberg expectations.

Fig. 1: Comparison of HUMFES/FPS allele frequencies

Table 1: HUMFES/FPS allele frequencies (n=451)

allele designation	frequency (%)
8	1.7
9	0.3
10a	23.4
10	3.3
11a	2.3
11	43.5
12	22.5
13	2.9
14	0.1

χ^2=9.76; df=10; 0.4<p<0.5
Mean exclusion chance (MEC) 0.48
Power of discrimination (PD)   0.86
Discrimination index (DI)   0.15

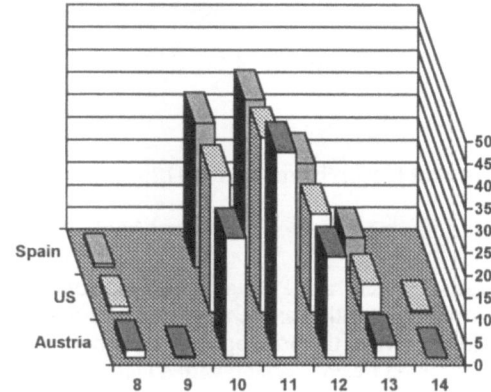

Austrian versus
    US Caucasians: χ^2= 15.88; df=6; 0.01<p<0.025
    Spanish Caucasians: χ^2= 22.21; df=6; 0.001<p<0.005

(to allow the comparison alleles 10a and 11a were counted with 10 and 11, respectively

When comparing the allelic distribution of our population to other Caucasian samples [Cabrero 1994, Hammond 1994], a statistically significant deviation in the distribution of alleles 10, 11 13 was observed (Fig.1).

Sequencing:

Sequence determination of 13 samples including all alleles was in perfect agreement with the already published data [Moeller 1994]. The allele 14 (sequence not published so far) showed just another reiteration of the core repeat and no transversion at position 34 of the 5' flanking region.

REFERENCES

Cabrero C, Diez A, Valverde E, Carracedo A, Alemany J: Allele frequency distribution of four PCR-amplified loci in the Spanish population. Forensic Science Int.71: 153-164 (1994)

Hammond HA, Jin L, Zhong Y, Caskey CT, Chakraborty R: Evaluation of 13 Short Tandem Repeat loci for use in personal identification applications. Am.J.Hum.Genet. 55: 175-189 (1994)

Moeller A, Meyer E, Brinkmann B: Different types of structural variation in STRs: HumFES/FPS, HumVWA and HumDS21S11. Int.J.Leg.Med. 106: 319-323 (1994)

Polymeropoulos MH, Rath DS, Xiao H, Merril RM: Tetranucleotide repeat polymorphism at the c-fes/fps proto-oncogene(FES). Nucleic Acids Res. 19: 4018 (1991)

Schwartz DWM., Jungl EM, Krenek OR, Mayr WR: Simple and rapid typing for VNTR polymorphisms using high resolution electrophoresis of PCR products on rehydratable polyacrylamide gels. Advances in Forensic Haemogenetics 5: 170-172, Springer, Berlin, FRG (1994)

ACKNOWLEDGEMENTS

The authors are grateful to B.Brinkmann for providing an allelic ladder for standardisation and to H.Gnauer for his excellent technical assistance.

ANALYSIS OF THE STR POLYMORPHISM VWA AND FES: ALLELE FREQUENCY AND FAMILY STUDIES IN AN ITALIAN POPULATION SAMPLE.

Ponzano E., Caenazzo L., Crestani C., Bonan G., Cortivo P.

Institute of Legal Medicine, University of Padova, Italy

System and locus: HumVWA31 (12p12-pter) and HumFES (15q25-qter)

Population and sample size: Veneto (Italy). N: 115

Methods: Primers and PCR amplification conditions(Urquhart et al.).
Electrophoretic methods: 8% native vertical polyacrilamide gel 25 cm the electrophoresis was stopped when the bromophenol blu front had reached the anodal end of the gel. Typing was performed by comparison with a ladder of known alleles.

Results:

HumVWA31 observed genotypes

gen.	obs.	gen.	obs.	gen.	obs.
14-14	2	15-16	2	17-17	16
14-15	2	15-17	12	17-18	11
14-16	6	15-18	2	17-19	9
14-17	9	15-19	4	18-18	5
14-18	2	16-16	7	18-19	1
14-19	1	16-17	13	18-20	1
15-15	5	16-18	5		

HumVWA31 Allele frequencies

Allele	frequency	allele	frequency	allele	frequency
14	0.1044	17	0.3740	19	0.0652
15	0.1391	18	0.1391	20	0.0043
16	0.1739				

$X^2 = 11.766$, d.f. 20, $P = 0.90$

HumFES observed genotypes

gen.	obs.	gen.	obs.	gen.	obs.
8-10	1	10-11	22	11-13	5
8-12	3	10-12	14	11-14	1
9-10	4	10-13	7	12-12	5
9-12	1	11-11	20	12-13	3
10-10	11	11-12	18		

HumFES Allele frequencies

Allele	frequency	allele	frequency	allele	frequency
8	0.0174	11	0.3740	13	0.0652
9	0.2170	12	0.2130	14	0.0043
10	0.3043				

$X^2 = 4.534$, d.f. 14, P = 0.991

Comments: 12 excluded paternity cases, were examined for exclusion with each of the two STRs: 50% were excluded with HumFES, while 66% were excluded by HumVWA31; 33% were excluded with both systems. The results of statistical analysis and the informativity derived from our results data demonstrate the efficency and suitability of this marker for routine application in forensic investigation.

References

1 Kimpton CP, Walton A, Gill P (1992) A further tetranucleotide repeat polymorphism in the VWA gene. Hum Mol Genet 1:287-289

2 Polymeropoulos MH, Rath DS, Xiao H, Merril CR (1991) Tetranucleotide repat polymorphism at the human c-fes/fps proto-oncogene (FES). Nucleic Acis Res 19:4018

3 Urquhart A, Kimpton K, Downes TJ Gill P (1994) Variation in short tandem repeat sequences a survey of twelve microsatellite loci for use as forensic identification markers. Int J Leg Med 107:13-20

Analysis of the short tandem repeat polymorphism D21S11 in German Caucasians

C.Seidl, O.Jäger, E.Seifried

Institute for Transfusion Medicine and Immunohematology, Red Cross Blood Donor Service Hessen, Sandhofstrasse 1, 60528 Frankfurt, Germany

INTRODUCTION

Short tandem repeat loci (STR) are polymorphic markers that can be used for human identification in forensic or paternity casework. We have investigated the polymorphism of the STR locus D21S11 in a german population sample.

SYSTEMS AND LOCUS: D21S11 (21q21)

POPULATION AND SAMPLE SIZE: Hesse (Germany)
N: 77

METHODS

Primersequences were choosen according to Sharma and Litt (1992). The 5' primer was labelled with HEX (6-carboxy-2',4',7',4,7-Hexachlorofluorescein, Perkin Elmer - ABD).
PCR amplification conditions: 95 C - 5 min; 28 cyles 95 C - 30 sec , 54 C 40 sec, 72 C 30 sec; 72 C 5 min. (Perkin Elmer 9600).
PCR reaction conditions: 10-100ng DNA, 5pmol 5'and 3' primer, 200 μmol dNTP's, 0,5 Units Taq DNA polymerase (Appligene) and the corresponding buffer (Appligene) in a final volume of 50 μl.
Electrophoretic methods: 6% polyacrylamide denaturing gel electrophoresis. The gels were run for 8h at constant power (30W) 1200V and 28mA on an ABD automated DNA seqencer 373A. Typing was performed by comparison with an ROX (6-carboxy-X-rhodamine) labelled internal standard generated from the vector pGL-2-Basic (Promega) using the Southern local method for fragment size assignement (GENESCAN software, Perkin Elmer - ABD).
Sequence analysis: Individual alleles were sequenced using the solid-phase sequence strategy. Analysis of sequence reactions was conducted on an ABD 373A automated DNA sequencer using the SEQUENCE NAVIGATOR software (Perkin Elmer - ABD).
Statistical analysis: The polymorphic information content (PIC) was calculated using the formula of Botstein (1980). The discrimination index (DI) and the matching probability (pM) were calculated by the method of Jones (1972). The sample gene diversity (geneD) (frequency of heterozygotes expected under Hardy Weinberg equilibrium was calculated as described by Kimpton (1993).

RESULTS

Observed genotypes

Gen.	Obs. (N)	Gen.	Obs.(N)	Gen.	Obs.(N)	Gen.	Obs.(N)
57 - 63	1	61 - 70	1	63 - 72	1	66 - 68	1
59 - 61	1	61 - 72	1	64 - 68	1	66 - 70	2
59 - 63	1	63 - 63	4	65 - 65	6	67 - 68	2
61 - 61	2	63 - 65	5	65 - 66	4	68 - 70	2
61 - 63	5	63 - 66	2	65 - 67	6	70 - 70	1
61 - 65	4	63 - 67	2	65 - 68	3	70 - 72	1
61 - 67	1	63 - 68	3	65 - 70	7		
61 - 68	3	63 - 70	3	66 - 66	1		

Allele frequencies

Allele (bp)	Frequency	Allele (bp)	Frequency	Allele (bp)	Frequency
57 (209)	0,007	64 (223)	0,007	68 (231)	0,097
59 (213)	0,013	65 (225)	0,266	70 (235)	0,117
61 (217)	0,13	66 (227)	0,071	72 (239)	0,026
63 (221)	0,201	67 (229)	0,071	73 (241)	0,02

COMMENTS

STR locus	HR	gene D	PIC	DI	pM	mean exclusion change
D21S11	0,818	0,838	0,819	0,99	0,012	68,12

The observed genotype distribution follows the Hardy Weinberg equilibrium (Chi-square value 0,368; df 65; p>0,99). The sequence analysis of alleles at the D21S11 locus reveals a tetranucleotide repeat structure that contains a hexanucleotide repeat in alleles with even repeat numbers leading to size differences of 2 base pairs. Allele assignement was done as proposed by Urquhart (1994) counting each tetra- or hexanucleotide repeat as two or three dinucleotide repeats respectively. Locus D21S11 can be easily analysed by PCR amplification. Using an internal size standard and fluorescence labelled primers proper allele assignment of allele fragments differing by only 2 bp could be performed. Computer generated band sizes of the different fragments observed in our population sample exhibited a maximum band size range of 0,3 bp (corresponding to ± 0,15 bp either side of the mean value).

REFERENCES

Botstein D, White RL, Skolnick M, Davis RW (1980) Construction of a genetic linkage map in man using restriction fragment lenght polymorphisms. Am.J.Hum.Genet. 32: 182-190

Jones DA (1972) Blood samples: Probability of discrimination. J.Forens.Sci.Soc., 12: 355-359

Kimpton CP, Gill P, Walton A, Urquhart A, Millican ES, Adams M (1993) Automated DNA profiling employing multiplex amplification of short tandem repeat loci. PCR methods and applications, 3: 13-22

Sharma V and Litt M (1992) Tetranucleotide repeat polymorphism at the D21S11 locus. Hum. Mol. Genetics,Vol 1, No.1: 67

Urquhart A, Kimpton CP, Downes TJ, Gill P (1994) Variation in short tandem repeat sequences - a survey of twelve microsatellite loci for use as forensic identification markers. Int.J.Leg.Med. 107: 13-20.

Population data of the VNTR loci D10S28, D4S139, D16S309 and D5S110 in German Caucasians

C.Seidl, U.Rabold, B.Brüggemann, M.Kilp, D.Teixidor, E.Seifried

Institute for Transfusion Medicine and Immunohematology, Red Cross Blood Donor Service
Hessen, Sandhofstrasse 1, 60528 Frankfurt, Germany

INTRODUCTION

Variable number of tandem repeat (VNTR) loci are highly polymorphic markers that are commonly used for paternity and forensic testing. The allele distribution of these markers however differs between ethnic groups. Therefore, proper calculation of paternity probability (PP) can only be conducted with frequencies obtained from population samples of the same ethnic origin as the individual tested. We have studied the allele distribution of four VNTR loci, D10S28, D4S139, D16S309 and D5S110 in a population sample of German Caucasians.

PROBE AND LOCUS: TBQ7 (D10S28)   (Bragg 1987)
                            PH30 (D4S139)   (Milner 1989)
                            MS205 (D16S309)   (Royle 1992)
                            LH1   (D5S110)   (Armour 1990)

POPULATION AND SAMPLE SIZE: Hesse (Germany)
                            N: 201 Individuals, (D10S28)
                            N: 133 Individuals, (D4S139)
                            N: 221 Individuals, (D16S309)
                            N: 147 Individuals, (D5S110)

METHODS

Restriction enzyme   HAEIII : D10S28 (TBQ7), D4S139 (PH30), D5S110 (LH1)
                          HINF I : D16S309 (MS205)

Electrophoretic methods: Fragments were separated by agarose gelelectrophoresis (24-26 hours at 0.8-1.0 V/cm). Electrophoresis conditions were chosen depending on the range of fragment sizes detected by the various DNA probes. Hybridisation, southern blot transfer to nylon membrans (Qiabrane from Qiagen Inc, Chatsworth, CA, USA) and chemiluminescence detection of probes was performed as recommended by the manufacturers (NICE™ MS205 ICI/CELLMARK, GenePrint Light™ TBQ7 Promega and ACES™ LH1/pH30 Gibco BRL). Fragments were analysed by an semiautomatic computerized system (DNA-Auswertungssystem Version 2.40 from Muche M. Immucor Medizinische Diagnostik GmbH, Rödermark, Germany).

RESULTS

MS205 Allele sizes and frequencies (0,1 kb Intervals)

Allele	Frequency	Allele	Frequency	Allele	Frequency	Allele	Frequency	Allele	Frequency
0,8	0,0045	1,7	0,0068	2,4	0,0566	3,1	0,0362	3,8	0,0158
1,1	0,0023	1,8	0,0091	2,5	0,0543	3,2	0,0566	3,9	0,0136
1,2	0,0045	1,9	0,0226	2,6	0,0452	3,3	0,0362	4,0	0,0091
1,3	0,0045	2,0	0,0339	2,7	0,0566	3,4	0,0204	4,1	0,0023
1,4	0,0091	2,1	0,0249	2,8	0,1041	3,5	0,0249	4,2	0,0023
1,5	0,0045	2,2	0,0498	2,9	0,0973	3,6	0,0317	4,3	0,0023
1,6	0,0158	2,3	0,0543	3,0	0,0520	3,7	0,0271	4,4	0,0091

PH30 Allele sizes and frequencies (0,1 kb Intervals)

Allele	Frequency	Allele	Frequency	Allele	Frequency	Allele	Frequency	Allele	Frequency
2,8	0,005	5,8	0,02	7,8	0,02	10,2	0,005	13,2	0,005
3,5	0,01	5,9	0,025	7,9	0,005	10,3	0,005	13,4	0,005
3,6	0,02	6,1	0,03	8,0	0,015	10,4	0,01	13,8	0,005
3,8	0,01	6,2	0,03	8,2	0,005	10,5	0,01	13,9	0,005
3,9	0,005	6,3	0,02	8,3	0,005	10,6	0,005	14,3	0,005
4,0	0,005	6,4	0,015	8,4	0,015	10,7	0,005	14,4	0,005
4,1	0,005	6,5	0,025	8,6	0,025	10,8	0,005	15,2	0,005
4,3	0,005	6,6	0,025	8,7	0,005	10,9	0,01	15,7	0,005
4,4	0,005	6,7	0,015	8,8	0,02	11,0	0,005	16,2	0,005
4,5	0,025	6,8	0,01	9,0	0,005	11,1	0,005	16,3	0,005
4,7	0,015	6,9	0,015	9,2	0,005	11,3	0,005	16,8	0,005
4,8	0,03	7,0	0,03	9,4	0,005	11,6	0,005	17,6	0,005
5,0	0,01	7,1	0,015	9,5	0,01	11,7	0,005	17,8	0,005
5,1	0,02	7,2	0,02	9,6	0,005	11,9	0,01	17,9	0,005
5,2	0,005	7,4	0,01	9,8	0,025	12,3	0,01	18,2	0,005
5,3	0,01	7,5	0,02	9,9	0,015	12,5	0,005	21,5	0,005
5,5	0,015	7,6	0,015	10,0	0,005	13,0	0,01	22,7	0,005
5,7	0,015	7,7	0,005	10,1	0,01	13,1	0,005		

TBQ7 Allele sizes and frequencies (0,1 kb Intervals)

Allele	Frequency	Allele	Frequency	Allele	Frequency	Allele	Frequency	Allele	Frequency
1,0	0,005	2,1	0,0473	3,2	0,00995	4,3	0,00746	5,5	0,00746
1,1	0,017	2,2	0,0423	3,3	0,0149	4,4	0,0124	5,6	0,0025
1,2	0,015	2,3	0,0124	3,4	0,00746	4,5	0,0174	5,7	0,0025
1,3	0,015	2,4	0,0249	3,5	0,0274	4,6	0,00498	5,9	0,005
1,4	0,0075	2,5	0,0149	3,6	0,0249	4,7	0,00995	6,0	0,00746
1,5	0,0522	2,6	0,0174	3,7	0,0174	4,8	0,0174	6,1	0,0025
1,6	0,0597	2,7	0,00995	3,8	0,00746	4,9	0,0174	6,5	0,005
1,7	0,0547	2,8	0,0398	3,9	0,0124	5,0	0,0025	7,1	0,0025
1,8	0,0547	2,9	0,0249	4,0	0,0249	5,1	0,00746	9,2	0,0025
1,9	0,0771	3,0	0,0448	4,1	0,0174	5,3	0,0025		
2,0	0,0323	3,1	0,0149	4,2	0,0124	5,4	0,0025		

LH1 Allele sizes and frequencies (0,1 kb Intervals)

Allele	Frequency	Allele	Frequency	Allele	Frequency	Allele	Frequency	Allele	Frequency
1,2	0,0102	2,4	0,0272	3,5	0,0442	4,6	0,0102	5,9	0,017
1,4	0,0034	2,5	0,0238	3,6	0,0544	4,7	0,0102	6,0	0,0068
1,5	0,0102	2,6	0,034	3,7	0,017	4,8	0,0102	6,1	0,0068
1,6	0,017	2,7	0,0204	3,8	0,0102	4,9	0,0034	6,5	0,0034
1,7	0,0238	2,8	0,0442	3,9	0,0306	5,0	0,0102	7,0	0,0102
1,8	0,0136	2,9	0,0578	4,0	0,0068	5,1	0,0068	7,2	0,0034
1,9	0,0272	3,0	0,0306	4,1	0,0204	5,2	0,0136	7,6	0,0034
2,0	0,0204	3,1	0,0374	4,2	0,0136	5,3	0,0068	7,7	0,0034
2,1	0,0442	3,2	0,0306	4,3	0,0136	5,4	0,0102	7,8	0,0034
2,2	0,034	3,3	0,0238	4,4	0,0204	5,7	0,0034	8,1	0,0034
2,3	0,0204	3,4	0,0442	4,5	0,0204	5,8	0,0034		

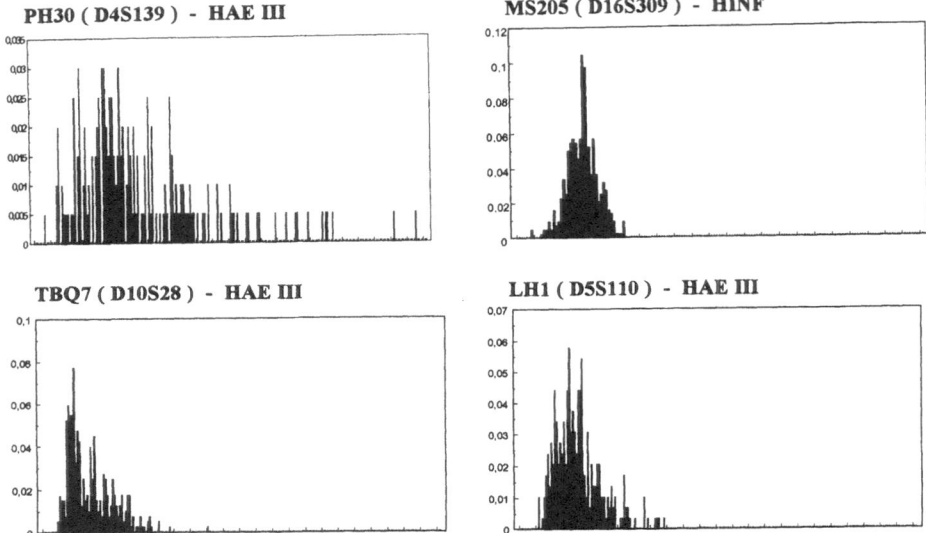

Figure 1: Allele sizes and frequencies of VNTR SLP polymorphisms in German Caucasians

COMMENTS

Chemiluninescence detection of these probes could be easily performed. Reproducibility of size measurement was performed by examining control DNA (K 562) on every gel. The allele distribution observed with the SLP's TBQ7, LH1 and MS205 did reveal frequent fragments lying close together in the lower kb region, whereas the SLP PH30 exhibited a more irregular distribution with 19,8% of fragments lying above 10 kb (Fig.1). Size determination of fragments above 10 kb is very often limited due to the reduced electrophoretic separation of these fragments. The range of the fragment size of individual alleles in this high molecular region can increase to more than $\pm$ 5% and thus the precise determination of identical fragments between to individuals is limited. In this respect, the information content of loci with wide spread allelic size ranges is reduced. Nevertheless, in cases of clear differences in the fragment sizes of alleles between two individuals these high molecular fragments can be very informative. In conclusion, the high heterozygosity rates and the extensive polymorphism of these SLP's are ideal for human identification testing.

VNTR loci	HR	VNTR loci	HR
D10S28 (TBQ7) - HAEIII	0,90	D16S309 (MS205) - HINFI	0,98
D4S139 (PH30) - HAEIII	0,97	D5S110 (LH1) - HAEIII	0,96

REFERENCES

Armour JA, Povey S, Jeremiah S, Jeffreys AJ (1990) Systematic cloning of human minisattelites from ordered array charomid libraries. Genomics, Vol. 8: 501-512
Bragg T, Nakamura Y, Jones C, White R (1987) Isolation and mapping of a polymorphic DNA sequence (cTBQ7) on chromosome 10 (D10S28). Nucleic Acids Research, Vol 16 (233): 11395
Milner ECB, Lotshaw CL, van Dijk KW, Concannon P, Schroeder HW (1989) Isolation and mapping of a polymorphic DNA sequence pH30 on chromosome 4 [HGM provisional no. D4S139] Nucl Acids Res, Vol 17 : 4002
Royle NJ, Armour JA, Webb M, Thomas A, Jeffreys AJ (1992) A hypervariable locus D16S309 located at the distal end of 16p. Nucl Acids Res, Vol 20 : 1164

A POPULATION STUDY OF 5 PCR GENETIC MARKERS, LDLR, GYPA, HBGG, D7S8 AND Gc, IN ITALY

Adriano Tagliabracci (*), Loredana Buscemi (**), Nicola Cucurachi (**), Roberto Mencarelli (*), Raffaele Giorgetti (**), and Santo Davide Ferrara (**)

Institute of Legal Medicine, Universities of Ancona (*) and Parma (**), Italy

The Amplitype® PM PCR Amplification and Typing Kit (Perkin Elmer Corporation, Norwalk, CT) permits multiplex PCR amplification of six loci:
1) low density lipoprotein receptor (LDLR) (Yamamoto et al. 1984), on chromosome 19, PCR product of 214 bp, 2 alleles (A and B);
2) glycophorin A (GYPA) (Siebert and Fukuda 1987), on chromosome 4, PCR product of 190 bp, 2 alleles (A and B) and other variants in African-American populations not distinguishiable using the above kit;
3) haemoglobin G-gammaglobin (HBGG) (Slightom et al. 1980), on chromosome 11, PCR product of 172 bp, 3 alleles (A, B and C);
4) D7S8 (Horn et al. 1990), on chromosome 7, PCR product of 151 bp, 2 alleles (A and B);
5) group-specific component (Gc) (Yang et al. 1985), on chromosome 4, PCR product of 138 bp, 3 alleles (A, B and C);
6) HLA-DQA1 (previously named HLA-DQa) (Gyllestein and Erlich 1988) on chromosome 6, PCR product of 239/242 bp, 6 alleles.
The amplification products of the first five loci can subsequently be typed simultaneously on the same nylon strip using a reverse dot blot method (Saiki et al. 1989), whereas the HLA-DQA1 PCR product hybridizes with the S specific probe which acts as control (Fig. 1b).
Validation studies on the suitability and forensic efficiency of this system were recently reported (Budowle et al. 1995; Fildes and Reynolds 1995) together with allele frequencies from several populations (Hochmeister et al. 1994; Budowle et al. 1995; Hausmann et al. 1995). However, further studies on allele frequencies from populations of various countries are desirable, to improve knowledge of the genetic profiles of these loci and to create a wide data-base. Since such information has not yet been reported for Italians, we investigated a suitable sample population with the aims of: 1) analysing the polymorphism of these 5 loci; 2) establishing a database of allele frequencies, in view of its application in forensic investigations, and 3) examining the performance of amplitype kit and problems arising from its use.

MATERIALS AND METHODS
DNA was extracted from samples of fresh peripheral blood from 98 healthy unrelated donors living in Northern (Parma= n. 46) and Central Italy (Ancona= n. 52), following the method suggested by Budowle and Baechtel (1990). In addition, 5 mother-child pairs were examined in the same conditions using the AmpliType® PM PCR Amplification and Typing Kit (supplied by Cetus Corporation). Amplification was carried out in a thermal cycler Gene Amp PCR System 2400 (Perkin Elmer) in the conditions suggested by the manufacturer, using quantities of DNA ranging from 10 to 50 ng. The PCR product was checked before hybridization by electrophoresis on a silver stained polyacrylamide gel (Fig. 1a). The frequency of alleles for each locus was calculated from the number of genotypes. The Hardy-Weinberg law was verified by the chi-square test between observed and expected genotype frequencies. The power of discrimination (PD) was calculated using Fischer's (1951) equation. A computer program kindly supplied by G. Carmody (Carleton University, Ottawa, Canada) was used to test for homogeneity between various population samples.

RESULTS AND DISCUSSION

The distributions of observed phenotypes and allele frequencies for the five PM genetic markers are shown in Tables 1 and 2. All five loci were polymorphic in our sample. The chi-square test did not detect any deviation from the Hardy-Weinberg expectations for the five loci. The combined PD was 0.994. The distribution of PM allele frequencies were found to be similar to those described for Caucasians (Hochmeister et al. 1994, Budowle at al. 1995, Hausmann et al. 1995) for all five loci (Table 3).

In our experience, care must be taken when interpreting the typing of the Gc locus. In one case of mother-child pair typing there was an apparent exclusion (mother A, child C), due to signal imbalance for the Gc B dot, which appeared less intense than the control. This problem was solved by adding EDTA after amplified product denaturation, to prevent primer extension which may mask the Gc B probe binding site on the strip (Reynolds, pers. com.).

REFERENCES

Budowle B, Lindsey JA, DeCou JA, Koons BW, Giusti AM, Comey CT (1995) Validation and population studies of the loci LDLR, GYPA, HBGG, D7S8, and Gc (PM loci), and HLA-DQa using a multiplex amplification and typing procedure. Journal of Forensic Sciences 40: 45-54

Fildes N, Reynolds R (1995) Consistency and reproducibility of Amplitype® PM results between seven laboratories: field trial results (1995). Journal of Forensic Sciences 40: 279-286

Fisher RA (1951) Standard calculations for evaluating a blood group system. Heredity 5: 95-102

Gyllensten UB, Erlich HA (1988) Generation of single-stranded DNA by the polymerase chain reaction and its application to direct sequencing of the HLA-DQ alpha locus. Proc Natl Acad Sci USA 85: 7652-7656

Hausmann R, Hantschel M, Lötterle J (1995) Frequencies of the 5 PCR-based genetic markers LDLR, GYPA, HBGG, D7S8, and Gc in a North Bavarian population. Int J Leg Med 107: 227-228

Hochmeister MN, Budowle B, Borer UV, Dirnhofer R (1994) Swiss population data on the loci HLA-DQa LDLR, GYPA, HBGG, D7S8, Gc and D1S80. Forensic Sci Int 67: 175-184

Horn GT, Richards B, Merrill JJ, Klinger KW (1990) Characterization and rapid diagnostic analysis of DNA polymorphisms closely linked to the cystic fibrosis locus. Clin Chem 105: 233-238

Saiki RK, Walsh S, Levenson CH, Erlich HA (1989) Genetic analysis of amplified DNA with immobilized sequence-specific oligonucleotide probes. Proc Natl Acad Sci USA 86: 6230-6234

Siebert PD, Fukuda M (1987) Molecular cloning of a human glycophorin B cDNA: nucleotide sequence and genomic relationship to glycophorin A. Proc Natl Acad Sci USA 84: 6735-6739

Slightom JL, Blechl AE, Smithies O (1980) Human fetal G-gamma- and A-gamma-globulin genes: complete nucleotide sequences suggest that DNA can be exchanged between these duplicated genes. Cell 21: 627-638

Yamamoto T, Davis CG, Brown MS, Schneider WJ, Casey ML, Goldstein JL, Russell DW (1984) The human LDL receptor: a cysteine-rich protein with multiple Alu sequences in its mRNA. Cell 39: 27-38

Yang F, Brune JL, Naylor SL, Cupples RL, Naberhaus KH (1985) Human group specific component (Gc) is a member of the albumin family. Proc Natl Acad Sci USA 82: 7994-7998

Fig. 1. Polyacrylamide gel electrophoresis of PCR amplified product (a) and probe strip typing (b) of PM loci

A

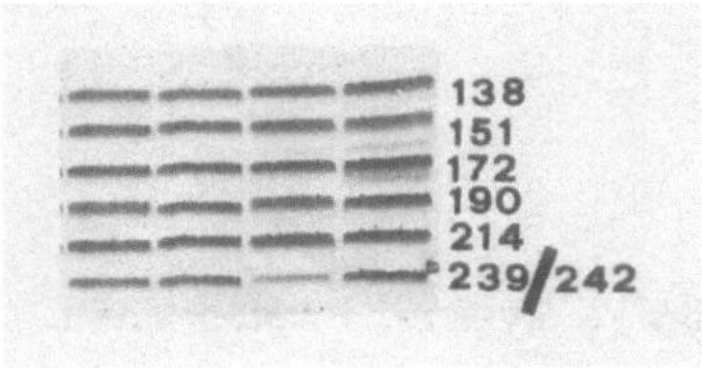

B

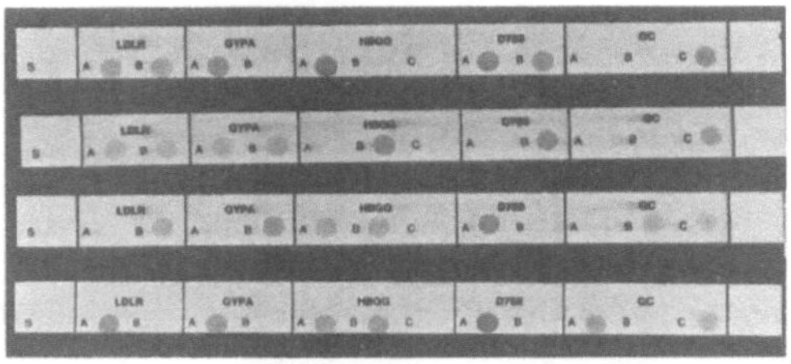

Table 1. Observed PM loci genotype frequencies in a sample of 98 Italians

Genotype	LDLR	GYPA	HBGG	D7S8	Gc
AA	0.133	0.378	0.245	0.286	0.051
AB	0.561	0.459	0.367	0.541	0.071
BB	0.306	0.163	0.357	0.173	0.031
AC	NG[a]	NG	0.010	NG	0.275
BC	NG	NG	0.021	NG	0.143
CC	NG	NG	0.000	NG	0.429

[a] NG, no genotype, there is no allele C.

Table 2. PM loci allele frequencies in a sample of 98 Italians

Allele	LDLR	GYPA	HBGG	D7S8	Gc
A	0.413	0.607	0.434	0.556	0.224
B	0.587	0.393	0.551	0.444	0.138
C	NA[a]	NA	0.015	NA	0.638

[a] NA, there is no allele C in AmpliType® PM kit

χ test	2.4240	0.1373	5.2799	0.8925	1.6023
Prob.	$0.10<P<0.25$	$0.50<P<0.75$	$0.10<P<0.25$	$0.25<P<0.50$	$0.50<P<0.75$
d.f.	$n = 1$	$n = 1$	$n = 3$	$n = 1$	$n = 3$

Table 3. Results of test for heterogeneity between Italians, Americans, North Bavarians and Swiss

	LDLR	GYPA	HBGG	D7S8	Gc
G-stat.	8.9407	5.7412	24.1789	2.5166	18.1277
Prob.	0.1810±0.0122	0.4480±0.0157	0.0490 ±0.0068	0.8710±0.0106	0.3000 ±0.0145

ALLELE FREQUENCIES OF THE HUMFES/FPS SYSTEM IN NORTHERN AND CENTRAL ITALY.

Tagliabracci A., Paoli M., Rodriguez D. (*)
Cucurachi N., Buscemi L., Ferrara S.D. (**)
Previderè C., Peloso G., Riva A., Pierucci G. (°)
Domenici R., Fornaciari S., Spinetti I., Nardone M., Bargagna M. (°°)

Universities of Ancona (*), Parma (**), Pavia (°), Pisa (°°)

INTRODUCTION

The tetrameric (ATTT) short tandem repeat HUMFES/FPS system, located on chromosome 15 (15q25-qter), displays a polymorphism (Polymeropoulos et al. 1991) which has been investigated for forensic purposes (Hammond et al. 1994). The aim of the present work was to study the polymorphism of this system in a large Italian population sample: 1) to verify allele frequency distribution, 2) to check whether allele frequencies show inter-regional differences, 3) to evaluate the effectiveness of this system for paternity testing and personal identification. For this purpose, collaborative research was performed on subjects from four Italian regions in laboratories of the Institutes of Legal Medicine of the Universities of Pavia (Lombardy), Parma (Emilia), Pisa (Tuscany) and Ancona (Marches).

MATERIALS AND METHODS

The study was carried out on fresh blood samples collected from healthy unrelated donors living in Pavia (n= 120), Parma (n=150), Pisa (n=162) and Ancona (n=159). The four laboratories conducted analyses according to the method described by Möller *et al.* (1994) with minor modifications; electrophoresis was carried out on a non-denaturing polyacryamide gel and the bands were visualized by silver staining (Budowle et al. 1991). Alleles were identified by side-to-side comparison with home-made ladders consisting of a cocktail of amplified products (fig. 1).

The 4 Italian population samples were tested for heterogeneity with an R x C contingency table using a computer program kindly supplied by G. Carmody (Carleton University, Ottawa, Canada). The results were verified by the chi-square test between observed and expected genotypes according to the Hardy-Weinberg law and by comparison of the observed and expected heterozygosity frequencies, the latter calculated as allele diversity (Nei et al. 1974). $\sqrt{[h(1-h)/N]}$ was the formula used to compute the standard error for H, where h was the expected heterozygote frequency and N the number of subjects examined.

The power of discrimination (PD) was calculated using Fischer's (1951) equation. The exclusion chance was calculated from allele frequencies (Garber and Morris 1983).

Table 1. HUMFES/FPS observed genotypes in 591 Italians from four regions.

Genotypes	Observed
8-10	2
8-11	2
8-12	2
9-11	1
10-10	45
10-11	122
10-12	92
10-13	20
10-14	2
11-11	89
11-12	115
11-13	28
11-14	5
12-12	38
12-13	20
12-14	3
13-13	4
13-14	1

Table 2. HUMFES/FPS allele frequency distribution from 591 Italians.

HUMFES/FPS Allele	Lombardy 120 subjects	Emilia 150 subjects	Tuscany 162 subjects	Marches 159 subjects	Combined data
8	0.013	0.007	–	0.003	0.005
9	–	0.003	–	–	0.001
10	0.27	0.26	0.287	0.289	0.277
11	0.387	0.387	0.358	0.396	0.382
12	0.25	0.277	0.278	0.236	0.261
13	0.058	0.06	0.068	0.072	0.065
14	0.020	0.007	0.009	0.003	0.009

Heterogeneity test: $\chi^2 = 15.9478$, P $= 0.6110 \pm 0.0154$;
G statistic $= 16.2560$, P $= 0.6380 \pm 0.0152$

a) H-W equilibrium expectation

$\chi^2 = 4.887$ P > 0.975   df = 21

b) Obs. Heterozy. = 0.70   *Exp. Heterozy. = 0.70* ± 0.018

c) PD = 0.86   *Mean excl. chance = 0.45*

RESULTS AND DISCUSSION

591 subjects living in 4 Italian regions were typed for STR system HUMFES/FPS. A total of 18 genotypes (Table 1) and the 7 common alleles (Table 2) identified by Hammond et al. (1994) were found and classified according to the repeat number. The two anodal variant alleles 10a and 11a, recently described by Möller et al. (1994), were pooled together with alleles 10 and 11, respectively.

The 4 samples showed similar distribution of allele frequencies when tested for heterogeneity (Table 2), so that they can be considered as a single Italian population sample.

The PD and mean esclusion chance were, respectively, 0.86 and 0.45, suggesting that the HUMFES/FPS system is a useful and powerful tool for forensic purposes.

REFERENCES

Budowle B, Chakraborty R, Giusti AM, Eisenberg AJ, Allen RC (1991) Analysis of the variable number of tandem repeats locus D1S80 by the polymerase chain reaction followed by high resolution polyacrylamide gel electrophoresis. Am J Hum Genet 48: 137-144
Fisher RA (1951) Standard calculations for evaluating a blood group system. Heredity 5: 95-102
Garber RA, Morris JW (1983) General equations for the average power of exclusion for genetic system of n codominant alleles in one-parent and no-parent cases of disputed parentage. In: Walker RH (ed) Inclusion probabilities in parentage testing. AABB, Arlington, VA, pp 277-280
Hammond HA, Jin L, Zhong Y, Caskey CT, Chakraborty R (1994) Evaluation of 13 short tandem repeat loci for use in personal identification applications. Am J Hum Genet 55: 175-189
Möller A, Meyer E, Brinkmann B (1994) Different types of structural variations in STRs: HumFES/FPS, HumVWA and HumD21S11. Int J Leg Med 106: 319-323
Nei M, Roychoudhury (1974) Sampling variances of heterozygosity and genetic distance. Genetics 76: 379-390
Polymeropoulos MH, Rath DS, Xiao H, Merril CR (1991) Tetranucleotide repeat polymorphism at the human c-fes/fps proto-oncogene (FES). Nucleic Acids Res 19: 4018

Fig 1. Silver-stained HUMFES/FPS system polyacrylamide gel of amplified fragments. Left to right: ladder (alleles 8,10,11,12,13,14): lane 1,4,7. HUMFES/FPS phenotypes: lane 2: 10-11; lane 3: 10-12; lane 5: 10-11; lane 6: 10-11.

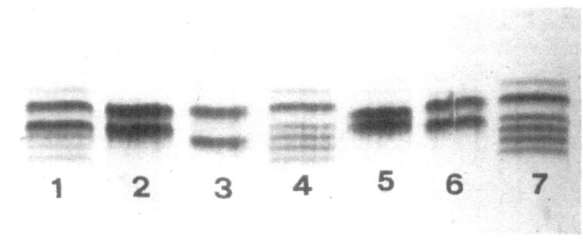

THE Y-LINKED LOCUS Y27H39 (DYS19), FREQUENCY DISTRIBUTION IN SOUTH BAVARIAN AND APPLICATION TO PATERNITY TESTING

G.M. Weichhold, W. Keil and B. Bayer

Institut für Rechtsmedizin der Universität München
Frauenlobstr. 7a, D-80337 München, Germany

Introduction

The short tandem repeat (STR) Y27H39 was discovered by Roewer et al. 1992 on the short arm of the Y-chromosome in 1992. It is based upon a (GATA)n repeat. Due to their heredity along male lines, Y-linked polymorphisms have a considerable potential in paternity expertises, especially in deficiency cases (Santos et al. 1993, Gomolka et al. 1994). We present a genetic population study based upon the analysis of a random sample of non-related men from southern Bavaria. The performance of the Y-linked polymorphism is demonstrated by means of a paternity case in which the two putative fathers were not available.

Materials and Methods

DNA-Preparation: DNA was isolated from whole blood samples using phenol/chloroform extractions (Manniatis et al. 1989). The amount of DNA was determined by comparison of the ultraviolet fluorescence of an aliquot of each sample with known quantities of lambda DNA.
RFLP-Analysis: 3-4 μg DNA were digested with HinfI and separated by electrophoresis in 0,8% garose gels. Single locus probes were provided labeled with the NICE system (ZENECA). Southern transfer and hybridisation were done by standard methods (Manniatis et al. 1989).
PCR-Analysis: PCR reactions were carried out using 1-5 ng of genomic DNA in a 50 μl reaction volume. Reaction mixtures consisted of 10 mM Tris(HCl) pH 8,3; 50 mM KCl; 1,5 mM $MgCl_2$; 200 μM dNTPs; 2,5 U Taq polymerase (Perkin Elmer, USA); 0,20 μM of each Primer. Primer sequences: HumTHO1 (TC11, Edwards et al. 1991), HumVWA31/A (VWA, Kimpton et al. 1992), D21S11 (Sharma et al. 1991), ACTBP2 (SE33, Polymeropoulos et al. 1992), Y27H29 (Roewer et al. 1992). Amplification was carried out a GeneAmp PCR System 9600 from Perkin Elmer Cetus. Temperature cycling conditions were as follows: 30 cycles of 95 °C for 20s, 58 °C (THO1, VWA, SE33, D21S11) or 56 °C (Y27H29) for 30s, 72 °C for 20s followed by a final 7 min incubation at 72°C.

RESULTS AND DISCUSSION

Five different alleles were obtained from a sample of 156 southern Bavarian non-related men. The frequencies of the respective alleles: allele A (186 bp) 16%, allele B (190 bp) 45%, allele C (194 bp) 17%, allele D (198 bp) 19% and allele E (202 bp) 3%. Upon examination of 35 proven father-son-exclusions, exclusive constellations existed in 28 cases (80%) when employing the Y27H39-polymorphism.

Figure 1:

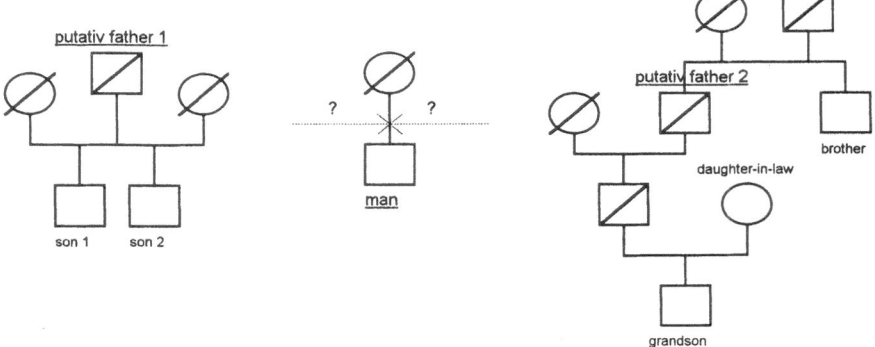

Table 1: Results of a deficienciy case.
Which putative father was the father of the "man"?

Probes	man	son 1	son 2
		putative father 1	putative father 1
MS43a	8,0 / 9,1	5,7 / 9,1	5,1 / 5,7
MS31	6,4	6,4 / 7,0	6,6 / 7,0
MS8	2,3 / 6,8	2,8 / 5,2	2,8 / 4,8
MS1	2,1 / 9,5	4,9 / 8,3	4,6 / 6,7
G3	3,4 / 7,1	7,1 / 2,1	5,0 / 2,1
Y27H39	4	2	2

Probes	man	brother putative father 2	grandson putativ father 2	daughter-in-law putative father 2
MS43a	8,0 / 9,1	9,1 / 5,9	9,6 / 8,2	8,2 / 8,9
MS31	6,4	6,0 / 6,4	8,6 / 7,0	7,0 / 5,8
MS1	2,1 / 9,5	10,2 / 12,4	2,8 / 2,4	2,4 / 5,5
G3	3,4 / 7,0	6,4	7,0 / 9,6	9,6
VWA	16 / 16	17 / 17	18 / 17	17 / 16
THO1	6 / 7	9 / 9,3	9 / 9	9 / 9,3
SE33 [a]	3 / 18	3 / 18	3 / 11	11 / 18
D21S11[a]	9 / 13,2	2 / 13,2	13,2 / 8	8 / 10
Y27H39	4	4	4	

a: Nomenclature like Kratzer A. et al. 1994.

Figure 1 shows the family tree of a deficiency case in which both supposed putative fathers were no longer available for paternity examinations. Two sons, half-brothers of another, were included on behalf of the first deceased putative father. The second putative father was substituted by a brother, a grandson and a daughter-in-law. Results of examinations centring on 4 single locus systems, 4 STR´s and the Y27H39 locus of the persons involved are summarised in table 1.
Constellations of exclusion in regard to putative father 1 could be shown in the Y27H39 and MS1 systems. It was assumed that the men A and B (fig. 1) factually are half brothers.
No exclusive constellation was found in regard to putative father 2. A paternity probability of W = 97,37% was calculated by M.P. Baur, Bonn, Germany.

SUMMARY

The allele distribution in the southern Bavarian population as seen by us as well as the paternity-related data emphasise the potential of the tetranucleotide repeats Y27H39, especially in regard to deficiency cases. In addition, this system lends itself to determination of sex as well as forensic trace analysis.

REFERENCES

Edwards A, Civitello A, Hammond HA, Caskey CT (1991) DNA typing and genetic mapping with trimeric and tetrameric tandem repeats. Am-J-Hum-Genet 49:746-756
Gomolka M, Hundrieser J, Nurnberg P, Roewer L, Epplen JT, Epplen C (1994) Selected di- and tetranucleotide microsatellites from chromosomes 7, 12, 14, and Y in various Eurasian populations. Hum Genet. 93:592 596
Kimpton C, Walton A, Gill P (1992) A further tetranucleotide repeat polymorphism in the vWF gene. Hum Mol Genet 1:287
Kratzer A, Gränacher A, Jamnicki M and Bär W (1994) Swiss population data for 3 STR-Systems, HLADQα and D1S80. In: Bär W, Fiori A, Rossi U (eds.) Advances in Forensic Haemogenetics Vol 5. Springer, Berlin, p 515-517
Manniatis T, Fritsch EF, Sambrock J (1989) Molecular cloning: A laboratory manual Cold Spring Harbor, University Press, New York
Polymeropoulos M H, Rath D S, Xiao H; Merri C R (1992) Tetranucleotide repeat polymorphism at the human beta-actin related pseudogene H-beta-Ac-psi-2 (ACTBP2). Nucleic Acids Res. 20:1432
Roewer L, Arnemann J, Spurr N K, Grzeschik K H, Epplen-J T (1992) Simple repeat sequences on the human Y chromosome are equally polymorphic as their autosomal counterparts. Hum Genet 89:389-394
Santos FR, Pena SD, Epplen JT (1993) Genetic and population study of a Y linked tetranucleotide repeat DNA polymorphism with a simple non isotopic technique. Hum Genet 90:655 656
Sharma V, Litt M (1992) Tetranucleotide repeat polymorphism at the D21S11 locus. Hum Mol Genet 1:67

STUDIES ON THE HUMACTBP2 (SE33)

G. M. Weichhold, W. Keil and B. Bayer

Institut für Rechtsmedizin der Universität München
Frauenlobstr. 7a, D-80337 München, Germany

INTRODUCTION

The short tandem repeat (STR) HumACTBP2 (human beta-actin related pseudogene) displays a highly variable polymorphism of length. Therefore it has a high information content in trace analysis and paternity examinations. The purpose of the study was to answer the question of how exact a determination of the alleles of the HumACTBP2 system may be obtained with the ABI 373A sequencer by means of a genetic population study involving 327 non-related persons of the greater Munich area. Apart from the internal standard GS350, an allelic ladder was added to each sample in order to increase the accuracy of allele determination. In addition, families with proven paternity were examined and scanned for mother/child or father/child mismatches.

MATERIALS AND METHODS

DNA was prepared from whole blood using the QIAmp Blood Kit, Qiagen or standard methods (Manniatis et al. 1989).
Amplification conditions: After quantification PCR reactions were carried out using 1-5 ng of genomic DNA in a 25 µl reaction volume. Reaction mixtures consisted of 10 mM Tris(HCl) pH 8,3; 50 mM KCl; 1,5 mM $MgCl_2$; 0,1% Tween 20; 200 µM dNTPs; 1,25 U Taq polymerase (Perkin Elmer, USA); 0,15 µM of each Primer (HumACTBP2/1 5´ AAT CTG GGC GAC AAG AGT GA 3´ labelled with "6-FAM" or with "HEX" (ABD) for the internal allelic ladder, HumACTBP2/2 5´ AAT CTG GGC GAC AAG AGT GA 3´, Polymeropoulos et al. 1992). Amplification reactions were carried out on a Perkin Elmer Cetus 9600 thermal cycler and consisted of 30 cycles of 95 °C for 20s, 59 °C for 40s, 72 °C for 20s followed by a final 7 min incubation at 72°C.
Detection: Aliquots of each amplification reaction were combined with the internal lane standard GS350 (ROX) and a HEX-labelled allelic HumACTBP2-ladder. Samples were loaded onto 6% denaturing gels (19:1, 24 cm well to read) and run in 1xTBE on an ABD 373A Sequencer for 7 h at constant power (30 Watts). Fragment sizes were determined using Genescan 672 Software employing the Local Southern method.
Taq-Cycle-Sequencing: After Etidiumbromid-staining DNA bands were cut from a 6% PAA gel, eluated using the "crush and soak" method (Maniatis et al. 1989) and

reamplified in a 100 µl reaction volume. Amplification products were desalted and concentrated using Microcon 50 (Amicon, Beverly, USA). Sequencing reactions were carried out using the Taq Dye-Deoxy-Terminator Cycle Sequencing Kit (ABD) with 100 - 300 ng template DNA and 6 pmol sequencing primer (5´AAT CTG GGC GAC AAG AGT GA 3´), 25 cycles total of 96 °C 15s, 58 °C 15s, 60 °C 4 min.

RESULTS

A genetic population study was carried out involving the STR-system HumACTBP2 of 327 non-related persons of the greater Munich area. In order to increase accuracy, an allelic ladder was added to all samples as additional internal standard. The frequency distribution obtained is shown in Fig. 1. Nomenclature from the allelic ladder followes Kratzer et al. 1994.

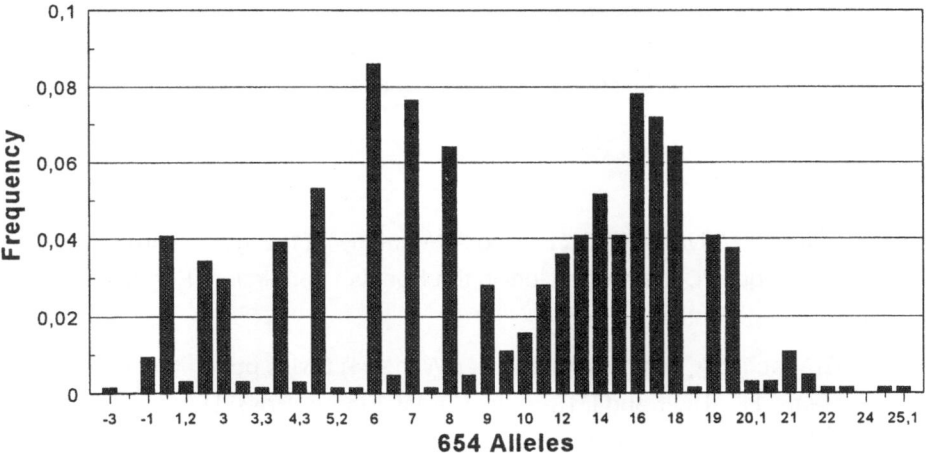

Fig. 1: Distribution of the HumACTBP2 Alleles

Using Genescan analysis in the 223 to 325 bp range 41 alleles with frequencies between 0,15% and 8,26% could be differentiated. Twenty of these alleles displayed an allele frequency of less than 1%. Data found in other examinations concerning population genetics let the discovery of additional alleles seem possible (Wiegand 1993 et al., Kratzer et al. 1994 Cabrero et al. 1995).
The power of discrimination of HumACTBP2 was 0,995 and heterocygosity was 0,938.

The alleles of the additional allelic ladder showed gel-to-gel differences between 0,8 and 2,3 bp, depending on allele size, in the 235 to 318 bp segment. Gel-to-gel differences bigger than 1% were found only in alleles larger than 250 bp. Lane-to-lane differences in gels with 24 or 36 tracks were less than 0,01 bp.

Examination of families with proven paternity showed one mutation per 176 meioses. A total of 2 mutations was found. After sequencing with the Taq Cycle sequencing reaction one (GAAA) repeat unit was lost in both cases respectively.

Sequencing of the allele 16 (291 bp, Genescan) shows a $(GAAA)_{11}(GAAAAA)$ $(GAAA)_{15}$ repeat with a total fragment length of 285 bp. The Allele coresponds to allel 27 from Möller et al. 1994.

SUMMARY

A genetic population study was carried out involving the STR-system HumACTBP2 of 327 non-related persons of the greater Munich area. We detected 41 different HumACTBP2 alleles with frequencies between 0,15% and 8,26%. Some of these alleles differing by as little as one base. Data found in other examinations concerning population genetics let the discovery of additional alleles seem possible.

REFERENCES

Cabrero C, Diez-A, Valverde E, Carracedo A, Alemany J (1995) Allele frequency distribution of four PCR-amplified loci in the Spanish population. Forensic Sci Int 71: 153-164

Kratzer A, Gränacher A, Jamnicki M and Bär W (1994) Swiss population data for 3 STR-Systems, HLADQα and D1S80. In: Bär W, Fiori A, Rossi U (eds.) Advances in Forensic Haemogenetics Vol 5. Springer, Berlin, p 515-517

Manniatis T, Fritsch EF, Sambrock J (1989) Molecular cloning: A laboratory manual Cold Spring Harbor, University Press, New York

Möller A, Brinkmann B (1994) Locus ACTBP2 (SE33) Sequencing data reveal considerable polymorphism. Int J Leg Med 106:262-267

Polymeropoulos M H, Rath D S, Xiao H; Merri C R (1992) Tetranucleotide repeat polymorphism at the human beta-actin related pseudogene H-beta-Ac-psi-2 (ACTBP2). Nucleic Acids Res 20:1432

Wiegand P, Budowle B, Rand S, Brinkmann B (1993) Forensic validation of the STR systems SE 33 and TC 11. Int J Legal Med 105:315-320

Hungarian population data for 11 PCR-based polymorphisms

J. Woller, S. Füredi and Z. Pádár

Institute for Forensic Sciences, P.O.Box 314/4, Budapest, Hungary

INTRODUCTION

Before introducing any new genetic marker into forensic casework, population surveys are needed in the relevant population samples. The legal DNA work requires highly informative polymorphic markers, and also requests sufficiently large database for the systems used. Considering these demands, we carried out population genetic surveys for 11 PCR-based polymorphic loci LDLR, GYPA, HBGG, D7S8, GC, HLA-DQα, D1S80, ApoB3', HUMVWFA31, HUMTH01, and HUMFES/FPS. In this study we present data for these systems in population samples of at least 244 unrelated Hungarian Caucasian individuals.

MATERIALS AND METHODS

DNA was obtained from whole liquid blood samples of 661 unrelated individuals. Amplification and typing of PM and HLA-DQα loci were performed according to the Perkin Elmer protocol. The rest of the systems were amplified in singleplex ways [1,2], and were analysed on horizontal non-denaturing/high-resolutional PAGE followed by silver staining except ApoB3', for which agarose gel electrophoresis and ethidium bromide staining was used [3]. The Hardy-Weinberg expectations (HWE) were checked by using the heterozygosity-test [4] and the χ^2-analysis, where the allele binning strategy [5] was applied for VNTRs and STRs.

RESULTS AND DISCUSSION

The allele frequency distributions for the 11 polymorphic loci are shown in Table 1. In Table 1 we also denoted the allele counts (n) for each system.

LDLR: We could observe all the 3 possible genotypes, the most common one was AB (50%). Statistical analyses were performed as follows: χ^2 (1df) = 0.186, P = 0.666; observed heterozygosity (h^{obs}) = 0.5000.

GYPA: All the 3 possible genotypes were found, the most common one was AB (48.8%). The results of statistical analyses: χ^2 (1df) = 0.066, P = 0.798; h^{obs} = 0.4877.

HBGG: We encountered 4 out of 6 possible genotypes with the genotype AB being the most frequent (47.1%). The statistics was calculated as follows: χ^2 (1df) = 0.441, P = 0.507; h^{obs} = 0.4877.

D7S8: All the 3 possible genotypes were detected, the most common one was AB (50%). The results of statistical calculations: χ^2 (1df) = 0.469, P = 0.493; h^{obs} = 0.5000.

GC: All the 6 possible genotypes were encountered with the genotypes AC and CC the most common ones (33.6% for both). Statistical analyses resulted as follows: χ^2 (3df) = 0.692, P = 0.875, h^{obs} = 0.5656. The 5 PM loci result a combined discrimination power (PD) of

0.994. Similarly, the combined chance of exclusion (CE) value for the 5 systems in the Hungarian Caucasian population is 0.692.

HLA-DQα: We observed all the 21 possible genotypes with the genotype 4-4 being the most frequent (11.8%). In the statistical computations we obtained the following results: χ^2 (14df) = 9.87, P = 0.772; h^{obs} = 0.793, PD = 0.930, CE = 0.602.

D1S80: We obtained 103 different genotypes and the genotype 18-24 was the most frequent (17.2%). Statistical analyses were performed as follows: χ^2 (10df) = 8.24, P = 0.606; h^{obs} = 0.8321; PD = 0.942, CE = 0.645.

ApoB3': 56 distinct genotypes could be typed in this survey. We noticed the genotype 35-37 most frequently (18%). The results of statistical analyses: χ^2 (6df) = 1.55, P = 0.956; h^{obs} = 0.7734, PD = 0.923, CE = 0.587.

HUMVWFA31: In this population sample we distinguished between 30 genotypes with the genotype 16-17 being the most common (13.2%). Statistical results: χ^2 (21df) = 11.30, P = 0.957; h^{obs} = 0.8151, PD = 0.935, CE = 0.621.

HUMTH01: In the TH01 analysis 22 different genotypes were detected. The genotype 6-9.3 was most frequently observed (14.4%). Statistical analyses were performed as follows: χ^2 (15df) = 12.13, P = 0.669; h^{obs} = 0.7847, PD = 0.917, CE = 0.575.

HUMFES/FPS: In the course of the typing for FES/FPS we did not distinguish between the alleles 10 and 10a as well as between the alleles 11 and 11a on non-denaturing PAGE, thus 17 distinct genotypes were counted. The most frequent genotype was 10-11 with 26.5%. The results of statistical analyses: χ^2 (10df) = 9.79, P = 0.460; h^{obs} = 0.6872, PD = 0.833, CE = 0.417.

There was no significant deviation from HWE for the 11 systems based on the χ^2-analysis and the heterozygosity-test. In a different survey [6] there was found little evidence for departures from expectations of independence of alleles across 7 loci (LDLR, GYPA, HBGG, D7S8, GC, HLA-DQα, D1S80) in a Hungarian population sample. Validation of the independence across all the 11 loci is under investigation. Since the high degree of polymorphisms of the 11 PCR-based markers led to a combined PD = 0.999999998 and a combined CE value of 0.998 in the Hungarian population, the joint application of these systems gives an extremely informative tool to the hand of the forensic scientist.

REFERENCES

[1] AmpliFLP™ D1S80 PCR Amplification Kit protocol. Perkin Elmer/Roche.

[2] Pestono C, Lareu MV, Rodríguez MS, Munoz I, Barros F, Carracedo A (1995) Int J Legal Med 107:283-290

[3] Schnee-Griese J, Teifel-Greding J. (1991) Forensic Sci Int 51:173-178

[4] Nei M, Roychoudhury AK (1974) Genetics 76:379-390

[5] Brenner C, Morris JW (1990) In: Proceedings for the International Symposium on Human Identification. Promega Corporation, Madison, USA, pp 21-53

[6] Budowle B, Koons B, Smerick J, Woller J, Füredi S, Pádár Z, Comey CT (1995) J Forensic Sci (submitted)

Table 1   Allele frequency distributions for 11 PCR-based loci in Hungarian Caucasian population samples

D1S80 Allele	(n=1322) Frequency	*ApoB3'* Allele	(n=1156) Frequency	*PM loci* Allele	(n=488) Frequency
14	0.0015	29	0.0009	LDLR A	0.4180
16	0.0023	31	0.0969	LDLR B	0.5820
17	0.0045	33	0.0580	GYPA A	0.6004
18	0.2451	35	0.2457	GYPA B	0.3996
19	0.0030	36	0.0026	HBGG A	0.5102
20	0.0257	37	0.3746	HBGG B	0.4816
21	0.0242	39	0.0450	HBGG C	0.0082
22	0.0424	41	0.0112	D7S8 A	0.6025
23	0.0106	43	0.0017	D7S8 B	0.3975
24	0.3404	45	0.0095	GC A	0.2766
25	0.0620	47	0.0597	GC B	0.1934
26	0.0166	49	0.0735	GC C	0.5840
27	0.0061	51	0.0147		
28	0.0620	53	0.0051		
29	0.0378	55	0.0009		
30	0.0113				
31	0.0620				
32	0.0061				
33	0.0045				
34	0.0023				
35	0.0015			*HLA-DQα* Allele	(n=726) Frequency
36	0.0083				
37	0.0121			1.1	0.1983
38	0.0008			1.2	0.1556
39	0.0008			1.3	0.0964
40	0.0030			2	0.1019
41	-			3	0.1185
>41	0.0030			4	0.3292

HUMVWFA31 Allele	(n=1136) Frequency	*HUMTH01* Allele	(n=734) Frequency	*HUMFES/FPS* Allele	(n=748) Frequency
13	0.0009	5	0.0041	8	0.0134
14	0.1039	6	0.2139	9	-
15	0.1206	7	0.1621	10	0.2500
16	0.1998	8	0.1158	11	0.4532
17	0.2879	9	0.1853	12	0.2313
18	0.1954	9.3	0.3106	13	0.0481
19	0.0757	10	0.0082	14	0.0040
20	0.0132				
21	0.0026				

Allele frequency distribution of the STR system ACBP2 (SE33) in a Population of Portugal (Central Area)

L. Souto and M. C. Vide

Institute of Legal Medicine. 3000 Coimbra. Portugal

System and locus: HUMACBP2 (SE33), chromosome 5.

Population and sample size: Portugal (Central Area). N: 144

Methods: Primers (Wiegand et al. 1993)
PCR amplification conditions: 94°C - 45", 60°C - 30 ", 72°C - 30"; 30 cycles.
Electrophoretic methods: 6% polyacrylamide denaturing gel electrophoresis. The gels were run for 6 h at constant power (30w), 2500 V and 40 MA on the ABI 373 A DNA Sequencer. Typing was performed using the internal standard Genescan Rox 2500 and an allelic ladder of 23 sequenced alleles (from the EDNAP trial for the STR system ACTBP2 (SE33), 1995.)

Results:

SE33

Observed genotypes

Gen.	Obs.	Gen.	Obs.	Gen.	Obs.	Gen.	Obs.	Gen.	Obs.
9-18	1	15-27	2	17-28	2	19-29	2	25-27	2
11-28	1	15-28	1	17-29	2	19-30	1	25-28	1
12-14	1	15-29	1	17-31	2	20-21	1	25-29	1
13-17	1	15-30	1	18-19	2	20-24	2	25-31	1
13-27	1	16-18	1	18-20	1	20-28	1	26-28	2
13-30	1	16-19	4	18-21	3	20-29	1	26-30	1
13-32	1	16-20	1	18-22	1	20-30	1	27-29	2
14-17	1	16-22	2	18-23	2	20-34	1	27-30	1
14-18	1	16-23	1	18-24	2	21-24	1	27-31	2
14-19	2	16-27	1	18-27	1	21-27	2	27-34	2
14-27	1	16-28	1	18-28	2	21-30	2	28-29	4
14-28	2	16-29	2	18-29	2	22-24	1	28-30	2
14-31	1	16-30	1	18-31	1	22-27	1	29-29	1
15-16	2	16-31	1	19-19	1	22-29	1	29-30	1
15-17	1	17-18	2	19-20	2	22-30	3	29-33	1
15-18	2	17-19	1	19-21	1	22-31	1	30-30	1
15-19	2	17-21	1	19-22	3	22-33	1	30-31	2
15-21	1	17-23	1	19-24	1	24-25	1	30-32	1
15-22	2	17-26	2	19-27	1	24-32	1	31-31	1
15-23	1	17-27	3	19-28	1	25-26	1		

Allele frequencies

Allele	Frequency	Allele	Frequency	Allele	Frequency	Allele	Frequency
9	0.0035	17	0.0660	24	0.0313	31	0.0451
11	0.0035	18	0.0833	25	0.0243	32	0.0104
12	0.0035	19	0.0868	26	0.0208	33	0.0069
13	0.0139	20	0.0382	27	0.0764	34	0.0104
14	0.0313	21	0.0417	28	0.0694		
15	0.0556	22	0.0556	29	0.0764		
16	0.0590	23	0.0174	30	0.0695		

Exact Test P=0.18

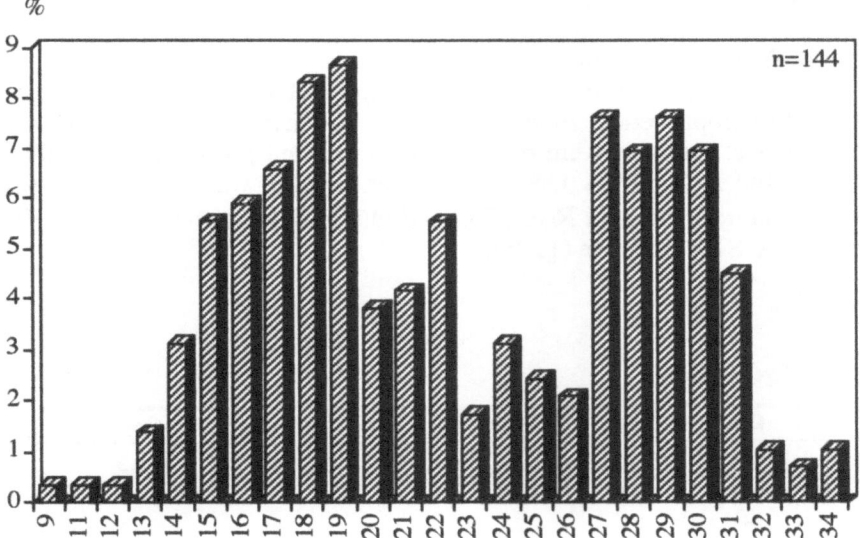

Comments: This study represents our preliminary results. Further devellopment of our database is required for such a complex system.
Nevertheless, the present data show good accordance with other published SE33 frequencies.
A total of 25 different alleles were found.
Family studies (45 families, results to be published) show, so far, no significant differences with Mendelian expectations.

References: Wiegand P , Budowle B, Rand S and Brinkmann B (1993) Forensic validation of the STR systems SE 33 and TC 11. Int J Leg Med 105:315 - 320.

Allele Frequencies in 4 Str's in a Population of Portugal (Central Area)

L. Souto, D. N. Vieira, F. Corte-Real and M. C. Vide

Institute of Legal Medicine. 3000 Coimbra. Portugal

Systems and loci: HUMTHO1 (11 pl. 5.5 - p 15); HUMVWA31 (12 p 12 - pter.); HUMF13A1 (6 p 25 - p 24); HUMFESFPS (15 q25 - q ter).

Population and sample size: Portugal (Central Area). N: 344.

Methods: Primers (Kimpton et al. 1995)

PCR amplification conditions: Kimpton et al. 1995 (quadruplex).

Electrophoretic methods: 6% polyacrylamide denaturing gel electrophoresis. The gels were run for 6 h at constant power (30w), 2500 V and 40 mA on the ABI 373 A DNA Sequencer. Typing was performed using the internal standard Genescan Rox 2500 and allelic ladders from the 2nd EDNAP Collaborative STR Exercise (1995).

Results:

TH01

Observed genotypes

Gen.	Obs.	Gen.	Obs.	Gen.	Obs.	Gen.	Obs.
6-6	14	7-7	4	8-8	5	9-9.3	37
6-7	19	7-8	11	8-9	17	9.3-9.3	34
6-8	28	7-9	23	8-9.3	25	9.3-10	2
6-9	30	7-9.3	24	8-10	2		
6-9.3	54	7-10	2	9-9	13		

Allele frequencies

Allele	Frequency	Allele	Frequency	Allele	Frequency
6	0.2311	8	0.1352	9.3	0.3052
7	0.1265	9	0.1933	10	0.0087

Exact Test P=0.86

FES

Observed genotypes

Gen.	Obs.	Gen.	Obs.	Gen.	Obs.	Gen.	Obs.
8-10	3	10-11	86	11-12	61	13-13	1
8-11	7	10-12	55	11-13	7		
8-12	3	10-13	6	12-12	21		
10-10	32	11-11	53	12-13	9		

Allele frequencies

Allele	Frequency	Allele	Frequency	Allele	Frequency
8	0.0189	11	0.3881	13	0.0349
10	0.3110	12	0.2471		

Exact Test P=0.82

VWA

Observed genotypes

Gen.	Obs.	Gen.	Obs.	Gen.	Obs.	Gen.	Obs.
13-16	1	15-15	1	16-19	11	18-19	8
14-14	4	15-16	21	16-20	1	18-20	1
14-15	13	15-17	20	17-17	24	18-21	1
14-16	17	15-18	20	17-18	39	19-19	3
14-17	26	15-19	3	17-19	12	19-20	1
14-18	14	16-16	19	17-20	3		
14-19	5	16-17	40	17-21	2		
14-20	1	16-18	24	18-18	9		

Allele frequencies

Allele	Frequency	Allele	Frequency	Allele	Frequency
13	0.0014	16	0.2224	19	0.0669
14	0.1221	17	0.2762	20	0.0102
15	0.1148	18	0.1817	21	0.0043

Exact Test P=0.84

F13

Observed genotypes

Gen.	Obs.	Gen.	Obs.	Gen.	Obs.	Gen.	Obs.
3.2-3.2	6	4-5	2	5-7	40	6-16	2
3.2-4	1	4-6	5	5-8	2	7-7	51
3.2-5	8	4-7	6	5-14	4	7-8	5
3.2-6	19	4-16	1	5-16	3	7-14	3
3.2-7	17	4-17	1	6-6	35	7-16	4
3.2-16	1	5-5	10	6-7	67	7-17	2
4-4	2	5-6	46	6-8	1		

Allele frequencies

Allele	Frequency	Allele	Frequency	Allele	Frequency
3.2	0.0843	6	0.3052	14	0.0102
4	0.0291	7	0.3575	16	0.0160
5	0.1817	8	0.0116	17	0.0044

Exact Test P=0.24

Statistical parameters (4 STRs)

	TH01	FES	VWA	F13	Comb
CE	0.5616	0.4216	0.6219	0.5078	0.9528
PD	0.9145	0.8436	0.9365	0.8885	0.9999
h	0.7764	0.6900	0.8086	0.7375	

CE, chance of exclusion; PD, power of discrimination; h, allelic diversity values

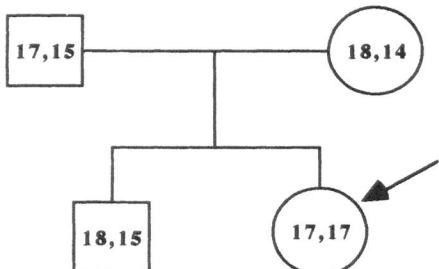

An odd exclusion of mother, in the VWA system, found in a family, under study.

Comments: Our sample was found to be in Hardy - Weinberg equilibrium. The other statistical parameters show that this 4-plex is a robust and discriminating combined system, very useful to routine forensic casework, namely in parentage analysis.

Family studies involving 120 families (data to be published) show no disagreement with Mendelian inheritance. However in one particulary family, we detected an exclusion of the mother, in the VWA system. Such an odd exclusion is in contradiction with data from 26 other ("classical" and PCR) systems, yet confirmed by singleplex amplification of the VWA system alone and by repeated analysis with different samples from the same individuals. This problem requires further and extensive investigation, still in progress at our laboratory.

Some modifications of Primer concentrations had to be done in order to get balanced allele signals from the different PCR systems. Each new batch of Primers must be tested prior to use in routine, and concentrations adjusted, if necessary.

References: Kimpton C et al.(1995). Report on the second EDNAP collaborative STR exercise. Forensic Sci Int 71 : 137 - 152.

DNA PROFILING: A GENETIC STUDY OF TWO VNTR LOCI IN THE EAST MIDLANDS

V.J. Stinton and S.S.Mastana

Human Genetics Laboratory, Department of Human Sciences,
Loughborough University of Technology, Loughborough, Leicestershire, England.

Introduction: DNA fingerprinting developed by Jeffreys, Thein and Wilson(1985) is the most discriminating technique used to identify an individual. It has proved to be a powerful tool in the legal world aiding in the identification of criminals and solving paternity disputes. In recent years DNA fingerprinting has been increasingly replaced by DNA profiling. A number of problems with the application of this powerful tool have recently been highlighted in United States courts(Joyce, 1990; Bown, 1993). One particular concern in the application of genetic typing is the use of general population databases to determine DNA profile probabilities. It has already been established that there are racial differences in allele frequencies(Gill et al, 1991; Buffrey et al, 1991). This had led to the construction of databases for different racial groups. However, it has recently been proposed that minisatellite allele frequencies are different within sub-populations of a major population(Lander, 1989; Lewontin and Hartl, 1991). Population stratification would have important implications for forensic and paternity work. General databases used to calculate forensic and paternity probabilities may not accurately represent sub-population diversity. To date, studies by Budowle and Monson(1994) and Budowle et al(1994) indicate that DNA profile probabilities may not be affected by using general databases. However, further research is required to clarify and support or disprove these findings.

Objectives: The main aim of this study was to establish the Federal Bureau of Investigation(FBI) fixed bin allele frequencies of MS1(D1S7) and MS43a(D12S11) minisatellite loci in the Caucasian East Midlands population. The allele frequencies of MS43a were compared with other UK Caucasian sub-populations, the Forensic Science Service(FSS) Caucasian and racial databases and other Caucasian populations world-wide to determine if the populations were heterogeneous. The heterozygosity, paternity(exclusion) and forensic(inclusion) calculations were conducted on the East Midlands data to determine the efficiency of using MS1 and MS43a probes in this population.

Population and sample size: Caucasian East Midlands. N:102

Methods: DNA extracted from random blood donor samples was digested with restriction enzyme Hinf1 and VNTR profile was established using standard Southern blotting methodology. NICE MS1 and MS43a probes (Cellmark Diagnostics) were used in this study along with MW100 probe as a Molecular Weight Marker. The log molecular weights of MS1 and MS43a alleles were binned into FBI fixed bins(Budowle and Monson, 1994). The allele frequency in each bin was calculated and used for comparative work.

Analysis of results: Comparisons of population FBI bin frequencies in different populations was done using heterogeneity chi square analysis. The heterozygosities of MS1 and MS43a were calculated. The probability of match(PM), discrimination probability(DP) and probability of exclusion(PE) using MS1 and MS43a independently and combined using the Caucasian East Midlands population database.

Results and discussion: Significant heterogeneity chi-square values for MS43a and MS1 were found in a large number of FBI bins in UK Caucasian, world Caucasian (US, Norway and Spanish) and UK racial population comparisons. MS1 studies are relatively limited and require further studies to evaluate subpopulation heterogeneity. However, of main interest is that the study's data indicates that population stratification may exist within the United Kingdom at the MS43a minisatellite locus (Table 1). The large number of significant population heterogeneity χ 2 values in comparisons of the East Midlands, Newcastle and FSS Caucasian databases highlight this. This emphasises that a general database such as the FSS may not represent the MS43a allele frequencies found in the East Midlands and Newcastle. The study's results also challenge the findings of Budowle and Monson(1994) and Budowle et al(1994) who claimed from their data that sub-population differences were small and hence irrelevant. The implies that geographical databases may be required in the UK as the present general database may underestimate/overestimate DNA probabilities. However, further investigation would be required to support the present study's findings.

Table 1: Population heterogeneity chi-square(χ2) values of five population comparisons of FBI fixed bin MS43a allele frequencies.

	A_1	B_2	C_3	D_4	E_5
FBI Fixed Bins (base Pairs)	Heterogeneity χ2	Heterogeneity χ2	Heterogeneity χ2	Heterogeneity χ2	Heterogeneity χ2
3330 - 3674		14.03***	37.39***	45.65***	40.04***
3675 - 3979		3.99*	15.60***		11.88***
3980 - 4323		3.99*	16.10***	75.15***	23.28***
4324 - 4821	3.31	0.28	4.51	8.95	0.27
4822 - 5219	0.38	0.15	0.44	5.93	3.22
5220 - 5685	1.8	6.10*	6.54*	33.15***	5.03*
5686 - 6368	6.08*	9.97**	40.48***	140.16***	14.24**
6369 - 7241	6.21*	48.39***	121.16***	228.86***	27.22***
7242 - 8452	0.01	2.37	2.71	40.79***	13.21***
8453 - 10093	16.07***	2.37	47.12***	66.21***	64.58***
10094 - 11368	9.07**	4.76*	57.53***	120.21***	36.56***
11369 - 12829	0.36		24.39***	49.83***	
12830 -	18.07***		43.42***	119.08***	

* Significant at 5% level; ** Significant at 1% level; *** Significant at 0.1% level.

Comparative analysis:
[1] East Midlands\Newcastle (Newcastle data obtained from Human Genetics Department , Newcastle university.)
[2] East Midlands/Caucasian FSS(FSS data from Forensic Science Service, Birmingham)
[3] East Midlands/Newcastle/Caucasian FSS.
[4] East Midlands/Newcastle/Caucasian FSS/US Caucasians/Norwegians/Spanish (US Caucasian, Norwegian, and Spanish data from Budowle and Monson(1994)).
[5] East Midlands/Afro Caribbean/Asian(Afro Caribbean and Asian data from FSS)

657

The heterozygosity of MS1 was 94.3% and MS43a 90.6%. These relatively high heterozygosities implies that both probes are suitable for forensic and paternity work. This is supported by the low PM(0.0016), high DP(0.9984) and high PE(0.9559) when the probes are combined(Table 2).

Table 2 - Table showing forensic and paternity probabilities of MS1 and MS43a using the Caucasian East Midlands database.

Probe	Forensic Inferences		Paternity Inferences
	Probability of Match	Discrimination Probability	Probability of Exclusion
MS1	0.0322	0.9678	0.8096
MS43a	0.0499	0.9501	0.7692
MS1 + MS43a	0.0016	0.9984	0.9559

Conclusions: This study has found that both MS1 and MS43a are efficient markers for forensic and paternity work. The study has shown that Caucasian population heterogeneity may exist within the United Kingdom at the MS43a locus. MS1 data also showed some significant differences but there are not many populations studied for this locus. This implies that present probability calculations for forensic and paternity work using general Caucasian population databases should be used with caution for MS43a probe. However, further research is required to clarify the findings.

Acknowledgements: Our sincere thanks to Mrs Alice Pacynko for technical help and Drs. S.Papiha and P.Gill for comparative data.

References:
Bown W (1993) DNA fingerprinting back in the dock. New Scientist 137:14-15.
Budowle B et al (1994) Evaluation of Hinf 1 generated VNTR profile frequencies determined using various ethnic databases. Journal of Forensic Science 39:988-1008.
Budowle B and Monson K L (1994) Greater differences in forensic DNA profile frequencies from racial groups than from ethnic subgroups. Clinica Chimica Acta 228:3-18.
Buffrey C et al (1991) Allele frequency distributions of four hypervariable number tandem repeat(VNTR) loci in the London area. Forensic Science International 52:53-64.
Gill P et al (1991) Population genetics of four hypervariable loci. International Journal of Legal Medicine 104:221-227.
Jeffreys A J, Wilson V and Thein S L (1985) Hypervariable "minisatellite" regions in human DNA. Nature 316:76 -79.
Joyce C (1990) High profile DNA in court again. New Scientist 127:24 -25.
Lander E S (1989) DNA fingerprinting on trial. Nature 339:501 - 505.
Lewontin R C and Hartl D L (1991) Population genetics in forensic DNA typing. Science 254:1745-1750.

COMPARISON OF TURKISH SUBPOPULATIONS USING TWO STR's

S. Atasoy, E. Abacı-Kalfoğlu, P. Wiegand, B. Brinkmann

Institute of Legal Medicine and Forensic Sciences, University of Istanbul
34303 Istanbul-Turkey
Institute of Legal Medicine University of Münster
48149 Münster-Germany

Abstract

The short tandem repeat (STR) systems HumTH01 and Hum VWA were used for PCR typing of two Caucasian subpopulations, one living in the Black sea area (northern Turkey), the other being a subpopulation from eastern Anatolia (eastern Turkey). The allele frequency data were compared with a turkish subpopulation from Adana area (southern Turkey) and a group of Turks living in Brussels (Belgium). The HumTHO1 data showed a significant difference in the Black Sea region compared to the 3 other groups while the subpopulation from the eastern Anatolia showed significant differences in Hum VWA system.

Introduction

STR polymorhisms represent a widely used method for linkage studies and human identification (Edwards et al. 1991), even on highly degraded DNA (Brinkmann 1992). This study was carried out with the systems HumTH01 and HumVWA (Kimpton et al. 1992) on two turkish subpopulations living in the Black Sea and Eastern Anatolia. The population genetic data were compared with a turkish subpopulation living in Brussels, (Belgium) since 1960 and another population living in southern Turkey (Adana area) (Alper et al., in press).

Materials and Methods

The blood samples were collected from unrelated individuals living in two provinces the Artvin province in the eastern Black Sea and the Elazığ province situated in eastern Anatolia. DNA was extracted from 200 µl blood, air dried on sterile cotton fabric. The extraction procedure was carried out using 150 µl Chelex 100 (Biorad, Germany) with the addition of 50 ml proteinase K (2 mg/ml) as previously described (Wiegand et al. 1993 a). The reaction assay, the amplification and electrophoresis conditions for both systems were carried out as previousyl described (HumTH01: primers according to Gill et al. 1992, amplification conditions and electrophoresis according to Wiegand et al. 1993 b, HumVWA: primers according to Kimpton et al. 1992, amplification and electrophoresis according to Möller et al. 1994).

The statistical analysis was performed with standard Chi square method the logarithmic likelyhood ratio (G) test, and the exact -test by random shuffling the observed alleles 5000 times (HWE analysis, version 3.0, C. Puers, Münster Germany). The mean paternity exclusion probability was calculated according to Brenner and Morris (1989); the polymorphic information content according to Botstein et al. (1980); the probability of match and the discrimination power according to Jones (1972). The frequency profile comparison between the populations was performed using a test for genetic heterogeneity (RXC contingency table; G. Carmody, Ottawa, Canada).

Results and Discussion

A total of 7 alleles in the Black Sea and 6 allels in easten Anatolian populations for HumTH01 system, and 8 and 7 alleles respectively for HumVWA system have been observed (Fig. 1a,b).

Due to allele number and distribution both systems showed relatively high forensic efficiency values (Table 1).

HumTH01 typing results for the Black Sea area showed significant differences in comparison to the other 3 subpopulations (p>0.05) while the eastern Anatolia population show no significant difference in their allele frequencies from the Adana and Brussels Turks. For HumVWA a contrary situation was found. The Black Sea population did not differ significantly from Adana and Brussel subpopulations while significant differences were found in eastern Anatolia. No significant deviation from Hardy Weinberg equilibrium could be detected (p>0.05).

Both subpopulations, each in its geographical position is considerably isolated. The differences found may be expected because these two subpopulations must have genetic diversity once they have geographical, ecological linguistic and cultural seperation (Andrews 1989). The sample size for eastern Anatolia was too small for a relable statistical evaluation. This part of the study is still under investigation.

References

Alper B., Wiegand P., Brinkmann B. Frequency profiles of 3 STRs in a Turkish population. Int. J. Legal Med. in press.

Andrews, P.A. (1989) Ethnic Groups in the Republic of Turkey, Wisbaden.

Botstein D., White RL., Skolnick M., Davis RW., (1980) Construction of a genetic linkage map in man using restriction fragment length polymorphisms. Am J Hum Genet 32:314-331

Brenner C., Morris J. (1990) Paternity index calculations in single locus hypervariable DNA probes:validation and other studies. In: Proceedings of the international symposium on human identification 1989, Promega Corporation, pp357-373.

Edwards A., Civitello A., Hammond H.A., Caskey C.T. (1991) DNA typing and genetic mapping with trimeric and tetrameric tandem repeats. Am J Hum Genet 49:746-756.

Gill P., Kimpton C.P., Sullivan K.M. (1992) A rapid polymerase chain reaction method for identifying fixed specimens. Electrophoresis 13:173-175.

Jones D.A. (1972) Blood samples: Probabilities of discriminations. J Forensic Sci Soc 12:355-359

Kimpton C., Walton A., Gill P. (1992) A further tetranucleotide repeat polymorphism in VWF gene. Hum Mol Genet 1:287

Möller A., Weigand P., Grüschow C., Seuchter S.A., Baur M.P., Brinkmann B. (1994) Population data and forensic efficiency values for the STR systems Hum VWA, Hum MBP and Hum FABP. Int J Leg Med. 106: 183-189

Wiegand P., Bajanowski T., BrinkmannB. (1993 a) PCR typing of debris from fingernails. Int J Legal Med. 106:81-84.

Wiegand P., Budowle B., Rand S., Brinkmann B. (1993 b) Forensic validation of the STR systems SE33 and TC11. Int. J. Leg. Med. 105:315-320

Table1. Forensic efficiency values for HumTH01 and HumVWA.

Group I - Black Sea region		
	TH01	**VWA**
	n = 174	*n = 228*
MEC	0.57	0.62
MEP	0.56	0.61
PIC	0.75	0.78
pM	0.09	0.07
D		
Group II - Eastern Anatolia region		
	n = 63	*n = 76*
MEC	0.61	0.54
MEP	0.62	0.51
PIC	0.78	0.71
pM	0.09	0.11
D	0.91	0.89

MEC = mean exclusion chance
MEP = mean exclusion probability
PIC = polymorphic information content
PM = match probability
D = discrimination power

THO1

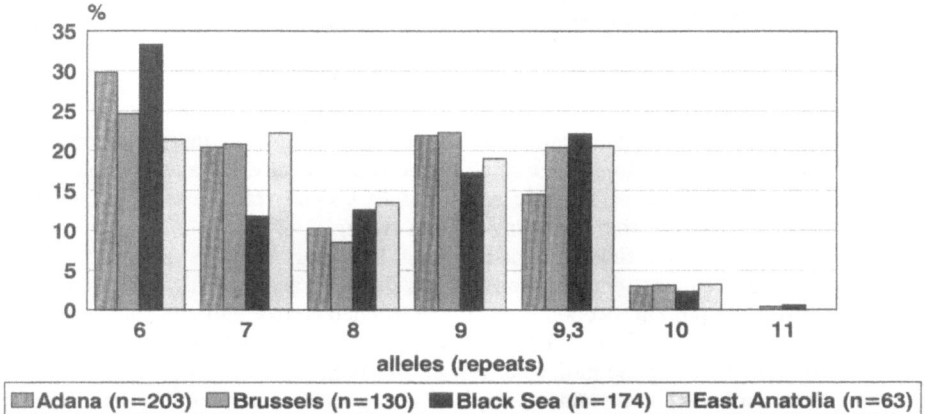

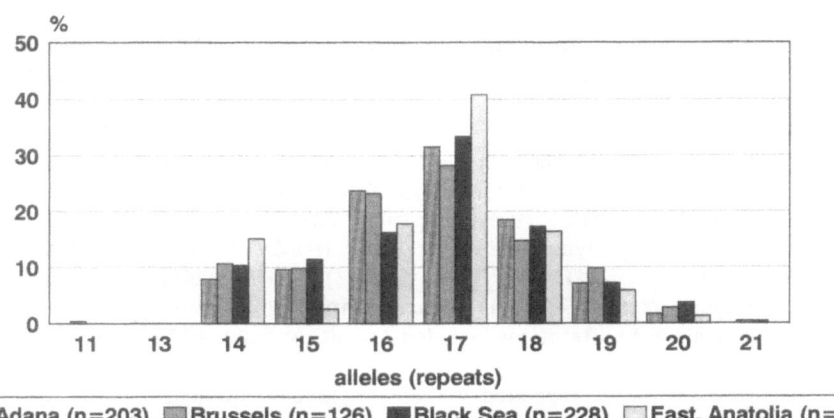

VWA

The Genetic Structure Of Four Argentine Ethnic Groups Reflected By The Analyses Of Ten Strs .

Sala, A[1].; Penacino, G[1].; Goycoechea, A[2].; Carnese, F[2].; Tomeo,[3] A. and Corach, D[1].

1-Servicio de Huellas Digitales Genéticas, Facultad de Farmacia y Bioquímica UBA. Junín 956, 1113-Buenos Aires.
2- Instituto de Antropología Facultad de Filosofía y Letras UBA,
3-Serv. Hemoterapia, Hospital de Clínicas UBA. Argentina

Introduction:

PCR tehniques have a distinct advantage over restriction fragment length polymorphism techniques due to their ability to analyze small amounts of partially degraded samples. These features broadened the field of forensic science with special references to personal and evidentiary material identification by means of DNA typing.

Beyond its aplicability in the field of gene mapping, hereditary diseases diagnosis, forensic investigation, human remains identification in mass disasters and paternity testing, the STR systems may offer a rapid and economic approach to characterize and compare the genetic structure of populations of different ethnic origins. The availability of a high number of STR systems allows a more complete molecular insight of the groups providing results that may contribute to a more accurate anthropological interpretation that could shed light on controversial topics such as migration.

The aim of this present study is to characterize four different ethnic groups from Argentina by means ot ten STR systems, two of them located on sex chromosomes and two on autosomal chromosomes. The information obtained allowed us to compare their genetic parameters and, as a by-product, to generate a local database to be used in forensic case-work.

Materials and Methods

Populations

Blood samples were obtained from unrelated donors belonging to the followings groups: 1) Caucasoid group: Buenos Aires City Metropolitan area population (average samples size n=175); 2)Aboriginal groups: a-Mapuches (n=55) Cerro Policía, SW Province of Río Negro , b-Wichis (n=35) Santa Victoria Este, NE Province of Salta and c-Tehuelches (n=28) Chalía, SW Province of Chubut. DNA was extracted by using a CTAB-based protocol (Corach, 1992, 1994).

PCR amplification of STR loci

PCR amplifications were performed in simplex or multiplex reactions. *Loci* D6S366 (Panzer,1993), Y27H39 (Roewer,1992), HUMRENA4 (Edwards,1992), HUMCSFPO (Hammond,1994) and HUMF13A (Polymeropoulos 1991b) were amplified in simplex reactions, HUMFES/FPS (Polymeropoulos,1991a) / HUMVWA (Kimpton,1992), were amplified as duplex and HUMTHO-1 (Edwards,1992) / HUMHPRTB (Edwards,1992) / HUMFABP (Polymeropoulos,1991c) as triplex. Amplifications were performed with a Perkin Elmer Thermal Cycler. Reactions included 0.02 μCi/sample α-dATP P[32] .

Amplicon detection

Amplification products were separated by electrophoresis through a 5% denaturing polyacrylamide sequencing gel. Electrophoresis was performed at 1500 V(constant voltage) in 1X TBE for three hours. Gels were then exposed to radiographic film.

Statistic analyses

Allele frecuency distributions and observed heterozigosity were established by counting, discriminative power and exclusion power were then calculated. In order to determine if the different groups fulfill the Hardy-Weinberg expectations, the test for H-W equilibrium was conducted by using a chi square test (Edwards,1992; Smouse,1986). For the investigation of the X-chromosome specific STR, HUMHPRTB only female samples were considered.

Results and Discussion

Data evaluation showed differential atributtes between the metropolitan area population, with a free gene flow, and the aboriginal groups, geographically isolated and with a restricted gene flow. Hardy-Weimberg equilibrium, evaluated by comparison of the observed and expected heterozygotes, denoted deviations in the HUMFES/FPS in Metropolitans, HUMHPRTB in Mapuches and Tehuelches, and HUMF13A1 in Tehuelches. Heterozigocity defficiency was observed in HUMFES/FPS-Tehuelches, HUMFABP-Mapuches and HUMTHO-1-Wichis and can be attributed to high endogamy levels.

Both caucasoid and the three aboriginal groups displayed differences in their allele distributions as may be seen in the histograms depicted in "Fig. 1". *Loci* HUMRENA4 and HUMFABP exhibited similar allele distribution and almost identical frequency for the most common alleles in the four populations. In contrast, at other *loci* the predominant alleles differ between populations as HUMTHO-1, HUMvWA, HUMHPRTB and Y27H39. In Wichis group, only one allele appears in the Y27H39 system (variant"A"). Table I shows the most common genotypes for all nine loci combined (P) and the probability of a match (P2).

The power of exclusion (PE) and discriminative power (DP) were calculated for each *locus* in the four populations. The PE ranged from 10.6% to 64.5%, the DP from 58.8% to 94%. The STR D6S366 showed the highest PE and DP in the three groups (Metropolitan, Mapuches and Tehuelches). Instead HUMF13A1 showed the highest PE and DP in the Wichis group.

TABLE I: MATCHING PROBABILITY of STR Loci

	Met	Map	Teh	Wich
THO-1	0,17	0,28	0,25	0,5
FABP	0,31	0,48	0,50	0,35
VWA	0,14	0,29	0,18	0,28
RENA4	0,61	0,54	0,76	0,51
FES/FPS	0,21	0,27	0,5	0,25
D6S366	0,14	0,11	0,25	0,28
HPRTB	0,16	0,26	0,36	0,33
CSF1PO	0,2	0,23	0,28	0,32
F13A1	0,19	0,17	0,15	0,23
P	8,04E-07	6,35E-06	3,23E-05	4,24E-05
P2	6,47E-13	4,03E-11	1,04E-09	1,80E-09

References

Corach D. A Reliable, Rapid and Simple Method for DNA Extraction from Frozen Sperm. Cells.Fingerprint News. Vol 3 (4):13, October 1991.

Corach D., Penacino G. and Sala A. (1994).Cadaveric DNA Extraction Protocol Based on Cetyl Trimethyl Amonium Bromide(CTAB). Medinae Legalis 1994 (In Press). Springer Verlag

Edwards A., Hammond H., Jin L., Caskey CT., Chakraborty R (1992). Genetic variation at five trimeric and tetrameric tandem repeat loci in four human population groups. Genomics 12: 241-253

Hammond HA., Jin L., Zhong Y., Caskey CT., and Chakraborty R. (1994). Evaluation of 13 ShortTandem Repeat Loci for Use in Personal Identification Applications. Am J Hum Genet 55: 175-189

Kimpton C., Walton A. and Gill P. (1992).A Futher Tetranucleotide Repeat Polymorphism in the vWF Gene Hum. Molec. Genet. 1: 287.

Panzer SW., Hammond HA., Stephens L., Chai A., Caskey CT. (1993) Trinucleotide repeat polynorphism at the D6S366 locus. Hum Mol Genet 2: 1511.

Polymeropoulos MH., Rath DS., Xiao H. Merril CR. (1991a) Tetranucleotide repeat polymorphism at the human c-fes/fps proto-oncogene (FES). Nucleic Acids Res 19: 4018.

Polymeropoulos MH., Rath DS., Xiao H. Merril CR. (1991b) Tetranucleotide repeat polymorphism at the human coagulation factor XIII A subunit gene (F13A1). Nucleic Acids Res 19: 4306.

Polymeropoulos MH., Rath DS., Xiao H. Merril CR. (1991c).Trinucleotide repeat polymorphism at the human fatty acid binding protein gene (FABP2). Nucleic Acids Res 18: 7198.

Roewer L., Armemann J., Spurr Grzeschik K.H., Epplen J.T. (1992). Simple Repeat Sequences on the Human Y Chromosome are Equally Polymorphic as Their Autosomal CounterpartsHum. Genet. 89: 389- 394

Smouse P. and Chakraborty R (1986). The use of restriction fragment length polymorphisms in paternity analysis. Am J. Hum Genet 38: 918-939

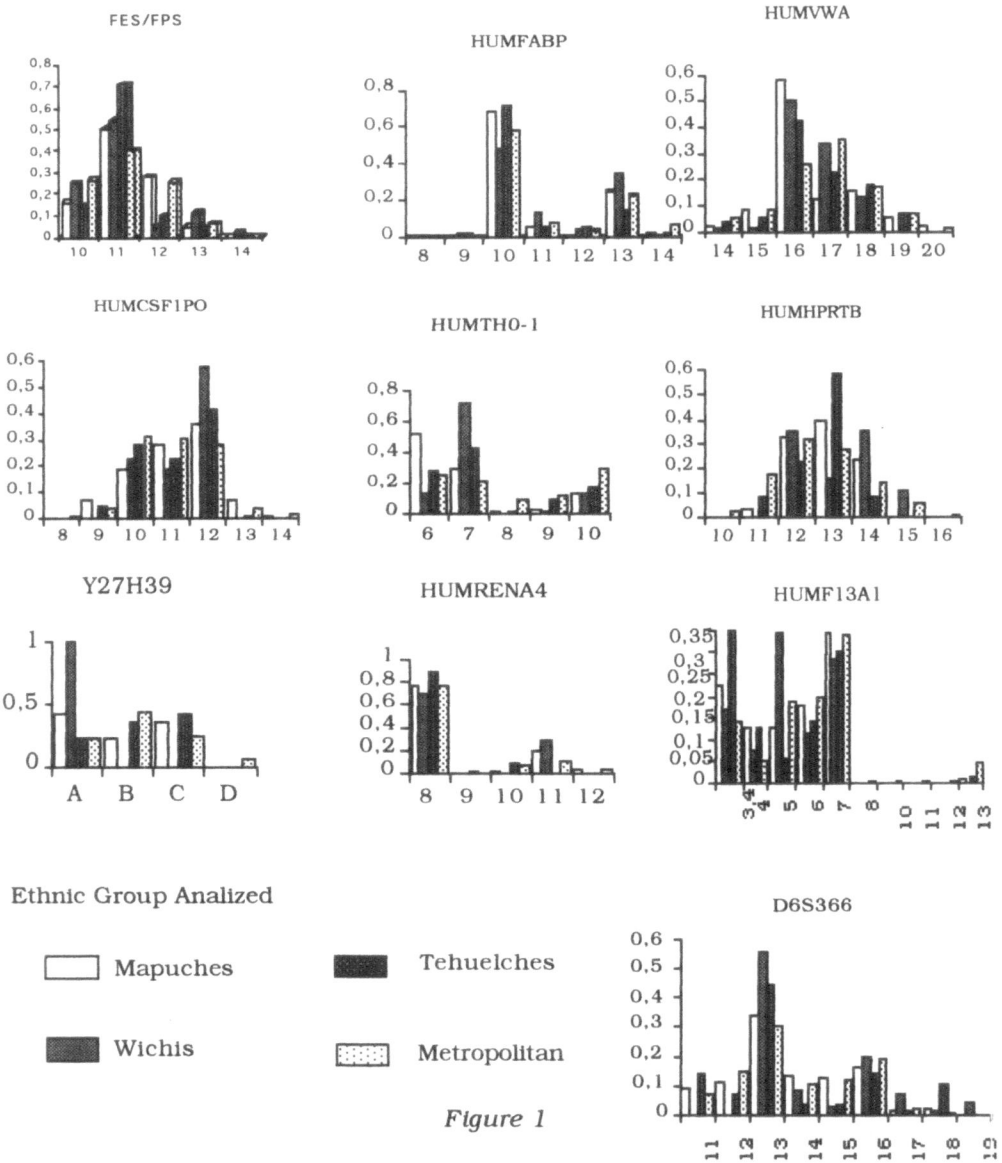

Figure 1

D1S80 AMP-FLP ATTRIBUTES IN TWO DIFFERENT ETHNIC GROUPS OF ARGENTINIAN POPULATIONS.

Penacino G[1]; Sala A[1]; Smerick J[2]; Perez Calvo J[3]; Baechtel S[2]; Budowle B[2] and Corach D[1]
1-Serv. de Huellas Dig. Genéticas, Fac. de Farm. y Bioquímica (UBA), ARGENTINA.
2-FBI Research and Training Center, Quantico Virginia, U.S.A..
3-Policía del Neuquén, ARGENTINA.

INTRODUCTION

The highly polymorphic *locus* D1S80 is the most investigated and used AMP-FLP system in the field of the molecular identification. This is, due in part, to the moderate to high number of alleles (25), the frequency distribution of the alleles, and even amplification of alleles in most samples, inspite of the considerable fragment length differences that range from 401 to 801 bp. Optimization of amplification protocols and amplicon detection systems has yielded high reproducibility of results, fullfiling basic requirements for forensic case work. Since a large number of studies have been performed in distantly located populations around the world, a great deal of genetic information, concerning this *locus*, is available for comparison.

The present study focused on the comparison of D1S80 allelic distributions exhibited by two distinct populations from Argentina: 1- a caucasian group and 2- an autochthonous population of Mapuche indians. Moreover , this study enabled the generation of a local database to be employed in forensic casework and paternity testing.

MATERIALS AND METHODS

Populations:

1- Caucasoids: 191 unrelated donors inhabiting the metropolitan area of Buenos Aires city (Argentina).

2- Aborigines: 61 unrelated Mapuche indians inhabiting three geographically closed communities: Cerro Policía, Aguada Guzmán and Loncovaca Arriba, all located in Río Negro province (Argentina).

DNA isolation:

DNA was extracted from 5 mm^2 blood stains spotted on watmann 3MM paper (about 200 µl/sample). After hydration and removal of paper debris, DNA was purified by means of a standard organic extraction procedure. Briefly: digestion with proteinase K /

SDS in TEC (10mM, 10mM, 100mM), incubation at 56°C overnight, phenol / chlorophorm / isoamyl alcohol (25:24:1) extraction, and washing and concentration with Microcon 100 (Amicon) concentrators.

DNA quantitation:

In order to obtain similar quantities of DNA samples to be amplified Slot-blot hybridization approach using the human probe D17Z1, was performed (ACES 2.0 Human DNA Quantitation System, GIBCO BRL).

PCR Amplification of *Locus* D1S80

Primer sequences: 1- 5' GAA ACT GGC CTC CAA ACA CTG CCC GCC G 3'
2- 5' GTC TTG TTG GAG ATG CAC GTG CCC CTT GC 3' .Reaction mix included:5 µl 10X PCR buffer (GeneAmp, Pekin Elmer Cetus), 4 ul 2.5 mM dNTP's, 1 µl 12.5 uM each primer, 2.5 units AmpliTaq DNA Polymerase (Perkin Elmer Cetus), 5 ng genomic DNA, and sterile water added to a final volume (50µl). Amplifications were carried out in a Perkin Elmer Cetus Thermal cycler GeneAmp PCR System 9600. Cycling was as follows: denaturation: 10 s, 95°C; annealing 10 s, 67°C; extension 30 s, 70°C, for a total of 27 cycles. PCR products were separated by electrophoresis in a discontinuous buffer system using ultrathin (0.4 mm) polyacrylamide gels (7.5 % T, 2 % C) with piperazine diacrylamide as the crosslinker. Gels contained 60 mM tris-formate buffer, pH 9. Gels were cast onto a gel support medium (19.5 x 37 cm, Gelbond, FMC). The trailing ion was 0.28 M tris borate, pH 9.0. Electrophoresis settings were 1000 v (mA and W values setted at maximun). An SA32 electrophoretic apparatus (BRL Life technologies, USA) was used. The separated amplification products were visualized by silver staining the gel using the method of Budowle et al. (1991).

RESULTS

The D1S80 locus met Hardy-Weinberg expectations in both sample populations. The allele frequency distributions of the two populations generally were similar. The absence of some alleles and the higher frequencies for alleles 25 and 31 (figure 1) in the Mapuche population might be due to sample size. Nevertheless, genotype frequency distributions showed the presence of very unusual allele combinations, such as 21-34 and 31-37 which were carried by 4.8% of the Mapuche individuals analyzed. These two genotypes were not previously reported in caucasian populations, such as Dutch (Kloosterman et al, 1993), Finns (Sajantila et al, 1992), US Caucasians (Budowle et al, 1991), Spanish (Alonso et al, 1993) Portuguese (Pontes et al, 1994) and Argentineans, representing a total of 1010 urelated individuals screened. This observation should be investigated further in order to determine the possible causes of the presence of such combinations.

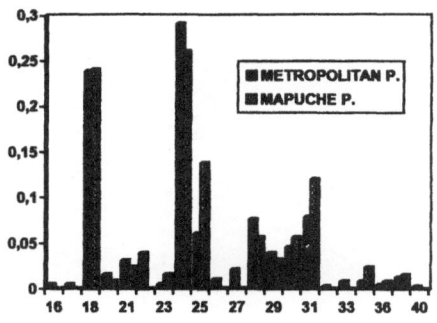

STATISTICAL PARAMETERS	Met.	Map.
Power of discrimination	95.70 %	93.90 %
Observed heterozygosity	82.72 %	87.06 %
Expected heterozygosity	84.22 %	83.97 %

Met.: Metropolitan population
Map.: Mapuche population

Figure 1

REFERENCES

Alonso A, Martin P, Albarran C, Sancho M (1993) Amplified fragment lenght polymorphism analysis of the VNTR locus D1S80 in Central Spain. Int. J. Leg. Med. 105: 311-314.

Budowle B, Chakraborty R, Giusti A, Eisenberg A, Allen R (1991) Analysis of the VNTR locus D1S80 by the PCR followed by high-resolution PAGE. Am J Hum Genet 48: 137-144.

Kloosterman A, Budowle B, Daselaar P (1993) PCR-amplification and detection of the human D1S80 VNTR locus. Int J Leg Med 105: 257-264.

Pontes M, Pinheiro M (1994) Study of D1S80 locus polymorphism in the North of Portugal. Adv. in For. Haemogenet. 5: 562-564.

Sajantila A, Budowle B, Strom M, Johnson V, Lukka M, Peltonen L, Ehnholm C (1992) PCR amplification of alleles at the D1S80 locus: comparison of a Finnish and a North American Caucasian population sample, and forensic casework evaluation. Am J Hum Genet 50: 816-825.

9 Standardization, Ethics

Ethical and Legal Aspects

Santiago Grisolía, M.D.

Fundación Valenciana de Estudios Avanzados
Pintor López, 7-1°. 46003-VALENCIA (Spain)

All living structures have a genome, which contains the "blueprint" that provides all the instructions necessary to make and maintain an organism. With the exception of the red blood cells, each of the various billions of cells which make up each individual, contains a complete genome. This consists of a double chain of deoxyribonucleic acid (DNA). The chromosomes are portions of DNA plus protein. Our genes, ca. 100,000, are a small part of the very long stretch of DNA which is composed of about 3 x 10 nucleotides, generally abbreviated as "bases". These bases contain the purines, adenine and guanine and the pyrimidines, cytosine and thymine. The double chain is so formed that whenever there is an adenine in a chain, there will be a thymine in the opposite chain and whenever there is a guanine in one there will be a cytosine in the other chain. A great portion, ca. 90%, of the nuclear DNA does not contain genes. On the other hand the very small DNA of the mitochondria is occupied entirely by genes, and is inherited entirely from the mother. This has a very important application in legal medicine as will be extensively covered in this encounter. In this regard, because of its historical interest I will refer to the work of Mary Clare King with the children of the Grandmothers of the Plaza de Mayo in Argentina. Also, I will discuss the Declarations of Valencia and of Bilbao. Because of its pioneer interest, the 2nd Declaration of Valencia is included.

All our DNA is subject to continuous changes, i.e. mutations, by a wide variety of agents. There are many mechanisms to correct mutations. It should be noted that the mutation rate is from 10 to 100 times higher in mitochondrial DNA than in nuclear DNA and that the mitochondria are not as well endowed to correct mutations as is the nuclear DNA. Indeed, because of this it has been suggested that aging is related to the higher mutation rate of mitochondria. In many cases mutations are not corrected in which case they may affect a gene or result in an extensive modification of the DNA, e.g. excessive multiple repeat copies of trinucleotides will give origen to a disease; these repetitions tend to increase in successive generations and thus the severity and frequency of the disease.

In a somewhat arbitrary way we can divide the medical applications resulting from the increased knowledge of the Human Genome into diagnostic and therapeutic. The latter could be divided into "direct" (gene therapy) and into "indirect" (gene oriented pharmacology). Of course the new predictive medicine, including genetic counseling should be included here.

Because of its novelty a major portion of this resume will be devoted to gene therapy and to brief considerations of ethic and legal issues.

The term human gene therapy came into use because it identified, as presumptively beneficent, technologies that might have provoked more opposition if called human genetic engineering. Particularly in the 1970s, when any development or means for altering the genetic capacity of human cells was hotly debated and bitterly opposed by some; the question, if asked, "What are the good uses of human genetic engineering? might have produced a negative response. Human gene therapy is and sounds benign.

On September 14th of 1990 a little girl four years old, with a deficiency of adenosine deaminase (ADA), was injected with millions of her own T cells in which had been inserted a normal ADA gene. This was done in the Childrens Unit of Intensive Care of the Clinical Center of the National Institutes of Health (NIH) in Bethesda, Maryland. That was the beginning of gene therapy in humans. Although gene therapy is a rational and logical treatment for certain types of diseases in humans, until rather recently the use of this type of technology was criticized as something very far in the future and almost science fiction. As a consequence, there was very extensive debate before the protocol for ADA deficiency was approved. Nevertheless, once it was shown to be possible, most people were favorably impressed. Thus, in spite of the few people who suffer from ADA deficiency in the whole world, the protocols used to correct this deficiency played a key role in the demonstration of the feasibility of gene therapy, and therefore established the first step towards a new Medicine. The Advisory Committee of the NIH (RAC) has approved some 90 protocols for several diseases, whereas the first gene therapy protocol of Anderson (1989) for ADA was reviewed 15 times by 7 different regulatory bodies. A mere six years later most protocols can be approved on a standard FDA review. Also Great Britain, France, Italy, Holland and China have started to use some 50 protocols in quite a number of patients, as of September of 1995. Interestingly the majority, 80%, are for cancer, or cancer related protocols.

This is not surprising since, indeed, it has become evident in the last two years that in addition to the approximatly 4000 monogenetic diseases known, potentially all diseases have a genetic origen. That is to say that many diseases have a polygenic origen, for example a large portion of persons affected with diabetes, and that the predisposition to a number of diseases also has a genetic basis. In all likelihood, a great deal of emphasis in the future will be given to treat the more common diseases, and precisely by their being more common they will be of more interest to society and thus to industry. This will have great benefits for many people including those of the 3rd World, but may carry the paradoxical danger of postponing or forgetting the treatment of certain monogenic deseases, particularly the less common ones, although these were the ones which originated gene therapy!.

Although the advances in Gene Therapy are impressive, it is necessary to advance much more, particularly in gene transference; it is also necessary to insure that treatments are not reserved for a few privileged persons or as a show for a few top hospitals. Ideally, there should be a great deal of emphasis in making possible the use of injection of genes, to avoid the need for large multidisciplinary groups as is the case now. There is a need to be able to integrate specific genes in the cell genome of the recipient so as to eliminate the risk, even if low, of initiating a cancer in the treated individual due to the possible integration of the new gene near an oncogene or near a gene dealing with tumor suppression. There is a need to regulate the expression of the new genes, particularly for the future and in the treatment of diseases such as diabetes in which the deficient genes necessitate a precise regulation. For the immediate future, gene therapy will be restricted to the treatment of somatic cells and it is unlikely that it will be extended soon to germinal cells. However, there will doubtless be much debate as soon as someone submits a protocol for germinal cells, since obviously any gene modification of these cells will be transmitted to future generations.

Although, gene therapy does not resemble any form of treatment previously used in medicine, it has, as any other experimental approach in medicine, the same restrictions based on ethical, scientific and safety principles. As in any treatment, we should make sure that the balance, risk-benefit, will be toward or in favor of the patient. Finally, society must have access to the facts related to protocols. The absolute clarity of information given to the public is the best guarantee of social responsibility and of the concern of the scientific community.

In short any major Scientific advance or program often generates new dilemmas. The notable advances in the Human Genome Project have without doubt presented new problems and brought back to light older ones. There is no doubt that public enthusiasm is great, but it is mixed with the fear of how the new knowledge will be used. The discussions about how new genetic knowledge is going to concern us all will increase in the coming years. Principles of bioethics elaborated recently in relation to people, benefits, autonomy and justice, must be included in legal protection of the people as well as of society. These principles will not be adequate to solve many of the complex questions and controversies resulting the advances in genetics. Certainly, ethical dilemmas will arise because of the conflicts between collective and individual interests.

So-called eugenics and racial hygiene were based on an erroneous belief in the improvement of the inheritance pool, leading to negation of individual decisions about having children, choosing mates, and, under nazi genocide, the right to life. Eugenics in terms of coercive social politics has not disappeared; it is alive in some countries in which there are still sterilization codes, and as ideology it is taken into consideration in some countries and is trying to appear in certain groups, e.g. American right-wing extremists. Investigations related to behavioral genetics and their results are easily misused, as we have often seen in the controversies about IQ tests, affective disorders and other mental diseases. The problems and dilemmas related to the use of eugenic information will not need special draconian measures, but we must be ready. For example, employers, personnel directors and insurance companies could discriminate against those whose genetic characteristics make them susceptible to certain diseases, premature death or disability. Without doubt there is a potential conflict between individual interest and those of society. However, no one chooses his or her genes, and the information given by them must be kept confidential. No one should be analyzed genetically without his knowledge, and the information obtained must not be released without the consent of its owner, unless it is necessary to avoid damage to other people.

The human genome project will increase and present new problems. For example if a genomic analysis can predict that a person will die still young of a serious genetic disease, which until now is without treatment; would anyone like to be analysed?. There are already examples of persons who do not want to know, and have the right not to know. What would be their attitude if he/she knows that such an analysis can imform them whether or not he will pass such a disease to his descendants. There will be more rapid developments of genetic probes to detect diseases than cures for such diseases!. Will the increased knowledge of the Human Genome increase the tolerance of society toward persons affected by disease or will it increase discrimination?. Present laws offer some protection but would they be able to cope in a just and reasonable way with the new information revealed by the increased knowledge of the human genome?.

II WORKSHOP ON INTERNATIONAL COOPERATION FOR THE HUMAN GENOME PROJECT: ETHICS. Valencia declaration on ethics and the Human Genome Project.

1.- We, the participants in the Valencia Workshop, affirm that a civilized society entails respect for human diversity, including genetic variations. We acknowledge our responsability to help ensure that genetic information is used to enhance the dignity of the individual, that all persons in need have access to genetic services, and that genetics programs abide by the ethical principles of respect for persons, beneficence, and justice.

2.- We believe that knowledge gained from mapping and sequencing the human genome will have great benefit for human health and wellbeing. We endorse international colaboration for genome research and urge the widest possible participation of countries throughout the world, within the resources and interests of each country.

3.- We urge coordination among nations and across disciplines in the conduct of research and the sharing of information and materials relating to the genomes of human beings and other organisms.

4.- Concerns about the use and misuse of new genetic knowledge have provoked debate in many quarters. In addition to discussions in professional circles, further public debate on the ethical, social, and legal implications of clinical, commercial, and other uses of genetic information is urgently needed.

5.- We support efforts to educate the public, through all means including the press and the schools, about genome mapping and sequencing, genetic diseases, and genetic services.

6.- In light of the great increase in prognostic and therapeutic information that will arise from the genome project, we urge greater support for training of genetic counselors and genetic education of other health professionals.

7.- As a general principle, genetic information about an individual should be ascertained or disclosed only with authorization from the individual or his or her legal representative. Any exceptions to this principle require strong ethical and legal justification.

8.- We agree that somatic cell gene therapy may be used for the treatment of specific human diseases. Germ-line gene therapy faces technical obstacles and does not command ethical consensus. we endorse further discussion of the technical, medical, and social issues on this topic.

THE DEVELOPMENT OF QUALITY ASSURANCE MEASURES IN FORENSIC DNA TYPING

LAWRENCE A. PRESLEY and JAMES L. MUDD, QUALITY ASSURANCE UNIT, FORENSIC SCIENCE RESEARCH AND TRAINING CENTER, FBI LABORATORY, FBI ACADEMY, QUANTICO, VIRGINIA 22135, USA

Introduction

The use of DNA analysis to assist in solving violent crimes has significantly impacted the criminal justice system. Because of the significant discriminating power of forensic Restriction Fragment Length Polymorphism (RFLP) and Polymerase Chain Reaction (PCR) DNA analyses, substantial attention has been directed to the proper use of these DNA technologies by the forensic community. In 1992, the National Academy of Sciences National Research Council stated (NRC,1992):

> "Laboratories involved in forensic DNA typing should move quickly to establish quality assurance programs. After a sufficient time for implementation of quality assurance programs has passed, courts should view quality control as necessary for general acceptance."

Quality control (QC) and quality assurance (QA) have been defined as two different and specific functions (ANSI 1978 and Kilshaw, 1986, 1987a, 1987b). The QC measures are designed to insure that the quality of the product, that is the DNA typing result, meets and satisfies specific criteria. The QA program should provide all concerned, primarily the courts in the forensic application, the criteria that can be used to establish with confidence that the QC functions are being performed acceptably.

The Technical Working Group on DNA Analysis Methods and the International Society of Forensic Haemogenetics

In November, 1988, the first meeting of the Technical Working Group on DNA Analysis Methods (TWGDAM) took place at the FBI Academy in Quantico, Virginia. TWGDAM has since produced guidelines for quality assurance in 1989, 1990, 1991 and 1995 (TWGDAM, 1989,1990,1991,1995), guidelines for quality audits in 1993 (TWGDAM, 1993) and guidelines for proficiency manufacturing and testing in 1994 (TWGDAM, 1994). The DNA Identification Act of 1994 has established the TWGDAM guidelines as interim standards for forensic DNA testing laboratories. United States crime laboratories using DNA analysis generated QA/QC guidelines which incorporated and paralleled the TWGDAM guidelines. The DNA Analysis Unit of the FBI Laboratory suggested an outline of quality control measures for casework in 1989 (Adams et al, 1989). State forensic laboratory directors were becoming increasingly aware of the requirements for detailed, specific and documented QA/QC guidelines (Ferrara, 1990). The DNA Commission of the International Society for Forensic Haemogenetics has also generated recommendations regarding QA/QC protocols for DNA typing of RFLP and PCR-based polymorphisms (ISFH Recommendations, 1989, 1992, 1992, 1995)

Published Validation Studies on Forensic DNA Applications

Since 1985, validation studies have repeatedly addressed specific issues related to forensic evidence samples, and these studies have provided valuable data in helping to establish meaningful quality assurance and quality control measures.

Quality Control Measures in Forensic DNA Analysis

For RFLP analysis, several control measures have been established and include: the K 562 control sample, restriction enzyme monitoring, use of appropriate size markers, DNA quantity estimates and the National Institute of Standards and Technology (NIST) Standard Reference Material (SRM) 2390.

For PCR analysis, control measures have included: positive and negative amplification controls, DNA quantity estimates, reagent blanks and appropriate size markers. Mitochondrial (mt)DNA analysis may require capillary electrophoresis controls as well as automated sequencer instrumental procedures which appropriately document the procedure.

Routine Forensic Casework Quality Assurance Measures

Routine casework will require appropriate written and photographic records, technical reviews and interpretational guidelines. Forensic DNA laboratories will also be required to participate in established proficiency testing programs which may include external and/or internal proficiency testing.

External Quality Assurance Measures for Forensic DNA Laboratories

Several external quality assurance measures may directly affect forensic DNA laboratories. Accreditation for forensic laboratories has been available from the American Society of Crime Laboratory Directors-Laboratory Accreditation Board(ASCLD-LAB) and the National Measurement Accreditation Scheme(NAMAS) in Great Britain. Professional certification in forensic biology is available from the American Board of Criminalistics (ABC). Both ASCLD-LAB and ABC require the court testimony and proficiency test monitoring of forensic DNA examiner/analysts.

Internal and external audits of forensic DNA laboratories are becoming an established measure for monitoring performance.

Conclusion

The forensic DNA community has voluntarily incorporated the concepts and practices of quality assurance and quality control measures and is continually striving to attain the highest quality forensic DNA analyses.

REFERENCES:

National Research Council, DNA Technology in Forensic Science,, National Academy Press, Washington, D.C. 1992, p. X.

American National Standard ANSI/ASQC A3-1978 (1978). Quality Systems Terminology. American Society for Quality Congrol, Milwaukee, Wisconsin.

Kilshaw, D., (1986) Quality Assurance. 1. Philosophy and basic principles,., 43: 377-381.Med. Lab. Sci., 43: 377-381.

Kilshaw, D., (1987a) Quality Assurance. 1. Internal quality control, Med. Lab. Sci., 44: 73-83.

Kilshaw, D., (1987b) Quality Assurance. 1. External quality assessment, Med. Lab. Sci., 44: 178-186.

Technical Working Group on DNA Analysis Methods (TWGDAM) 1989, Guidelines for a Quality Assurance Program for DNA Restriction Fragment Length Polymorphism Analysis, Crime Lab. Digest, 15 (4): 109-113.

Technical Working Group on DNA Analysis Methods (TWGDAM) 1990, Guidelines for a Proficiency Testing program for DNA Restriction Fragment Length Polymorphism Analysis, Crime Lab. Digest, 17 (3): 50-60.

Technical Working Group on DNA Analysis Methods (TWGDAM) 1991, Guidelines for a Quality Assurance Program for DNA Analysis, Crime Lab. Digest, 18 (2): 44-75.

Technical Working Group on DNA Analysis Methods (TWGDAM) 1995, Guidelines for a Quality Assurance Program for DNA Analysis, Crime Lab. Digest, 22 (2): 21-43.

Technical Working Group on DNA Analysis Methods (TWGDAM) 1993, A Guide for Conducting a DNA Quality Assurance Audit, Crime Lab. Digest, 20 (1): 8-18.

Technical Working Group on DNA Analysis Methods (TWGDAM) 1994, Guidelines for DNA Proficiency Test Manufacturing and Reporting, Crime Lab. Digest, 21 (2): 27-32.

Adams, D.E., Presley, L.A., Deadman, H.A. and Lynch, A.L., (1989) "DNA Analysis in the FBI Laboratory," Proceedings of the International Symposium on the Forensic Aspects of DNA Analysis, U.S. Government Printing Office, Washington, D.C., pp. 173-178.

Ferarra, P.B., (1990) Forensic Laboratory Manager's Responsibility for Quality Assurance in DNA Analysis, Crime Lab. Digest, 17 (2): 40-42.

ISFH-Editorial-Recommendations of the International Society for Forensic Haemogenetics concerning DNA Polymorphisms. Forensic Science International, (1989) 43: pp. 109-111.

ISFH-Editorial-1991 Report concerning recommendations of the DNA Commission of the International Society for Forensic Haemogenetics relating to the use of DNA polymorphisms. Forensic Science International, (1992) 52: pp. 125-130.

ISFH-Editorial-Recommendations of the DNA Commission of the International Society for Forensic Haemogenetics relating to the use of PCR-based polymorphisms. Forensic Science International, (1992) 52: pp. 1-3.

ISFH, March, 1995 Newsletter.

THE AMERICAN ASSOCIATION OF BLOOD BANKS INSPECTION AND ACCREDITATION PROGRAM FOR PARENTAGE TESTING LABORATORIES

R. H. Walker

American Association of Blood Banks
Bethesda, MD, USA

INTRODUCTION

The Parentage Testing Inspection and Accreditation (PT-I&A) Program of the American Association of Blood Banks (AABB) was conceived and created by the AABB Committee on Parentage Testing in 1984. Although implementation of the program was originally the responsibility of the Parentage Testing Committee, in 1993 the AABB Board of Directors separated the PT-I&A program from the committee and merged it with the AABB National I&A Program for Blood Banks and Transfusion Services which is where it remains today.

The PT-I&A is a voluntary program based upon Standards for Parentage Testing Laboratories (Standards), now in its second edition. The Standards address code of conduct, general policies, identification of the parties, specimen collection, all phases of commonly used methods in laboratory testing for parentage determination, statistical evaluation and the contents of the final report. The Standards are promulgated by the Committee on Parentage Testing after they have been circulated to the parentage testing community for comment.

OBJECTIVES

The primary purpose of the PT-I&A program is to foster the improvement of parentage testing laboratories and their policies and procedures as they relate to services to tested individuals and clients. Adherence to the Standards assists laboratory directors and their staff in providing high quality performance. The AABB PT-I&A Program is designed to assist directors of parentage testing laboratories in determining whether methods, procedures, personnel, equipment and physical plant meet established requirements. It is also a means for detecting problems in practice and provides, when needed, consultation for their correction. The I&A Program provides recognition through accreditation to those facilities functioning in accordance with existing published requirements of the AABB. Accreditation by the AABB is required by many states for contract recipients. The AABB Committee on Parentage Testing has worked closely with the Office of Child Support Enforcement in order to assure that laboratory reports and interpretations have credibility and substance in courts of law. Basic minimum requirements for accreditation of parentage testing laboratories are embodied in the AABB Inspection Report Form (IRF) for Parentage Testing Laboratories. These requirements are based primarily on the text of the Standards.

ORGANIZATION OF PROGRAM

The PT-I&A Program is under the immediate administration of the National Committee on Inspection and Accreditation, members of which are appointed by the Association's President subject to approval by the Board of Directors. The National Committee is composed of a national chair, six vice chairs and three parentage testing area chairs together with liaisons from other related AABB committees, the College of American Pathologists, the FDA, Office of Biologics, the Centers for Disease Control and the US Armed Services Blood Program.

Implementation of the PT-I&A Program is handled by the I&A area chairs with clerical assistance provided through the AABB National Office. Each I&A area chair is responsible for I&A activities in a designated area of the United States (Eastern, Central, and Western).

Serving under the three I&A area chairs are 16 inspectors, all with advanced academic degrees and experience. All of these individuals contribute their time and talents to the program and receive no monetary compensation. Only the inspection-related out-of-pocket expenses incurred by assigned inspections are reimbursed, upon request, by the AABB.

All parentage testing laboratories are urged to seek AABB accreditation. Inspection must be requested by the director responsible for the parentage testing laboratory. Prior to inspection, the director is provided with a copy of the IRF. The IRF indicates most of the questions to be asked and items that will be reviewed by the inspector during the on-site visit. The IRF is partially completed by the director in accordance with the instructions printed on the front page. The IRF is then forwarded to the National Office along with three copies of the laboratory Procedure Manual and all of the records, films and documents relating to four parentage test cases (selected at random by the AABB).

INSPECTION PROCEDURE

The I&A area chair assigns an inspector to complete the inspection within 30 days of receipt of the above materials. The inspector will review all of the submitted documents (IRF, Procedure Manual, and four cases) prior to the on-site inspection.

During the inspector's visit, there will be a detailed review of technical proficiency and quality control procedures; quality assessment program; reports and recording methods; equipment and its functions; and physical plant adequacy. The inspector completes those parts of the IRF applicable to the facility and forwards the report to the I&A area chair.

Any deficiencies found at the time of inspection, or, even subsequently when the I&A area chair reviews the IRF, facility's records and cases, will be reported in writing to the director by the I&A area chair. The report may include recommendations for improvements and means for correcting deficiencies.

The director of the inspected facility sends details of corrective action directly to the I&A area chair. If the stated corrections are satisfactory, the I&A area chair will recommend that accreditation be granted. If the deficiencies noted at the time of the inspection are major and/or numerous, the I&A area chair may inform the director that a reinspection is necessary after the deficiencies have been corrected. In that event, an inspector will return for a second review. Any deficiencies found upon reinspection must be corrected following the above procedure.

ACCREDITATION

AABB accreditation is for a two-year period. The procedures for renewal inspections are the same as for initial inspections except that only new or recently revised procedures are submitted prior to the inspection.

EVALUATION OF THE PROGRAM

The I&A Program is continuously in review. Comments and constructive criticism are sought from all those inspected, through the use of a Post-inspection Questionnaire which provides an opportunity to evaluate all aspects of pre-inspection, on-site inspection and the post-inspection process. Letters of response to criticisms and comments, when appropriate, are initiated by the national chair or by the responsible I&A area chair, or both. Resolution of individual problems is attempted. Criticisms and comments often influence long-range planning, as they are critiqued at the annual meeting of the Inspection and Accreditation Committee-at-Large.

In addition, there are periodic workshops presented by I&A area chairs for the inspectors. The workshops provide an opportunity to discuss and review the I&A Program and result in a more uniform application of AABB requirements during the inspection process.

EDUCATIONAL ASPECTS OF THE PROGRAM

AABB inspections provide an educational experience for all participants. A detailed review of the facility's physical plant, procedures, record forms and techniques and an assessment of compliance with the Standards and I&A accreditation requirements can be an enlightening experience for those who actively participate in the inspection process. Educational benefits are derived from the analysis and feedback provided by the AABB inspectors and I&A area chairs. Additionally, valuable knowledge is gained through letters from I&A area chairs to directors relating deficiencies and recommendations, comments and suggestions on how to correct these deficiencies, thus improving service to the establishment of paternity and to child support. Finally, the process of correcting deficiencies often necessitates a reassessment of the level and quality of practice. This frequently results in greater interaction and cooperation between the facility director and personnel. It often leads to increased communication and awareness within the facility.

Parentage Testing Survey Program of the College of American Pathologists: Red Cell Antigens, Serum Proteins and Red Cell Enzymes Testing Results

H Polesky*, D Endean, CR Harrison, J Morris, R Roby, R Walker

*Memorial Blood Centers of Minnesota, 2304 Park Avenue, Minneapolis, Minnesota, 55404, USA

Since its inception in 1993, results from seven mailings of the joint American Association of Blood Banks/College of American Pathologists parentage testing survey program, PI, have been analyzed. Results were reported in six red cell antigens (RCA), 14 serum proteins (SP) and 11 red cell enzymes (RCE) genetic systems. The total number of laboratories reporting results, the number of results reported and the number of non-consensus answers are listed in Table 1.

	1993 A	1993 B	1993 C	1994 A	1994 B	1994 C	1995 A
Total labs reporting	51	58	60	85	89	93	125
RCA							
No. of labs	33	39	36	49	50	54	49
Total results	534	537	561	702	678	726	693
Non-consensus	4	1	5	1	2	1	3
SP							
No. of labs	8	14	12	22	20	17	21
Total results	102	114	105	171	141	165	186
Non-consensus	1	1	1	4	4	2	1
RCE							
No. of labs	11	20	18	32	36	29	34
Total results	108	216	171	321	303	339	369
Non-consensus	0	0	2	11	4	8	9

Results in the following systems were reported by more than 10 participants: ABO, Rh, MNSs, Kell, Duffy, Kidd, Gc, Hp, AK, ADA, PGM1, ACP, ESD and GLO. In the Gc and PGM1 systems, results were reported with both electropheresis and isoelectric focusing techniques. The number of laboratories reporting by each technique is listed in Table 2.

	1993	1994	1995 PI-A
Gc	5	9	11
Gci	6	11	10
PGM1	6	13	14
PGM1i	11	20	20

In one mailing, PI-A 1994, the alleged father was unrelated to the mother and child. Among the RCA/SP/RCE genetic systems testing, only PLG, PGM1i and ACP demonstrated an exclusion.

When considering only the genetic systems where a consensus can be established and assuming that three concurring laboratories establish a consensus, the following overall rate of error can be calculated: RCA 0.004; SP 0.02; RCA 0.02. This demonstrates good consistency between laboratories performing genetic testing with conventional systems.

The Parentage Testing Proficiency Survey Program of the College of American Pathologists

CR Harrison*, D Endean, J Morris, H Polesky, R Roby and R Walker

*Department of Pathology, University of Texas Health Science Center at San Antonio, 7703 Floyd Curl Drive, San Antonio, Texas, 78284-7750, USA

External proficiency testing is a requirement for accreditation of parentage testing laboratories by the American Association of Blood Banks (AABB). In 1993 the College of American Pathologists (CAP), in collaboration with the AABB, created a joint parentage testing proficiency survey program, PI, to replace the PSP program of the AABB.

This program consists of three yearly mailings of three ACD whole blood samples from a mother, child and alleged father trio. Participants report their results and information on the methodology used. The results are collated and summarized anonymously and a summary of responses is returned to the participants. This program allows for testing and reporting of genetic systems in red cell antigens, red cell enzymes, serum proteins and DNA polymorphisms by RFLP or PCR. HLA testing by serological methods cannot be performed on the samples.

The enrollment and rate of response for each survey mailing is depicted in Table 1.

	1993			1994			1995
	A	B	C	A	B	C	A
Enrolled	62	77	79	105	110	113	125
Responses	51	58	60	85	89	93	91
% Response	82	75	76	81	81	82	73

Of the laboratories responding, an average of 81.5% perform parentage testing. The remaining laboratories report performing either forensic testing or monitoring for engraftment of bone marrow transplantation.

All the trios tested so far included the biological father of the child except for one (PI-A 1994) where the alleged father was unrelated to the mother and child. In this latter case none of the red cell antigen systems tested and only three (PLG, PGMi, ACP) of the serum protein and red cell enzyme systems tested excluded the man. Of the 26 DNA-RFLP loci tested, five did not demonstrate an exclusion and only 9 out of 18 DNA-PCR loci tested revealed an exclusion. Of the 80 laboratories reporting an overall interpretation, 61 excluded the tested man, 10 did not exclude, 6 requested additional testing, and three reported an indeterminate result. It is likely that many of the laboratories unable to exclude the tested man would normally perform HLA typing by serological methods as part of their routine group of tests.

This survey program provides participating laboratories with a mean to compare their testing results with those of others in the field and to assess current techniques and methodologies used in parentage testing. It is anticipated that in the future grading criteria will be instituted in order for participants to receive individual evaluation for all systems where a consensus result can be established.

A REVIEW OF THE 1991-1994 PATERNITY TESTING WORKSHOPS OF THE ENGLISH SPEAKING WORKING GROUP

D Syndercombe Court and P Lincoln for the English Speaking Working Group of the International Society for Forensic Haemogenetics

Department of Haematology, The London Hospital Medical College, Turner Street, London E1 2AD, UK

INTRODUCTION

The ability of any laboratory offering paternity tests to correctly assign relationship is an essential attribute that needs to be tested by a quality control programme. Such a programme could involve regular internal laboratory testing of blinded samples and involvement in an external testing programme. Since 1991 members of the English Speaking Working Group (ESWG) of the International Society for Forensic Haemogenetics (ISFH) have organised and participated in an annual Paternity Testing Workshop that fulfils the latter requirement in part. The exercise was not intended, however, to be concerned only with proficiency, but also to provide a forum for the discussion of paternity related topics, whether it be current and developing methodology, anomalous results or measurement variation, at the annual ESWG meeting. On behalf of the ESWG we present below a report of the last four workshops.

METHODS

Blood samples from a 'family' were sent to participating laboratories in the Spring of each year, from 1991 to 1994, with the request that they perform a paternity investigation and make a report in their usual manner. In addition laboratories were asked to complete a questionnaire to provide more detailed information on their current routine methodology and what additional testing might be carried out if a laboratory found it difficult to resolve the case. Nine laboratories were approached for the initial workshop in 1991; since then ten other laboratories who came to the first paternity workshop forum, or who had heard about the workshop, have asked to participate. Although samples were not presented blind, only the two named authors were aware of the true family relationships and did not participate in the testing process.

Workshop Families

1991: Two possible fathers, mother and child. One of the possible fathers was a sibling of the other but information about this relationship was not provided to the testers.

1992: Two possible fathers and child. One of the possible fathers was a sibling of the mother, who had not been presented for testing, but again this information was withheld from the testers.

1993: One possible father, mother and child. The possible father was a sibling of the true father (information not provided to testers).

1994: One possible father, mother and child.

RESULTS

The number of participating laboratories has increased from 9 (1991) to 13 (1992), 16 (1993) and 19(1994). All laboratories performed some form of DNA testing, with around 75% using DNA single locus probes (SLP). About 40% of laboratories reporting SLPs have continued to report other conventional test systems (red cell and white cell antigens, red cell enzymes and serum protein polymorphisms). Since 1993 the small number of laboratories using multi-locus probe (MLP) testing as their main testing process have also used other test systems as 'back-up', principally SLPs. YNH24, MS43a, MS31 and G3 have remained the most popular probes in use throughout, followed by MS1, which has decreased in popularity, and MS205 which has increased in popularity. Eight other probes have been used routinely, with pMLJ14, MS8 and TBQ7 being the most popular. Chemiluminescent labelled probes have increased in popularity. In 1991 only radioactively labelled probes were used but in 1992 over 50% of laboratories were using chemiluminescent systems and that increased significantly to around 80% in 1993 and 85% in 1994. Hinf I was the restriction enzyme favoured by around 70% in 1991, increasing to 80% in 1994. Others use Alu I or Hae III. Since 1992 there has been an increase in the number of laboratories developing PCR based systems (under 10% in 1992 to over 40% in 1994), with short tandem repeat (STR) systems gaining in popularity over other PCR based systems. No laboratories were reporting PCR systems as part of their routine paternity investigation up to 1994.

Four 'families' have been tested and reported, all without conflicting conclusions. The 1991 case, in which the two possible fathers presented were brothers, proved difficult to resolve with one laboratory only obtaining a single exclusion after seven SLP probes and no laboratory found exclusions on more than two SLP test systems. About 80% of the laboratories also suggested that the two men were related. Since 1991 all laboratories who provided a report came to the same conclusion about the paternity of the men tested. Over 80% of laboratories, in writing their report, provide the raw results on which their conclusion is based; the remainder provide either their conclusion alone, or indicate fragment size rank only.

The variation between laboratories has been examined with time, comparing fragment sizes provided by laboratories using the same restriction enzyme and the four most popular probes (YNH24, MS43a, MS31 and G3). Figure 1 presents the range of coefficient of variation results for each fragment reported. There is a highly significant inverse correlation between the year of testing and coefficient of variation (Spearman's Rank Order correlation = -0.65, p<0.000001), with the decrease in coefficient of variation being highly significant between 1992 and 1993 (Scheffé's Post-Hoc Test, p<0.001). The maximum coefficient of variation fell from around 7% in 1991 to under 2% in 1994 when we observed a percentage difference in fragment size measurements, between laboratories, of 1.6% to 5.0%, dependent on fragment size. The measurements from one laboratory providing results in 1994 were excluded from this analysis since the fragment sizes given were highly discrepant (about 1-2 kb) away from the consensus for the majority of the test systems used.

DISCUSSION

This review of the activities of the ESWG in paternity testing illustrates the continuing popularity of DNA SLP testing, with conventional systems frequently being used in addition. MLP testing seems no longer to be performed in isolation and frequently SLP tests are used to support the MLP interpretation. Four probes (YNH24, MS43a, MS31 and G3) have maintained their popularity. MS1 usage has decreased, probably because of the high rate of mutations found, but use of MS205, a newer probe, is becoming more common. More laboratories are experimenting with PCR based systems and it is

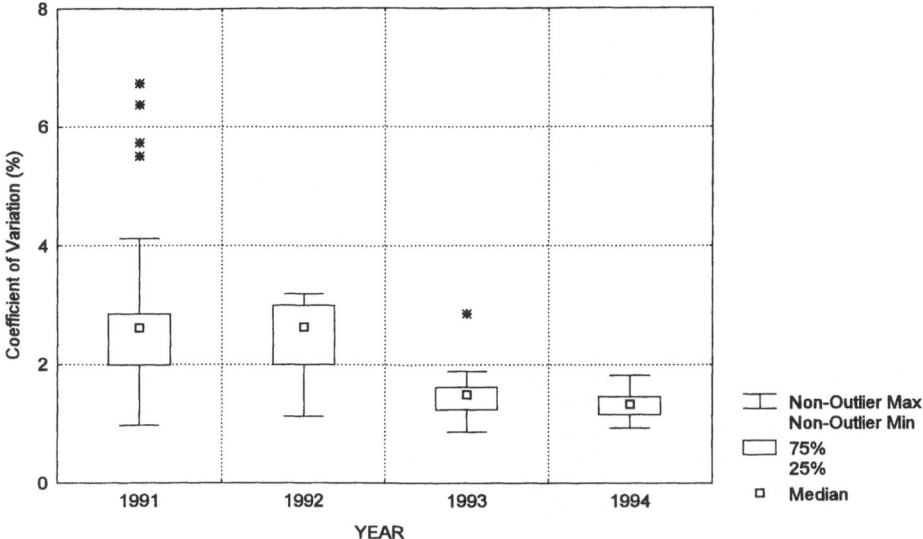

Figure 1: Box and whisker plot showing median, interquartile range, non-outlier range and outliers (*) of measures of coefficient of variation, between laboratories, for each fragment measured in any particular test year.

possible that we will see such systems being used routinely in the future. The general decreased variability in fragment size measurement seen between laboratories over the four years is likely to be due principally to the increased use of chemiluminescent techniques, providing much clearer band patterns and enabling more precise measurements to be made, but increased experience may also be important. Although one family proved particularly difficult to resolve, consensus concerning the conclusion was achieved in all cases that were reported and the meetings have proved a useful forum for discussion of paternity related matters, particularly in relation to the methodologies being applied. Comparison of different laboratory's results, whether it be DNA SLP fragment sizes or other genetic markers, can provide independent quality criteria for laboratories. Laboratory identity is kept anonymous to encourage participation in the exercises. Participation in external quality tests is also an important feature of many accreditation schemes and The English Speaking Working Group Paternity Workshop has proven itself both useful in this aspect and inexpensive to run.

Particular thanks are due to the staff of the following participating laboratories: Cellmark Diagnostics, Abingdon; Central Laboratory of the Netherlands Red Cross Blood Transfusion Service, Amsterdam; Institut National de Criminalistique, Bruxelles; Institute of Forensic Genetics, Copenhagen; Police Forensic Science Laboratory, Dundee; Institut für Blutgruppenforschung, Düsseldorf; Institut de Médecine Légale, Genève; Dr med Jan H Bartel, Heidelberg; Institut de Médecine Légale, Lausanne; Céntre Regional de Transfusion Sanguine, Lille, Statens Rättserologiska Institut, Linköping; The London Hospital Medical College, London; University Diagnostics Limited, London; Institut für Rechtsmedizin, Mainz; Division of Human Genetics, Newcastle; Rettsmedisinsk Institutt, Oslo; Institut National de Transfusion Sanguine, Paris; The Forensic Science Service, Wetherby; Institut für Rechtsmedizin, Zurich.

DNA LEGISLATION IN THE NETHERLANDS

H.J.T. Janssen, A.D. Kloosterman

Forensic Science Laboratory of The Ministry of Justice
Volmerlaan 17, 2288 GD Rijswijk, The Netherlands

INTRODUCTION

The Forensic Science Laboratory in The Netherlands started DNA investigation in casework in 1989. The use of DNA evidence as exculpatory evidence was admitted by the Dutch Supreme Court in 1990. Despite the fact that DNA investigation offered enormous possibilities especially in sexual assault cases, the application of DNA profiling was sometimes prevented by the existing legislation. The willingness of a suspect to give a bloodsample or other bodily material for DNA-investigation became an obstacle in an increasing number of cases.
Thereupon the Dutch Minister of Justice proposed a bill regarding the DNA investigation in crimecases in December 1991. The bill was a response to the report of a commission which studied the renewal of the penal code, including the use of DNA investigation. The proposals were passed into law almost without alternation and legislation came into force on the first of September 1994.

The new DNA-legislation is characterised by a number of elements:
- the compulsory sampling of bodily material
- the role of the investigating judge
- the role of the prosecutor
- the right of the defendant to have a second DNA test
- the construction of a database of DNA profiles
- the chain of evidence

These elements will be discussed below.

THE COMPULSORY SAMPLING OF BODILY MATERIAL

According to the new law, only the Investigating Judge can require to give bodily material, when a suspect refuses to give a sample voluntarily. However, the compulsory sampling is restricted to crimes liable to a penalty of eight years or more of imprisonment. The warrant can also be given if it concerns certain specific offences with a maximum punishment of at least six years of imprisonment, such as serious kinds of maltreatment, public violence and fornication. It is necessary that facts and circumstances indicate serious charges against the suspect and DNA investigation is necessary in the pursuit of truth. The compulsory sampling of bodily material has to be performed by a surgeon.

THE ROLE OF THE INVESTIGATING JUDGE

As mentioned it is only the Investigating Judge who can order the compulsory sampling of bodily material from a suspect. When biological evidence has been found in a crime, he can order to determine the amount of DNA in crime scene samples. This part of the investigation is restricted to the Forensic Science Laboratory. When a report states that there is enough DNA for two or more DNA tests, mostly this will result in a continuation of the order to start a DNA profiling. The Forensic Science Laboratory reports when the investigation will take place and when the results are available. The suspect can exercise the right to have a second expert present at this first DNA investigation. If there is not enough material available for a second DNA test, the suspect has a choice to which laboratory the DNA test is granted. Besides the Forensic Science Laboratory only one other independent laboratory in The Netherlands is allowed to perform forensic DNA analysis. In case of two or more suspects there is no individual right for a suspect to point a laboratory.

THE ROLE OF THE PROSECUTOR

The power to order a DNA investigation in a crime without a suspect is given to the Prosecutor and is not limited to certain serious cases. The Prosecutor can independently demand the Forensic Science Laboratory to start a DNA investigation of the biological evidence in order to determine the origin. In the near future DNA profiles of biological samples can be compared to DNA profiles of suspects in prior criminal cases and biological crime scene samples in a database. A match has to be reported to the Prosecutor. The suspect, when become known in a later stage, will have the right for a second DNA test if enough material is left for a second investigation.

THE RIGHT OF A SECOND DNA TEST

An important element of the DNA legislation is the right of the suspect to demand a second DNA test. Within fourteen days after the suspect has been informed by the Investigating Judge or the Prosecutor about the results of the first DNA test, the suspect can request a second test. If the suspect has used the right to have a second expert present at the first DNA investigation, he is not entitled to have a second DNA test. The new law lays down that a minimum of material has to be used for DNA investigation. Using the PCR technique as a standard technique in the Forensic Science Laboratory meets this requirement. At least half of the stain material is retained, especially for a second DNA test. For privacy reasons no information about the identity of the involved persons may get known to the independent laboratory. Reference cell material of an individual is transferred under a unique number. Therefore the results of the second DNA test are send to the Forensic Science Laboratory, which completes the report by adding the identity of the individuals before sending the report to the investigating judge. Remaining stain and reference material from the second DNA test has to be returned to the Forensic Science Laboratory.

THE CONSTRUCTION OF A DATABASE OF DNA PROFILES

DNA legislation allows the Forensic Science Laboratory to set up a database. This database contains DNA profiles from cell material of suspects in prior criminal cases and DNA profiles of samples detected at loci delicti. The aims of the database are the identification of repeated offenders, deceased persons, persons who are unable to identify themselves and to get statistical information on allele and genotype frequencies. The database is administered by the Forensic Science Laboratory and the consultation is stick to strong regulations. By order of the Prosecutor the DNA-profile of a suspect has to be deleted immediately in case the registered person was suspected wrongly. DNA profiles of suspects will be deleted after a period of thirty years, those of samples detected at loci delicti after a period of eighteen years.

CHAIN OF EVIDENCE

To guarantee that forensic DNA investigations will be performed carefully, the legislation contains very detailed procedures. Forensic working procedures for police officers and surgeons have been drawn up: the sampling of liquid blood, buccal cell or hair roots by surgeons, the sampling of bloodstains, bloodstained items, semen stains and saliva stains by police officers. Special sets for sampling bloodsamples, buccalcell samples or a hair sample have been developed by the Forensic Science Laboratory. Regulations are given for the preservation and the expedition of goods to the Forensic Science Laboratory. To ensure the chain of evidence, all secured reference material and goods have to be provided with numbered seal. A seal with the same number is found on the official police report of the seizure of goods. During the course of the analysis this unique seal number is the identification of the stain.

CONCLUSION

The extension of the Dutch Code of Criminal Procedure with provisions on behalf of forensic DNA investigations has enlarged the possibilities of forensic investigations enormously.
Under the new law a compulsory sample can be taken from a suspect and a right of a second DNA test has been created. Very detailed procedures ensure the chain of evidence and the quality of the DNA investigation. In practice the execution of the procedures is very time-consuming and not always useful. Therefore it is necessary to reconsider the effectiveness of the procedures in the next future.

REFERENCE

Kampen P van, Nijboer H (1994) DNA fingerprinting in the Dutch Code of Criminal Procedure. Expert Evidence, 3(2):70-74

SCIENCE AND CONSCIENCE: REGULATION OR GUIDELINES FOR FORENSIC HAEMOGENETICS?

M. Lorente[1], J.A. Lorente[1], B. Budowle[2] & E. Villanueva[1]

[1]University of Granada, Dept. of Forensic Medicine, Granada, Spain

[2]FSRTC - Research Unit. Laboratory Division. FBI Academy. Quantico, Va, USA

INTRODUCTION

Since the earliest endeavors by man, there has been confrontation between the advances of science and the views and opinions of society. History is replete with examples of conflict between science (or scientists) and society, e.g., Socrates and the Athenian government, Galileo and the Church, and the use of atomic energy and the implications of world destruction. Usually technical questions are resolved, after some debate and discussion, when a general consensus is reached by the relevant scientific community. However, social opinions remain unresolved for longer periods of time and can vary substantially among peoples. These apparent conflicts are not necessarily bad, but they do pose questions for one to consider.

It is in this atmosphere that one should consider the use of DNA typing technologies for exculpating or inculpating individuals associated with crime scene evidence samples or for resolving paternity matters. On one hand, DNA technology is going to be employed to resolve criminal and parentage matters; it would be a shame if innocent people could not avail themselves of such a powerful tool and if society could not use the DNA typing methods to assist in identifying perpetrators of henious acts. On the other hand, society needs to be concerned about potential abuses of the use of DNA typing tools and results that may infringr on the rights of individuals. Some of the problems between these points of view can be resolved by better educating the lay public. Some of the issues are generally not part of science, but are judicial, legal, religious, ethical, and/or philosophical. However, scientists also have a responsibility to promote the necessary discussions and to reflect on the pertinent social implications.

The forensic analytical investigation is carried out in a scientific frame (e.g., with the use of validated protocols and/or standard operating protocols, and under QC/QA guidelines) wich is contained within the legal systems of society. The interaction between the analytical aspects and the legal system of society. As a general framework for discussion in this paper for the use of DNA analysisis within the criminal justice systme(s) in Europe, one can refer to the Recommendation No R(92) of the Council of Europe, Committee of Minister.

We believe that the elements that should be considered by domestic legal systems are:

i) Means: human and technical considerations for standardization of DNA analysis methods and National and/or International levels.

ii) Evidence and samples should be collected and handled according to domestic laws maintaining scientific and legal guarantees.

iii) People involved: suspect in a criminal investigation and the information related to group people.

As an example, one may have to consider obtaining a reference sample from a suspect where consent may be an issue. In some legal systems the rights of the individual might be compromised, if acquiring a sample may deny liberty of movement, physical security, no self-incrimination, and presumption of innocence. There is some debate in some jurisdictions whether or not samples from suspects can be taken by use of force, or by consent, or by invoking probable cause, or being able to obtain samples at all. Some have circumvented these issues by obtaining samples in an indirect manner from hairs, a toothbrush, biological materials left in aprison cell, or indirectly from relatives. Others have suggested obtaining DNA from clinical samples, if they exist, that originated from the suspect.

There will be limits to resolving issues such as obtaining reference samples that may fall under ethical rules, not just under legal rules. Ruiz Vadillo, Judge of the Spanish Supreme Court, stated that *"Truth is not an absolute principle that has to be investigated at any price"*. Moreover, Roxin affirmed that *"an exhaustive and unlimited clarification of what has happened could pose a danger for many social and personal values. For these reasons the investigation of the truth is not an absolute value, rather the investigation is within the hierarchy of ethical and judicial values of the State"*.

Genetic databanks - Three types of **genetic databases** that may be considered for forensic identification are:

i) General - involving the whole population with no distinction for obtaining samples.

ii) Risky professions - wich may include such occupations as airplane pilots and military personnel.

iii) Criminal - wich may include convicted offenders, suspects, victims, profiles from unsolved cases, and profile to resolve missing children cases.

Issues regarding wich of these groups, such as general databases or suspects who have not been convicted, can be typed and their profiles stored may have to be considered.

DNA profile satabases is the collection of people in the databank, wich in actually is a sum of individuals, and the individual rights of these people versus the right of society will have to be weighed. Generally, there are little problems to be encountered when using DNA profile data from the types of genetic markers used in forensic that might infringe upon and individuals rights (Recommendation 3 of the Council of Europe). However, there should be safeguards that the information (or DNA samples) maintained in the databases is not used in a manner other than the legitimate aims or scope of the databanks.

Scientific reflections - Scientists, at times, tend to have difficulty accepting the fact that some lawyers may attempt to confuse issues or present false arguments. However, as stated well by James R. Wooley *"Defendants have an absolute right to attempt to obscure or hide the truth about DNA testing in criminal cases"*. While the courtromm may be where some of the immediate contact issues are made, society may have additional concerns (whether or not the concern are legitimate). These may include:

i) physycal harm

ii) genetic manipulation

iii) potentail associations with disease

iv) standards versus standardization

v) regulation and safeguards of abuses

vi) what types of people (convicted felons, suspects, etc.) should be in a databank.

It is apparent that domestic laws and commissions will have to define what is the legal framework for DNA tyuping. All decisions may have to be tempered based on ethical standards as well. Perhaps scientists could make an effort to educate the lay person regarding science, as well as educate themselves on the concerns of considering the use of DNA typing for human identification. Despite these attempts there will always be debates and resolutions that will affect the progress of science, the rights of the individual, and the rights of society.

REFERENCES

McEwen JE, Reilly PR (1994) A review of State legislation on DNA forensic databank. Am J Hum Genet 54: 941-958

Council of Europe. Committee of Minister. Recommendation No. R(92)1. - On the use of analysis of DNA within the framework of the criminal justice systems.

HumTH01 ALLELE FREQUENCIES IN ITALY - REPORT OF THE GEFI COLLABORATIVE STUDY

E. d'Aloja* and R. Domenici✦ editors

(*) Immunohematology laboratory, Istituto Medicina Legale, Università Cattolica, Largo F.Vito,1, 00168 Roma, Italy; (✦) Istituto Medicina Legale, Università di Pisa

INTRODUCTION

In order to achieve an harmonisation among protocols for STRs typing and create a national database, since 1991 the GEFI (Gruppo Ematologi Forensi Italiani) promotes (Pascali 1994, Presciuttini 1994) every two years an inter-laboratory exercise to identify the polymorphic loci more suitable for exchange and comparison of forensic data.

In 1993 two markers of different classes were chosen (namely, D1S80 as a Variable Number of Tandem Repeats, VNTR, and HumTH01 as a Short Tandem Repeats, STRs) according with the aim to investigate the reproducibility of several typing procedure.

Participants were asked to use the typing methodology currently employed in their labs in forensic casework and to identify two bloodstains at both loci investigated.

A comparison of the different methods and the allele frequencies resulted for HumTH01 locus (11p15,5-p15) (Edwards 1991) are here reported.

MATERIALS AND METHODS

Twenty-two laboratories were invited to this experiment covering almost all the area of Italian Peninsula, with the only exclusion of Sardinia.

Each participating laboratory was asked to analyse at least 50 unrelated individuals, resident in the region, and was supplied with two "unknown" samples, an HumTH01 allelic ladder (containing all the alleles from 6 to 11 but 9.3) and the relevant primers (according to Edwards).

Laboratories were set free to use whichever methods for amplification, electrophoresis and detection they had chosen for routine analysis.

However a basic protocol of amplification (Edwards with minor modifications) and separation (PAGE 8% T and 5% C) was suggested by the group responsible for the allelic ladder supply.

Allele designation was achieved by side to side comparison with the allelic laddder supplied.

All groups involved in paternity analysis were aldo asked to give information about the mutation rate at this locus.

RESULTS

Results are shown in table n.1 and in Fig.1 as the following allele frequencies were ascertained.

The allelic designation given by the participating labs was not always uniform due to the fact that 5 out 15 laboratories pooled togheter the 9.3 and 10 allele frequencies. In the present table only results concerning 1305 individuals were considered, representing the population sample typed for all the eigth major alleles.

Observed genotypes

Gen	Obs	Gen	Obs	Gen	Obs	Gen	Obs
6 - 6	63	6 - 7	103	7 - 8	55	8 - 10	5
7 - 7	29	6 - 8	89	7 - 9	70	9 - 9.3	120
8 - 8	17	6 - 9	149	7 - 9.3	122	9 - 10	9
9 - 9	46	6 - 9.3	148	7 - 10	11	9.3 -10	6
9.3-9.3	87	6 - 10	13	8 - 9	60	9.3 - 11	1
10 -10	1	6 - 11	1	8 - 9.3	98	5 - 9.3	2

Allele frequencies

Allele	Frequency	Allele	Frequency
5	0.001	9	0.192
6	0.242	9.3	0.257
7	0.160	10	0.018
8	0.131	11	0.001

COMMENTS

Results were returned by fifteen laboratories for a total number of 1611 unrelated individuals and over 200 meiosis.

A number of different electrophoresis and detection systems were utilised by the participants. The majority of laboratories employed native polyacrilamide gel as electrophoretic system and silver staining as detection (86%); denaturing polyacrilamide gels using either an automated laser fluorescent apparatus (7%) or radioactive detection (7%) were also employed.

Eight alleles, ranging from allele five (two observations) to the one containing eleven repeats (two observations), were detected although not all the laboratory showed the same ability to clearly identify allele 9.3 and 10, mainly due to the choice of the native separation method employed.

All GEFI laboratories participating in this exercise successfully typed the DNA from the two 'unknown' stains at the HumTH01 locus. This was achieved despite variation in the amplification, electrophoresis and detection systems utilised by individual laboratories. The results demonstrate that this simple STR locus is ideal for standardisation in the forensic community, where different laboratories have varying resources.

REFERENCES

Edwards A, Civitello A, Hammond HA, Caskey CT (1991). DNA typing and genetic mapping with trimeric and tetrameric tandem repeats. Am. J. Hum. Genet. 49:746-756.

Pascali VL, Domenici R (1994) Garda1 (D2S44 SBA) - Harmonization of protocols and a collaborative database. In: W. Bar, A. Fiori, U. Rossi (eds.) Advances in Forensic Haemogenetics 5. Springer-Verlag, Berlin Heidelberg New York pg 545.

Presciuttini S, De Stefano F (1994) An Italian collaborative study on the HLA-DQA1 locus (GEFI's "Garda 1" project). In: W. Bar, A. Fiori, U. Rossi (eds.) Advances in Forensic Haemogenetics 5. Springer-Verlag, Berlin Heidelberg New York pg 438.

Fig. 1: HumTH01 Italian Sample Population - Allele frequencies

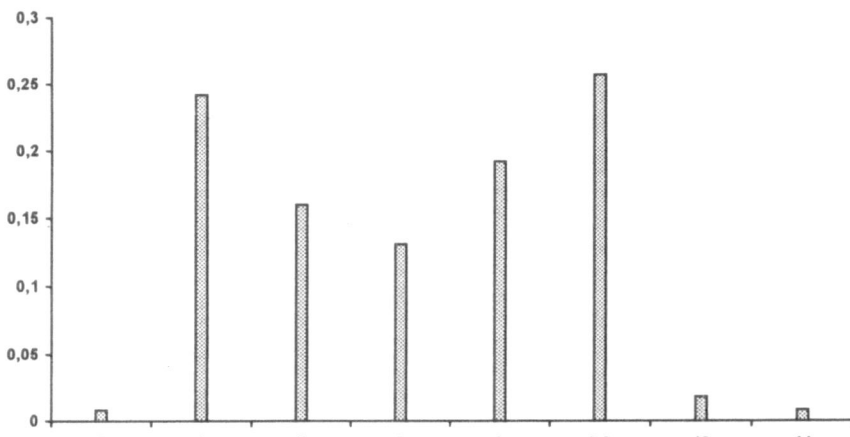

List of participating laboratories

Istituto di Medicina Legale, Università di **Ancona**; Istituto di Medicina Legale, Università di **Bologna**; Istituto di Medicina Legale, Università di **Brescia**; Istituto di Medicina Legale, Università di **Catania**; Istituto di Medicina Legale, Università di **Genova**; Istituto di Medicina Legale, Università di **Modena**; Istituto di Medicina Legale, Università di **Padova**; Istituto di Medicina Legale, Università di **Parma**; Istituto di Medicina Legale, Università di **Pavia**; Istituto di Medicina Legale, Università di **Pisa**; Istituto di Medicina Legale, Università di **Roma UCSC**; Istituto di Medicina Legale, Università di **Roma "La Sapienza"**; Istituto di Medicina Legale, Università di **Perugia** (sezione distaccata di **Terni**); Istituto di Medicina Legale, Università di **Trieste**; Istituto di Medicina Legale, Università di **Verona**.

A REVIEW OF THE COLLABORATIVE EXERCISES OF THE SPANISH AND PORTUGUESE ISFH WORKING GROUP

J.Gómez and A. Carracedo* for the Spanish and Portuguese Working Group of the ISFH

Sección de Unidad de Garantía de Calidad. Instituto Nacional de Toxicología. Mº de Justicia e Interior. Madrid
*Instituto de Medicina Legal. Facultad de Medicina. 15705 Santiago de Compostela. (Spain)

1.- Introduction

The Spanish and Portuguese working group of the ISFH comprises a total of 22 Laboratories from Spain, Portugal and some South American countries. Practically all the casework in forensic genetics in Spain (15 Labs) and Portugal (5 labs) is carried out in these laboratories. Since 1990 the group have organized collaborative exercises in DNA polymorphisms with the aim of progresion in standarization and for the discussion of technical and statistical problems as a first step towards a quality control program in Spain and Portugal.

Three exercises have been carried out up to now. In all these exercises 6 bloodstains were sent to different laboratories for DNA extraction and DNA polymorphism analysis. The systems used in the first exercise (1991-1992) were two SLPs (YNH24 and MS43a) and two PCR- based systems (HLADQA1 and D1S80). HUMTH01 was added in the second exercise (1993-1994). In the last exercise (1994-1995) Polymarker, HMVWA31, HMF13A1 and HUMFES were added to the above mentioned systems. In this exercise 15 labs have participated with very satisfactory results.

The main aim now of the Spanish and Portuguese labs is now to organize a quality control program for both countries.

This quality control program is planned for December 1995 toghether with the 4th collaborative exercise of the group. For this next trial a statistical exercise has been designed in addition to the standard exercise.

These collaborative exercises together with other activities of the group (statistics, legal regulation in Spain and Portugal) have proved to be extremely valuable and have clearly improved the quality of the medical-legal work in forensic genetics in Spain and Portugal.

2.- Materials and methods

The exercise scheme

A total of six bloodstains were distributed to participants. Each bloodstain was made with whole blood placed on a cotton cloth and air dried.
Laboratories were free to use any method of electrophoresis and detection, but each laboratory was requested to inform about the methodology used in the analysis of SLP's as well as PCR-based system.
The exercises were organized once a year.
Each laboratory was given a code in order to preserve anonimate.
Participants in the exercise were supplied with a data sheet, which included methodological questions for the loci included on each exercise (primers, ladders, buffers, gel characteristics, detection system, etc.)

DNA systems included on each exercise

The number of DNA polymorphisms included increased : 4 in the first exercise, 5 in the second and 9 in the third.
      1: YNH24 / Hinf I, MS43 / Hinf I, HLADQA1, D1S80
      2: YNH24 / Hinf I, MS43 / Hinf I, HLADQA1, D1S80, HUMTH01
      3: YNH24 / Hinf I, MS43 / Hinf I, HLADQA1, PM, D1S80, HUMTH01, HUMF13A01, HUMVWA, HUMFES

Participant laboratories

10 laboratories expressed an interest in participating in the first exercise, 16 in the second and 17 in the last exercise. 10 laboratories returned results in the first exercise, 10 in the second and 15 in the last one.

3.- Results

As the third exercise is the most significative due to the greater number of participating laboratories and DNA loci included, in this section we are going to include only the methodology used and the results obtained in this last exercise.

3.1.- PCR

HLADQ1 and PM:

The amplification and typing of the HDLA-DQA1 and PM systems were performed using the AmpliType HLA-DQA1 and PM Forensic DNA Amplification and Typing Kits (Perkin Elmer Corporation, Norwalk,CT) for all laboratories.

D1S80:

All participant laboratories performed the D1S80 amplification using the AmpliFLPD1S80 Amplification Kits (Perkin Elmer Corporation, Norwalk,CT). The typing of the PCR products was carried out by diferent electrophoretic systems.

10 laboratories used native PAGE and silver stain, 2 laboratories used SDS- PAGE and silver stain, 1 laboratory used agarose (2% Metaphor) and ethidium bromide, and 1 laboratory used Hydrolink gel and an authomatic sequencer.

All the laboratories, except one, classified the alleles by comparison with the commercial D1S80 ladder of 27 alleles (Perkin Elmer Corporation, Norwalk,CT).

STR SYSTEMS:

The amplification of STR loci was performed using different primers and detection systems depending of the laboratories. Basically, the laboratories can be classified as those that used the primers included in the GenePrint STR System (Pomega Corporation, Madison, WI, USA) or similar lab-synthesized primers and silver stain detection (10 lab.) and those that used primers of the EDNAP exercise and authomatic detection (4 lab.)

12 laboratories used denaturing PAGE (1 lab used Hydrolink) electrophoresis followed by silver stain or authomatic detection and 2 laboratories used native PAGE electrophoresis for the analysis of PCR products.

The classification of the alleles was performed with commercial ladders (GenePrint STR Systems, Promega Corporation) (5 lab.), lab-made ladders (4 lab) or internal standards (3 lab).

3.2. -Single locus probes

The fragments sizes for YNH24 and MS43 and deviation from the mean for each laboratory are shown in Table 1. In Table 2 the percentage of deviation from the mean is presented

The table can be used to determine the "bin" size needed for 2 laboratories to compare results. For example, laboratories 1 and 3 need a bin of 2,64 % to match the high molecular weight fragment (10408 y 10135 bp respectively).

Table 1. FRAGMENT SIZES (YNH24 AND MS43) AND DEVIATION FROM THE MEAN FOR EACH LABORATORY

Laboratories							Mean	SD	CV (%)
1	3	5	6	8	11	13			
10408	10135	10280	10328		10221	10511	10313,8	133,9	1,30
10166	9807	9974	10091		10221	10511	10128,3	238,7	2,36
10286	9992	10065	10015		10077	10117	10092	105,0	1,04
9870	9673	9888	9938		9938	10029	9889,3	119,5	1,21
9528	9293	9403	9297		9306	9563	9398,3	121,5	1,29
9230	9094	9261	9258		9309	9693	9307,5	202,4	2,17
9230	9173	9122	9119		9079	9178	9150,2	53,8	0,59
8522	8542	8480	8448		8463	8443	8483	40,6	0,48
7941	7980	7953	7887		7907	7981	7941,5	38,3	0,48
7659	7505	7548	7487		7497	7562	7543	64,1	0,85
5509	5447	5493	5496	5250		5534	5454,8	104,3	1,91
5279	5211	5237	5143		4885	5238	5165,5	144,6	2,80
4999	4972	4961	4915		4990	4958	4965,8	29,6	0,60
4637	4575	4603	4591	4400		4570	4562,7	83,2	1,82
3737	3706	3701	3682	3625		3727	3696,3	40,0	1,08
3465	3458	3471	3448	3400		3464	3451	26,2	0,76
3053	3078	3068	3047	3000		3039	3047,5	27,2	0,89
3062	3039	3062	3060	3000		3040	3043,8	24,0	0,79
3034	2967	2979	2938	2925		2949	2965,3	38,8	1,31
2968	2942	2969	2976	2925		2945	2954,2	19,9	0,67
2723	2700	2732	2729	2700		2716	2716,7	14,0	0,52
2668	2650	2660	2625	2650		2635	2648	15,8	0,60
2641	2589	2614	2565	2550		2575	2589	33,5	1,30
2441	2414	2426	2426	2400		2417	2420,7	13,8	0,57
							Mean CV		1,14

FRAGMENT SIZES ARE RANKED IN DESCENDING ORDER

Table 2. DEVIATION FROM THE MEAN (%)

Laboratories							Range (%)
1	3	5	6	8	11	13	
0,91	-1,73	-0,33	0,14		-0,90	1,91	3,71
0,37	-3,17	-1,52	-0,37		0,91	3,78	7,18
1,92	-0,99	-0,27	-0,76		-0,15	0,25	2,94
-0,20	-2,19	-0,01	0,49		0,49	1,41	3,68
1,38	-1,12	0,05	-1,08		-0,98	1,75	2,91
-0,83	-2,29	-0,50	-0,53		0,02	4,14	6,59
0,87	0,25	-0,31	-0,34		-0,78	0,30	1,66
0,46	0,70	-0,04	-0,41		-0,24	-0,47	1,17
-0,01	0,48	0,14	-0,69		-0,43	0,50	1,19
1,54	-0,50	0,07	-0,74		-0,61	0,25	2,30
0,99	-0,14	0,70	0,75	-3,76		1,45	5,41
2,20	0,88	1,38	-0,44		-5,43	1,40	8,07
0,67	0,12	-0,10	-1,02		0,49	-0,16	1,71
1,63	0,27	0,88	0,62	-3,57		0,16	5,39
1,10	0,26	0,13	-0,39	-1,93		0,83	3,09
0,41	0,20	0,58	-0,09	-1,48		0,38	2,09
0,18	1,00	0,67	-0,02	-1,56		-0,28	2,60
0,60	-0,16	0,60	0,53	-1,44		-0,13	2,07
2,32	0,06	0,46	-0,92	-1,36		-0,55	3,73
0,47	-0,41	0,50	0,74	-0,99		-0,31	1,74
0,23	-0,61	0,56	0,45	-0,61		-0,02	1,19
0,76	0,08	0,45	-0,87	0,08		-0,49	1,64
2,01	0,00	0,97	-0,93	-1,51		-0,54	3,57
0,84	-0,28	0,22	0,22	-0,85		-0,15	1,71
Mean lab.deviation:							
0,87	-0,39	0,22	-0,24	-1,58	-0,63	0,64	3,22

FRAGMENT SIZES (YNH24 AND MS43) RANKED IN DESCENDING ORDER FOR EACH LABORATORY

5.- Conclusion

The number of DNA Markers used and the number of laboratories participating increased and in spite of this results remained satisfactory.

Most of the laboratories used the EDNAP electrophoresis protocol for SLP analysis and the uniformity of results is excellent.

For STRs despite the different primers and methods used for detection there is a general agreement in ladders and nomenclature and the correlation of results is also excellent. Other PCR-bases polymorphisms were studied using commercially available kits also with good results.

Only a few isolated errors were found in the last exercise. No errors were reported in the following systems : HLA-DQA1, LDLR, D7S8, GC, HUMTH01, HUMF13A01 and HUMFES.

Laboratories participating in these exercises

Cátedra de Medicina Legal y Toxicología. Granada
Cátedra de Medicina Legal, Facultad de Medicina. Alicante
Departamento de Biología Molecular, Pharma Gen S.A. Madrid
Dpto. de Medicina Legal y Toxicología. Facultad de Medicina. Universidad Complutense, Madrid
Dpto de Medicina Legal, Cátedra de Medicina Legal y Toxicología. Facultad de Medicina. Zaragoza
Dpto. de Biología Celular y C.C Morfológicas. Facultad de Medicina y Odontología. Leioa (Vizcaya)
Instituto de Medicina Legal de Coimbra (Portugal)
Instituto de Medicina Legal de Lisboa (Portugal)
Instituto de Medicina Legal do Porto (Portugal)
Instituto de Medicina Legal, Facultad de Medicina. Santiago de Compostela
Laboratorio de la Policia Científica. Lisboa (Portugal)
Laboratorio Policia País Vasco, Lab U.T.A.P, Dep. del Interior. Gobierno Vasco. Bilbao
Sección de Biología. Instituto Nacional de Toxicología. Departamento de Sevilla
Sección de Biología. Instituto Nacional de Toxicología. Departamento de Barcelona
Sección de Biología.Instituto Nacional de Toxicología. Departamento de Madrid
Servicio Central de Policía Científica, 2ª Sección Criminalística I, Laboratorio de Biología
Servicio de Huellas Digitales Genéticas Facultad de Farmacia y Bioquímica. Buenos Aires (Argentina)

Comparability of RFLP Results Between Laboratories: AABB/ CAP Survey Data

C. Harrison, R. Allen, D. Endean, J. Morris, H. Polesky, R. Roby, R. Walker

College of American Pathologists, Resource Committee on Parentage Testing
325 Waukegan Road, Northfield , Illinois 60093, USA

INTRODUCTION

The American Association of Blood Banks (AABB) and the College of American Pathologists (CAP) jointly sponsor a proficiency testing program for parentage and forensic laboratories. This report summarizes data on band size (Kb) and paternity index based on RFLP analysis.

METHOD

Results from seven quarterly mailings of three whole blood samples collected in ACD were evaluated to determine variability in band size reported by laboratories testing the same locus with similar probe/enzyme combinations. Extraction method, restriction condition, electrophoresis, hybridization , and detection system varied depending on the laboratories routine for testing samples. Standard deviation (SD) and coefficient of variation (CV) were determined for combinations with multiple responses. Each laboratory was requested to provide results on K562 controls, bin limits and frequency, database source, delta value, and the paternity index for the system tested.

RESULTS

Tables 1 shows that laboratories using the same probe/enzyme combination for testing at the D2S44 locus have comparable results. With the exception of the B-93 survey the CV for the results has been below 3.2%. On all of the seven surveys conducted between January 1993 and May of 1995, band size variation has been less than 100 base pairs. Table 2 shows the results from 17 laboratories reporting on the trio mailed in March of 1995. These results are representative of what has been observed with a large number of other probe/enzyme combinations. In all cases the SD and CV of the band size are very similar regardless of the reporting laboratory. As in table 2, it has been observed that the variation in reported band size increases as the marker detected is bigger. Table 3 shows examples of the range of values for the paternity index reported for various probe/enzyme combinations. The widely divergent values reported for similar test results is representative of all the AABB/CAP surveys evaluated to date. There is no apparent correlation of this variation with the databases used, the reported delta values, or the bin limits.

CONCLUSION

Inter laboratory comparison of RFLP testing on seven trios tested by similar probe/enzyme combinations show that band sizes reported by multiple laboratories are very similar. The observed SD and CV are small although there is an increase in the variability as the band size increases. In contrast to the comparability of band size, the paternity index values reported on similar RFLP results show wide variability.

TABLE 1

Comparability of RFLP Allele Sizes

D2S44/YNH 24, Hae III

Survey (n)	$\overline{X}$ (Kb)	SD (Kb)	CV (%)
A -93 (15)	2.98	0.064	2.16
B -93 (11)	1.14	0.081	7.13
C -93 (17)	1.99	0.062	3.13
A -94 (30)	2.81	0.057	2.02
B -94 (24)	3.08	0.096	3.1
C -94 (26)	1.56	0.024	1.6
A -95 (28)	2.91	0.084	2.9

TABLE 2

RFLP Results: 17 Laboratories

PI -A 95 (Locus/Enz: D4s139/Hae III)

Band	Size (Kb)*	SD (Kb)	CV (%)
Mother	4.89	0.043	0.88
AF	7.66	0.104	1.36
Mother	7.81	0.147	1.88
M/Ch	7.83	0.132	1.68
AF/Ch	8.6	0.163	1.9
AF	8.61	0.159	1.84

*Mean

TABLE 3

Reported Paternity Index: PI -A95

Marker	Enzyme (*)	Low	High
D2S44	Hae III (21)	2.53	11.36
	Hinf1 (4)	4.25	6.43
D4S163	*Pst1* (7)	16.67	34.94
D7S22	**Hinf1 (5)**	4.83	8.65
D10S28	Hae III (17)	7.94	80.83
D12S11	**Hinf1 (6)**	12.11	21.84
	Pst1 (6)	10.84	28.8

* **Number of participants**

PROFICIENCY TESTING IN FORENSIC DNA ANALYSIS

A S Riordan, M Parker and G Rysiecki

Cellmark Diagnostics, Blacklands Way, Abingdon Business Park, Abingdon, Oxfordshire, OX14 1DY, UK.

INTRODUCTION

Quality assurance systems are now essential in any laboratory and a fundamental part of such systems is regular participation in an external quality assessment scheme. External quality assessment addresses variation in the results produced by different laboratories when analysing identical samples. The results are reported to all participants, providing a mechanism by which laboratories can assess their proficiency and the accuracy of their systems, thereby identifying areas for improvement. In the forensic setting, quality assessment allows laboratories to compare the results of their analysis of mock crime cases with those of other laboratories. This is particularly important when using new and rapidly-developing technologies such as DNA testing where reproducibility between laboratories and competence of individual members of staff must be demonstrated. In some countries participation in external proficiency testing schemes is now a requirement for laboratory accreditation. The International Quality Assessment Scheme (IQAS), in operation since April 1991, has examined and compared forensic DNA testing carried out in 58 laboratories in 16 countries using a range of different methodologies.

METHODS

IQAS is operated in accordance with guidelines issued by the American Society of Crime Laboratory Directors (ASCLD) and the Technical Working Group on DNA Analysis Methods (TWGDAM) (ref1). A mock case is distributed once every three months. Samples are chosen to reflect real forensic casework and each distribution contains a mock scene of crime sample, three control blood stains and a blank control for the crime sample as well as a brief description of the case. Participants are asked to analyse the samples using their normal laboratory methods, to record their results for each sample on the standard forms provided, and to return these within 16 weeks of receipt, identifying which of the control samples matches the mock crime sample. A questionnaire is also completed to provide details of the testing systems used. Results are collated into a report which is distributed to all participants. Participating laboratories remain anonymous and are identified only by code numbers. Details of the amount of DNA extracted from each sample, band sizes calculated for each single locus probe (VNTR) and alleles identified in PCR tests by each laboratory, are all included in the report.

RESULTS

Since 1991 17 IQAS distributions have been sent out to a total of 78 participants in 58 laboratories and 614 sets of results have been returned and reported.

Methodologies used have included DNA profiling using both HaeIII and HinfI with a range of single locus probes (VNTR's), HLA DQα and PolyMarker (AmpliType®, Perkin Elmer), AMFLP D1S80 and short tandem repeat (STR) analysis (see Tables 1 and 2). Table 3 contains a sample of the DNA profiling results returned from distribution 9501. 38 participants analysed HaeIII digested K562 genomic control DNA with YNH24 and all allele sizes reported fell within ±1.2% of the sample mean allele sizes. The standard deviations calculated for the two alleles were 13.66 and 9.67 base pairs respectively. 39 participants analysed the mock crime sample (semen on a cotton wool swab) using HaeIII and YNH24. All allele sizes reported fell with ±2.5% of the sample mean allele sizes while the standard deviations calculated for the two alleles were 29.22 and 20.06 base pairs respectively. Similar results were reported by laboratories using HinfI (see Table 3). More than 600 sample matches have been reported to date using the various techniques and none has ever been incorrect.

DISCUSSION

Participation in proficiency testing schemes allows individual forensic scientists to compare the quality of their systems and the results they produce with those of their peers. This allows the rapid identification and correction of problems and poor performance as well as highlighting areas for improvement. Increasingly laboratories are being asked by courts and defence lawyers to demonstrate the quality of their work and the reproducibility of the technology itself. External proficiency testing results are invaluable in answering such questions.

REFERENCES

1.   Guidelines for DNA Proficiency Test Manufacturing and Reporting. Crime Laboratory Digest, 1994 Vol 21, No 2, P27-32.

Table 1. Different methods reported by participants in IQAS distribution 9501 (March 1995)

METHOD OF ANALYSIS	NUMBER OF PARTICIPANTS
Single locus probing (VNTR's)	51
- using HaeIII	41
- using HinfI	10
PCR - HLA DQα	20
- PolyMarker	16
- STR's	7
- AMFLP D1S80	8

Table 2. Loci analysed by participants in IQAS distribution 9501 (March 1995)

SINGLE LOCUS PROBES		STR'S AND AMFLP'S
D2S44 (YNH24)	D4S139 (PH30)	HUMvWFA31/A
D1S7 (MS1)	D17S79 (V1)	HUMTHO1
D10S28 (TBQ7)	D5S110 (MS621,LH1)	HUMF13A01
D12S11 (MS43A)	D5S43 (MS8)	HUMFES/FPS
D7S21 (MS31)	D7S467 (PAC415)	HUMACTBP2
D16S309 (MS205)	D14S13 (CMM101)	D1S80
D7S22 (G3)	D17S26 (EFD52)	HPRTB

Table 3. *Example of Results Returned in Distribution 9501* (March 1995)

RESTRICTION ENZYME	PROBE	SAMPLE	DATA	ALLELE 1 (bp)	ALLELE 2 (bp)
Hae III	YNH24	KS62 Genomic Control	n mean range SD	38 2916 2880 - 2950 (98.8 - 101.2% of mean) 13.66	38 1794 1777 - 1820 (99 - 101.x% of mean) 9.67
	YNH24	Mock Crime Sample	n mean range SD	39 3364 3305 - 3414 (98.8 - 101.1% of mean) 23.22	39 2270 2205 - 2347 (97.5 - 101.8% of mean) 20.06
Hinf I	MS31	KS62 Genomic Control	n mean range SD	8 7983 7862 - 8150 (98.9 - 102.3% of mean) 95.07	8 7060 6975 - 7150 (98.8 - 101.3% of mean) 64.76
	MS31	Mock Crime Sample	n mean range SD	9 8630 8360 - 8780 (96.9 - 101.7% of mean) 127.5	9 6829 6720 - 6930 (98.4 - 101.5% of mean) 58.95

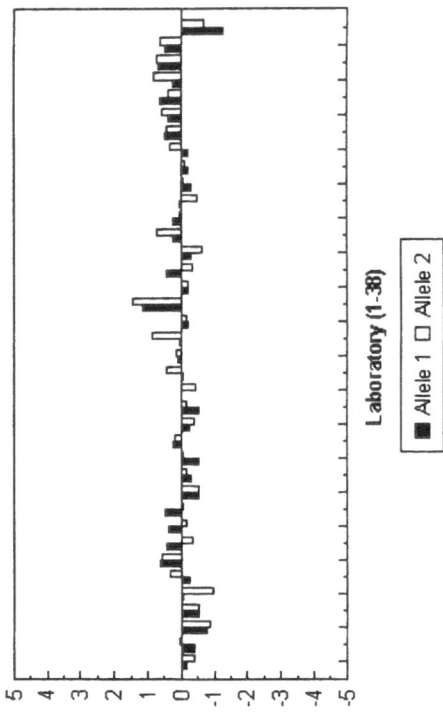

% Size Deviation from the Mean

Laboratory (1-38)

■ Allele 1   □ Allele 2

FIGURE 1. *Variation in allele sizes returned by 38 laboratories in Distribution 9501*